Anterior Segment THE REQUISITES IN OPHTHALMOLOGY

SERIES EDITOR

Jay H. Krachmer, MD
Professor and Chairman
Department of Ophthalmology
University of Minnesota Medical School
Minneapolis, Minnesota

OTHER VOLUMES IN THE REQUISITES IN OPHTHALMOLOGY SERIES

Glaucoma

Neuro-Ophthalmology

Pediatric Ophthalmology and Strabismus

Oculoplastic Surgery

Pathology, Physiology, and Refraction

Retina, Choroid, and Vitreous

Visit our website at **www.mosby.com**

Anterior Segment

THE REQUISITES

IN OPHTHALMOLOGY

CHRISTOPHER J. RAPUANO, MD
Associate Professor of Ophthalmology
Thomas Jefferson University
Cornea Service
Wills Eye Hospital
Philadelphia, Pennsylvania

JODI I. LUCHS, MD
Assistant Clinical Professor
Department of Ophthalmology and Visual Sciences
Long Island Jewish Medical Center
Albert Einstein College of Medicine
Bronx, New York

TERRY KIM, MD
Assistant Professor of Ophthalmology
Cornea and External Disease
Duke University Eye Center
Durham, North Carolina

Mosby

St. Louis Baltimore Boston Carlsbad Chicago Minneapolis New York Philadelphia Portland
London Milan Sydney Tokyo Toronto

Mosby
Dedicated to Publishing Excellence

Assistant Editor: Kimberly Cox
Senior Managing Editor: Kathryn H. Falk
Project Manager: Patricia Tannian
Production Editor: Richard Hund
Design Manager: Gail Morey Hudson

THE REQUISITES™
THE REQUISITES
THE REQUISITES
THE REQUISITES
THE REQUISITES

NOTICE
Pharmacology is an ever-changing field. Standard safety precautions must be followed, but as new research and clinical experience broaden our knowledge, changes in treatment and drug therapy may become necessary or appropriate. Readers are advised to check the most current product information provided by the manufacturer of each drug to be administered to verify the recommended dose, the method and duration of administration, and contraindications. It is the responsibility of the treating physician, relying on experience and knowledge of the patient, to determine dosages and the best treatment for each individual patient. Neither the publisher nor the editor assumes any liability for any injury and/or damage to persons or property arising from this publication.

Mosby, Inc.
A Harcourt Health Sciences Company
11830 Westline Industrial Drive
St. Louis, Missouri 63146

Printed in the United States of America

Library of Congress Cataloging in Publication Data

Rapuano, Christopher J.
The requisites in ophthalmology : anterior segment / Christopher J. Rapuano, Jodi I. Luchs, Terry Kim.
p. cm.—(Requisites in ophthalmology series)
Includes bibliographical references and index.
ISBN 0-323-00173-4
1. Anterior segment (Eye)—Diseases. I. Luchs, Jodi I. II. Kim, Terry. III. Title. IV. Title: Anterior segment. V. Series.
[DNLM: 1. Anterior Chamber—injuries. 2. Anterior Chamber—physiopathology. 3. Corneal Diseases—therapy. 4. Iris Diseases—therapy. WW 210 R221r 2000]
RE334.R36 2000
617.7—DC21
DNLM/DLC
for Library of Congress

99-35199
CIP

99 00 01 02 03 GW/MVY 9 8 7 6 5 4 3 2 1

To my wife, Sara, for her constant love, support, and encouragement.
To my children, Michael, Patrick, Daniel, and Megan, for reminding me what life is really about.
To my parents, Cathie and Al, for all they have done over the years.

C.J.R.

To my wife, Stacy, my sons, Ethan and Evan, and my father, Saul, for their love, patience, and endless support.

J.I.L.

With great love and appreciation, I dedicate this book to:
My wife, Ellie.
My daughter, Ashley.
My parents, Kyung Hwae and Hyun Sim.
My sister and brother, Suzanne and Michael.

T.K.

Preface

The goal of this book, and the Requisites Series in general, is to provide the reader with the essential knowledge to take excellent care of patients. When writing a textbook, there is a tendency to include encyclopedic information about each topic. We have tried hard to limit the information to what is most clinically relevant. The reader will not find footnotes or references in the body of the text, but rather Selected Readings at the end of each chapter. Also at the end of each chapter are Major Points, which highlight the "take-home" messages from the chapter. We have included a large number of black and white photographs throughout the text to depict the subject matter. Color photographs, grouped together in color plates, are used to highlight conditions where color is especially important. Black and white copies of these color plates appear sequentially in the text, with a note to alert the reader that the photograph also appears in the color plates. Many diagrams of surgical techniques can be found in the last two chapters on surgery and trauma.

While this book was written as a comprehensive anterior segment text, beginning with conjunctival and external disease, proceeding through corneal abnormalities and ending with surgery and trauma, each chapter can also stand alone. There is an outline at the beginning of each chapter to aid the reader in locating topics of particular interest. Additionally, the book can be used as a reference text because it has an extensive index.

Among our many mentors, we are particularly indebted to Jay H. Krachmer, MD, Peter R. Laibson, MD, and Elisabeth J. Cohen, MD, who have not only taught us a great deal in the fields of anterior segment, cornea, and external disease but also fine-tuned our clinical thinking process. They have graciously reviewed and provided invaluable help in the writing and editing of this book. Dr. Krachmer is the editor of this Series and was the fellowship preceptor for Christopher Rapuano, MD. Dr. Rapuano is in practice with Dr. Laibson and Dr. Cohen, with whom Jodi Luchs, MD, and Terry Kim, MD, completed their fellowships. We are extremely grateful to the three of them for their superb teaching, support, and friendship both during and since our fellowships.

Naturally we could not have completed the enormous job of writing this book without tremendous support at home. To put some extra stress into the mix, all three of us had children born during the writing of this book. We are eternally thankful to our wives Sara, Stacy, and Ellie and our children for putting up with us during this process. We are thrilled with the final product and hope you will find it as interesting as we find our subspecialty.

Christopher J. Rapuano, MD

Jodi I. Luchs, MD

Terry Kim, MD

Acknowledgments

It is with great pleasure and gratitude that we acknowledge many of the people who helped make this book possible. While most of the clinical photographs came from our own patients (and by extension, the photo archives of Jay H. Krachmer, MD, Elisabeth J. Cohen, MD, and Peter R. Laibson, MD), several other people generously supplied photos to us including Ira J. Udell, MD, George O. Waring, III, MD, R. Doyle Stulting, MD, PhD, Ralph C. Eagle, Jr., MD, Guy F. Webster, MD, PhD, James D. Auran, MD, Elizabeth L. Affel, MS, Deborah BenArosh, COA, and Carol L. Shields, MD. Dr. Shields also graciously reviewed the sections on iris cysts and iris tumors and Edward J. Holland, MD reviewed the section on limbal stem cell transplants. We are grateful to Bob Curtin, Jack Scully, and Roger Barone of the Audio-Visual Department at Wills Eye Hospital for all their help and expertise with our photography needs. Kathy Falk at Mosby and Marcia Craig at Graphic World Publishing Services were extremely helpful in the editing and final production of this text. We would also like to thank all of our residents and fellows, past and present, as they encourage us to continue learning each and every day. Last, but certainly not least, we are extremely lucky to have had the immense talents of Birck Cox, one of the finest medical illustrators around. His artwork has added enormously to this text.

Contents

CHAPTER 1

Conjunctiva and External Disease

This chapter describes a wide array of conditions involving the conjunctiva and its surrounding external adnexa. An attempt has been made to categorize these disorders according to specific underlying etiologies (infections, allergies) to facilitate organization and understanding. When examining a patient with an inflammatory disorder of the conjunctiva, reviewing all the categories of disorders can help the clinician to form a useful differential diagnosis with the goal of making the correct diagnosis and instituting the proper therapy.

CONJUNCTIVA

Anatomy

The conjunctiva is the continuous mucous membrane lining of the anterior surface of the eye as well as the posterior surface of the eyelids. It starts at the corneoscleral limbus and covers the anterior globe (bulbar conjunctiva), extends into the superior and inferior fornices (forniceal conjunctiva), forms the inner surface of the eyelids (palpebral conjunctiva), and ends at the upper and lower eyelid margins (Fig. 1-1). The conjunctiva is comprised of two layers: stratified, nonkeratinized squamous epithelium and underlying stroma known as substantia propria. The squamous epithelium is unique because it contains mucus-secreting goblet cells, whereas the substantia propria is composed of fibrovascular tissue containing blood vessels, lymphatics, and nerves.

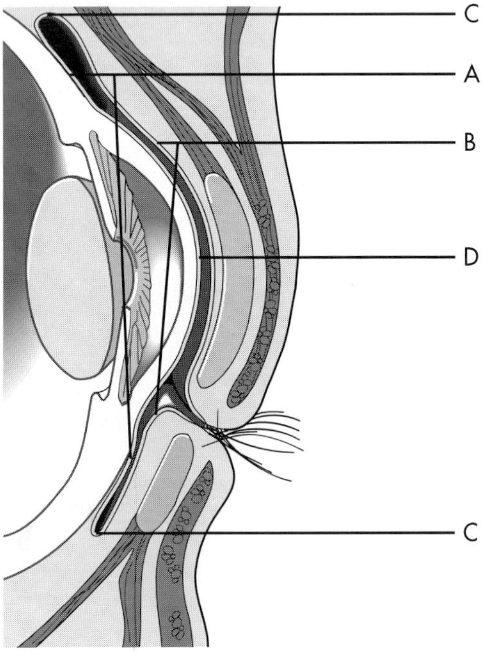

Fig. 1-1 Conjunctival anatomy diagram. The external ocular lining consists of bulbar conjunctiva (**A**), palpebral conjunctiva (**B**), conjunctival fornix (**C**), and corneal epithelium (**D**).

Inflammatory Responses

The inflammatory response in the conjunctiva can be categorized according to its onset and duration. Acute conjunctivitis generally refers to a relatively rapid onset of inflammation that typically lasts up to 4 weeks. Chronic conjunctivitis implies gradual, persistent inflammation lasting more than 4 weeks. Hyperacute conjunctivitis indicates the sudden presence of severe inflammation. These time frames merely designate the chronicity of an inflammatory disorder and are not meant to define strict time measures of a disease process. Therefore one may find adenoviral conjunctivitis as either an acute or a chronic process, depending on the disease duration.

Symptoms and signs of conjunctival inflammation may be nonspecific, but they do help guide the clinician in a general direction for diagnosing the underlying condition. For example, itchy and watery eyes are often symptoms of an allergic or a viral disorder, whereas a red eye with mucopurulent discharge usually indicates a bacterial infection. The conjunctival inflammatory response may manifest itself with several distinct signs (Box 1-1). The pattern, character, and location of these clinical features may be of great diagnostic value.

Conjunctival injection Conjunctival injection, or hyperemia, merely relates to conjunctival blood vessel dilatation (Fig. 1-2). Although hyperemia is a nonspecific sign of conjunctival inflammation, close attention to its characteristics can distinguish conjunctivitis from other ophthalmic conditions. Conjunctival injection located circumferentially around the limbus (called *ciliary injection*) usually suggests acute iritis, especially when accompanied by photophobia and anterior chamber inflammatory cells. Episcleral/scleral vessel injection (indicative of episcleritis/scleritis) is often mistaken for conjunctival injection, an error that can lead to confusion and mismanagement (Fig. 1-3). Conjunctival injection should be distinguished from episcleral and scleral injection (anesthetized conjunctiva moves readily with a cotton-tip applicator; additionally, conjunctival and episcleral, but not scleral, blood vessels blanch after the application of topical phenylephrine). Dilated episcleral

Box 1-1 Clinical Features of Conjunctival Inflammation

Hyperemia/hemorrhage
Chemosis
Discharge
Papillae
Follicles
Membrane/pseudomembrane
Granuloma

vessels (rarely from an underlying uveal melanoma, polycythemia vera, leukemia, or cavernous sinus thrombosis) may also mimic conjunctival hyperemia. Deeper levels of injection (such as those seen with episcleritis and scleritis) are generally not associated with discharge. Finally, vascular lesions of the conjunctiva, such as angiomas and Kaposi's sarcoma, should be considered when viewing areas of conjunctival injection.

Subconjunctival hemorrhage Conjunctival vessels can bleed leading to subconjunctival hemorrhage (Fig. 1-4). This entity often looks more ominous than it actually is (Fig. 1-5). The collection of blood under the conjunctiva results in the dramatic appearance of confluent redness on an area of the globe. Patients may report recent blunt or sharp trauma; sometimes they relate a history involving Valsalva maneuvers such as coughing or vomiting, though subconjunctival hemorrhages are usually spontaneous. Patients who undergo ophthalmic procedures (such as cataract extraction, strabismus surgery, scleral buckle, vitrectomy, etc.) often have subconjunctival hemorrhage as a result of surgery. However, if a patient has a history of recurrent subconjunctival bleeding, the possibility of a bleeding diathesis either from medication or from a clotting disorder should be suspected, especially in the presence of easy skin bruising, bleeding from the gums, or nosebleeds. Patients should always be questioned about the use of anticoagulants such as aspirin or warfarin. Other systemic illnesses such as malignant hypertension can also be associated with subconjunctival hemorrhage and should be appropriately worked up and treated (Box 1-2). Although these other causes are important to consider, trauma is by far the most frequent cause of subconjunctival hemorrhage.

Chemosis Chemosis refers to conjunctival edema resulting from the leakage of transudate from capillaries in the conjunctiva (Fig. 1-6). If the condition is severe

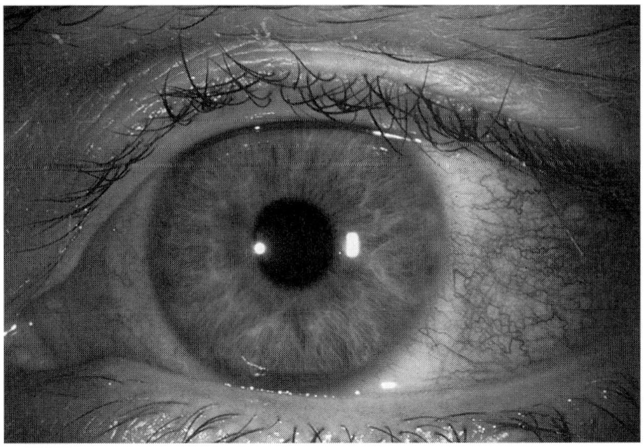

Fig. 1-2 Conjunctival injection. Diffuse conjunctival injection is present in this eye with mild viral conjunctivitis.

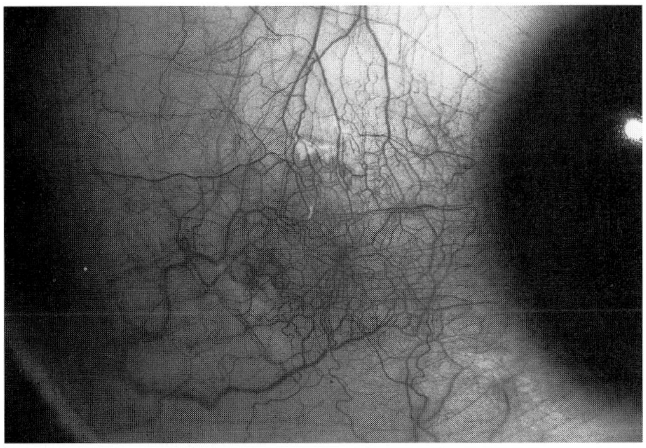

Fig. 1-3 Episcleral injection. Nodular episcleritis can mimic conjunctivitis. Note the deeper, more confluent involvement in this eye than is usually seen in simple conjunctivitis. (See color plate.)

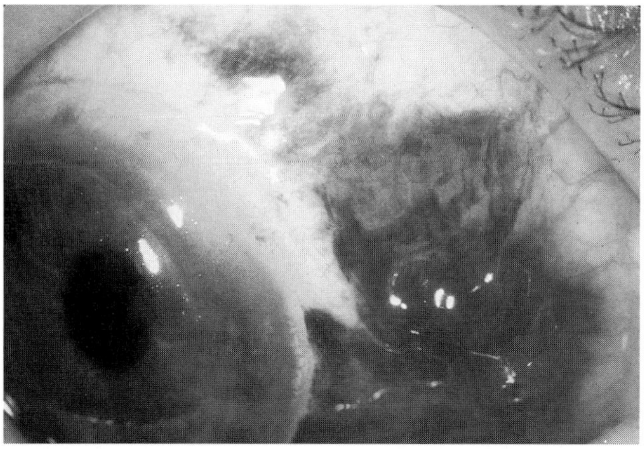

Fig. 1-4 Subconjunctival hemorrhage. Most likely the localized subconjunctival hemorrhage in this eye began inferiorly and tracked superiorly.

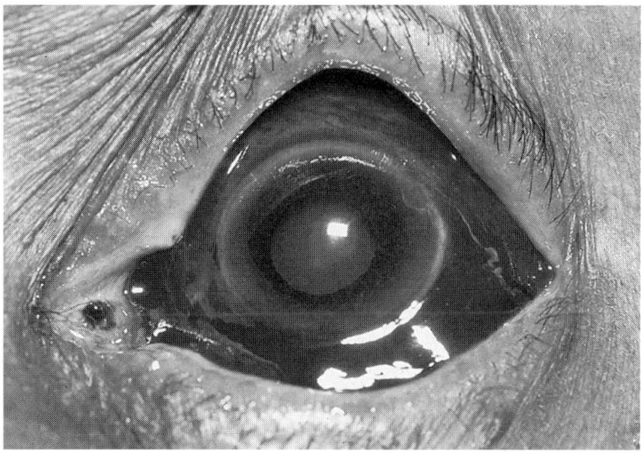

Fig. 1-5 Subconjunctival hemorrhage. A total subconjunctival hemorrhage can seem alarming, but it typically resolves without sequelae within a few weeks. (See color plate.)

Box 1-2 Causes of Subconjunctival Hemorrhage

SPONTANEOUS

TRAUMA (BLUNT OR SHARP)

VALSALVA MANEUVERS (E.G., COUGHING, VOMITING, CONSTIPATION)

SYSTEMIC DISORDERS
Bleeding Diathesis

1. Medications (e.g., aspirin, warfarin, heparin, ticlopidine)
2. Clotting disorders (e.g., hemophilia, von Willebrand disease, vitamin K deficiency, protein C deficiency, uremia, disseminated intravascular coagulation [DIC], myeloma, macroglobulinemia)

Microvascular Disorders (e.g., Hypertension, Diabetes Mellitus)

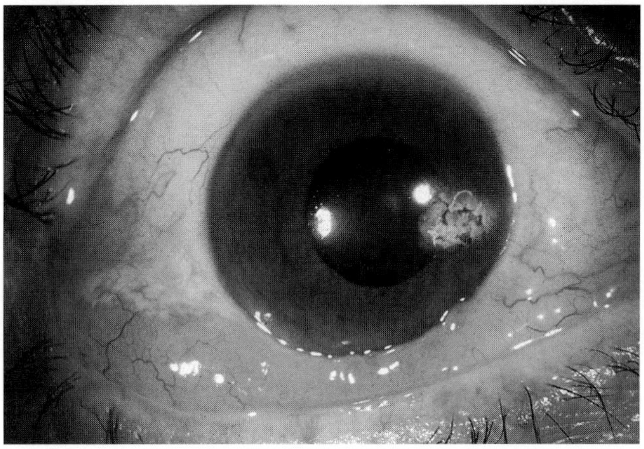

Fig. 1-6 Conjunctival chemosis. Conjunctival edema is prominent inferiorly. It is severe enough to protrude slightly through the palpebral fissure on eye closure. Nasally, there is an old calcified corneal scar.

enough, white, swollen conjunctival tissue may protrude through the interpalpebral fissure. It is usually mild and transient, however, and it alerts the clinician to an allergic response. Trauma and surgery can also cause chemosis. Rarely is it severe and chronic enough to require frequent lubrication or even tarsorrhaphy to prevent damage from exposure.

Conjunctival discharge Conjunctival discharge is a general term used to describe the exudate elicited from the conjunctiva during an infectious or inflammatory process (Fig. 1-7). Descriptions of its nature can help the clinician determine its cause. For instance, a watery discharge is often associated with allergic or viral conjunctivitis, whereas a mucopurulent discharge is commonly a result of a bacterial conjunctivitis.

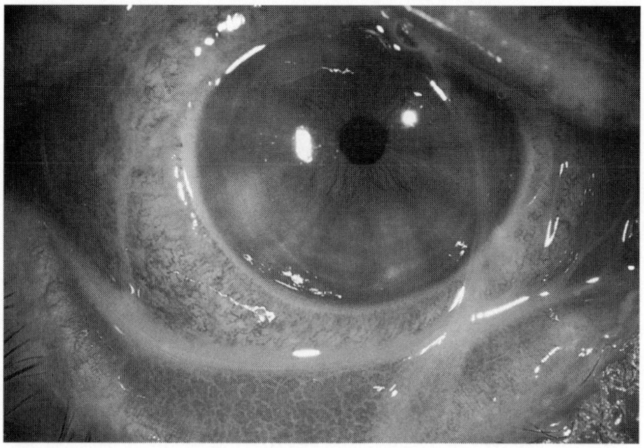

Fig. 1-7 Conjunctival discharge. Mucopurulent discharge is evident in this eye with bacterial conjunctivitis.

Papillae and follicles Papillae and follicles are inflammatory changes seen primarily in the palpebral tarsal conjunctiva (Fig. 1-8). Papillae are small conjunctival elevations distinguished by a central vascular core. They form as a result of edema and inflammatory cell infiltration of the tissue surrounding small conjunctival capillaries. Their presence commonly indicates bacterial or allergic conjunctivitis. Size and shape are determined by the connective tissue septa that anchor and restrict this inflammatory change to the fibrovascular core, with each papilla measuring less than 1 mm. These anchoring septa can become weakened and stretched from chronic and severe inflammation, leading to the formation of large, polygonal mounds, with each papilla measuring more than 1 mm. When they reach this size, they are referred to as giant papillae and can have a distinctive cobblestone appearance. This specific type of conjunctivitis (known as giant papillary conjunctivitis or GPC) (Fig. 1-9) is discussed later in this chapter.

Follicles are round elevations in the conjunctiva that represent collections of lymphocytes. These lymphoid follicles have no central fibrovascular core and actually obscure the underlying capillary vessels (Fig. 1-10). They can vary in size and typically appear in the inferior, and occasionally in the superior, palpebral conjunctiva, but rarely do they appear on the bulbar conjunctiva. Their presence commonly indicates viral or toxic conjunctivitis. There are many causes of acute and chronic follicular conjunctivitis (Box 1-3).

Pseudomembrane or membrane Various severe inflammatory disorders can cause a fibrinous response in the conjunctiva that results in pseudomembrane (Fig. 1-11) or membrane formation (Fig. 1-12). The difference between the two is qualitative and is based on severity. True membranes are more adherent and tend to bleed when they are stripped, whereas pseudomembranes are less adherent and generally do not bleed much when removed. Severe membranes can eventually lead to sig-

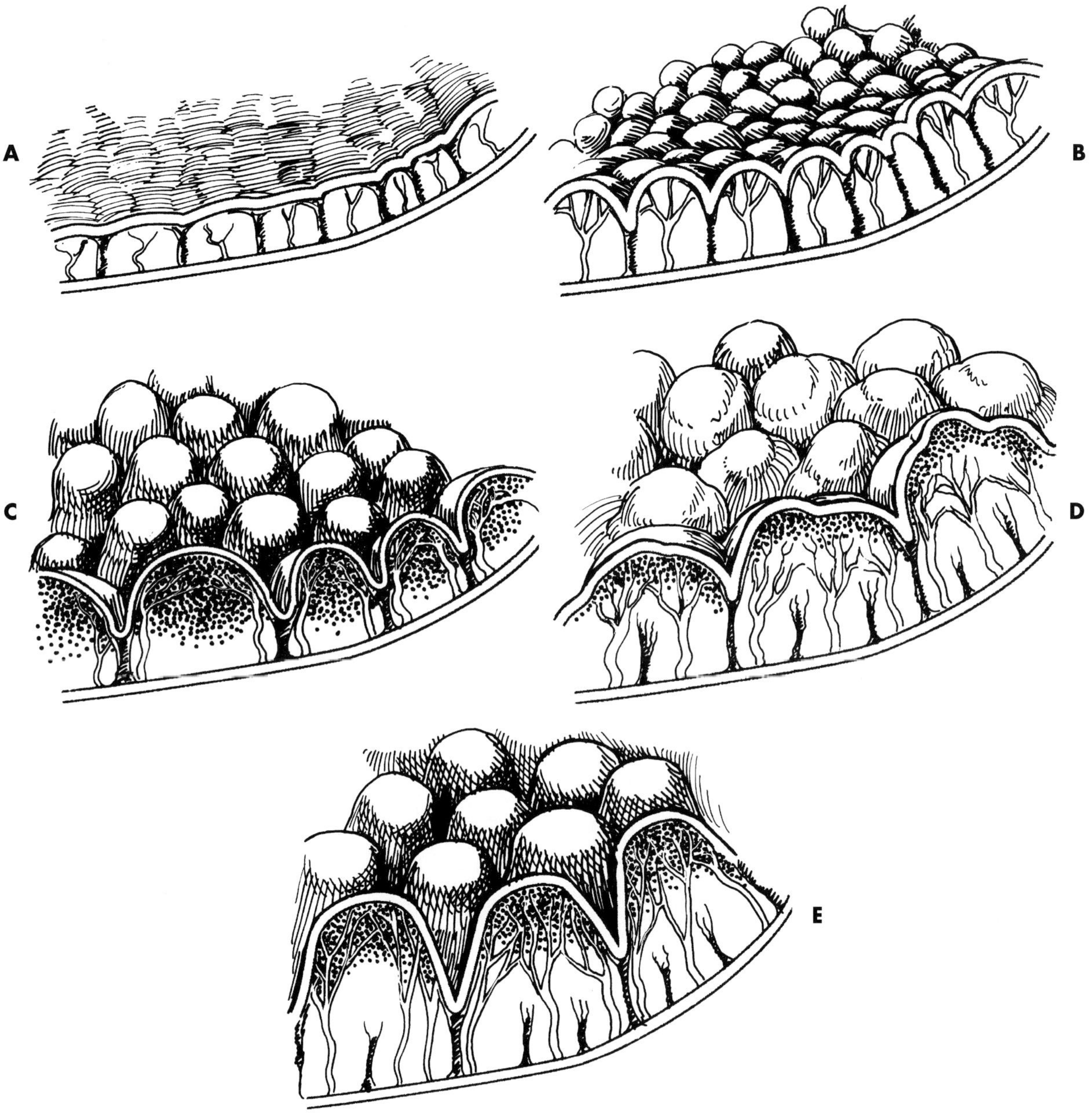

Fig. 1-8 Conjunctival papillae and follicles diagram. **A,** Normal conjunctiva demonstrates a smooth surface. **B,** Conjunctival papillae have a central vascular core. **C,** Conjunctival follicles have a clear center with tiny vessels at the edge. **D,** Giant papillae develop when the anchoring fibrils break. **E,** Large flat-topped cobblestone papillae are an extreme form of giant papillae.

nificant subepithelial fibrosis and scarring (Fig. 1-13). The conditions typically associated with a pseudomembrane or membrane are listed in Box 1-4.

Conjunctival granuloma Conjunctival granulomas signal the presence of chronic granulomatous inflammation of the conjunctiva. They vary in size from small nodules to large elevations (Fig. 1-14). These granulomas consist of mononuclear and giant cells with surrounding fibrovascular proliferation. They are relatively uncommon and, when associated with preauricular lymphadenopathy, are referred to as oculoglandular syndrome (see the section on Parinaud's oculoglandular syndrome in this chapter). They can also be found in patients with other conditions, such as sarcoidosis.

INFECTIOUS CONJUNCTIVITIS

Ophthalmia neonatorum Ophthalmia neonatorum, or neonatal conjunctivitis, is a general term used to refer to any form of conjunctivitis acquired at birth or within the first 2 to 3 weeks of life. Its causes are usually infectious (Table 1-1). The only exception is

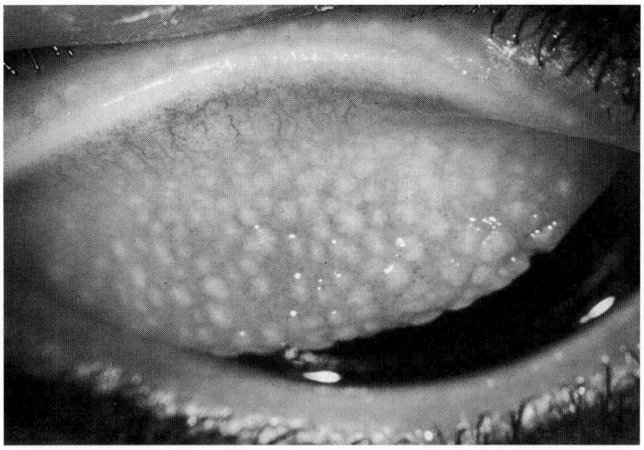

Fig. 1-9 Giant papillary conjunctivitis. Giant papillae are seen under the upper eyelid as a result of protein buildup on contact lenses.

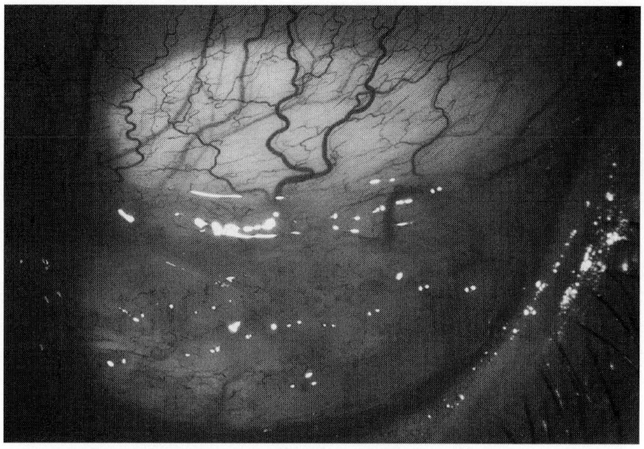

Fig. 1-10 Conjunctival follicles. Inferior conjunctival follicles are apparent in the eye of a patient allergic to bacitracin ointment.

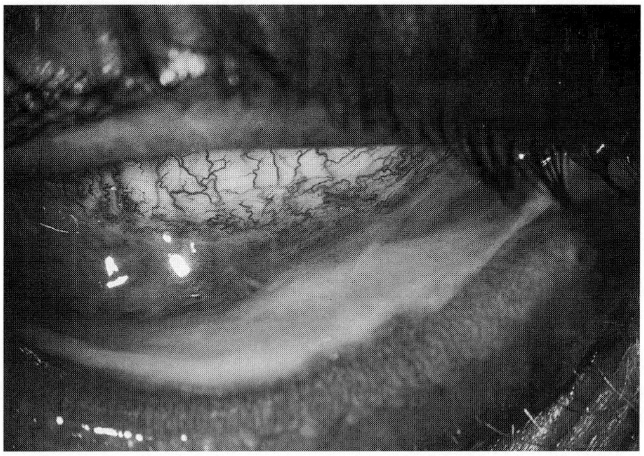

Fig. 1-11 Conjunctival pseudomembrane. When a fibrinous membrane is mildly adherent to the conjunctiva, it is considered a pseudomembrane.

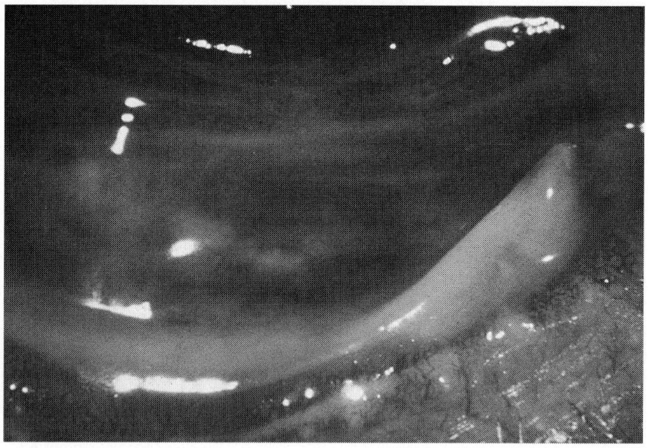

Fig. 1-12 Conjunctival membrane. When a fibrinous membrane adheres to the conjunctiva and bleeds on removal, it is considered a membrane. Severe viral conjunctivitis developed in this eye.

Box 1-3 Common Causes of Acute and Chronic Follicular Conjunctivitis

ACUTE	CHRONIC
Adenovirus	Inclusion conjunctivitis
Herpes simplex (primary and recurrent)	Molluscum contagiosum
Herpes zoster (early)	Toxicity
Inclusion conjunctivitis	Parinaud's oculoglandular syndrome
Picornavirus	Moraxella
	Pediculosis
	Trachoma

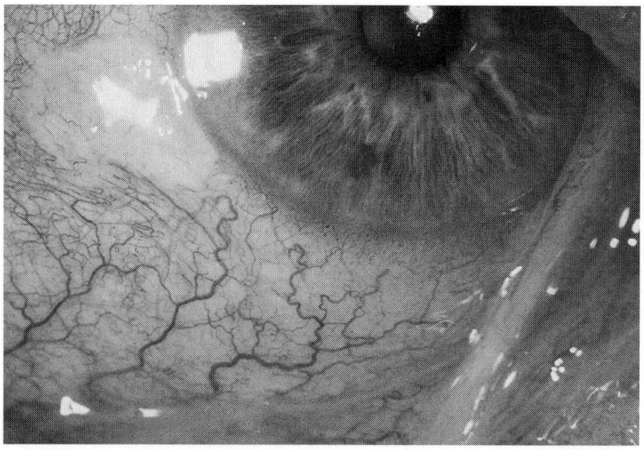

Fig. 1-13 Conjunctival subepithelial fibrosis. The eye in Fig. 1-12 that had a conjunctival membrane healed with moderate conjunctival scarring.

chemical or toxic conjunctivitis, caused by the instillation of a prophylactic agent at birth (usually silver nitrate) that lasts only 24 to 36 hours. Ophthalmia neonatorum should be suspected whenever diffuse conjunctival injection is discovered in one eye or both eyes of an infant, especially with associated mucopurulent discharge. Although various organisms may cause neonatal infectious conjunctivitis, the two most important ones are *Neisseria gonorrhoeae* and *Chlamydia trachomatis.*

N. gonorrhoeae causes severe, aggressive hyperacute neonatal conjunctivitis, which typically appears in the first several days of life. This type of conjunctivitis is

Box 1-4 Inflammatory Disorders Associated with Conjunctival Pseudomembranes or Membranes

Adenoviral conjunctivitis
Gonococcal conjunctivitis
Chemical burns
Stevens-Johnson syndrome
Ocular cicatricial pemphigoid
Seasonal conjunctivitis (vernal and atopic)
Diphtheroid conjunctivitis
Chlamydia in children
Beta-hemolytic streptococci
Ligneous conjunctivitis

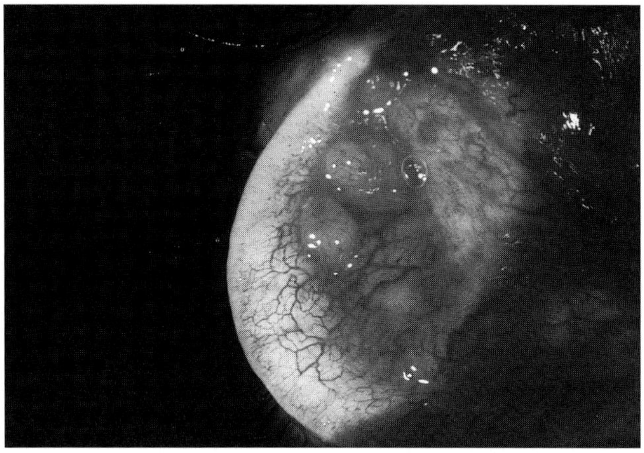

Fig. 1-14 Conjunctival granuloma. Several large conjunctival granulomas were noted in the inferior palpebral conjunctiva. Biopsy specimen showed that they were positive for sarcoidosis.

Table 1-1 Causes and features of ophthalmia neonatorum

Causes	Time of onset	Clinical features	Laboratory findings	Treatment
Chemical	1st-2nd day	Diffuse injection Scant discharge	None	Observation
Neisseria gonorrhoeae	1st week	Copious mucopurulent discharge Conjunctival injection, chemosis, and membrane Eyelid edema	Gram-negative intracellular diplococci in polymorphonuclear leukocytes on Gram stain	125 mg Ceftriaxone IM or 25-50 mg/kg Cefotaxime IV or IM every 8-12 h for 7 d and 12.5 mg/kg Erythromycin PO or IV every 6 h for 14 d plus Topical bacitracin ointment
Chlamydia trachomatis	2nd week	No follicles Conjunctival membrane Mucopurulent discharge	Basophilic intracytoplasmic inclusion bodies in conjunctival epithelial cells on Giemsa stain	12.5 mg/kg Erythromycin PO or IV every 6 h for 14 d plus Topical erythromycin ointment
Other bacteria	1st week	Conjunctival injection with variable mucopurulent discharge	Staphylococci, streptococci, gram-negative species on Gram stain	Bacitracin ointment qid
Herpes simplex virus	1st week	Corneal/conjunctival dendrites Eyelid vesicles	Multinucleated giant cells on Giemsa stain	Topical vidarabine 5×/day plus Systemic antiviral medication prescribed by pediatrician

Table 1-2 Causes of bacterial conjunctivitis

Organism	Laboratory findings	Severity	Onset
Neisseria spp (*N. gonorrhoeae, N. meningitidis*)	Gram-negative intracellular diplococci	Severe	Hyperacute (less than 24 h)
Hemophilus spp (*H. influenzae*)	Gram-negative coccobacilli	Moderate	Acute/subacute (hours to days)
Streptococcus spp (*S. pneumoniae*)	Gram-positive cocci	Moderate	Acute/subacute (hours to days)
Staphylococcus spp (*S. aureus*)	Gram-positive cocci	Mild-moderate	Acute/chronic (hours to weeks)
Moraxella spp (*M. lacunata*)	Gram-negative rods	Mild	Chronic (days to weeks)

characterized by copious mucopurulent discharge that reaccumulates soon after it is wiped away. It is usually accompanied by marked conjunctival injection and chemosis, conjunctival membranes, and eyelid edema. Laboratory stains and cultures showing gram-negative intracellular diplococci (shaped like coffee beans) from a conjunctival swab can help confirm the diagnosis. Any suspicion of this type of conjunctivitis warrants prompt diagnosis and treatment because of its rapid progression to corneal ulceration, perforation, and endophthalmitis. Disseminated gonococcal infection is rare but can lead to infant death. Neonates are also particularly susceptible to concomitant chlamydial infection causing meningitis, pneumonitis, and otitis media. The mainstay of treatment for gonococcal conjunctivitis is systemic antibiotic therapy. The current recommendation for neonates is a single injection of either 125 mg ceftriaxone intramuscularly (IM) or 25 to 50 mg/kg cefotaxime intravenously (IV) or IM every 8 to 12 hours for 7 days and 12.5 mg/kg erythromycin by mouth (PO) or IV every 6 hours for 14 days to cover for chlamydia. Local therapy consists of copious irrigation of the eye with normal saline and frequent administration of topical bacitracin ointment. Close follow-up is required to ensure that the cornea does not become involved.

C. trachomatis is an obligate intracellular bacterium that causes neonatal conjunctivitis. It may occur within days of birth in severe cases or it may not appear until several weeks after the neonate is born. It differs in several ways from adult inclusion conjunctivitis, most notably by the absence of follicles. Additional discussions of chlamydial conjunctivitis are addressed in a later section of this chapter. When chlamydial infection is suspected because of the clinical appearance of the patient, the conjunctiva should be swabbed for specific chlamydial stains, such as MicroTrak, and cultures. In addition, routine culture and Gram and Giemsa staining should be performed to confirm the presence of a *Chlamydia* sp and to rule out possible infection with a *Neisseria* sp or another bacterium. Although neonatal chlamydial infections usually respond to topical erythromycin ointment, systemic erythromycin therapy (12.5 mg/kg PO or IV every 6 hours for 14 days) should be instituted to prevent potential associated pneumonitis and otitis media. Parents of babies with infectious conjunctivitis should also be evaluated and treated.

Bacterial conjunctivitis Numerous microorganisms may cause bacterial conjunctivitis that ranges in onset and severity (Table 1-2). However, bacterial conjunctivitis is fairly uncommon; it accounts for only approximately 5% of all cases of conjunctivitis. Clinical signs include variable degrees of conjunctival injection, papillae, and mucopurulent discharge with no preauricular adenopathy (Fig. 1-15), except in hyperacute cases. Definitive diagnosis is based on stains and cultures after swabbing the conjunctiva. With the exception of hyperacute *Neisseria* spp, other bacterial infections are treated with a topical broad-spectrum antibiotic solution (e.g., trimethoprim/polymyxin B, ciprofloxacin, ofloxacin) or an antibiotic ointment (e.g., bacitracin, erythromycin, polymyxin B, ciprofloxacin) four times a day (qid) for approximately a week. *Hemophilus influenzae* conjunctivitis in children should be treated with oral amoxicillin/clavulanate potassium because of occasional nonocular involvement such as otitis media, pneumonitis, and meningitis.

Hyperacute bacterial conjunctivitis *N. gonorrhoeae* is the primary cause of hyperacute conjunctivitis in the adult, though *Neisseria meningitidis* can also cause severe conjunctivitis. These species may be distinguished from each other in the laboratory through their sugar fermentation patterns. *N. gonorrhoeae* ferments glucose, whereas *N. meningitidis* ferments glucose and maltose. Clinically, *Neisseria* spp conjunctivitis presents with a rapid, hyperacute onset of marked conjunctival chemosis associated with a massive purulent discharge and preauricular adenopathy (Figs. 1-16 and 1-17). When suspected, it is imperative that immediate Gram staining

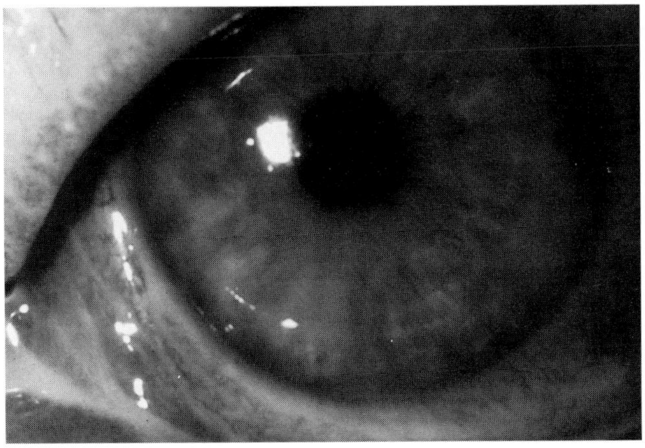

Fig. 1-15 Bacterial conjunctivitis. A moderate mucopurulent discharge can be seen in this eye with *Staphylococcus aureus* conjunctivitis.

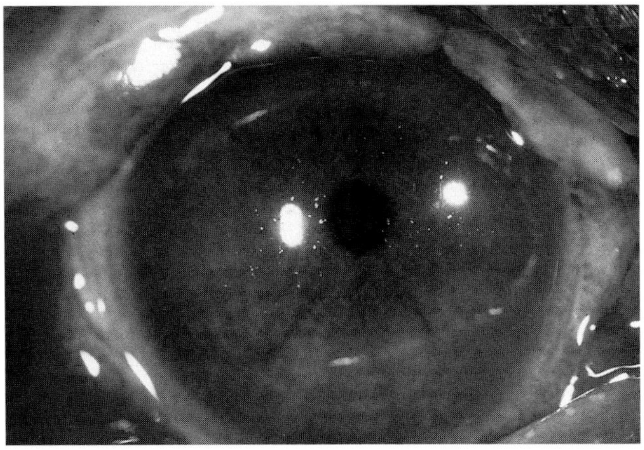

Fig. 1-17 *Neisseria gonorrhoeae* conjunctivitis. This eye with *N. gonorrhoeae* conjunctivitis had significant injection and chemosis. Purulent discharge could be seen at the superior limbus.

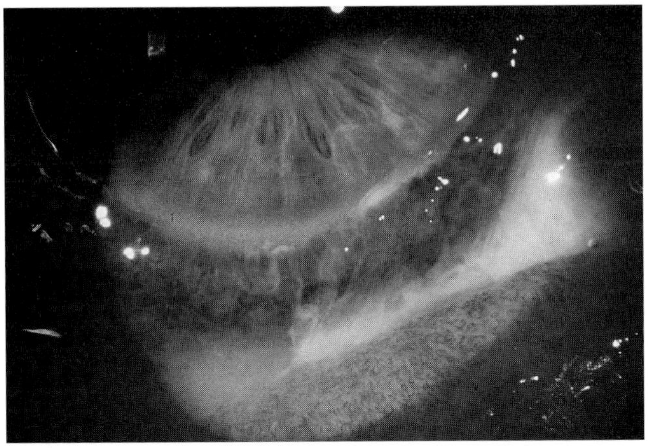

Fig. 1-16 *Neisseria gonorrhoeae* conjunctivitis. Diffuse conjunctival injection was observed in this eye with *N. gonorrhoeae* conjunctivitis. Significant reaccumulation of a purulent discharge occurred soon after it was wiped away.

be performed. Gram-negative intracellular diplococci are diagnostic for this condition. Untreated gonococci can penetrate an intact corneal epithelium and produce rapid stromal ulceration, necrosis, and perforation as early as 24 to 48 hours after infection. Treatment with systemic antibiotics is required. The organism must be cultured on chocolate agar maintained in a 10% carbon dioxide environment. The recommended treatment is 1 g ceftriaxone IM once for conjunctivitis and 1 g IM or IV every 12 hours for 3 to 5 days for corneal involvement. Ciprofloxacin and spectinomycin are alternatives for patients allergic to penicillin/cephalosporin. Topical treatment alone with medications such as ciprofloxacin is insufficient, though it may be a helpful adjunct. Frequent irrigation with saline may be required to remove the copious purulent discharge. Patients should be tested for other sexually transmitted diseases, including syphilis and human immunodeficiency virus (HIV); concurrent treatment with oral doxycycline, tetracycline, or erythromycin should be considered for chlamydial infection.

Viral conjunctivitis By far the most common cause of viral conjunctivitis is adenovirus (Table 1-3). Important clues in the patient's history include the spread of conjunctivitis from one eye to the other (with the first eye the more severely affected), recent upper respiratory tract infection, and contact with someone with a red eye. Besides redness (Fig. 1-18), symptoms of adenoviral conjunctivitis include itching and watery discharge. The classic sign on examination is conjunctival follicles, but subconjunctival hemorrhage (Fig. 1-19) and conjunctival membranes/pseudomembranes may also exist (Fig. 1-20). These patients usually have a tender, palpable preauricular node. If there is corneal involvement, symptoms and signs may include decreased vision, photophobia, foreign-body sensation, and pain, and epithelial and subepithelial infiltrates may be evident on examination. In severe cases, corneal erosion, pseudomembrane/membrane, or both may develop, as may residual scarring. The diagnosis of adenoviral conjunctivitis is clinical. Two commonly reported adenoviral syndromes are epidemic keratoconjunctivitis (EKC—serotypes 8, 11, 19, and 37) and pharyngoconjunctival fever (PCF—serotypes 3, 4, and 7). The incubation period is 5 to 12 days, and patients are infectious for approximately 2 weeks after onset. Treatment is supportive and consists of cold compresses, artificial tears, and rarely topical antihistamines and vasoconstrictors. Topical corticosteroids have been advocated for severe pseudomembranes/membranes and late-onset corneal infiltrates that reduce vision. Patients should be advised to take strict hygiene precautions (i.e., frequent handwashing, use of separate towels, and

Table 1-3 Causes and features of viral conjunctivitis

Causes	Clinical features	Treatment
Adenovirus	Inferior conjunctival follicles Punctate subconjunctival hemorrhages Membrane/pseudomembrane Palpebral preauricular node	Cold compresses Artificial tears Occasionally topical antihistamines and vasoconstrictors Rarely topical corticosteroids
Herpes simplex	Eyelid/skin vesicles Bulbar conjunctival dendrite Conjunctival follicles Palpable preauricular node	Topical trifluorothymidine drops or vidarabine ointment 5×/day
Picornavirus (enterovirus 70, coxsackievirus A24)	Acute subconjunctival hemorrhage in bulbar/palpebral conjunctiva Eyelid ecchymosis	Same as adenovirus
Molluscum contagiosum	Molluscum lesions on eyelid	Simple excision, incision and curettage, cautery, or cryotherapy of lesions

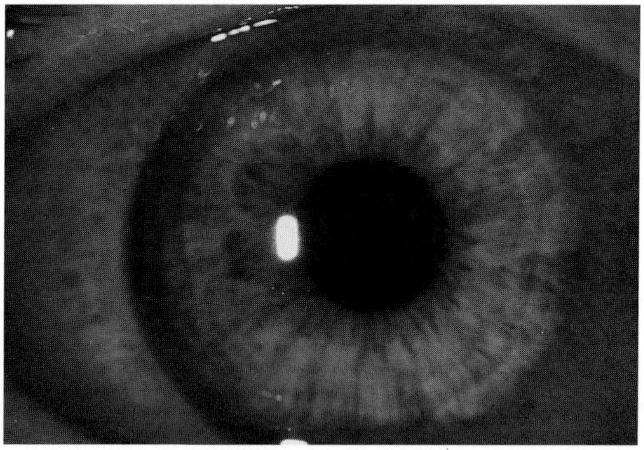

Fig. 1-18 Viral conjunctivitis. A diffusely injected conjunctiva is typical of a viral conjunctivitis.

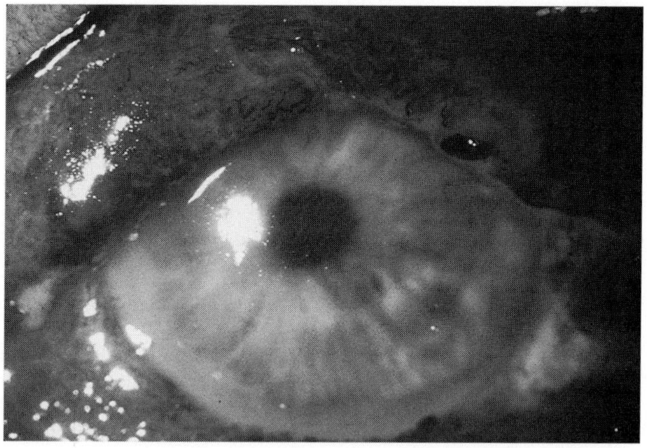

Fig. 1-19 Viral conjunctivitis. Beefy injected conjunctiva is apparent in this eye with severe viral conjunctivitis. Multiple small subconjunctival hemorrhages can be seen. (See color plate.)

avoidance of physical contact with other persons) because adenoviral infections are extremely contagious, especially in the first week or two (as long as the eye is red). Patients can expect symptoms to worsen for the first few days after onset and to be resolved in 2 to 3 weeks. Often the fellow eye becomes involved a few days after the first eye, though usually not as severely. Subepithelial infiltrates may develop after the first week or two. They are generally central rather than peripheral and may number from a few to many (Fig. 1-21). If the infiltrates are severe, patients may be treated with a slow taper of weak topical corticosteroids such as 0.1% fluorometholone. Long-term sequelae of severe adenoviral conjunctivitis include subconjunctival fibrosis and symblepharon formation (Fig. 1-22) with punctal or canalicular occlusion.

Picornaviruses, including enterovirus 70 and coxsackievirus A24, can cause an impressive infection known as acute hemorrhagic conjunctivitis, which is extremely contagious and may lead to epidemic spread. It is more common in warm climates. The incubation period is shorter than that for adenovirus, typically 1 to 4 days. It is characterized by unilateral or bilateral acute subconjunctival hemorrhages with follicles, chemosis, and marked mucopurulent discharge (Fig. 1-23). Eyelid edema, ecchymosis, and preauricular adenopathy are commonly observed (Fig. 1-24). The course is self-limited and lasts fewer than 7 to 12 days. Patients are infectious for approximately 7 days after onset. As with adenovirus, treatment is mainly supportive.

Although herpes simplex virus typically causes keratitis, infection may be limited to the conjunctiva. The patient often has a history of cold sores, fever blisters, or previous herpes simplex virus keratitis. On external examination a palpable preauricular lymph node and her-

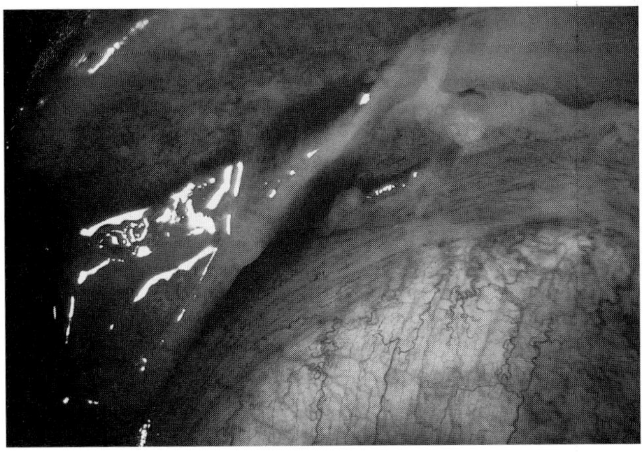

Fig. 1-20 Viral conjunctivitis membrane. A superior conjunctival membrane is present in this eye with viral conjunctivitis. It has been partially peeled, resulting in a small degree of hemorrhage.

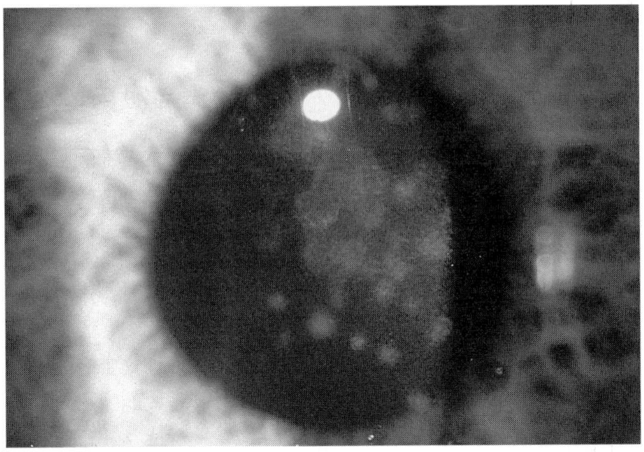

Fig. 1-21 Viral conjunctivitis subepithelial infiltrates. Multiple subepithelial infiltrates are seen centrally in this eye several months after an episode of adenoviral conjunctivitis.

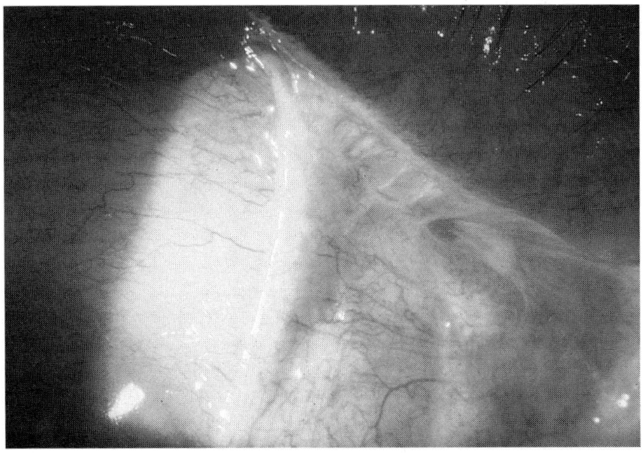

Fig. 1-22 Viral conjunctivitis scarring. Superior conjunctival scarring resulted after the patient had the severe viral conjunctivitis seen in Fig. 1-19. The upper eyelid margin was adherent to the bulbar conjunctiva.

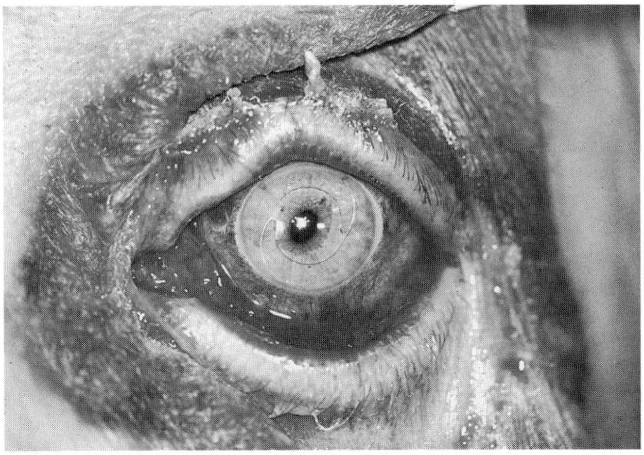

Fig. 1-23 Acute hemorrhagic conjunctivitis. Significant crusted discharge, conjunctival injection, and subconjunctival hemorrhage are evident in this eye with acute hemorrhagic conjunctivitis. An anterior chamber intraocular lens can be seen.

petic vesicles on the eyelids or the periocular skin may be found. The most common finding is a follicular conjunctival reaction. Occasionally, a dendrite that stains brilliantly with fluorescein is seen on the bulbar conjunctiva, confirming the diagnosis of herpes simplex conjunctivitis (Fig. 1-25). Slit-lamp examination reveals a follicular reaction alone or in addition to corneal changes from past or recurrent disease (see Chapter 4). Treatment for eyelid margin/conjunctival involvement includes topical antiviral therapy with 1% trifluorothymidine drops or 3% vidarabine ointment 5 times a day. Patients should be closely monitored for the development of corneal involvement.

Chlamydial conjunctivitis *C. trachomatis*, with its various serotypes, causes three distinct conjunctivitis syndromes: trachoma (serotypes A to C), adult inclusion conjunctivitis (serotypes D to K), and lymphogranuloma venereum (serotypes L1 to L3). Trachoma is endemic to North Africa, the Middle East, and other regions in which poor hygiene and poor sanitation remain a problem. The condition is spread from eye to eye by vectors such as the common housefly. Symptoms vary and include redness, tearing, and foreign body sensation. Early signs of conjunctival involvement include a severe follicular reaction involving the superior tarsal conjunctiva and the limbus (Fig. 1-26). These limbal follicles later scar to form depressed areas known as Herbert's pits (Fig. 1-27). Other late changes involve linear scarring of the superior tarsal conjunctiva (known as Arlt's line) (Fig. 1-28) and the eyelid margin causing cicatricial entropion, and trichiasis (Figs. 1-29 and 1-30). Corneal findings are both primary and secondary to the surrounding conjunctival/eyelid

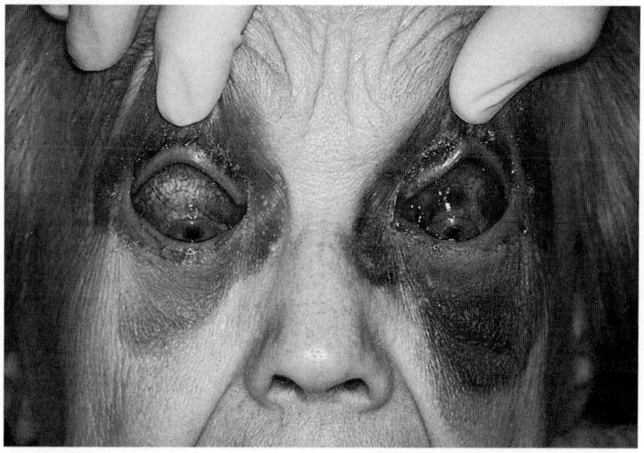

Fig. 1-24 Acute hemorrhagic conjunctivitis. Bilateral eyelid ecchymoses, conjunctivitis, and conjunctival hemorrhage are seen. This infection began in the left eye, which was more severely affected, and moved to the right eye within 1 day. (See color plate.)

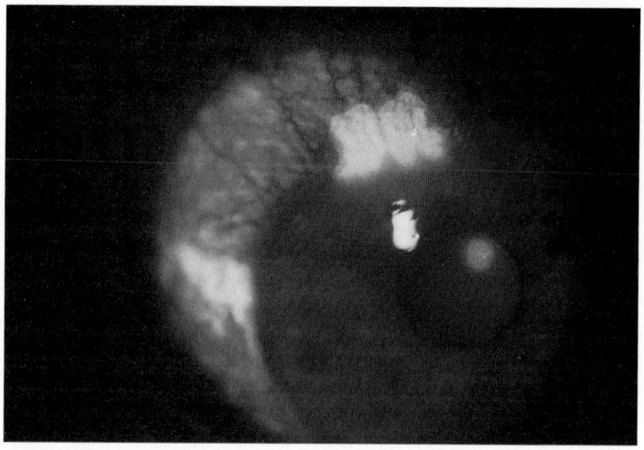

Fig. 1-25 Herpes simplex virus conjunctivitis. Two limbal conjunctival herpes simplex virus dendrites are seen in this patient with acquired immunodeficiency syndrome. The dendrites stain brilliantly with fluorescein. (See color plate.)

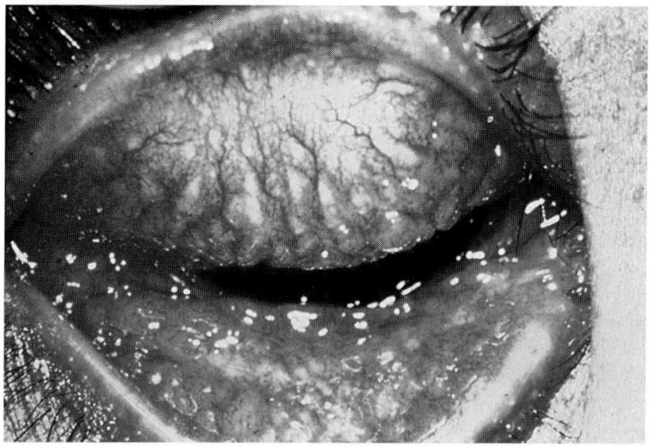

Fig. 1-26 Trachoma. Superior tarsal follicles are a prominent feature of trachoma. (Courtesy of George O. Waring III, M.D.)

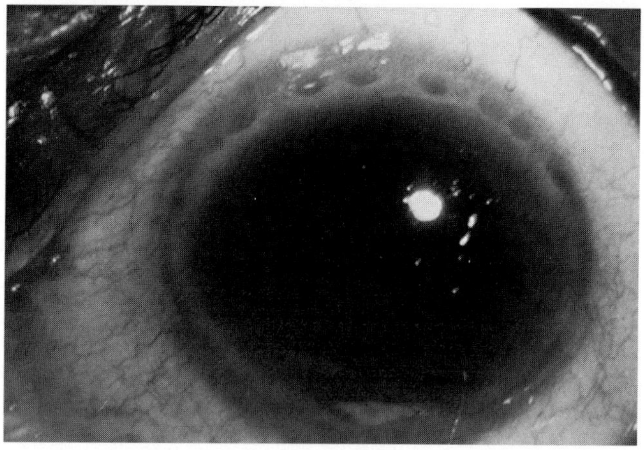

Fig. 1-27 Herbert's pits in trachoma. Multiple small, depressed areas of peripheral corneal scarring are visible at the superior limbus after scarring of limbal follicles.

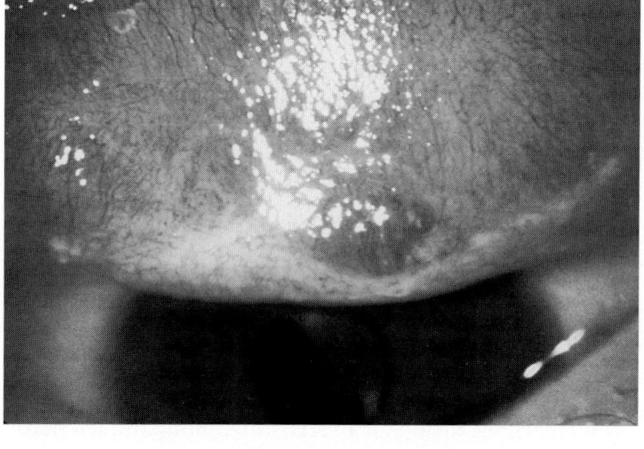

Fig. 1-28 Arlt's line in trachoma. A linear scar in the tarsal conjunctiva of the upper eyelid as a result of trachoma.

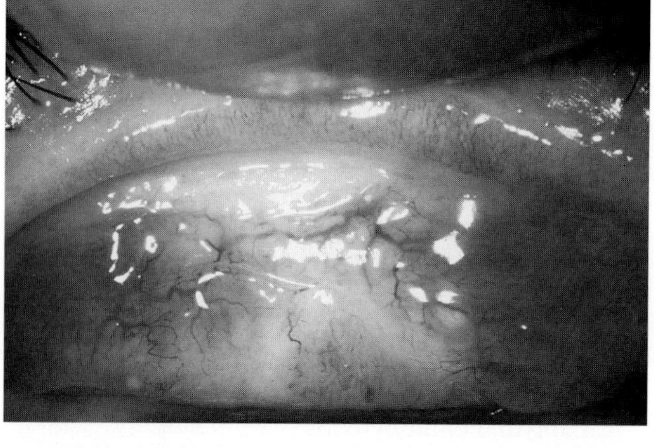

Fig. 1-29 Conjunctival scarring in trachoma. The superior tarsal conjunctiva can become diffusely scarred from trachoma.

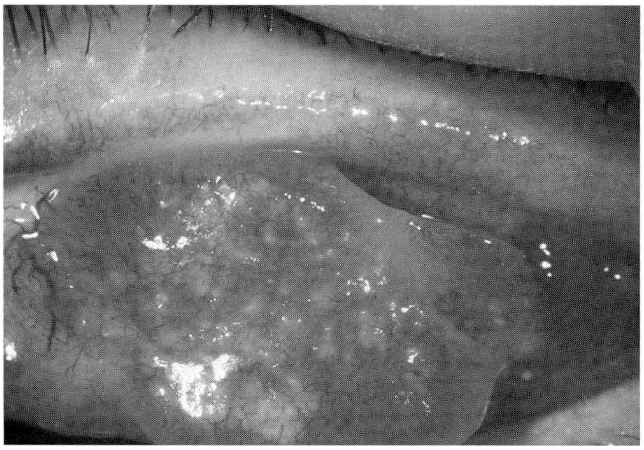

Fig. 1-30 Conjunctival scarring in trachoma. The fellow eye of the patient in Fig. 1-29 has a severe, elevated hypertrophic scar in the upper tarsal conjunctiva.

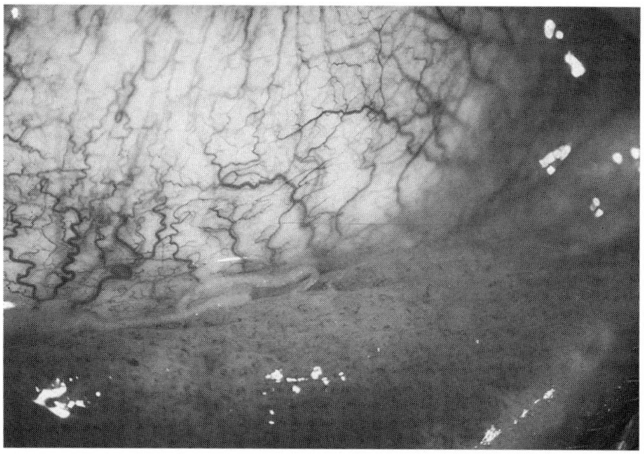

Fig. 1-31 Adult inclusion conjunctivitis. A stringy mucoid discharge can be seen along with small confluent inferior conjunctival follicles in this patient with *C. trachomatis* conjunctivitis.

Box 1-5 World Health Organization Classification of Trachoma

Follicles—severe conjunctival follicles
Inflammation—diffuse conjunctival inflammation
Scarring—tarsal conjunctival scarring
Trichiasis
Opacification—corneal opacification

Table 1-4 Neonatal versus adult chlamydial conjunctivitis

Clinical features	Neonatal form	Adult form
Follicular response	−	+++
Conjunctival membrane	+	−
Mucopurulent discharge	+++	+
Intracytoplasmic inclusions (on Giemsa stain)	+++	+
Response to topical medication (but requires systemic treatment)	+++	+

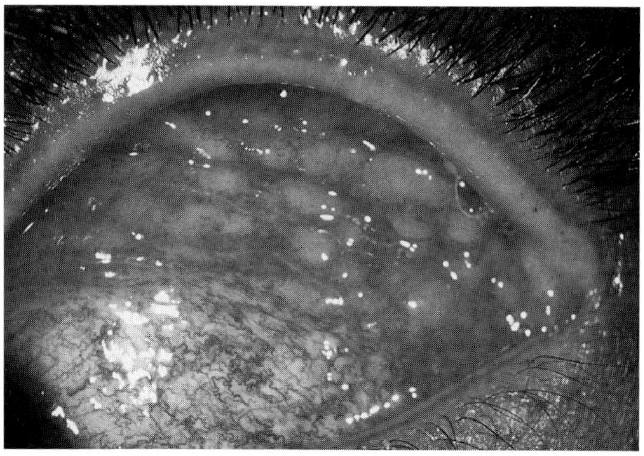

Fig. 1-32 Adult inclusion conjunctivitis. Although inferior follicles are almost always present, superior conjunctival follicles can also be seen in a patient with severe chronic *C. trachomatis* conjunctivitis.

scarring and usually result in a superficial fibrovascular scar in the superior cornea. The signs of trachoma are progressive, and various health groups have organized them according to severity. One useful classification schema, proposed by the World Health Organization (WHO), is outlined in Box 1-5. Trachoma is treated topically and systemically. Topical erythromycin ointment (twice a day [bid] to qid) and oral tetracycline or erythromycin (250 to 500 mg qid) should be administered for at least 1 month. Reinfection, however, is common if hygienic conditions do not improve.

Adult inclusion conjunctivitis is a sexually transmitted disease found typically in teenagers and young adults. Patients frequently are sexually active and may or may not have concomitant urethritis or cervicitis. Additionally, many patients have had a new sexual partner within the past 6 months. The characteristics are different from those of neonatal chlamydial conjunctivitis (Table 1-4). In adults the infection results in chronic follicular conjunctivitis most prominent in the inferior palpebral and forniceal conjunctivae (Figs. 1-31 and 1-32). Scant mucopurulent discharge, preauricular adenopathy, and superior or peripheral corneal epithelial and subepithelial infiltrates or both are other signs (Fig. 1-33). The appearance of adult inclusion conjunctivitis can mimic that of

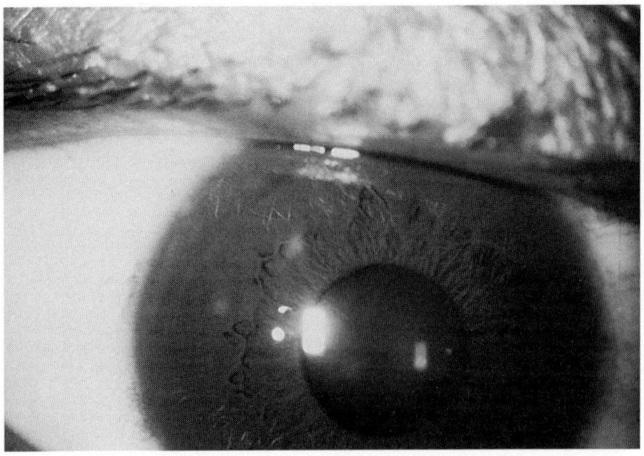

Fig. 1-33 Adult inclusion conjunctivitis. Several mid-peripheral subepithelial infiltrates are present in this eye with *C. trachomatis* conjunctivitis.

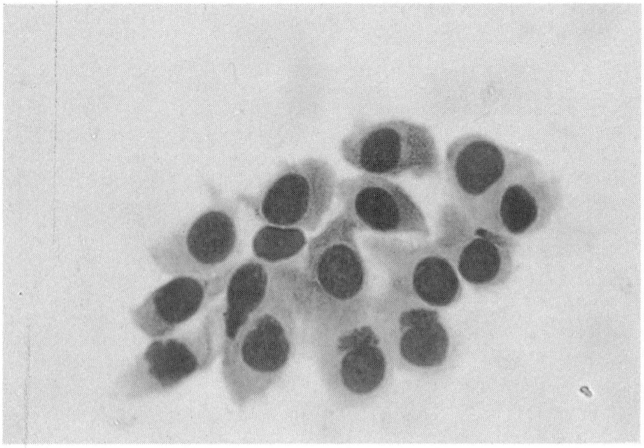

Fig. 1-34 Adult inclusion conjunctivitis. A Giemsa stain of a conjunctival scraping reveals intracytoplasmic basophilic inclusion bodies adjacent to the nuclei in these epithelial cells. (See color plate.)

Table 1-5 Adult inclusion versus adenoviral conjunctivitis

Clinical features	Adult inclusion	Adenovirus
Conjunctival follicles	Yes	Yes
Conjunctival discharge	Scant mucopurulent	Watery
Conjunctival membrane	No	Yes
Subepithelial infiltrates	Superior More peripheral	Central
Corneal pannus	Superior	None
Preauricular node	Yes	Yes

adenoviral conjunctivitis especially because each causes a follicular reaction. Certain clinical features can help differentiate the two (Table 1-5). Definitive diagnosis can be achieved through conjunctival scrapings for Giemsa staining (Fig. 1-34), chlamydial cultures, and direct chlamydial immunofluorescence tests. Recommended treatment is oral tetracycline (250 mg qid), oral erythromycin (500 mg qid), or oral doxycycline (100 mg bid) for 3 to 6 weeks. Equally important is the treatment of sexual partners. Patients and their sexual contacts should also be evaluated for other sexually transmitted diseases such as syphilis, gonorrhea, and HIV.

Lymphogranuloma venereum is a sexually transmitted chlamydial infection characterized by large and painful inguinal lymphadenopathy. Nonspecific constitutional symptoms include fever, headache, malaise, and arthralgia. Ocular involvement is rare and results in features seen with Parinaud's oculoglandular syndrome (see next section). Treatment for this condition is the same as that for adult inclusion conjunctivitis.

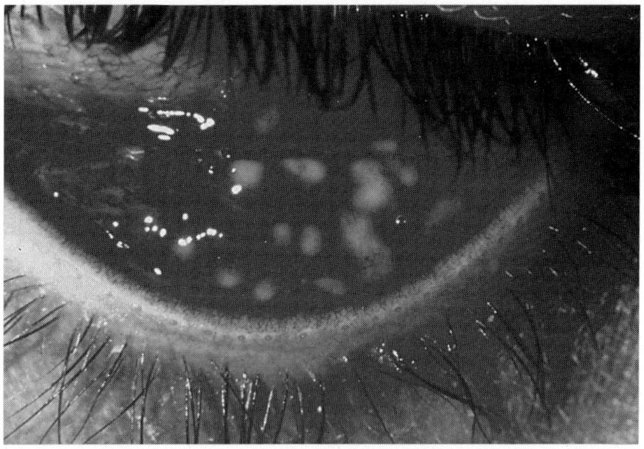

Fig. 1-35 Parinaud's oculoglandular syndrome. Multiple palpebral conjunctival granulomas are present inferiorly. (Courtesy of George O. Waring III, M.D.)

Parinaud's oculoglandular syndrome As indicated by its name, Parinaud's oculoglandular syndrome consists of granulomatous conjunctivitis associated with lymphadenopathy. The symptoms are nonspecific and include redness, foreign body sensation, and mucopurulent discharge. Palpebral conjunctival granuloma (Fig. 1-35) with marked swollen preauricular or submandibular lymph nodes or both on the same side are the clinical diagnostic signs (Fig. 1-36). The condition is usually unilateral and may be accompanied by fever, skin rash, and conjunctival follicles. Numerous causes have been cited, with cat scratch disease the most common (Table 1-6). The suspicion for cat scratch disease is heightened if the patient has been licked or scratched by a cat or kitten within 2 weeks of the onset of symptoms. Contact with rabbits, wild animals, or ticks suggests tu-

Table 1-6 Causes of Parinaud's oculoglandular syndrome

Causes	Organism	Treatment
Cat scratch disease	*Bartonella henselae*	250 mg Tetracycline PO qid or
	Afipia felis	500 mg Ciprofloxacin PO bid for 2 w
		Topical erythromycin ointment for 2 w
Tularemia	*Francisella tularensis*	1 g Streptomycin IM bid for 7 d
		Topical gentamicin every 2 h for 1 w and then 5×/d until resolved
		Medical consult
Tuberculosis	*Mycobacterium tuberculosis*	Medical consult for systemic antituberculous treatment
Sporotrichosis	*Sporotrichum schenckii*	Oral iodides (e.g., potassium iodide)
Syphilis	*Treponema pallidum*	Topical tetracycline ointment
		Medical consult for systemic penicillin

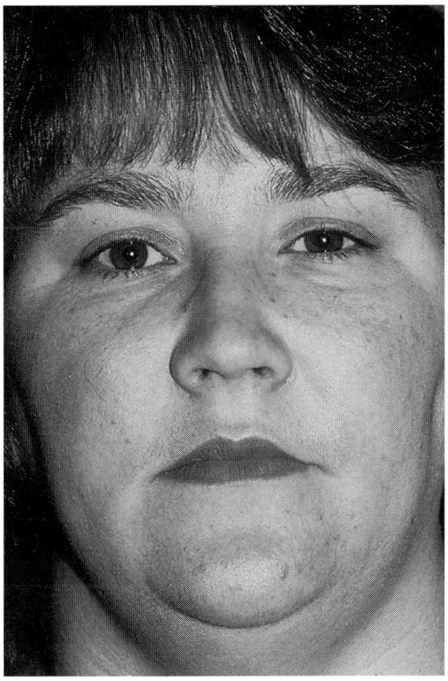

Fig. 1-36 Parinaud's oculoglandular syndrome. This patient with Parinaud's oculoglandular syndrome has submandibular lymphadenopathy.

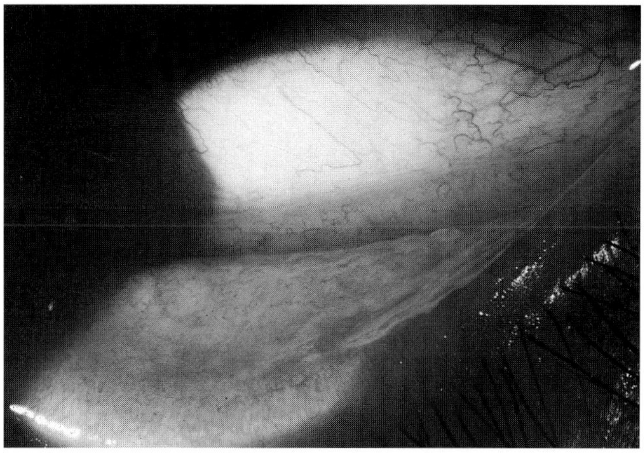

Fig. 1-37 Pediculosis. This patient with pediculosis has prominent follicular conjunctivitis.

laremia, whereas trauma involving vegetable matter could indicate sporotrichosis. When no specific cause is suggested, a general workup should be instituted that includes conjunctival biopsy specimens for Gram, Giemsa, and acid-fast staining and blood agar, Sabouraud's dextrose agar, thioglycolate broth, and Löwenstein Jensen culture medium. Serologic tests should include complete blood count, rapid plasmin reagent test, fluorescent treponemal antibody absorption test, blood culture (if the patient is febrile), and titers for tularemia. A chest x-ray, purified protein derivative test, and anergy panel should be taken to rule out tuberculosis. Besides the specific treatment outlined in Table 1-6, warm compresses for the lymph nodes and antipyretics should be started. Removal of the cat is not necessary if the patient has cat scratch disease.

Pediculosis Pediculosis refers to an infestation of pubic lice (almost always from sexual contact) and can result in acute or chronic conjunctivitis. The inciting organism is an arthropod crab louse known as *Phthirus pubis*. Adult lice and their eggs (called nits) reside on the eyelashes, causing infectious blepharitis and follicular conjunctivitis (Fig. 1-37). Blood-tinged debris on the eyelids and eyelashes is common (Fig. 1-38). Patients have redness and irritation of the eyes and often are sexually active. Close examination of the eyelid margins and eyelashes is necessary because the lice and eggs are often difficult to see (Figs. 1-39 and 1-40). Treatment involves the mechanical removal of all lice (Fig. 1-41) and eggs with fine forceps or their suffocation with topical ointments (e.g., erythromycin ointment three times a day [tid] for 10 days; 0.25% physostigmine ointment has been recommended in the past, but it has adverse ocular side effects). Additional therapy with antilice lotions and shampoos (e.g., lindane, permethrin) should be initiated

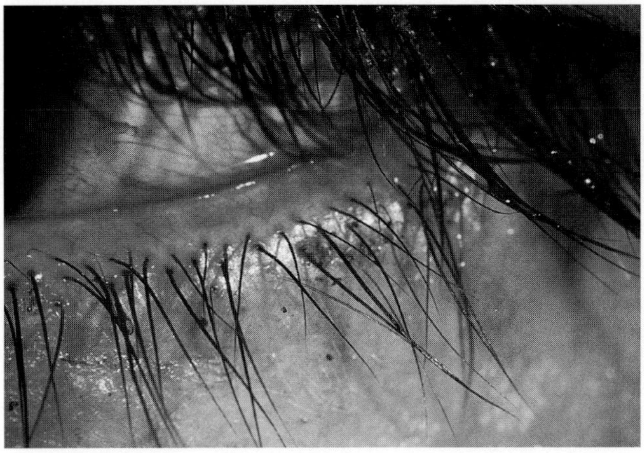

Fig. 1-38 Pediculosis. Blood-tinged debris can be seen along the lower eyelid margin.

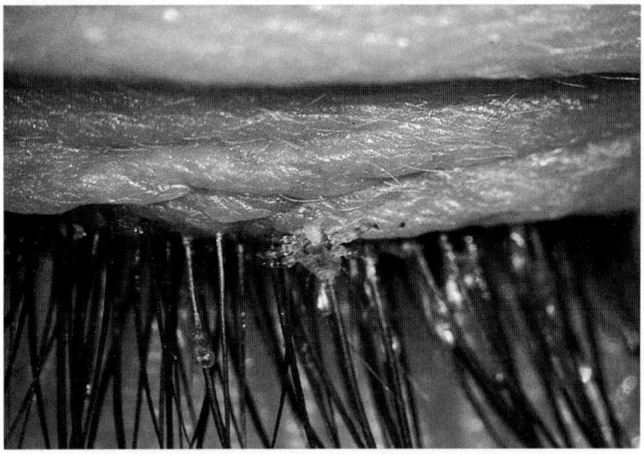

Fig. 1-39 Pediculosis. Several nits (eggs) are visibly attached to the eyelashes. A live louse can be seen at the base of an eyelash centrally.

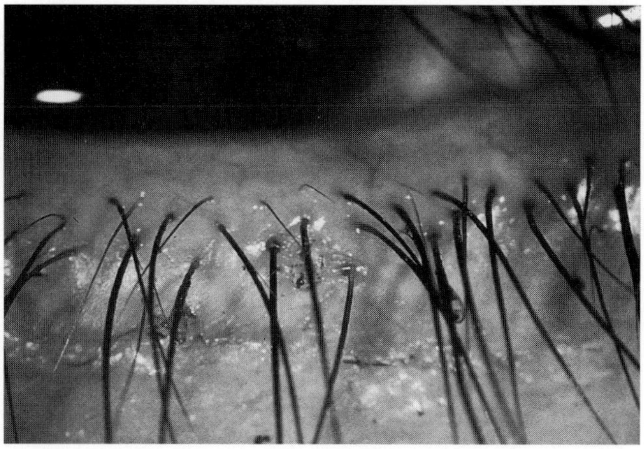

Fig. 1-40 Pediculosis. A crab louse is found embedded in the eyelid skin, attached to two cilia.

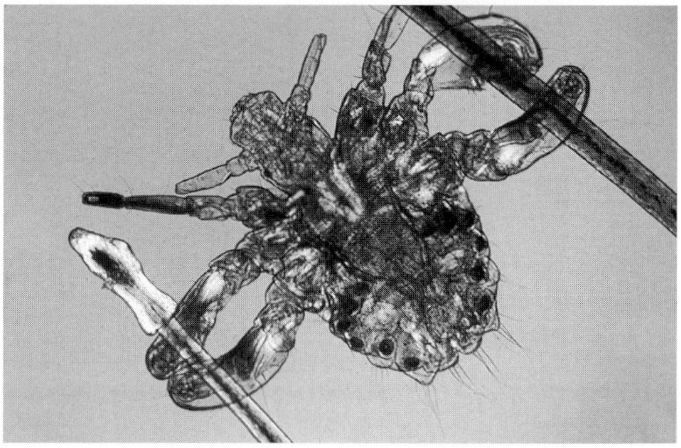

Fig. 1-41 Pediculosis. A crab louse is seen firmly gripping two cilia. Note the dark colored "breathing" holes on the sides of the posterior aspect of the thorax. Clogging these holes with ointment causes suffocation. (Courtesy of Ralph C. Eagle, Jr., M.D.)

on nonocular areas for the patient and sexual partners. All clothes, towels, and linens should be thoroughly washed and heat dried.

Allergic Conjunctivitis

This group of disorders comprises a varying spectrum of allergic ocular diseases, all mediated by a type I immunoglobulin (IgE) hypersensitivity reaction.

Hay fever conjunctivitis Hay fever conjunctivitis is an IgE-mediated allergic reaction to the same airborne allergens that cause hay fever (e.g., ragweed, pollen). Patients have red, itchy, watery eyes. Examination reveals bilateral conjunctival injection, chemosis, and papillae (Fig. 1-42). The condition is usually seasonal, occurring in the spring and fall, and is exacerbated by increased levels of these airborne allergens. Treatment consists of cool compresses, artificial tears, and topical antihistamines several times a day for mild cases. Patients with severe and chronic hay fever can be treated with topical mast cell stabilizers (e.g., 4% cromolyn sodium qid, lodoxamide qid, or olopatadine bid) and with topical and systemic antihistamines (e.g., levocabastine or emedastine drops qid, 25 mg diphenhydramine PO qid). Topical nonsteroidal antiinflammatory agents (e.g., ketorolac qid) can be used if a patient has significant itching. Low-potency corticosteroids (e.g., 0.2% loteprednol qid) may be useful for patients with severe allergic conjunctivitis, but they must be monitored for corticosteroid-induced side effects. Patients are advised to limit their exposure to the outdoors when pollen and other allergen counts are high.

Vernal keratoconjunctivitis Vernal keratoconjunctivitis is a bilateral, severe seasonal allergy that usually affects boys. Patients have marked itching, photophobia, and tearing with thick, ropy mucoid discharge in the

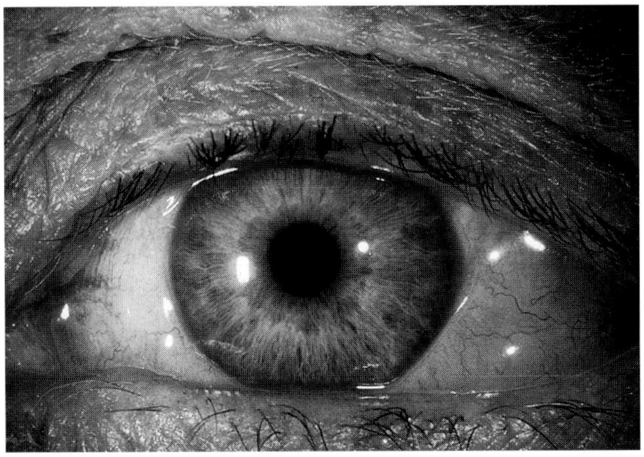

Fig. 1-42 Hay fever conjunctivitis. Significant conjunctival chemosis is evident in this patient with hay fever conjunctivitis.

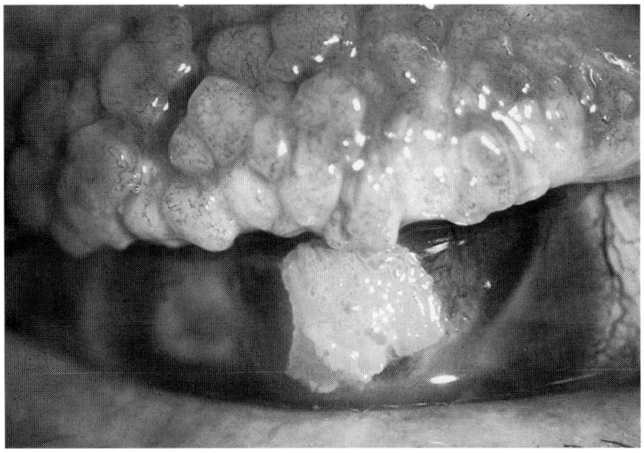

Fig. 1-44 Vernal conjunctivitis. A "shield ulcer" in the central cornea and large papillae on eyelid eversion can be seen in this patient with vernal conjunctivitis.

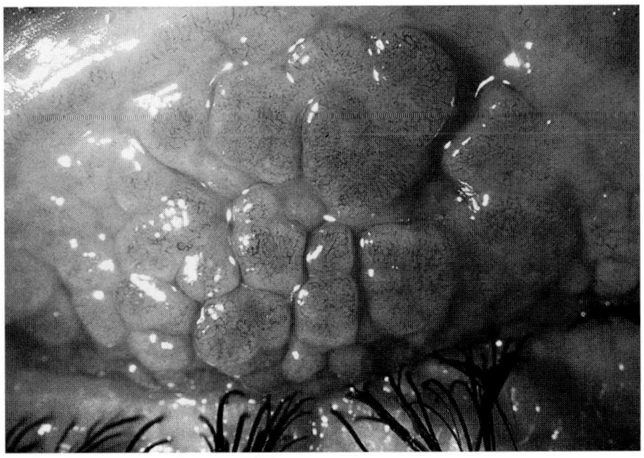

Fig. 1-43 Vernal conjunctivitis. Multiple large cobblestone papillae are present under the upper eyelid in this patient with severe vernal conjunctivitis.

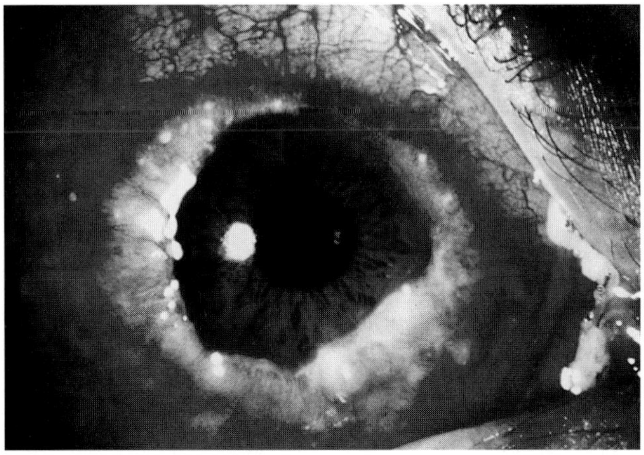

Fig. 1-45 Vernal conjunctivitis. Giant gelatinous papillae along the limbus are present in this limbal variant of vernal conjunctivitis. (Courtesy of George O. Waring III, M.D.)

spring, summer, and fall. The condition manifests itself in palpebral and limbal forms. In the palpebral form, patients have diffuse giant papillae that are more prominent on the upper than the lower palpebral conjunctiva. These giant papillae look like cobblestones with polygonal sides and flat tops (Fig. 1-43). They may be associated with sterile corneal ulceration (known as a shield ulcer), typically located in the upper half of the cornea (Fig. 1-44). Other corneal changes include punctate epithelial keratopathy and corneal vascularization. The limbal variant of vernal keratoconjunctivitis occurs predominantly in boys of African and Asian descent. In this form, giant papillae develop along the limbal margin to produce thickened, gelatinous nodules (Fig. 1-45). Raised white lesions composed of degenerated eosinophils may also appear amid the giant papillae and are termed Trantas dots (Fig. 1-46). Elements of both forms of vernal keratoconjunctivitis may appear together along with diffuse conjunctival hyperemia and chemosis. Besides supportive therapy, treatment is centered on suppressing the inflammatory process. Topical corticosteroids (e.g., fluorometholone or 1% prednisolone acetate qid) are effective in treating the acute inflammation until topical mast-cell stabilizers (e.g., lodoxamide or 4% cromolyn sodium qid or olopatadine bid) have a chance to work. Topical and systemic antihistamines (e.g., levocabastine or emedastine drops qid, 25 mg diphenhydramine PO qid) may also alleviate some of the symptoms. The initiation and duration of these medications should be based on the patient's history of this disease. Those patients who have regular seasonal exacerbations can be started on topical mast cell stabilizers 2 weeks before the anticipated onset of symptoms, whereas those with continuous disease can be maintained on this therapy all year long. Recent reports have also shown topical cyclosporine (2% or 4% cyclosporin A qid) to be effective in the management of severe or refractory cases of vernal and atopic keratoconjunctivitis. However, the topical form of cyclosporine is irritating and is not commercially available; it must be prepared by an experienced pharmacist.

Atopic keratoconjunctivitis Patients with atopic keratoconjunctivitis almost always have a history of atopy, including atopic dermatitis, asthma, or allergic rhinitis. Atopic keratoconjunctivitis has features similar to those of vernal keratoconjunctivitis with several distinguishing exceptions (Table 1-7). Most notably, patients with atopic keratoconjunctivitis exhibit more eyelid and periorbital skin involvement (Fig. 1-47). The inferior conjunctiva is also primarily affected (Fig. 1-48), and extensive corneal and conjunctival scarring and anterior and posterior subcapsular cataracts may develop. The treatment is the same as that for vernal keratoconjunctivitis.

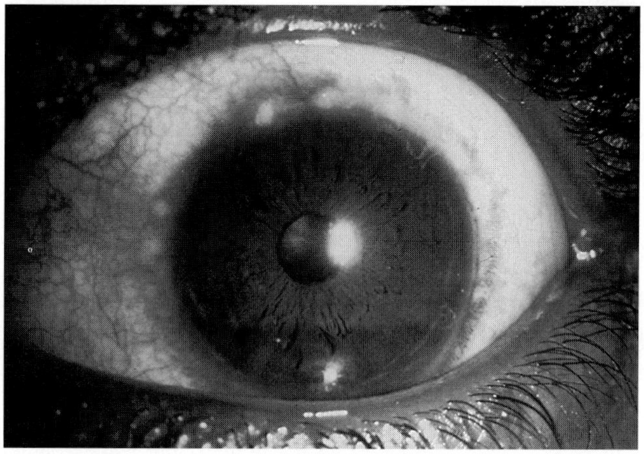

Fig. 1-46 Vernal conjunctivitis. Multiple raised, white lesions along the limbus, containing degenerated eosinophils, are termed Trantas dots.

Topical corticosteroid cream (e.g., 0.05% dexamethasone cream tid) can be used on the eyelid skin if it is severely inflamed. Intraocular pressure must be monitored routinely in all patients who use corticosteroid medications on the eyelids.

Giant papillary conjunctivitis Not to be confused by its name, GPC is considered a separate and distinct entity from other allergic conditions that may include giant conjunctival papillae. GPC refers to a condition in which foreign materials that come in contact with the eyelids produce a hypersensitivity response in patients. The most common precipitant is contact lenses, but others include ocular prostheses and exposed sutures. The condition occurs more frequently in wearers of soft contact lenses (incidence as high as 10% to 15%) and less frequently in wearers of rigid gas permeable and polymethylmethacrylate lenses (incidence, 1% to 5%). Patients have variable itching and mucous discharge, and numerous giant papillae appear on the superior tarsal conjunctiva that are immediately visible on upper eyelid eversion (Fig. 1-49). Treatment for the various precipitants is outlined in Box 1-6. Symptoms generally respond rapidly after removal of the inciting agent. However, it is important to know that the signs of GPC can persist long after symptoms have resolved (sometimes as long as months to years). Patients are generally instructed to return to contact lens and ocular prosthesis wear based on the clinician's evaluation of improvement. Specific steps to prevent future exacerbations among wearers of soft contact lenses include decreasing wearing time, switching to daily or biweekly disposable lenses, disinfecting with hydrogen peroxide systems, and using enzyme tablets more frequently. If the condition persists, patients may have to use rigid gas permeable lenses. Topical mast-cell stabilizers (e.g., lodoxamide or 4% cromolyn sodium qid or olopatadine bid) may be helpful.

Table 1-7 Features of vernal and atopic keratoconjunctivitis

Feature	Vernal	Atopic
Seasonal changes	Definite seasonal exacerbation	Little or no seasonal exacerbation
Itching	More prominent itching	Some itching
Papillae	Giant papillae greater in the upper than the lower palpebral conjunctiva	Small to medium papillae in upper and lower palpebral conjunctiva
Eyelid changes	Minimal external eyelid changes	Eczematous changes on eyelids
Chemosis	Minimal	Moderate milky, boggy conjunctival edema
Corneal scarring	Less corneal scarring	Extensive corneal scarring and vascularization
Conjunctival scarring	Less conjunctival scarring	More conjunctival scarring with symblepharon formation
Lens changes	No associated lens changes	Associated anterior and posterior subcapsular opacities
Eosinophils on cytologic examination	Numerous	Few

Mechanical Conjunctivitis

Disorders characterized as mechanical conjunctivitis have been grouped together because some type of mechanical phenomenon is thought to play a role in their pathophysiology.

Superior limbic keratoconjunctivitis Superior limbic keratoconjunctivitis (SLK) is an interesting disorder in which, as the name implies, the clinical manifestations occur at the superior limbus. The condition is thought to result from abnormal mechanical trauma involving the superior bulbar and palpebral conjunctivae. Patients often have unilateral or bilateral symptoms of dry eyes (redness, burning, foreign body sensation, photophobia, and tearing). Although associated dry eye symptoms may occur, the corneal surface is usually normal and basic tear secretion test results are normal. Instead, slit-lamp examination reveals radial injection limited to the superior bulbar conjunctiva and punctate epithelial keratopathy

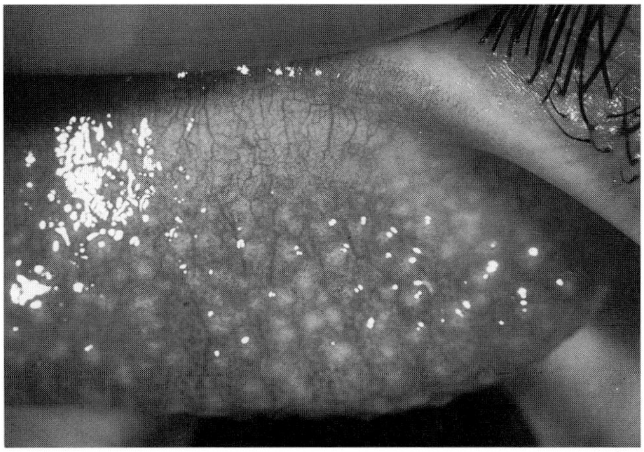

Fig. 1-49 Giant papillary conjunctivitis. Prominent giant papillae are seen on upper eyelid eversion in this wearer of extended-wear contact lenses. Small white scars may appear on the apexes of the papilla, which are smaller and rounder than the giant cobblestone papillae seen in vernal conjunctivitis.

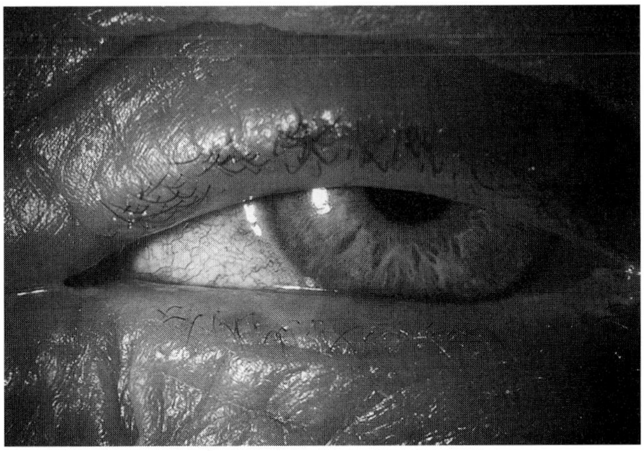

Fig. 1-47 Atopic conjunctivitis. Redness and thickening of the eyelid skin are prominent features of atopic ocular disease.

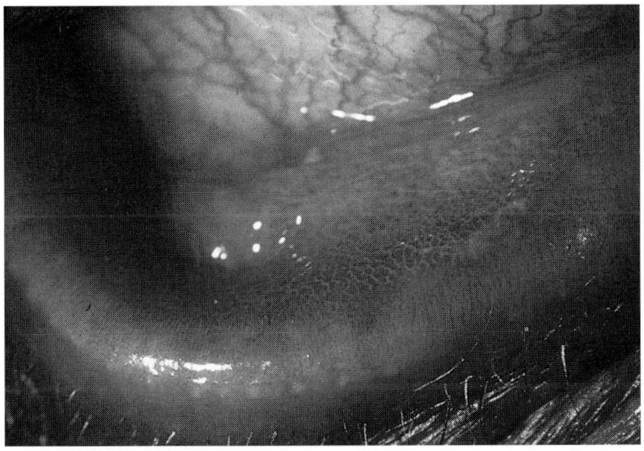

Fig. 1-48 Atopic conjunctivitis. Chronic mixed papillofollicular conjunctival reaction can be seen inferiorly in this patient with atopic conjunctivitis.

Box 1-6 Treatment Regimen for Giant Papillary Conjunctivitis

CONTACT LENSES

Mild Cases

1. Replace with new contact lenses if current lenses have been worn longer than recommended time or if they contain deposits
2. Decrease wearing time
3. Change from extended-wear to daily-wear lenses (frequent replacement or single use)
4. Increase cleaning frequency with appropriate cleaners, enzymes, and solutions
5. Start mast-cell stabilizer (e.g., 4% cromolyn sodium or lodoxamide qid)

Severe Cases

1. Discontinue contact lens wear temporarily
2. Start mast-cell stabilizer (e.g., 4% cromolyn sodium or lodoxamide qid)

OCULAR PROSTHESES

1. Replace prosthesis if old
2. Clean prosthesis more frequently
3. Consider special coating of prosthesis (e.g., Biocoat)
4. Start mast-cell stabilizer (e.g., 4% cromolyn sodium or lodoxamide qid)

EXPOSED SUTURE

1. Trim or remove exposed suture(s)
2. Topical bacitracin, erythromycin, polymyxin, or ciprofloxacin ointment bid for 4 days
3. Start mast-cell stabilizer (e.g., 4% cromolyn sodium or lodoxamide qid)

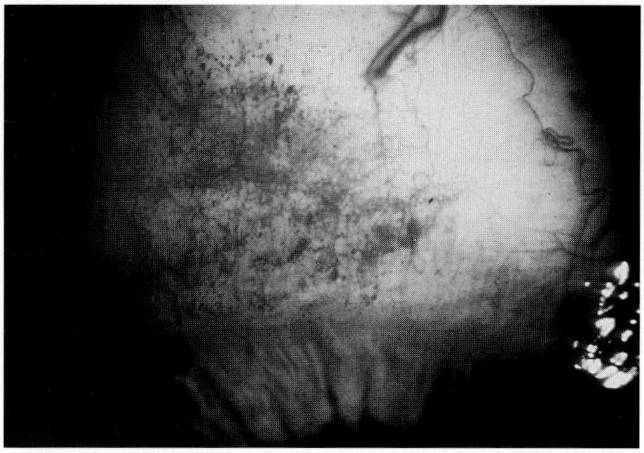

Fig. 1-50 Superior limbic keratoconjunctivitis. Significant rose bengal staining involving the superior bulbar conjunctiva is apparent. The eyelid must be held up on the patient's downgaze to evaluate the area. (See color plate.)

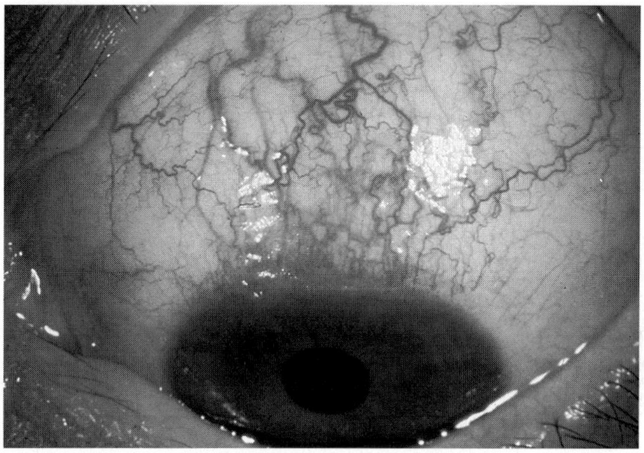

Fig. 1-51 Superior limbic keratoconjunctivitis. The superior bulbar conjunctiva is thickened and injected. This abnormality is most prominent at the limbus.

evident on fluorescein and rose bengal staining (Fig. 1-50). Other findings include fine papillae on the superior tarsal conjunctiva (seen on upper eyelid eversion) and superior bulbar conjunctival thickening (especially at the limbus) (Fig. 1-51). Although these changes may seem obvious, the diagnosis of SLK is frequently missed by ophthalmologists simply because the superior conjunctiva (obscured by the upper eyelid) is not carefully inspected during the examination. An easy and reliable way to avoid missing SLK is to examine the superior bulbar conjunctiva with the naked eye in a well-lit room while holding both upper eyelids up as the patient looks downward. This technique often helps differentiate true conjunctival injection from the normal state of conjunctival vessels (something that is difficult to do under high magnification with a slit-lamp biomicroscope!). Patients with SLK also have associated filamentary keratopathy (incidence, 50%) and thyroid disease (incidence, 30% to 50%). The treatment of this condition should be approached in a step-wise manner with management progressing from conservative to aggressive measures (Box 1-7 and Fig. 1-52). Patients are informed of the chronic course of the condition with its exacerbations and remissions. They progress through the staged treatment options until a therapeutic response is observed. They should be advised to consult a medical internist and to undergo thyroid function testing.

Box 1-7 Treatment Regimen for Superior Limbic Keratoconjunctivitis

1. Increase lubrication
   a. Preservative-free artificial tears 4-8 times a day
   b. Preservative-free ointment at bedtime
   c. Punctal plugs
2. Conduct trial of various topical agents
   a. Vasoconstrictors (e.g., naphazoline HCl qid)
   b. Mast-cell stabilizers (e.g., 4% cromolyn sodium or lodoxamide qid)
   c. Corticosteroids (e.g., 1% prednisolone acetate qid)
   d. Vitamin A drops and ointment
   e. 10% Acetylcysteine qid (for filaments)
3. Silver nitrate 0.5%-1% solution (**NOT silver nitrate cautery sticks**) on a cotton-tip applicator applied to the superior bulbar and palpebral conjunctiva for 10-20 seconds after topical anesthesia
   a. May have to be repeated once or twice on a weekly basis
   b. Should be treated with erythromycin ointment at bedtime after procedure for 1 week
4. Bandage contact lenses
5. Thermal cauterization of the superior bulbar conjunctiva (performed with a handheld thermal cautery unit in a PRP-like pattern after administration of topical and subconjunctival anesthesia)
6. Resection/recession of the superior bulbar conjunctiva (performed in the operating room)

Note: Conduct workup for thyroid disease and treat if present.

Floppy eyelid syndrome Patients with floppy eyelid syndrome complain of unilateral redness and irritation that is worse on awakening. Typically obese, these patients are frustrated by the chronic, recurrent nature of their symptoms. The diagnosis of floppy eyelid syndrome is often missed and mistaken for other causes of chronic red, irritated eye (e.g., chronic bacterial, adenoviral, or allergic conjunctivitis). The proposed mechanism for this condition is the spontaneous eversion of a lax upper eyelid during sleep, causing the eye to open and the superior palpebral conjunctiva to rub against the

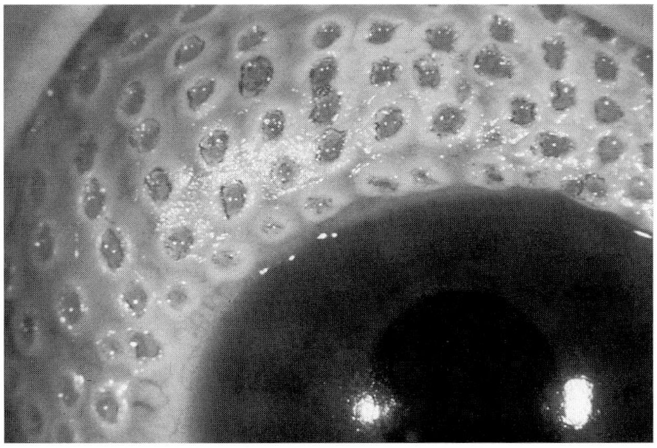

Fig. 1-52 Superior limbic keratoconjunctivitis. After the administration of local anesthesia, this patient with SLK was treated with local conjunctival cautery to the superior bulbar conjunctiva.

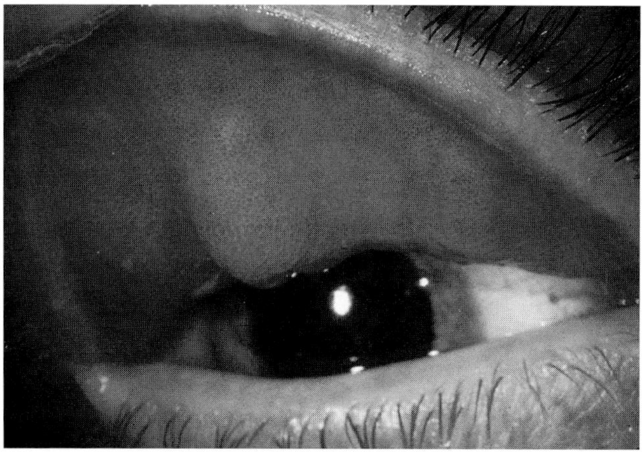

Fig. 1-53 Floppy eyelid syndrome. This extremely lax upper eyelid was everted simply by holding the eyelashes. Note the rubbery appearance and the diffuse fine papillary conjunctival reaction. (See color plate.)

bed sheets. Patients should be asked which side they generally sleep on and whether this side correlates with the affected eye. Examination should focus on the presence of lax upper eyelids that are easily everted with minimal force (ask patient to look down and then raise the eyelid with a finger or a cotton-tip applicator). Other signs include a red, rubbery upper tarsal plate and a fine papillary reaction on the upper palpebral conjunctiva (Fig. 1-53). Chronic corneal neovascularization and scarring may develop (Fig. 1-54). Treatment is centered on preventing eversion of and mechanical trauma to the upper eyelid. This situation can be achieved by taping the eyelid shut or by applying a hard plastic shield over the eye during sleep. Additional lubricants such as viscous artificial tears and ointments may also be used. Ultimately, patients with severe laxity of the eyelid may require a horizontal eyelid tightening procedure.

Mucus fishing syndrome Mucus fishing syndrome is a rare and peculiar disorder that is caused by inadvertent self-induced mechanical trauma to the ocular surface. The condition starts when patients experience excess mucus production because of nonspecific and variable ocular irritation (e.g., foreign body, allergic conjunctivitis, keratoconjunctivitis sicca). Because of the persistent irritation, the frustrated patient then develops a behavior pattern of "fishing" or removing the mucus from the eyes with a finger or a cotton-tip applicator. This action inevitably causes mechanical trauma to the ocular surface, further worsening the ocular irritation and responsive mucus production. This pattern of events results in a vicious cycle whereby the ocular surface undergoes repetitive self-induced trauma. Mucus fishing syndrome can be difficult to diagnose and involves keen suspicion and examination skills on the ophthalmologist's part. When questioned directly, patients commonly admit inserting their fingers in their eyes to remove the

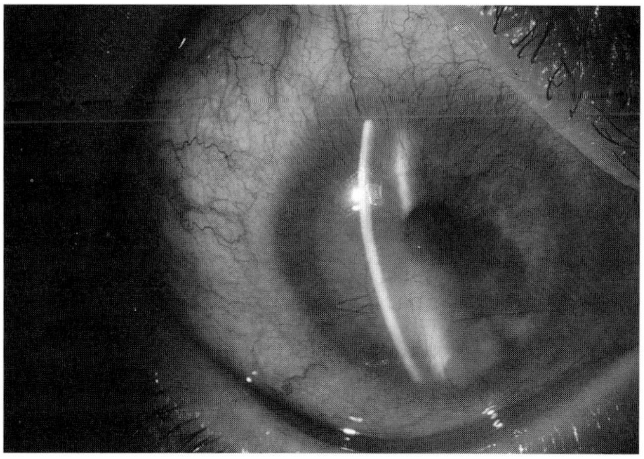

Fig. 1-54 Floppy eyelid syndrome. Corneal scarring and neovascularization have developed in this patient with chronic floppy eyelid syndrome.

mucus. Simple slit-lamp examination and fluorescein staining often reveal an apparently normal ocular surface. It is only with rose bengal staining that traumatized epithelium is detected (Fig. 1-55). The most common locations for ocular surface damage include the nasal and inferior bulbar conjunctiva (including the caruncle and plica). Therapy consists of educating the patient on the need to refrain from touching the eyes and of treating the underlying disorder. Symptoms and signs resolve once this pattern is broken.

Factitious keratoconjunctivitis Factitious keratoconjunctivitis should always be considered whenever a patient has a baffling case of persistent and unusual conjunctivitis. When secondary gain is identified, the term *malingering* is used. Although some patients induce intentional and voluntary mechanical or chemical damage, others are often psychologically disturbed or neurologi-

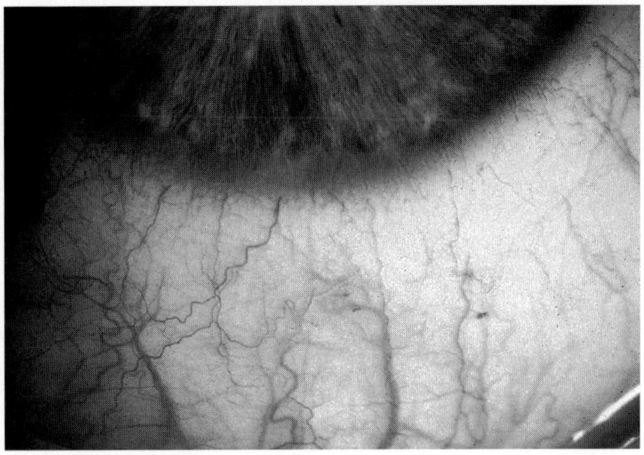

Fig. 1-55 Mucus fishing syndrome. An area of discrete conjunctival injection can be seen. Such areas often demonstrate localized fluorescein or rose bengal staining, which increases the suspicion for mucus fishing syndrome.

cally abnormal and have no knowledge of self-destructive behavior. Clinical signs are variable. Therapy consists of treating the damaged ocular surface with lubricants and antibiotics but often requires the assistance of a psychiatrist, psychologist, or neurologist.

Toxic Conjunctivitis

Toxic conjunctivitis results from a toxic reaction to the conjunctiva and usually is manifested as chronic follicular conjunctivitis.

Medicamentosa In general, toxic conjunctivitis occurs after the chronic application of various topical ophthalmic medications or solutions. Although certain medications are notorious for this condition, it should be noted that many contact lens solutions may cause similar reactions. The active ingredient of the medication is often responsible, but preservatives may also cause this toxic response (Box 1-8). Topical anesthetic abuse may also cause chronic conjunctivitis before the more classic neurotrophic-type keratitis (Fig. 1-56). Toxic conjunctivitis should always be suspected in any patient taking topical ophthalmic medications who has chronic follicular or papillary conjunctivitis. Clinical signs consist of follicles and papillae most prominently in the inferior palpebral and forniceal conjunctiva, bulbar and palpebral conjunctival injection (Figs. 1-57 and 1-58), and punctate epithelial changes in the conjunctiva and cornea (Figs. 1-59 and 1-60). Contact-type dermatitis may also develop (Fig. 1-61). Treatment is based on the discontinuation of the causative medication(s) and the institution of preservative-free lubricating tears and ointments. It is important to tell patients that severe cases may take weeks to months to resolve.

Molluscum contagiosum Molluscum contagiosum is a DNA poxvirus that produces single or multiple white, pearly, dome-shaped lesions with umbilicated centers on the eyelids and the surrounding periocular skin (Figs. 1-62 and 1-63). These lesions contain and shed active viral products that in turn elicit a toxic follicular reaction in the surrounding conjunctiva (Fig. 1-64). Ac-

Box 1-8 Common Medications Causing Toxic Conjunctivitis

ANTIVIRALS

- Idoxuridine
- Trifluorothymidine
- Vidarabine

ANTIGLAUCOMA AGENTS

- Apraclonidine
- Carbachol
- Dipivefrin
- Echothiophate
- Epinephrine
- Pilocarpine
- Cycloplegics
- Atropine
- Homatropine

PRESERVATIVES AND CONTACT LENS CLEANERS AND SOLUTIONS

- Thimerosal
- Benzalkonium chloride
- Chlorhexidine
- Hydrogen peroxide
- Polyvinyl alcohol
- Proteolytic enzymes (i.e., pancreatin, subtilisin)

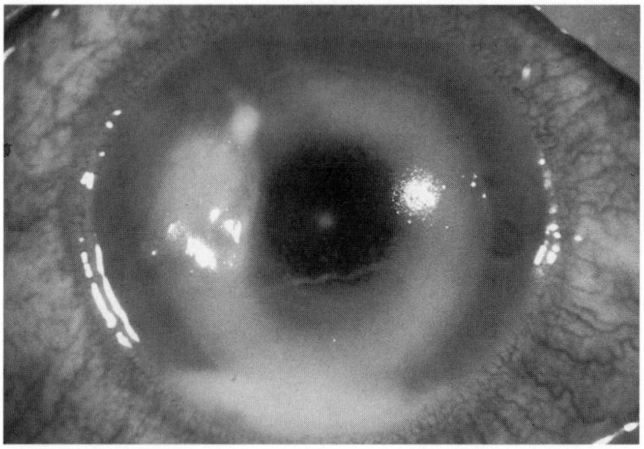

Fig. 1-56 Medicamentosa. During this patient's treatment for a small fungal keratitis in the corneal midperiphery from the 8 o'clock position to the 10 o'clock position, he obtained and abused a topical anesthetic, which led to the large ring infiltrate and hypopyon. It was not until late in the course of the disease that the patient admitted to the anesthetic abuse. Once it was stopped, the cornea slowly but steadily healed.

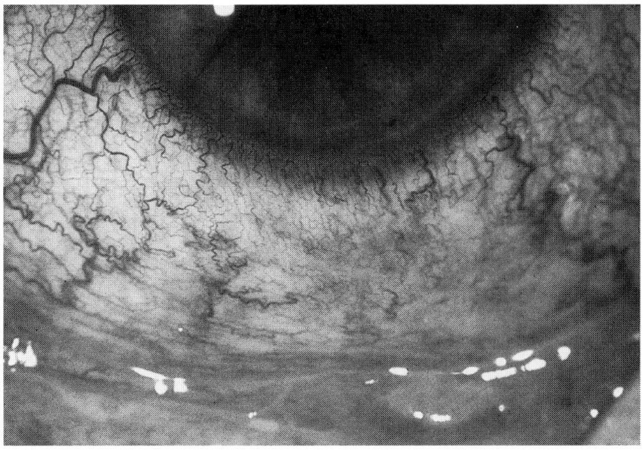

Fig. 1-57 Medicamentosa. Significant inferior conjunctival injection is seen in this patient on long-term topical gentamicin treatment.

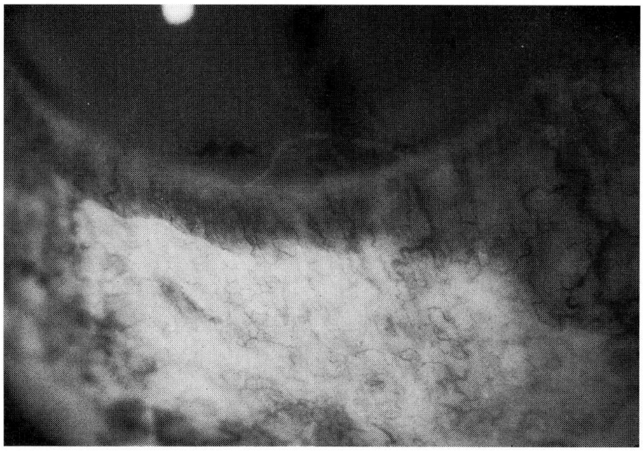

Fig. 1-58 Medicamentosa. Significant inferior conjunctival fluorescein staining is apparent in the eye seen in Fig. 1-57 treated with long-term topical gentamicin therapy. (See color plate.)

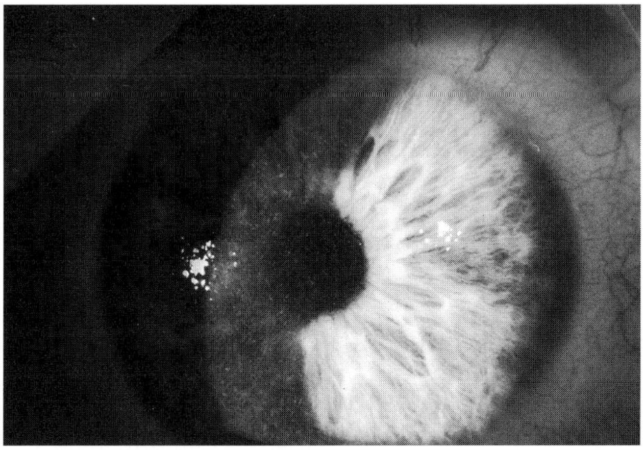

Fig. 1-59 Medicamentosa. Diffuse punctate fluorescein staining of the cornea can be seen in this patient on long-term topical trifluorothymidine treatment.

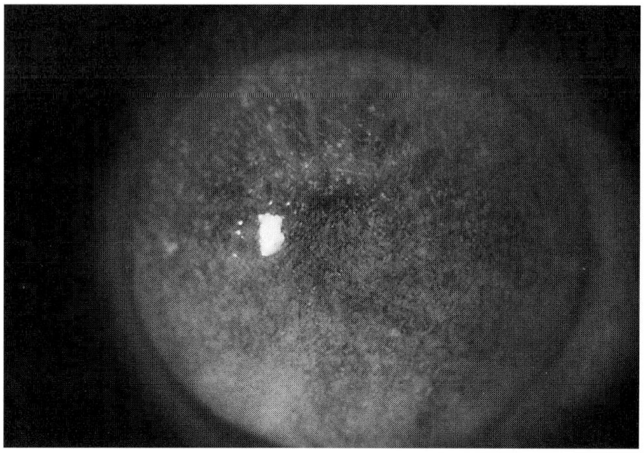

Fig. 1-60 Medicamentosa. Diffuse punctate fluorescein staining of the cornea is highlighted by the cobalt blue light in the patient seen in Fig. 1-59 on long-term topical trifluorothymidine. (See color plate.)

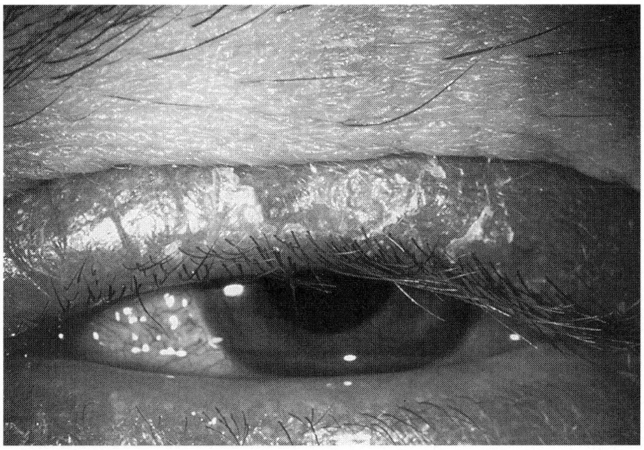

Fig. 1-61 Medicamentosa. Scaling, contact-type dermatitis may develop as a result of topical medications.

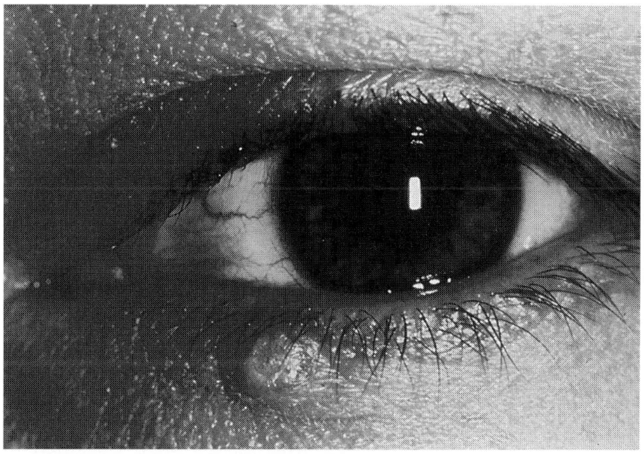

Fig. 1-62 Molluscum contagiosum. A large molluscum lesion with an umbilicated center appears on the lower eyelid skin.

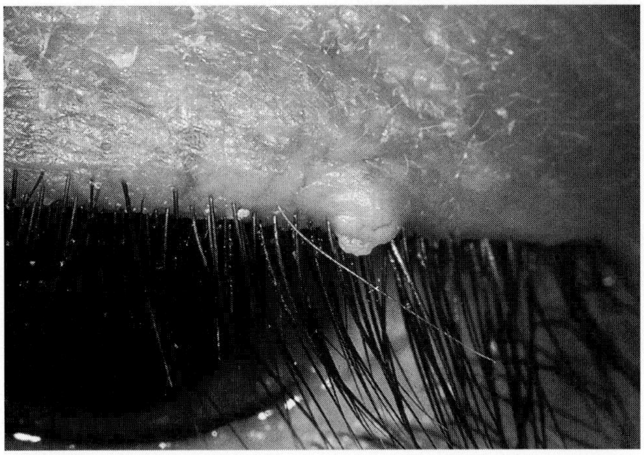

Fig. 1-63 Molluscum contagiosum. A small molluscum lesion, partially hidden by the eyelashes, can be seen along the upper eyelid margin.

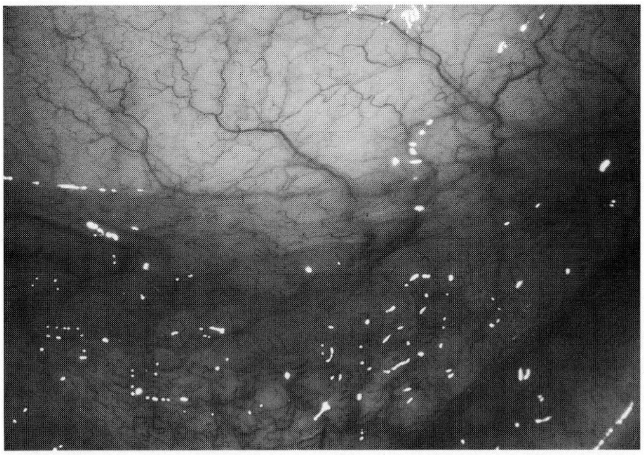

Fig. 1-64 Molluscum contagiosum. Significant follicular conjunctivitis has developed as a result of an eyelid margin molluscum lesion.

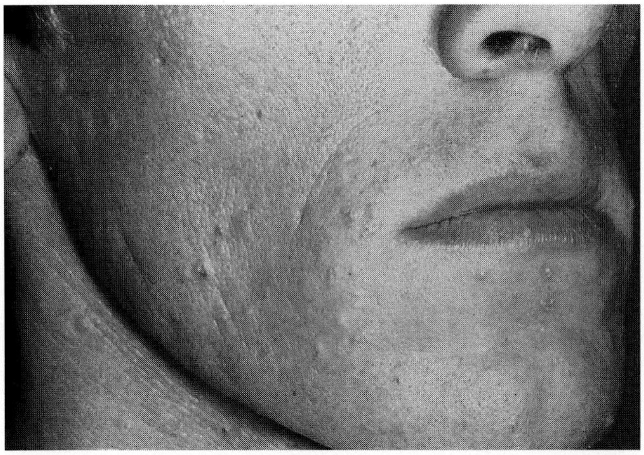

Fig. 1-65 Molluscum contagiosum. Multiple molluscum lesions of the facial skin are present in this patient with human immunodeficiency virus. (Courtesy of George O. Waring III, M.D.)

companying corneal changes include a punctate epithelial keratopathy and pannus. Molluscum lesions are often missed because they can be inconspicuous and hidden from view by eyelashes. Clinical diagnosis is therefore based on a careful inspection of the eyelid margins. In immunocompromised patients, the lesions are often large and numerous (Fig. 1-65), but the conjunctival reaction is less prominent. Molluscum contagiosum is generally a self-limited condition requiring several months to years for spontaneous resolution. Therefore, treatment is usually initiated and is centered on the removal of the toxic viral products. Various methods of accomplishing this task involve complete lesion excision, cryotherapy or cautery to the lesion, or incision and curettage of the umbilicated center of the lesion.

Membranous Conjunctivitis

Ligneous conjunctivitis

Ligneous conjunctivitis is a rare and peculiar disorder that usually develops during childhood. It appears to have an autosomal dominant inheritance pattern. Ocular findings include a characteristic "woody," thick, white membrane that is usually found on the upper tarsal conjunctiva (Fig. 1-66). Diagnosis is aided by the detection of similar lesions in other mucous membranes, such as the nasopharynx and the buccal mucosa. Cervical and middle ear involvement have also been described. Although the pathogenesis of this condition is unclear, various topical medications (e.g., corticosteroids, mucolytic agents, hyaluronidase, alpha-chymotrypsin) have been used to treat this disorder with limited success. For the past decade, the literature has shown some encouraging results with the use of topical cyclosporin A. Bulky lesions that are refractory to medical treatment can be excised surgically, but they often quickly recur. Recently, a neonate who had homozygous plasminogen deficiency and in whom ligneous conjunctivitis and nasopharyngeal and pulmonary symptoms developed soon after birth was successfully treated with lys-plasminogen replacement therapy; all ocular and respiratory problems resolved.

Cicatrizing Conjunctivitis

Essentially any form of conjunctivitis that causes membrane or pseudomembrane formation (see Box 1-4) may result in conjunctival scarring. However, Stevens-Johnson syndrome and ocular cicatricial pemphigoid are two disorders that deserve special attention and elaboration because symblepharon formation is the hallmark of these disorders.

Stevens-Johnson syndrome (erythema multiforme major) Stevens-Johnson syndrome and erythema multiforme major are synonymous terms used to refer to a

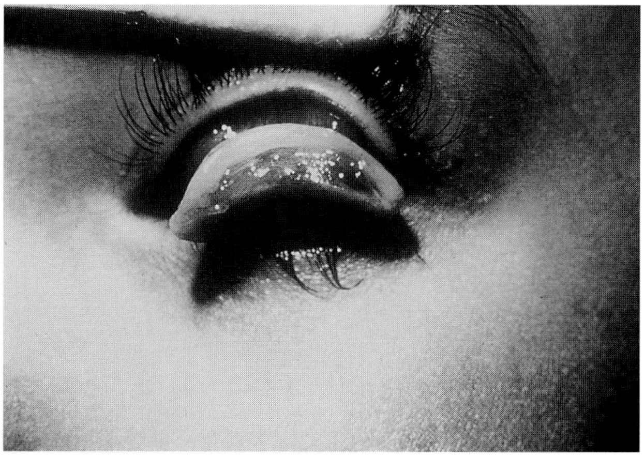

Fig. 1-66 Ligneous conjunctivitis. A thick, gray-white, "woody" membrane is seen attached to the superior tarsal conjunctiva.

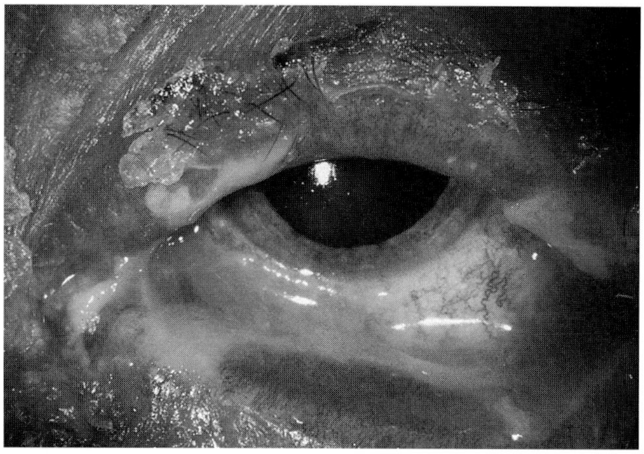

Fig. 1-68 Stevens-Johnson syndrome. The left eye of the patient seen in Fig. 1-67 shows severe membranous conjunctivitis.

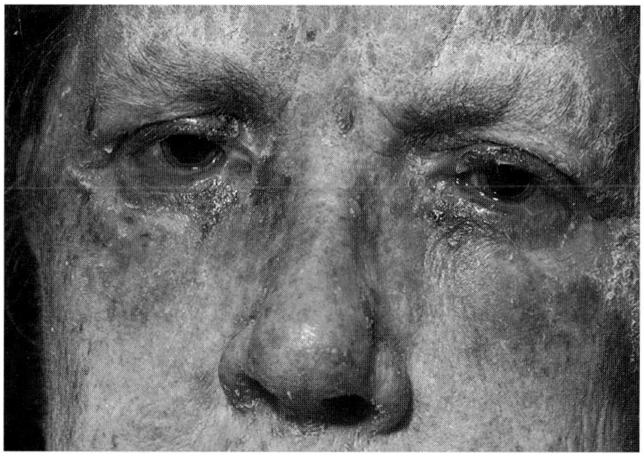

Fig. 1-67 Stevens-Johnson syndrome. This patient has Stevens-Johnson syndrome as a result of phenytoin. Prominent bullous changes of the facial skin are apparent.

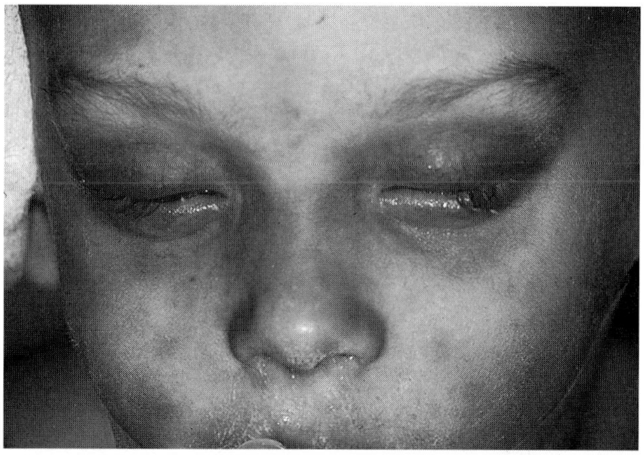

Fig. 1-69 Stevens-Johnson syndrome. Stevens-Johnson syndrome developed 1 month earlier in this patient as a result of amoxicillin treatment. The eyelid and skin lesions are beginning to resolve.

hypersensitivity disorder involving the skin and mucous membranes. Erythema multiforme minor denotes a more common but milder form of the disease affecting the skin only and sparing the mucous membranes, including the eyes. The major form can be devastating and life threatening. It occurs more frequently in women, children, and young adults. Systemic symptoms are nonspecific and include acute fever with associated headache, cough, arthralgia, and malaise. After a few days, red vesicles surrounded by a pale ring and then a red ring (hence the term *target* lesions) appear on the skin. Mucous membranes (primarily in the mouth and the eyes) undergo severe vesicular and bullous change that can progress to necrosis and scarring (Fig. 1-67). Ocular findings include initial mucopurulent conjunctivitis with membrane formation that later results in diffuse conjunctival scarring and symblepharon formation (Fig. 1-68). Corneas often undergo neovascularization and sterile and infectious ulceration (Figs. 1-69 and 1-70). The eyelids are often involved, and cicatricial entropion/ectropion formation and trichiasis develop (Figs. 1-71 and 1-72). The major form is active for approximately 6 weeks, and the mortality rate ranges from 10% to 33%. The pathogenesis of this disorder is unclear but seems to involve immune complex deposition in the skin and mucous membranes. Various drugs and infectious microorganisms have been identified as inciting agents (Box 1-9). The main differential diagnosis is ocular cicatricial pemphigoid, which produces many of the same changes but generally in a more slowly progressive fashion.

Treatment for Stevens-Johnson syndrome is mainly supportive. The patient should be admitted to the hospital, and care should be coordinated with the appropriate subspecialties (i.e., dermatology, infectious diseases). Patients with severe disease may have to be cared for in a burn unit. If the causative agent is a medication, it

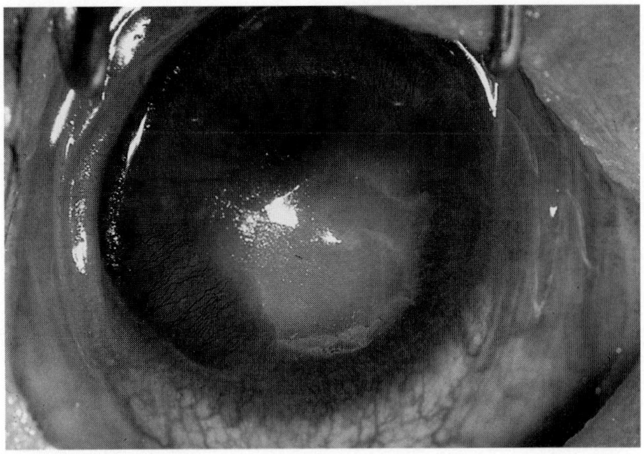

Fig. 1-70 Stevens-Johnson syndrome. The left eye of the patient seen in Fig. 1-69 shows conjunctival scarring and symblepharon superiorly. Significant corneal neovascularization and a dense corneal scar with an epithelial defect have also developed, perhaps because of chronic exposure during the 1-month illness.

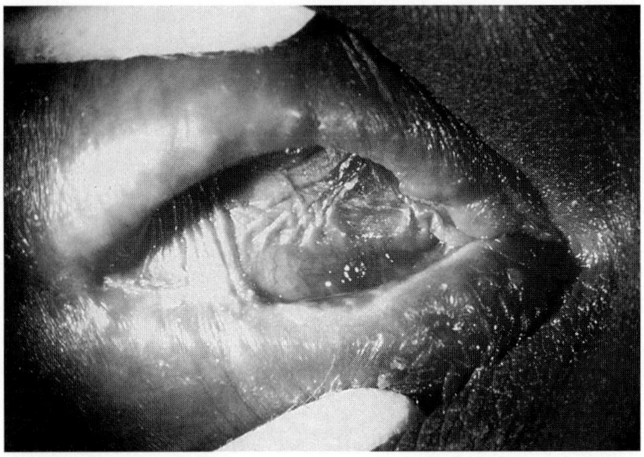

Fig. 1-72 Stevens-Johnson syndrome. Obliteration of the conjunctival fornices, severe trichiasis, and keratinization of the entire bulbar surface can be seen in end-stage Stevens-Johnson disease. (Courtesy of R. Doyle Stulting, M.D., Ph.D.)

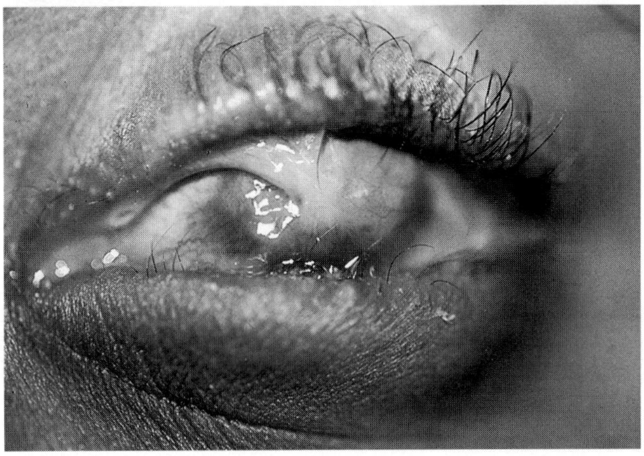

Fig. 1-71 Stevens-Johnson syndrome. Extensive symblepharon formation and corneal scarring have developed after an episode of Stevens-Johnson syndrome.

Box 1-9 Most Common Inciting Agents for Stevens-Johnson Syndrome

MEDICATIONS

Antibiotics
- Penicillins
- Sulfonamides
- Tetracyclines

Anticonvulsants
- Barbiturates
- Phenytoin

Isoniazid

Chlorpropamide

Codeine

Salicylates

Thiazide Diuretics

INFECTIOUS ORGANISMS

Bacteria (e.g., streptococci, mycoplasma)
Viruses (e.g., herpes simplex adenovirus)
Fungi

should be discontinued; if it is a microorganism, it should be treated appropriately. Ocular therapy for the acute phase is centered on providing copious lubrication and preventing secondary infection. Depending on the severity, frequent preservative-free artificial tears and ointments may not suffice and the patient may require punctal occlusion, moisture chambers, and ultimately tarsorrhaphy. Topical antibiotics (e.g., erythromycin or bacitracin ointment four to six times a day) should also be started. Topical corticosteroids (e.g., 1% prednisolone acetate four to eight times a day) and cycloplegic agents (e.g., 0.25% scopolamine tid) are usually necessary to control acute inflammation. However, long-term topical corticosteroid use should be avoided. Systemic corticosteroids are controversial because of the increased risk for systemic infection. Once cicatricial changes are noted, daily lysing of symblepharon and adhesions with a glass rod after topical anesthesia may help minimize permanent scarring. When the disease has quieted and regressed, the chronic complications of conjunctival, corneal, and eyelid scarring may be treated surgically. Unfortunately, severe cases often require extensive reconstruction of the ocular surface with only limited success. Corneal transplants have a poor success rate, often necessitating a concomitant limbal stem cell transplant procedure and systemic immunosuppression. A permanent keratoprosthesis should be considered for

Box 1-10 Stages of Ocular Cicatricial Pemphigoid

STAGE 1

- Conjunctival inflammation
- Mucoid discharge
- Rose bengal staining of the conjunctiva
- Subepithelial fibrosis

STAGE 2

- Conjunctival shrinkage
- Foreshortening of the inferior fornix

STAGE 3

- Symblepharon formation

STAGE 4

- End-stage disease:
  - Ocular surface keratinization/dryness
  - Corneal opacification/vascularization
  - Ankyloblepharon

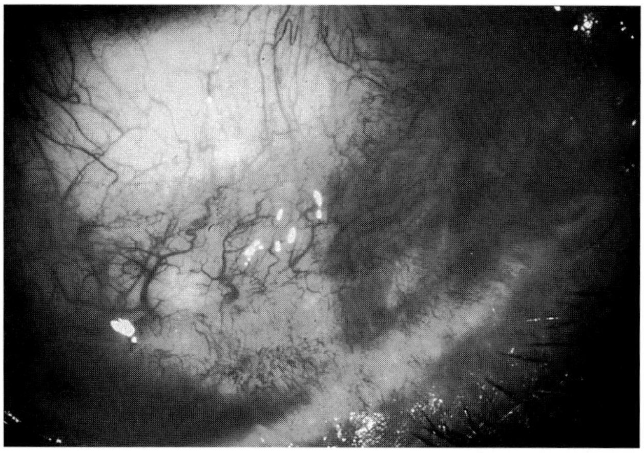

Fig. 1-73 Ocular cicatricial pemphigoid. In the early stages of ocular cicatricial pemphigoid, subepithelial fibrosis and fine conjunctival scarring can be seen. (Courtesy of George O. Waring III, M.D.)

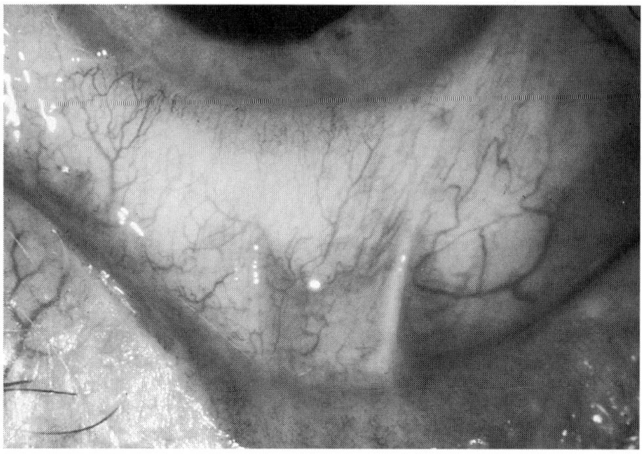

Fig. 1-74 Ocular cicatricial pemphigoid. As ocular pemphigoid progresses, forniceal foreshortening becomes more apparent.

patients with end-stage disease when macular and optic nerve function are preserved.

Ocular cicatricial pemphigoid/linear immunoglobulin A disease Unlike most cases of Stevens-Johnson syndrome, ocular cicatricial pemphigoid is a chronic cicatrizing conjunctivitis that typically affects women older than 55 years of age. It does resemble Stevens-Johnson syndrome in that it affects the skin and mucous membranes, such as the mouth, oropharynx, and genitalia, with no clear cause. However, it should not be confused with pemphigus, a dermatologic condition that rarely affects the eyes.

The onset of ocular cicatricial pemphigoid is typically insidious, with patients noting gradual redness, irritation, foreign body sensation, and tearing. Patients usually have recurrent bouts of nonspecific conjunctivitis with occasional associated mucoid discharge, edema, and ulceration. A typical early finding is trichiasis. It is important to examine the conjunctival fornices for foreshortening and symblepharon in all patients with trichiasis. Ocular findings are usually bilaterally asymmetric and are classified in various stages (Box 1-10). In stage 1, transient conjunctival bullae rupture (rarely seen) and lead to subepithelial fibrosis, which may be visible as fine gossamerlike strands or striae (Fig. 1-73). Stages 2 and 3 are distinguished by forniceal foreshortening (Fig. 1-74) and symblepharon formation, the classic feature of the disease (Fig. 1-75) (detected by pulling the lower eyelids down while the patient fixates in upgaze). Finally, stage 4 represents end-stage disease with severe destruction of goblet cells and lacrimal gland ducts and drainage channels, ultimately leading to abnormal, deficient tear production and profound ocular surface scarring and keratinization (Figs. 1-76 and 1-77). Examination (with the help of an experienced dermatologist) should include a thorough dermatologic evaluation to detect characteristic skin and mucous membrane lesions that could help support the diagnosis of pemphigoid. Definitive laboratory diagnosis can often (but not always) be achieved with a conjunctival biopsy specimen showing positive immunofluorescent staining of the basement membrane.

The typical clinical course for ocular cicatricial pemphigoid is slowly progressive deterioration marked by remissions and exacerbations. It is important to remember that cicatricial pemphigoid is a systemic disorder that requires systemic treatment, often coordinated with an internist, a dermatologist, or both. Treatment approaches vary, but a general regimen is outlined in

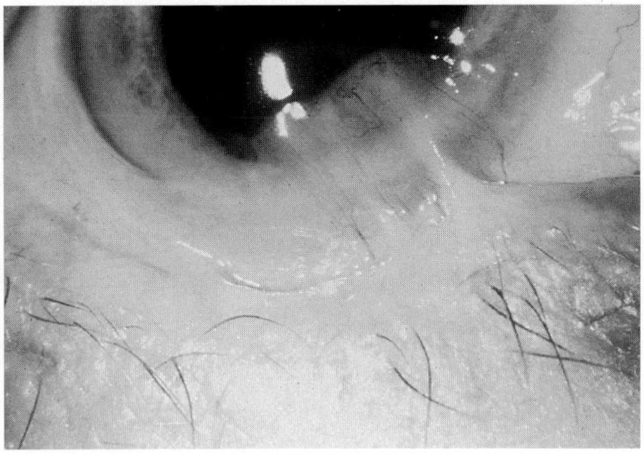

Fig. 1-75 Ocular cicatricial pemphigoid. Significant symblepharon formation, with the eyelid skin adherent to the cornea, signals advanced disease.

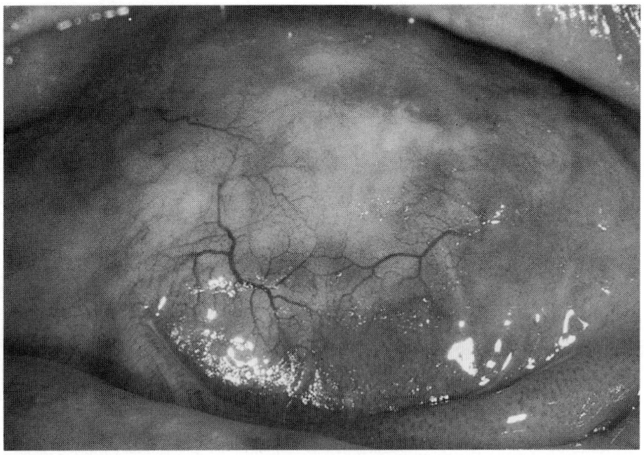

Fig. 1-76 Ocular cicatricial pemphigoid. Severe destruction of the conjunctival goblet cells and obliteration of the conjunctival fornices lead to corneal neovascularization and scarring.

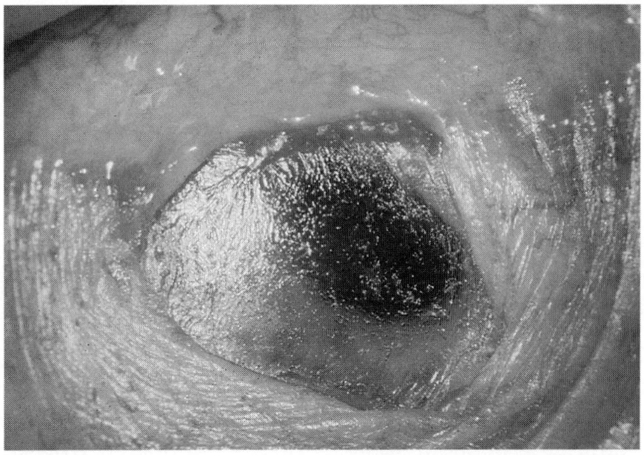

Fig. 1-77 Ocular cicatricial pemphigoid. In end-stage ocular cicatricial pemphigoid, the entire ocular surface becomes scarred and keratinized.

Box 1-11. Even with treatment, the prognosis regarding the vision for many of these patients remains poor because of the limited success of corneal transplantation and keratoprostheses.

Linear IgA disease, or dermatosis, is another rare skin disorder that has ocular findings identical to those of cicatricial pemphigoid. It is considered a close relative of pemphigoid and is treated in the same manner.

Pseudopemphigoid Pseudopemphigoid, or drug-induced pemphigoid, is a form of cicatrizing conjunctivitis associated with the chronic use of various topical ophthalmic medications (Box 1-12). It is manifested by conjunctival scarring that is clinically and histologically indistinguishable from that of true ocular cicatricial pemphigoid. Factors that differentiate this condition from cicatricial pemphigoid are outlined in Table 1-8. Because pseudopemphigoid is attributed to the chronic application of topical medications, treatment consists of discontinuing the offending agent(s), which usually halts further progression of the disease.

Box 1-11 Treatment Regimen for Ocular Cicatricial Pemphigoid

1. Frequent administration of preservative-free artificial tears and ointments
2. Punctal occlusion and moisture chamber goggles as necessary
3. Topical corticosteroid (e.g., 1% prednisolone acetate qid) as needed for acute exacerbations (long-term use should be avoided because of risk of corneal melting)
4. Systemic corticosteroids (e.g., 60 mg prednisone PO daily) with appropriate taper to suppress acute exacerbations
5. 25-100 mg Dapsone PO daily with appropriate increases and decreases according to clinical response (contraindications include patients with glucose-6-phosphate dehydrogenase deficiency and sulfone allergies; initial and follow-up blood tests should include complete blood count with reticulocyte count and glucose-6-phosphate dehydrogenase level because dapsone can cause dose-related hemolysis)
6. Various immunosuppressive medications as necessary (the side effects of these medications vary and can be very dangerous; patients should be appropriately informed and followed)
   a. Cyclophosphamide
   b. Methotrexate
   c. Azathioprine
7. Surgical reconstruction of the ocular surface and eyelids (once the disease has quieted for an adequate period of time; patients should be warned that any surgery can provoke further scarring and exacerbations)

Nutritional Disorders Involving the Conjunctiva

Vitamin A deficiency Vitamin A plays an important role in the generation of visual pigments, and its deficiency leads to xerophthalmia (dry eyes) and nyctalopia (night blindness). Vitamin A deficiency can result from decreased dietary intake or malabsorption. Although decreased vitamin A intake is primarily a problem in developing countries, it is seen in industrialized countries among persons who have eating disorders or who follow peculiar diets and among those who are alcoholic or homeless. A host of malabsorption disorders can account for vitamin A deficiency: cystic fibrosis, chronic pancreatitis and hepatitis, inflammatory bowel disease, and intestinal bypass surgery (for morbid obesity). The earliest symptom is the gradual onset of nyctalopia. Other symptoms are ocular dryness and foreign-body sensation. External ocular findings consist of diffuse punctate epithelial keratopathy and keratinization of the conjunctival and corneal surfaces (Fig. 1-78) evident with fluorescein and rose bengal staining. A superficial, foamy, gray-white triangular area known as Bitot's spot can be seen on the nasal or temporal bulbar conjunctiva near the limbus (Fig. 1-79). This spot is characteristic of vitamin A deficiency and is composed of keratinized epithelial and inflammatory cells that have a foamy appearance because of the metabolic reactions of *Corynebacterium xerosis*. Other signs include a diminished or nonexistent tear meniscus and markedly reduced results on tear secretion tests. Severe cases can produce sterile corneal ulcerations that progress to perforation (Fig. 1-80). Diagnostic workup should consist of a thorough ophthalmologic examination and a determination of the serum vitamin A level (<20 to 80 µg/dl is considered abnormal). Treatment involves vitamin A and other protein-calorie supplements. Vitamin A palmitate in oil (200,000 IU) may be given orally for 2 days and may be followed by an additional dose 1 month later. An equivalent dose may be given intramuscularly for patients in whom absorption is a problem. Topical treatment should involve intensive lubrication with preservative-free artificial tears and ointments (as often as every 15 minutes) and with vitamin A ointment two to four times a day (Fig. 1-81). Long-term treatment of the underlying disorder is required. Corneal scarring may require that the patient undergo penetrating keratoplasty.

Box 1-12 Most Common Topical Medications Associated with Pseudopemphigoid

ANTIVIRAL AGENTS

Idoxuridine

ANTIGLAUCOMA AGENTS

Demecarium Bromide
Echothiophate Iodide
Epinephrine
Pilocarpine
Timolol

Conjunctival Degenerations

Pingueculae/pterygia Pingueculae are degenerative lesions of the conjunctiva that probably result from environmental (e.g., sun, dust, wind), especially actinic, exposure. They occur more frequently in warm climates and among persons whose occupations keep them outdoors (e.g., farmers, lifeguards, sailors). It makes sense that pingueculae are found in the most exposed areas of the conjunctiva: the nasal and temporal bulbar conjunctiva adjacent to the corneoscleral limbus (nasal greater than temporal). They are white-yellow elevated fleshy lesions that vary in size and shape (Fig. 1-82). Histopathologically, these lesions are described as having elastoid or elastotic degeneration but are not considered elastic tissue. They may occasionally be associated with inflammation (termed *pingueculitis*), causing redness and irritation (Fig. 1-83). Rarely do they enlarge to interfere with contact lens wear or to become a cosmetic concern. Otherwise, they are asymptomatic. Episodes of inflam-

Table 1-8 Differentiating features of pseudopemphigoid and true pemphigoid

Feature	Pseudopemphigoid	True pemphigoid
Cause	Topical medications	Unknown (probably autoimmune)
Laterality	Unilateral and bilateral	Asymmetrically bilateral
Systemic involvement	None	Skin and other mucous membranes
Clinical course	Nonprogressive with discontinuation of offending topical agent(s)	Progressive
Immunofluorescent staining	Negative or nonspecific	Often positive

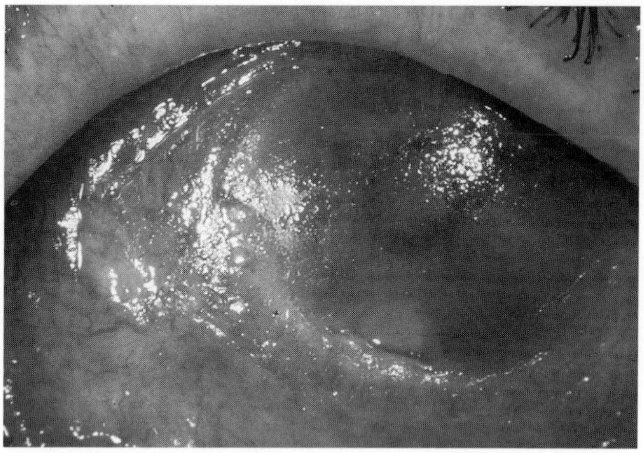

Fig. 1-78 Vitamin A deficiency. Severe conjunctival dryness and inflammation are apparent in this patient with malnutrition-induced vitamin A deficiency. Both the cornea and the conjunctiva have lost their natural luster. A small peripheral corneal infiltrate is seen inferiorly.

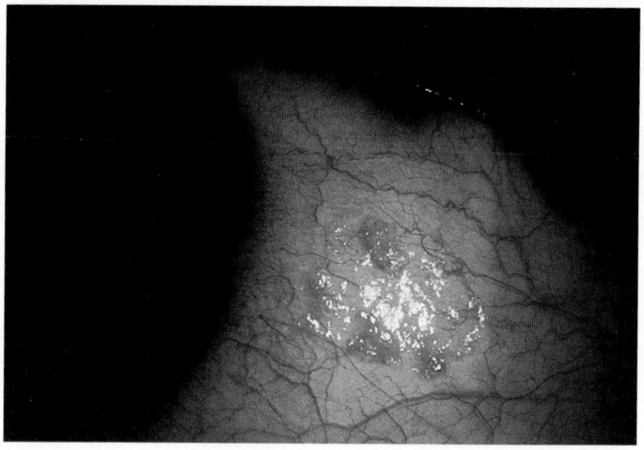

Fig. 1-79 Vitamin A deficiency Bitot's spot. A triangular area of keratinized conjunctival epithelium, called a *Bitot's spot,* can be seen at the limbus.

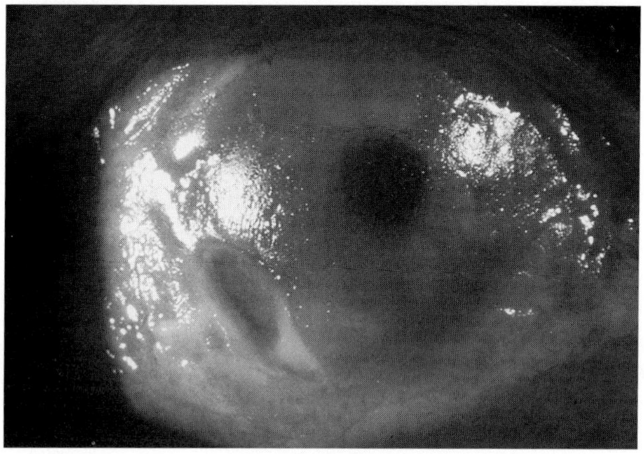

Fig. 1-80 Vitamin A deficiency. The fellow eye of the patient in Fig. 1-78 has a deep corneal ulceration, which is at risk for perforation.

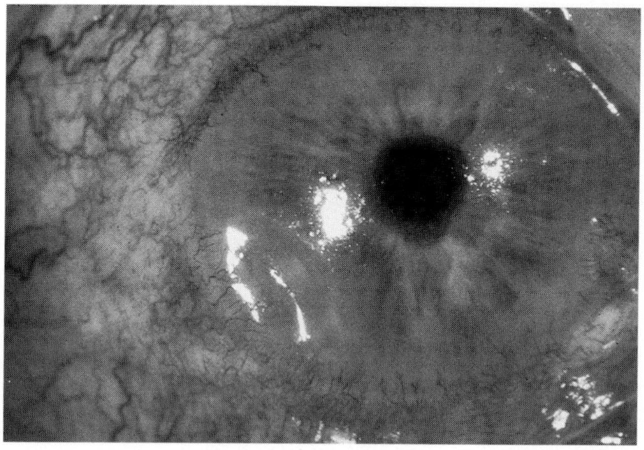

Fig. 1-81 Vitamin A deficiency. After 1 week of topical and systemic treatment, the eye of the patient in Fig. 1-80 has healed dramatically. The corneal ulceration has completely reepithelialized, and the natural corneal and conjunctival luster is returning.

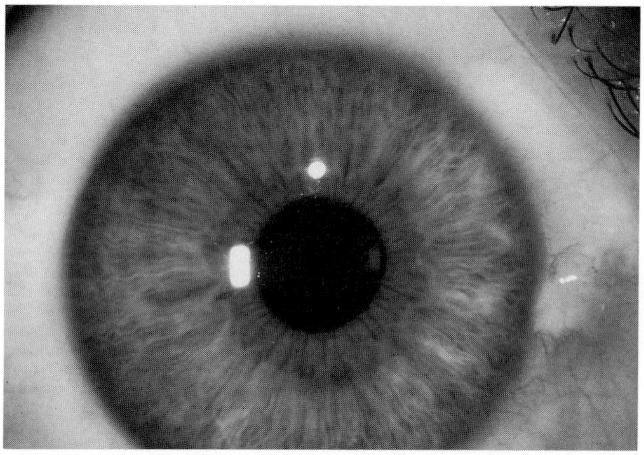

Fig. 1-82 Pinguecula. A small, slightly elevated pinguecula is present on the limbal sclera at the 3 o'clock position.

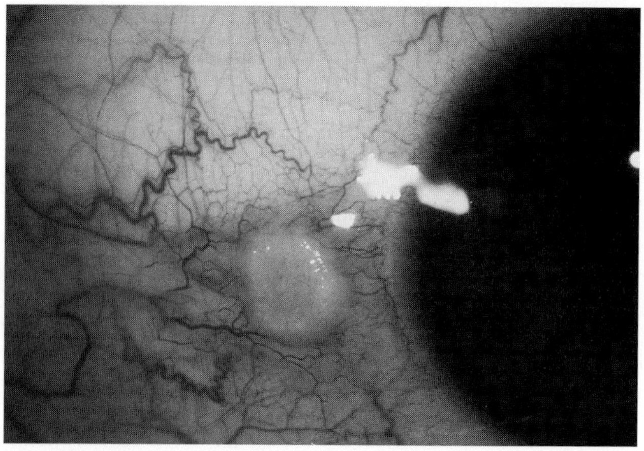

Fig. 1-83 Pinguecula. This inflamed, adherent, elevated, circular scleral lesion underwent biopsy and proved to be an inflamed pinguecula.

mation, redness, or foreign body sensation are treated with topical lubricants and vasoconstrictors (e.g., naphazoline qid for 1 to 2 weeks). Topical nonsteroidal anti-inflammatory medications (e.g., diclofenac or ketorolac qid) may be helpful. Short courses of mild topical corticosteroids (e.g., 0.1% fluorometholone qid) are sometimes necessary to control severe or prolonged inflammation. Patients should be advised to protect their eyes from the environment with eyewear that gives adequate ultraviolet protection. The indications for surgery are summarized in Box 1-13. If surgery is considered, the lesion should be sent for histopathologic examination, and the conjunctiva should be closed primarily.

A pterygium is a distinctive wing-shaped fibrovascular tissue growth in the interpalpebral bulbar conjunctiva that extends onto the cornea to varying degrees (Fig. 1-84). It often develops from the extension of a pinguecula onto the cornea. Although they are usually found nasally, pterygia may be located temporally or even nasally and temporally in the same eye (Fig. 1-85). At times, an iron line (called Stocker's line) can be seen in the corneal epithelium at the leading edge or "head" of the pterygium. The same causative factors described above are thought to be responsible for causing a pinguecula to progress to a pterygium. These lesions may enlarge and advance with time to cause decreased vision either from induced astigmatism or from invasion into the visual axis. They are also more apt than pingueculae to cause irritation, redness, and foreign body sensation. When indicated (see Box 1-13), these lesions can be removed. There are many surgical options available for pterygium excision, and the recurrence rates and complications vary according to the procedure. These procedures are discussed in Chapter 10. Whatever the surgical option, patients should be forewarned that pterygia can recur and that recurrent pterygia are often more aggressive and difficult to treat.

Box 1-13 Indications for Surgical Treatment of Pingueculae/Pterygia

PINGUECULAE	PTERYGIA
Recurrent or chronic inflammation	Decreased vision (from induced astigmatism or obliteration of visual axis)
Interference with contact lens wear	Progression that threatens visual axis
Cosmetic concern (rare)	Recurrent or chronic inflammation
	Interference with contact lens wear
	Cosmetic concern

Amyloidosis Amyloidosis is a degenerative disorder in which the noncollagenous protein amyloid is deposited either primarily or secondarily in the conjunctiva and other ocular tissues (e.g., cornea, uvea, eyelids, orbital adnexa). This protein is easily identified by its distinguishing traits on histopathologic examination, including positive Congo red dye staining, and dichroism and birefringence on examination with polarized light. It appears as a waxy, yellow-red deposit, typically in the palpebral conjunctiva, and resembles large follicles. It may occur as a mass lesion on the bulbar conjunctiva (Fig. 1-86). Various classification schema have divided amyloid deposition into four types (Box 1-14). The categories denote primary (idiopathic) or secondary (caused by chronic disease) deposition as well as the presence or absence of systemic involvement in addition to ocular involvement. Although the diagnosis and sys-

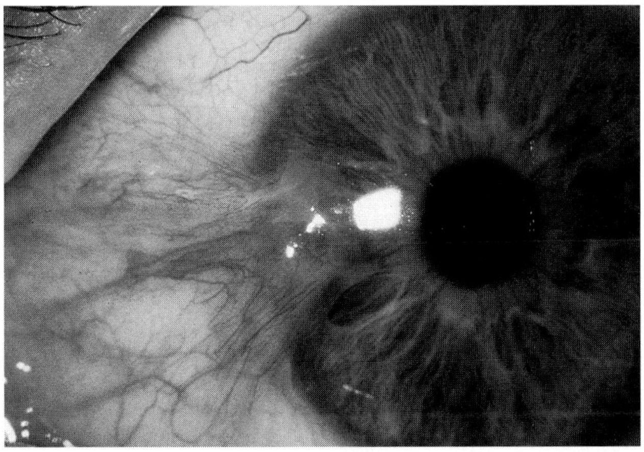

Fig. 1-84 Pterygium. A moderately sized pterygium can be seen extending several millimeters onto the cornea.

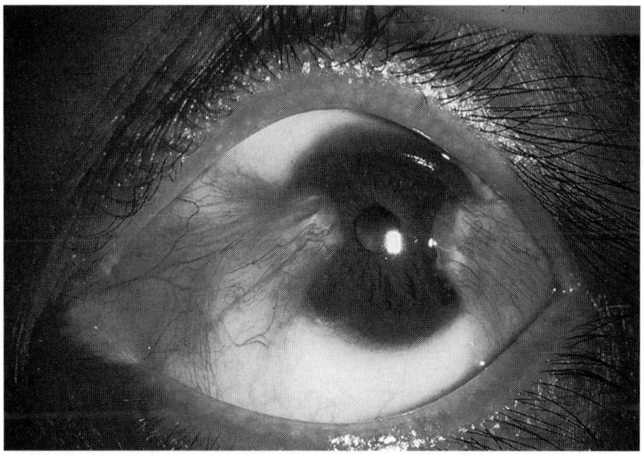

Fig. 1-85 Pterygium. This patient has large nasal and temporal pterygia in the same eye.

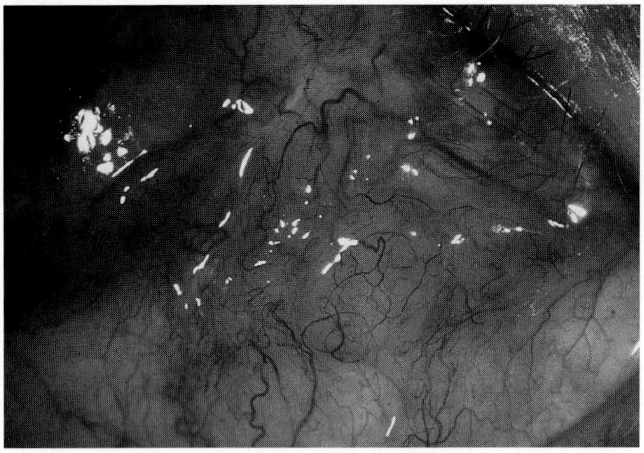

Fig. 1-86 Amyloidosis. Histopathologic examination of this creamy yellow conjunctival mass reveals amyloid.

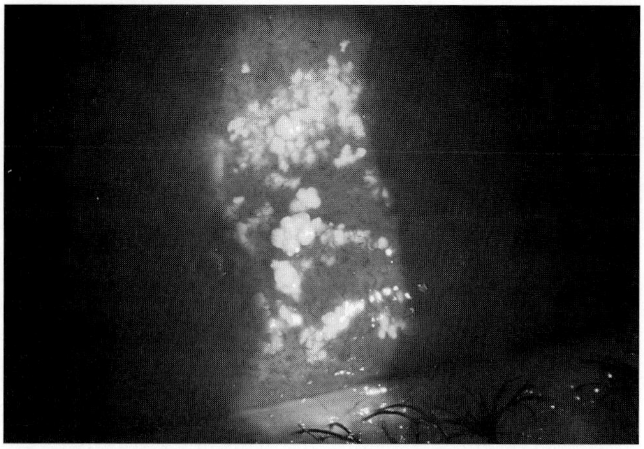

Fig. 1-87 Calcium concretion. Numerous calcium concretions are evident in the upper tarsal conjunctiva on eyelid eversion.

Box 1-14 Classification and Features of Amyloidosis

PRIMARY LOCALIZED AMYLOIDOSIS

Most common form
Deposition involving conjunctiva and occasionally central cornea (referred to as gelatinous drop-like dystrophy)
May be associated with systemic lymphoma

PRIMARY SYSTEMIC AMYLOIDOSIS

Deposition involving vitreous, eyelids, orbit, and extraocular muscles
Often present with weakness, fatigue, and abdominal pain
Patient may have congestive heart failure and renal disease
More common in males
Possible autosomal dominant inheritance

SECONDARY LOCALIZED AMYLOIDOSIS

Conjunctival and corneal deposition
Secondary to chronic ocular inflammation (e.g., trachoma, interstitial keratitis)

SECONDARY SYSTEMIC AMYLOIDOSIS

Associated with rheumatoid arthritis, leprosy, Mediterranean fever, and bronchiectasis
Eyelids less commonly affected than in primary systemic amyloidosis

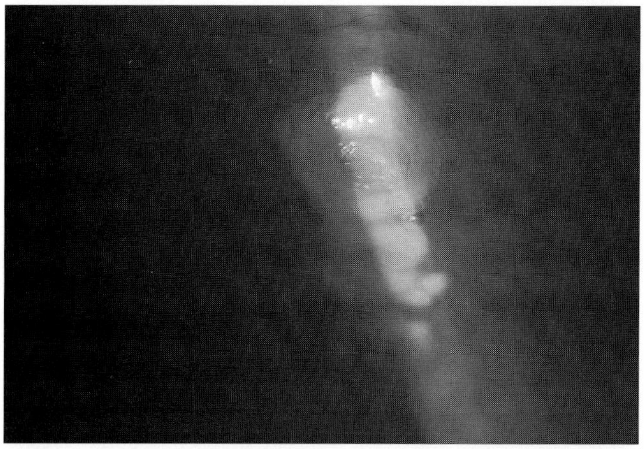

Fig. 1-88 Calcium concretion. This large calcium concretion has an overlying conjunctival epithelial defect that stains with fluorescein. It is often straightforward to shell out the concretion during slit-lamp examination.

temic workup are important, generally no ocular treatment exists for this disorder.

Calcium concretions Calcium concretions are yellow-white calcium deposits that appear embedded in the surface of the palpebral and forniceal conjunctiva. These lesions may be solitary or multiple, may vary in size, and are distributed randomly in the upper and lower palpebral conjunctiva (Fig. 1-87). Histologically, they are shown to be epithelial inclusion cysts that become secondarily calcified. If no calcification occurs, they are found to consist of epithelial and keratin debris and are then simply referred to as conjunctival concretions. Patients rarely have symptoms, but calcium concretions may cause a foreign body sensation if they erode through the conjunctival epithelium to abrade the bulbar surface. Applying fluorescein stain can help detect these eroded concretions, which are otherwise difficult to distinguish from concretions with an intact epithelium (Fig. 1-88). If patients do have symptoms, they can be treated with lubrication, either artificial tears and ointments or antibiotic ointments, or with simple expression of the concretion with a jeweler's forceps after topical anesthesia.

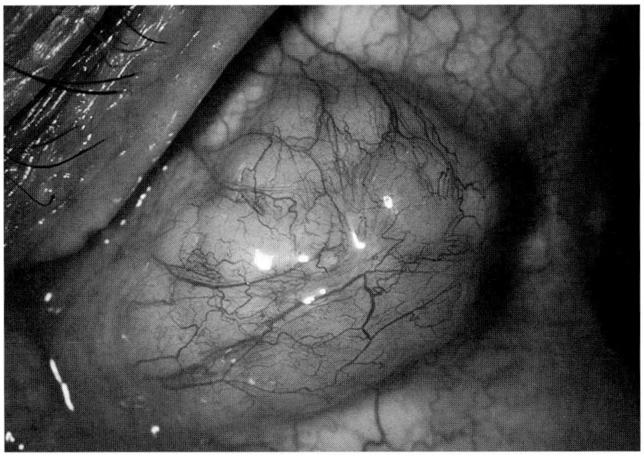

Fig. 1-89 Conjunctival cyst. A large conjunctival cyst causes chronic foreign body symptoms.

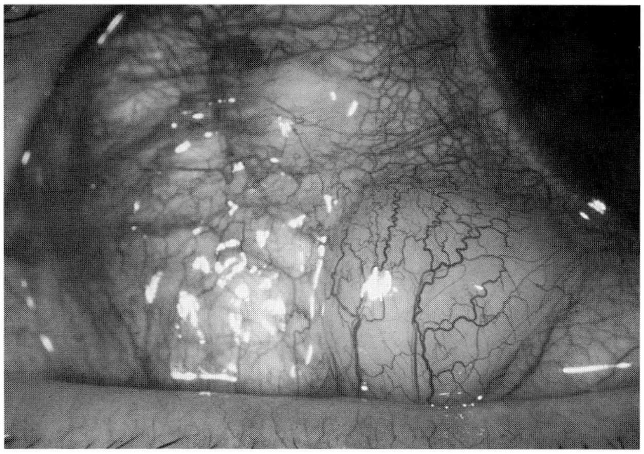

Fig. 1-90 Conjunctival cyst. This medium-sized conjunctival cyst is adjacent to the limbus at the 7 o'clock position but is freely mobile.

Conjunctival Tumors

Epithelial conjunctival tumors

Conjunctival cyst By definition, conjunctival cysts are lined with epithelium and appear as clear sacs anywhere on the conjunctiva (Fig. 1-89). They arise after trauma or inflammation but can develop congenitally. These lesions are benign, tend not to enlarge, and rarely cause any symptoms. They may be relatively firmly attached or freely mobile under the conjunctiva (Figs. 1-90 and 1-91). Surgical treatment is indicated only if a patient experiences significant foreign body sensation or if the cosmetic appearance is unacceptable. Curative treatment can only be achieved with complete excision or marsupialization of the epithelial cyst wall. Simple puncture or incomplete excision of the cyst leads to rapid recurrence.

Papilloma Conjunctival papillomas are benign squamous tumors of the epithelium that have either a viral or a neoplastic cause, each with different characteristics (Table 1-9). Viral papillomas are often caused by the human papillomavirus and appear in a pedunculated form generally on the palpebral conjunctiva (though they may appear elsewhere, including the caruncle and the lacrimal sac) (Figs. 1-92 and 1-93). They occur in younger patients, are often multiple (Fig. 1-94), and frequently recur after attempted excision.

The neoplastic variant usually is a sessile, solitary lesion on the bulbar conjunctiva near the limbus (Fig. 1-95). It occurs in older patients and tends not to recur after complete excision. These lesions should undergo complete excisional biopsy with supplemental cryotherapy of the base and remaining edges.

Pseudoepitheliomatous hyperplasia Pseudoepitheliomatous hyperplasia refers to a benign, reactive inflammatory lesion possibly caused by actinic exposure. Although it is usually seen on the eyelids, it rarely occurs in the conjunctiva and may be found overlying a pinguecula or pterygium.

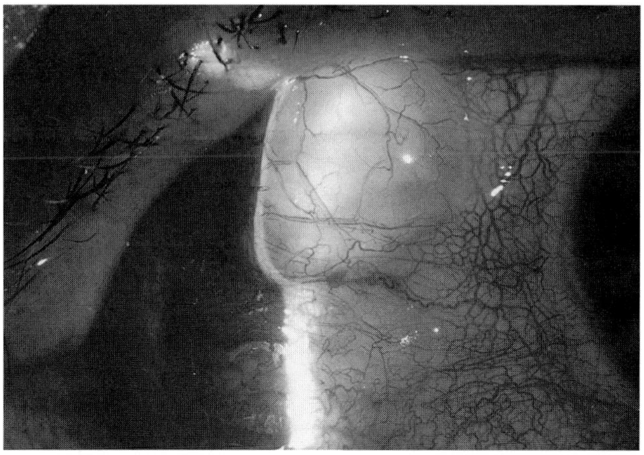

Fig. 1-91 Conjunctival cyst. The same cyst seen in Fig. 1-90 was easily moved to this location seen at the 10 o'clock position.

Hereditary benign intraepithelial dyskeratosis Hereditary benign intraepithelial dyskeratosis or HBID is a rare but interesting disorder found in the Haliwa Indian tribes of North Carolina. The name of this condition defines and summarizes its characteristics. It is thought to be a benign disorder dominantly inherited through many generations of this tribe. The lesions have a striking clinical appearance with marked conjunctival and episcleral vessel injection. They consist of whitish plaques of acanthotic and dyskeratotic epithelial cells and appear most often in the nasal and temporal interpalpebral conjunctiva (Fig. 1-96). Although these lesions have a distinctive appearance, they are frequently misdiagnosed as pingueculae or pterygia or as squamous cell carcinoma because of their location and vascularized configuration. Most of the lesions involve the conjunctiva only, but se-

Table 1-9 Characteristics of conjunctival papillomas

Feature	Viral	Neoplastic
Age of patient	Younger age	Older age
Cause	Viral (human papillomavirus)	Neoplastic
Base of lesion	Pedunculated	Sessile
Number of lesions	Usually multiple	Usually solitary
Corneal involvement	No corneal involvement	Limbal involvement
Location	Usually on palpebral conjunctiva	Usually at the limbus May extend to bulbar conjunctiva, cornea, or both
Recurrence rate	High after excision	Low after excision
Potential	May resolve spontaneously	May undergo malignant transformation

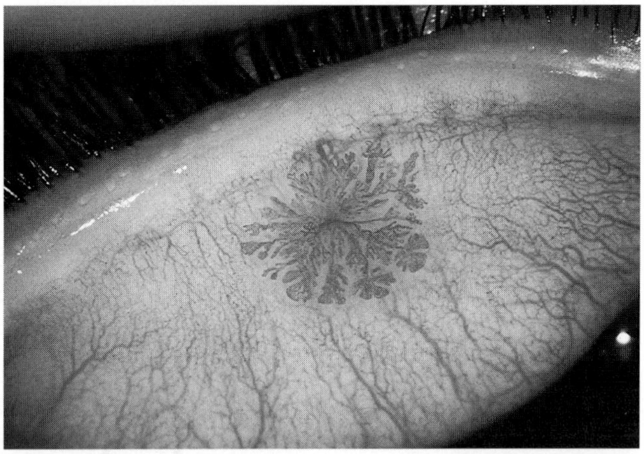

Fig. 1-92 Conjunctival papilloma. A small, pedunculated, stellate papilloma is seen on eversion of the upper eyelid.

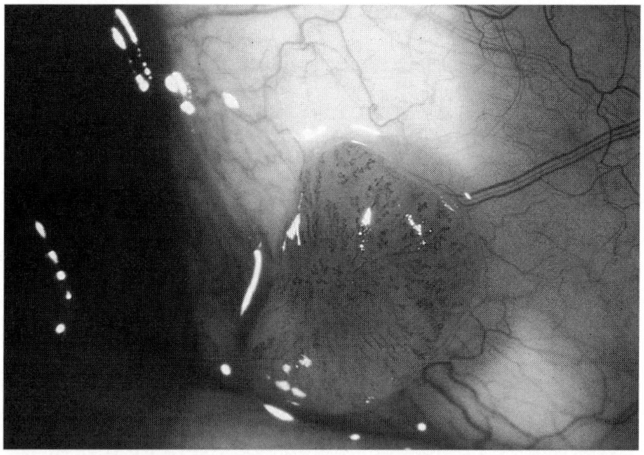

Fig. 1-93 Conjunctival papilloma. A large, pedunculated papilloma is present in the inferior fornix.

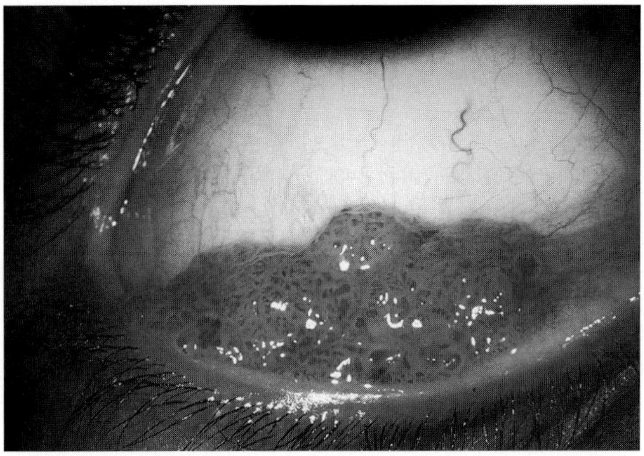

Fig. 1-94 Conjunctival papilloma. Multiple confluent papillomae are present in the fornix of this 4-year-old girl.

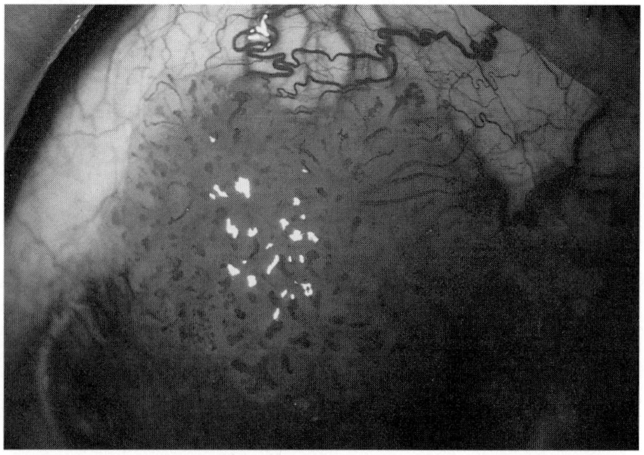

Fig. 1-95 Conjunctival papilloma. This large sessile papillomatous lesion developed in an elderly man. It was removed, and the histopathologic diagnosis was conjunctival intraepithelial neoplasia. (See color plate.)

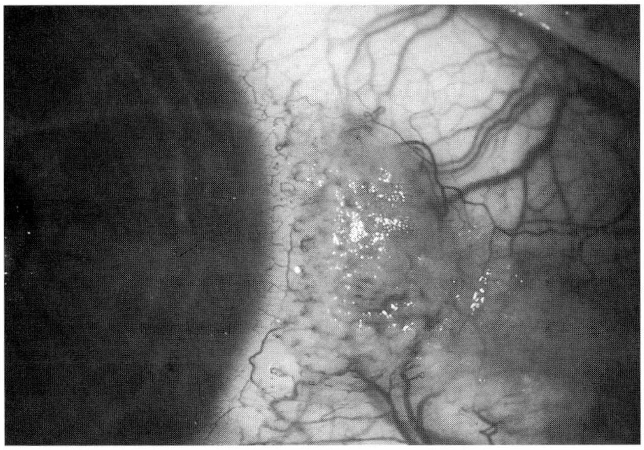

Fig. 1-96 Hereditary benign intraepithelial dyskeratosis. A whitish plaque of dyskeratotic conjunctival epithelial cells is seen at the 3 o'clock limbus. (See color plate.)

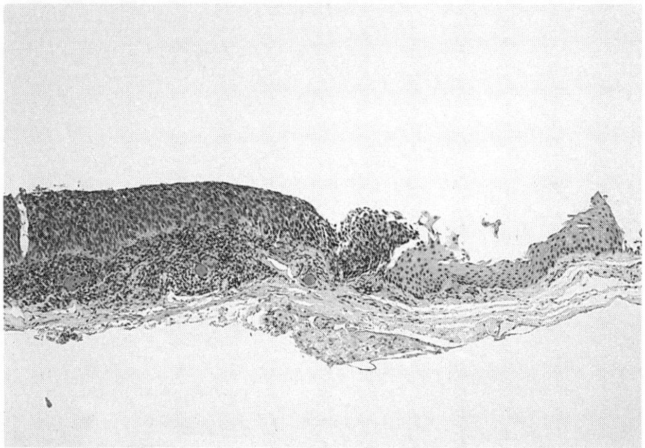

Fig. 1-98 Carcinoma in situ. Histopathologic evaluation of a conjunctival biopsy revealed carcinoma in situ with moderate to severe epithelial dysplasia. Note the abrupt transition from the normal epithelium on the right to the dysplastic epithelium on the left. The tumor does not extend through the basement membrane. (Courtesy of Ralph C. Eagle, Jr., M.D.) (See color plate.)

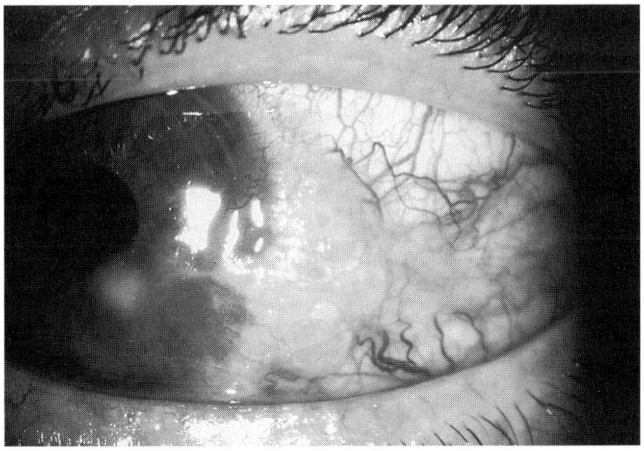

Fig. 1-97 Hereditary benign intraepithelial dyskeratosis. An extensive area of limbal involvement is associated with corneal scarring and neovascularization.

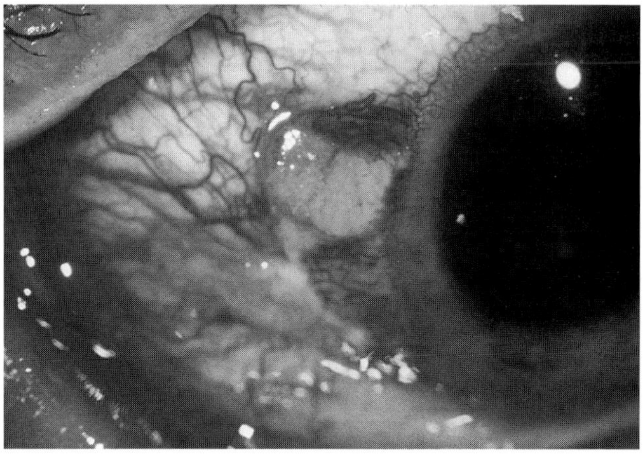

Fig. 1-99 Carcinoma in situ. An hourglass-shaped white carcinoma in situ gelatinous lesion is seen at the limbus.

vere cases can be associated with corneal scarring and neovascularization (Fig. 1-97). Similar lesions have been found on the oral mucosa. Excisional biopsy with adjunctive cryotherapy has been recommended for severe conjunctival lesions, but no curative treatment for this disorder has yet been identified.

Carcinoma in situ Carcinoma in situ, or conjunctival intraepithelial neoplasia, is defined as severe dysplasia and anaplasia that extends throughout the full-thickness conjunctival epithelium but does not extend through the epithelial basement membrane (Fig. 1-98). It is considered a premalignant lesion typically seen in middle-aged to elderly adults. Clinically, conjunctival intraepithelial neoplasia is usually found at the limbus and appears as a white-gray gelatinous lesion often with fingerlike fronds. They may become leukoplakic (Fig. 1-99). The lesion commonly spreads to adjacent cornea and occasionally invades deep to the basement membrane to become invasive squamous cell carcinoma. However, this transition can only be determined by histopathologic examination showing frank extension of the tumor beneath the basement membrane. Therefore, the recommended therapy involves obtaining a complete excisional biopsy specimen with wide conjunctival margins and conducting supplemental cryotherapy. Encouraging short-term results have been reported using topical mitomycin C for this disorder.

Squamous cell carcinoma As mentioned above, squamous cell carcinoma is designated by the invasion of neoplasm through the epithelial basement membrane of the conjunctiva or by metastasis to distant sites. Typically, squamous cell carcinoma is locally invasive (ex-

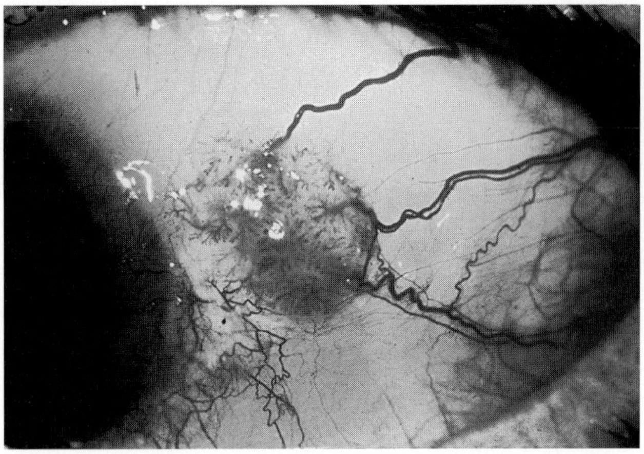

Fig. 1-100 Squamous cell carcinoma. A relatively small conjunctival mass with papillomatous fronds develops adjacent to the limbus.

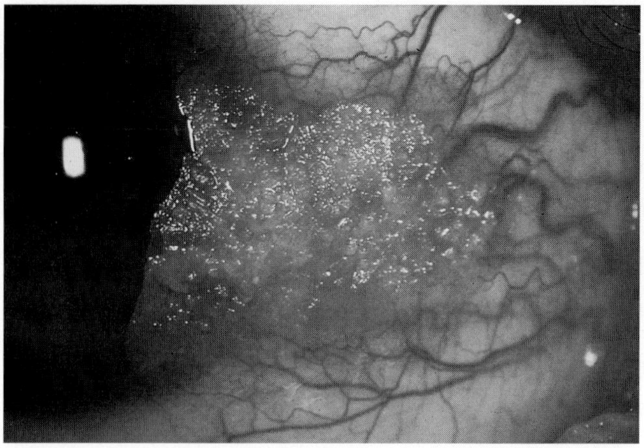

Fig. 1-101 Squamous cell carcinoma. A moderate-sized squamous cell carcinoma lesion involving the conjunctiva and the cornea is seen. Mild leukoplakia develops.

tending into the eye or to surrounding orbital tissue) with distant metastasis occurring only rarely. These lesions tend to occur in fair-skinned persons with a history of significant actinic exposure. They grow slowly and are rarely symptomatic until their gross appearance is noticed by the patient. Similar to conjunctival intraepithelial neoplasia, they have an amorphous, gelatinous appearance with papillary fronds and can develop a leukoplakic surface (Fig. 1-100). If left untreated squamous cell carcinoma frequently involves the underlying sclera and the adjacent cornea (Fig. 1-101). Recommended therapy involves complete excisional biopsy with wide conjunctival margins and supplemental cryotherapy using a double freeze-thaw technique. Depending on the extent of involvement, lamellar dissection into sclera, cornea, or both, or even irradiation and orbital exenteration, may be required (Fig. 1-102).

Mucoepidermoid carcinoma Mucoepidermoid carcinoma, a variant of squamous cell carcinoma, is known for its aggressive behavior and frequent intraocular and intraorbital invasion. Its name refers to the malignant goblet cells that accompany the malignant epithelial cells. It is more prevalent in persons older than 60 years and is treated in the same manner as is squamous cell carcinoma.

Melanocytic conjunctival tumors

Nevus Conjunctival nevi are benign hamartomatous lesions consisting of nests of modified melanocytes. The location of these nevus cells determines the classification as junctional, subepithelial, or compound. Junctional nevi have nevus cells located deep in the epithelium and along the substantia propria border. They are rare, typically found in childhood, and may be difficult to distinguish from primary acquired melanosis. With increasing age, these cells can migrate into the substantia propria to become subepithelial nevi. Subepithelial nevi are located in the substantia propria and are relatively inactive. Compound nevi are a transitional form with features of both junctional and subepithelial nevi. Clinically, compound nevi nearly always develop on the bulbar conjunctiva and have variable pigmentation, ranging from dark brown to tan (amelanotic nevus) (Fig. 1-103). Conjunctival nevi (particularly subepithelial and compound nevi) are frequently associated with small epithelial inclusion cysts that help distinguish them from other pigmented conjunctival lesions (Fig. 1-104). These cysts can secrete mucin and cause the nevi to enlarge, especially during puberty, thus giving a false impression of malignancy. Only rarely do these benign lesions undergo increased junctional activity and lead to malignant transformation. When signs of enlargement and color change are noted, these suspicious lesions should undergo excisional biopsy with supplemental cryotherapy to rule out

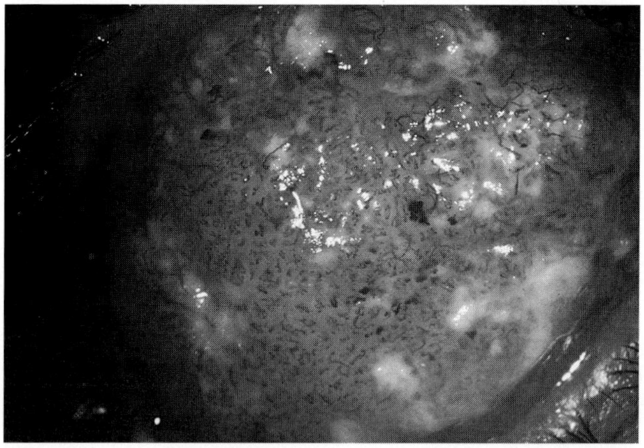

Fig. 1-102 Squamous cell carcinoma. Advanced squamous cell carcinoma involving the entire bulbar surface is evident. Confluent areas of papillary fronds can be seen. (See color plate.)

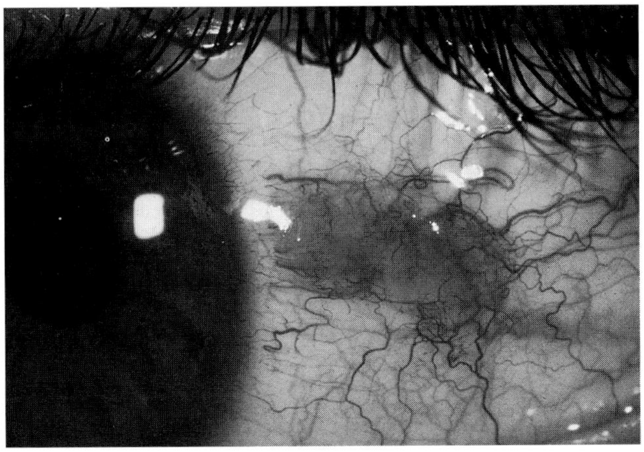

Fig. 1-103 Conjunctival nevus. An amelanotic compound nevus of the conjunctiva can be seen.

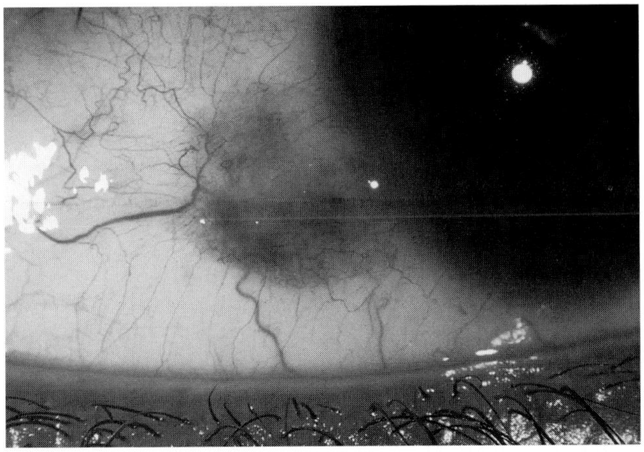

Fig. 1-104 Conjunctival nevus. A pigmented conjunctival nevus with small cysts has developed at the limbus.

malignant change. Otherwise, they should be observed regularly (every 6 to 12 months) with slit-lamp measurements, photographs, or both to document stability.

Ocular melanocytosis Ocular melanocytosis is not a true conjunctival lesion but is mentioned here because it is frequently mistaken as one. Manipulation of the conjunctiva with an anesthetized cotton-tip applicator helps confirm the absence of conjunctival involvement. Ocular melanocytosis is actually a unilateral, congenital blue nevus of the episclera and sclera characterized by multiple slate-gray patches of the episclera and sclera and sometimes deep conjunctiva (Fig. 1-105). It is associated with increased pigmentation of the uveal tract, involving the iris and the choroid. When the periocular skin is involved, the condition is usually unilateral but can be bilateral, and it is designated as oculodermal melanocytosis or nevus of Ota. These lesions are more common in African-American, Hispanic, and Asian populations. When found in white patients, the risk for malignant

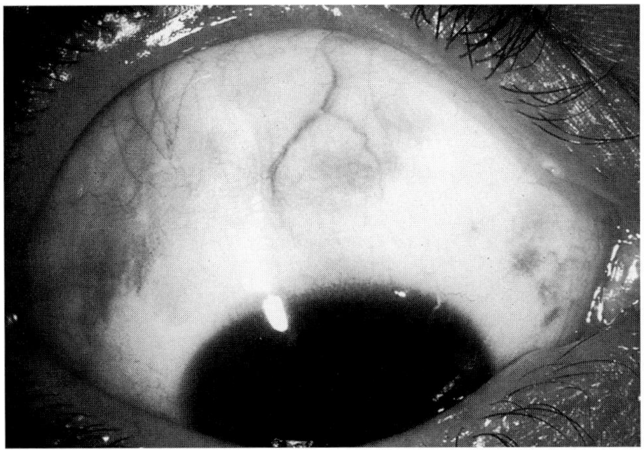

Fig. 1-105 Ocular melanocytosis. Multiple slate-gray patches of episcleral and scleral tissue are seen. In this patient the periocular skin was also involved, called *nevus of Ota*. (Courtesy of Carol L. Shields, M.D.)

transformation (of the skin, uvea, conjunctiva, orbit, and brain) rises dramatically.

Racial melanosis Racial melanosis refers to acquired pigmentation of the conjunctiva associated with populations that have dark or increased pigmentation (e.g., African-Americans, Hispanics). Brown pigmentation is usually distributed on the bulbar conjunctiva in a ring around the limbus and appears shortly after birth (Fig. 1-106). Racial melanosis rarely occurs in the fornices or on the palpebral conjunctiva. The condition is benign and has an extremely low potential for malignancy. Observation, however, is recommended.

Primary acquired melanosis Primary acquired pigmentation of the bulbar conjunctiva can occur, usually in middle-aged white patients. These pigmented patches consist of proliferating intraepithelial melanocytes and are usually unilateral, multiple, flat, and brown (Figs. 1-107 and 1-108). They can occur in the palpebral or bulbar conjunctiva. Pigmented areas in the fornix or palpebral conjunctiva should be regarded with high suspicion for primary acquired melanosis (PAM). It is important to identify these lesions because they have a high rate of transformation into malignant melanoma (as high as 20% to 30%). Signs that may indicate malignant transformation include change in size, shape, or elevation and evidence of increased vascularity. Suspicious PAM lesions should be treated with excisional biopsy and supplemental cryotherapy to rule out atypia or frank malignancy. Topical mitomycin C may also have a role in treatment.

Malignant melanoma Malignant melanoma of the conjunctiva typically occurs in middle-aged to elderly patients and has the potential for distant metastasis and death. It usually occurs in the bulbar conjunctiva (rarely in the palpebral conjunctiva) and can arise from three sources according to the "rule of thirds": nevi (approxi-

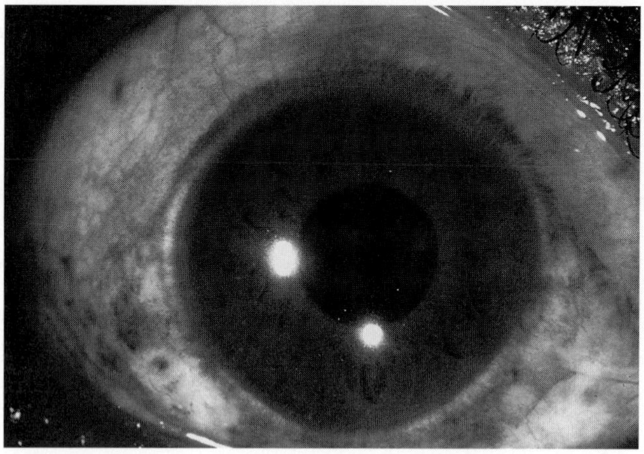

Fig. 1-106 Racial melanosis. There are large areas of conjunctival pigmentation, especially around the limbus, in this African-American patient.

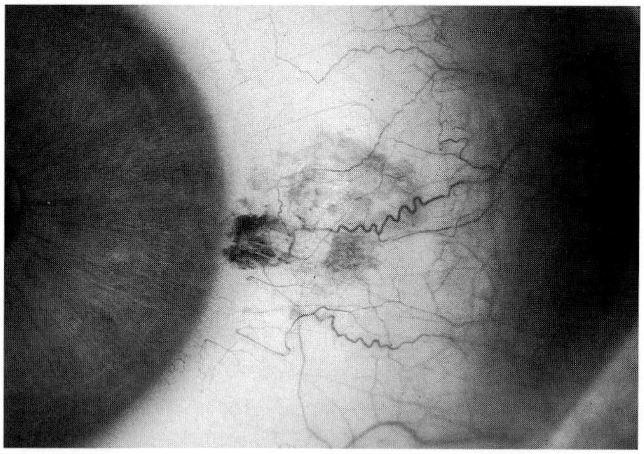

Fig. 1-107 Primary acquired melanosis. A small area of patchy conjunctival pigmentation can be seen at the limbus. Biopsy specimen revealed primary acquired melanosis with mild atypia.

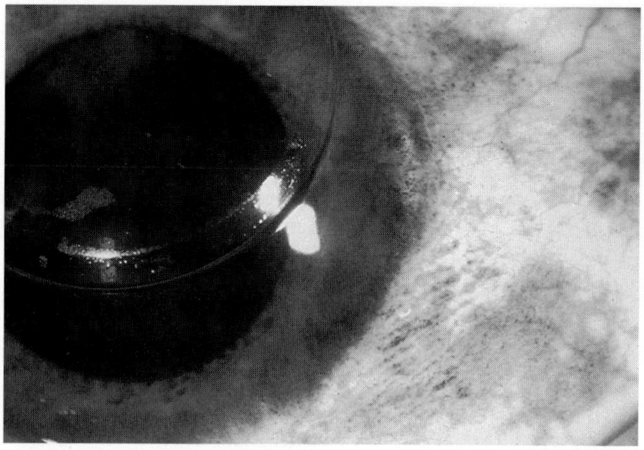

Fig. 1-108 Primary acquired melanosis. Several large areas of conjunctival and corneal pigmentation are seen in this patient. Biopsy specimen yielded primary acquired melanosis with moderate atypia that was successfully treated with topical mitomycin C.

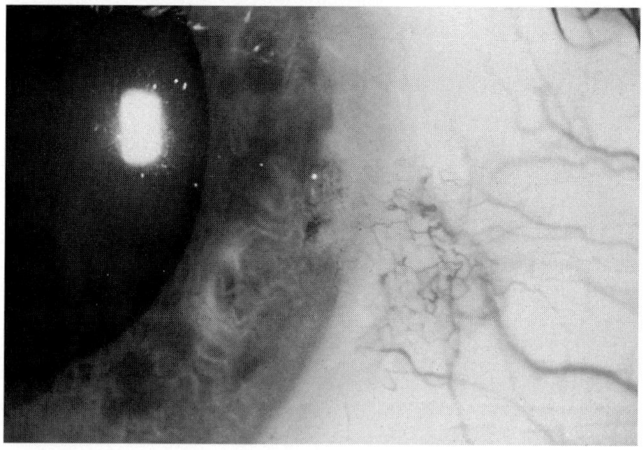

Fig. 1-109 Conjunctival malignant melanoma. A small area of conjunctival injection adjacent to a focal area of corneal pigmentation proved to be malignant melanoma.

mately 33%), PAM (approximately 33%), and de novo (approximately 33%). Each source has its own mortality rate: nevi (20%), PAM (40%), and de novo (40%). Clinically, these lesions have an amorphous, nodular, elevated shape with variable pigmentation, though most are brown (Fig. 1-109). They are usually associated with increased conjunctival/episcleral vascularization with an occasional large conjunctival feeder vessel (Figs. 1-110 and 1-111). Examination should include a dilated fundus evaluation, scleral transillumination, and B-scan ultrasonography to rule out underlying ciliary body melanoma. Although these tumors portend a better prognosis than cutaneous melanomas, they certainly have the capability of intraocular and orbital extension and of distant metastasis, primarily to the liver. Treatment consists of complete excisional biopsy with supplemental beta-irradiation or cryotherapy using a double freeze-thaw technique. Patients with advanced disease may require enucleation or orbital exenteration. Some research has shown a possible role for topical alkylating agents such as mitomycin C. Patients with conjunctival melanoma should undergo the appropriate metastatic workup by an oncologist.

Lymphoid conjunctival tumors

Benign reactive lymphoid hyperplasia Benign reactive lymphoid hyperplasia typically occurs in middle-aged adults and refers to the benign accumulation of various monocytes and polymorphonuclear lymphocytes. Its cause is unclear, but it seems to be a localized reaction to an irritative or antigenic stimulus. Benign reactive lymphoid hyperplasia appears as a light pink or salmon-colored lesion anywhere in the bulbar or forniceal conjunctiva and is clinically indistinguishable from conjunc-

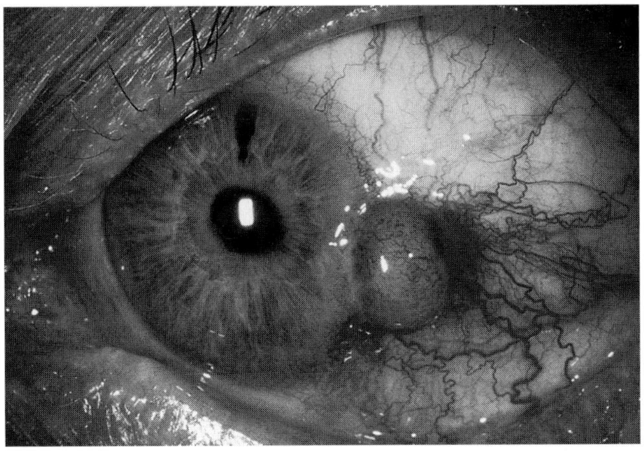

Fig. 1-110 Conjunctival malignant melanoma. A large elevated conjunctival mass with two small areas of pigmentation is evident at the limbus. Excisional biopsy revealed malignant melanoma.

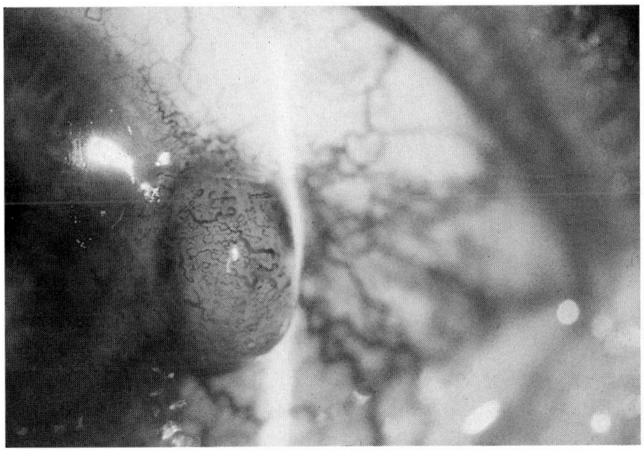

Fig. 1-111 Conjunctival malignant melanoma. A slit-beam view of the malignant melanoma seen in the patient in Fig. 1-110 reveals its elevated nature.

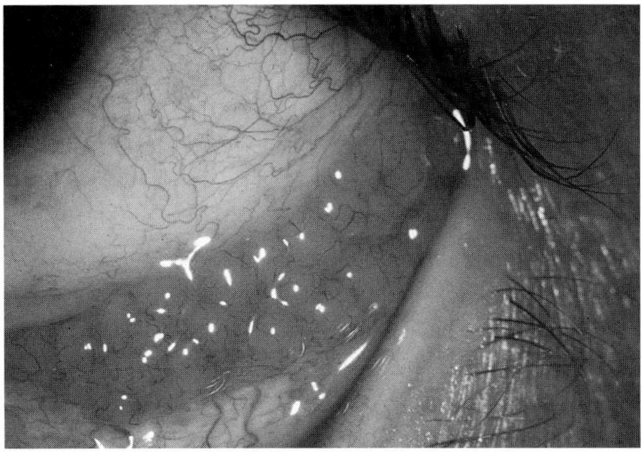

Fig. 1-112 Conjunctival benign reactive lymphoid hyperplasia. A prominent conjunctival salmon-colored follicular mass can be seen in the inferior fornix.

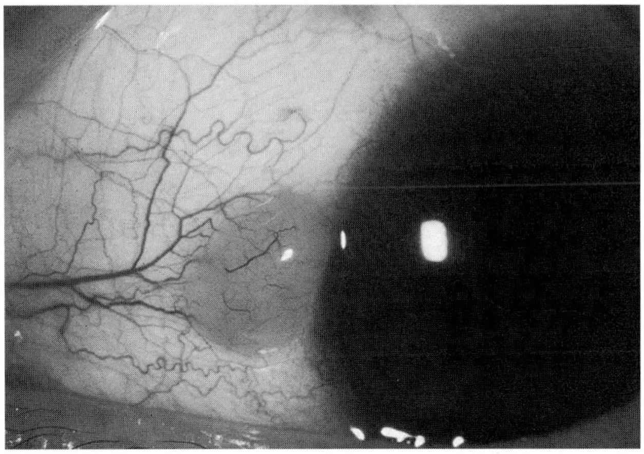

Fig. 1-113 Conjunctival lymphoma. Biopsy examination reveals that a small localized conjunctival mass was lymphoma.

tival lymphoma (Fig. 1-112). Hence, incisional or excisional biopsy is recommended with the appropriate tissue handling for special immunohistochemical studies. If it is benign, the lesion can be treated with complete excision, low-dose radiation, or topical corticosteroids.

Lymphoma Lymphomas are neoplastic lesions of the conjunctiva with characteristics similar to those of benign reactive lymphoid hyperplasia. Some consider the two entities to be representative of the same disorder with different potential for malignancy. Lymphomas lie on the malignant side of the spectrum and consist of a monotonous array of monoclonal B-cells. They may appear alone or in conjunction with systemic malignant lymphoma, and they may have the same clinical appearance as benign reactive lymphoid hyperplasia (Figs. 1-113, 1-114, and 1-115). Patients should undergo complete excisional biopsy with immediate referral to an oncologist for systemic evaluation. Depending on the extent of disease, local irradiation and systemic chemotherapy may be indicated. Leukemic conjunctival infiltrates, though rare, are clinically similar to lymphomas.

Vascular conjunctival tumors

Kaposi's sarcoma Kaposi's sarcoma, a malignant tumor, has become more prevalent because it occurs in approximately one third of all patients with AIDS. Histologically, it consists of proliferating capillaries, vascular endothelial cells, and pericytes that lie in the conjunctival stroma. Kaposi's sarcoma appears clinically as a nodular or diffuse red to purple subepithelial conjunctival lesion frequently mistaken for a subconjunctival hemorrhage (Fig. 1-116). In general, lesions involve the forniceal and bulbar conjunctiva and the eyelids. A careful history should help elucidate the diagnosis because these tumors progress slowly and do not resolve gradually with time. In addition, patients should be questioned about

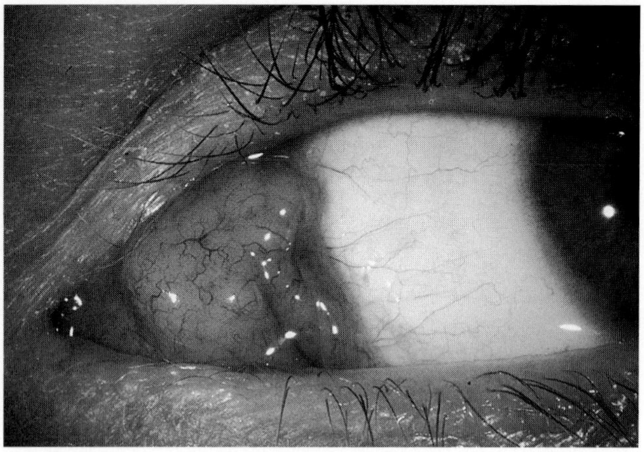

Fig. 1-114 Conjunctival lymphoma. This large conjunctival mass adjacent to the caruncle was also lymphoma.

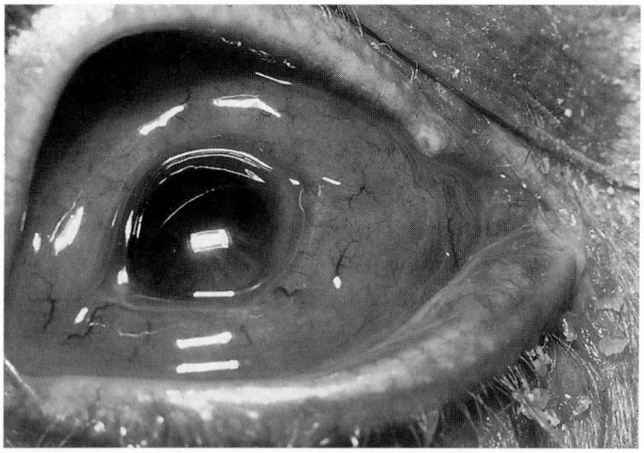

Fig. 1-115 Conjunctival lymphoma. This diffuse conjunctival mass was diagnosed as lymphoma.

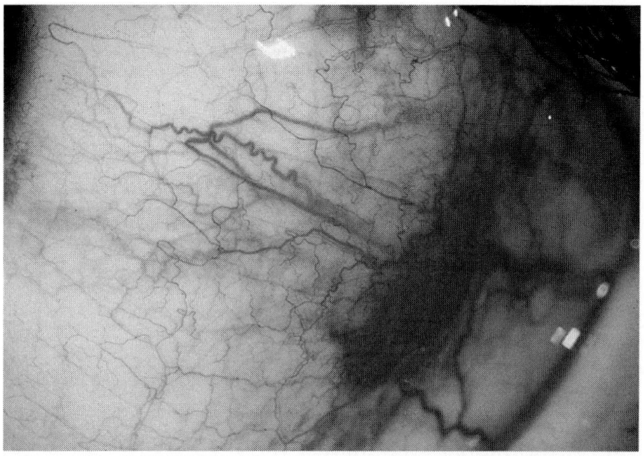

Fig. 1-116 Kaposi's sarcoma. An ill-defined bright red conjunctival mass seen in this patient with acquired immunodeficiency syndrome is Kaposi's sarcoma. (See color plate.)

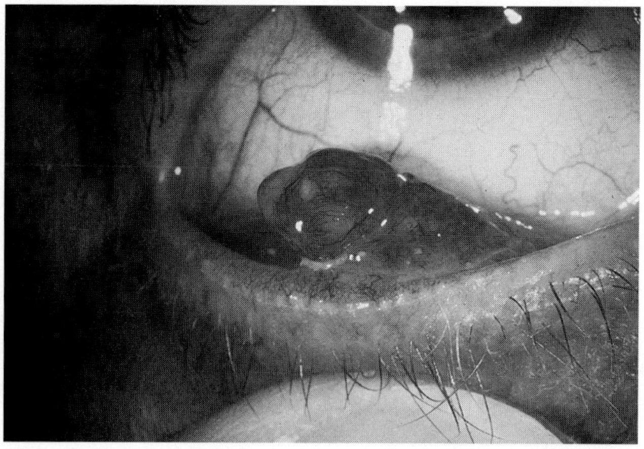

Fig. 1-117 Conjunctival pyogenic granuloma. A large pyogenic granuloma occurred soon after a chalazion developed in this area of the lower eyelid.

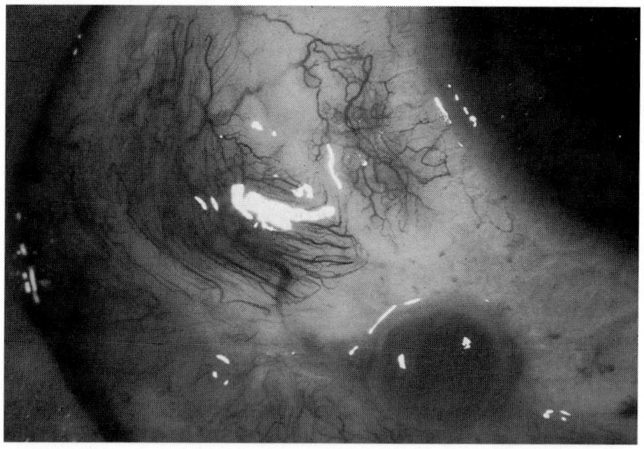

Fig. 1-118 Conjunctival pyogenic granuloma. A small round pyogenic granuloma developed in an area of bare sclera soon after excision of a large conjunctival tumor. It responded rapidly to topical corticosteroids.

possible symptoms or signs of HIV infection because Kaposi's sarcoma can be a presenting manifestation of AIDS. Although rarely invasive, treatment is initiated when these lesions cause discomfort, obstruction of vision, or eyelid-related problems such as entropion and ectropion. Treatment options include simple excision, cryotherapy, radiation therapy, chemotherapy, and immunotherapy with alpha-interferon. Success rates vary because of recurrent tumors.

Pyogenic granuloma A pyogenic granuloma is a fleshy, well-circumscribed, vascularized mass lesion of the conjunctiva (Fig. 1-117). Pyogenic granuloma is a misnomer because it is associated with neither purulent discharge nor granulomatous inflammation. It is considered a subset of a capillary hemangioma that often arises as a result of a chalazion or because of a conjunctival defect, such as after ocular surgery (Fig. 1-118).

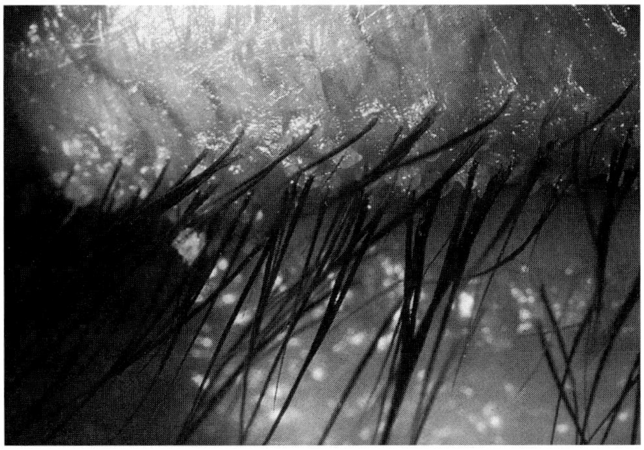

Fig. 1-119 Blepharitis. Significant crusting is visible at the base of the eyelashes in this patient with anterior blepharitis.

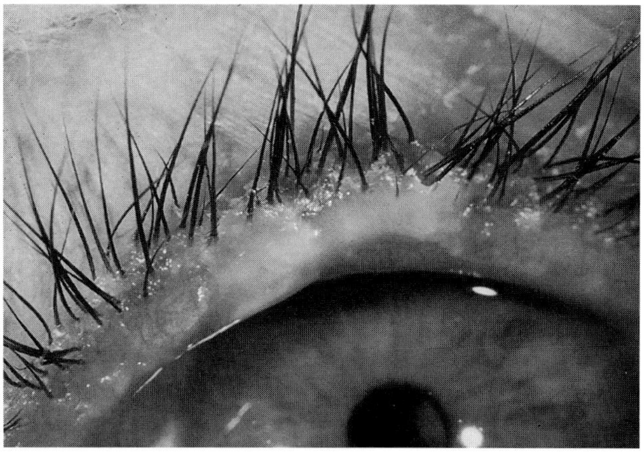

Fig. 1-120 Blepharitis. Eyelid margin ulceration is present in this patient with severe blepharitis.

EXTERNAL DISEASE

Disorders of external disease involve the surrounding ocular adnexa, including the eyelids and periocular skin. Because of their proximity, the conjunctiva, cornea, or both are often affected.

Blepharitis

Blepharitis is inflammation of the eyelid margins. One of the most common external diseases, it may primarily involve the anterior eyelid margin (anterior blepharitis) or the posterior eyelid margin (posterior blepharitis or meibomianitis). Anterior blepharitis may have an infectious or a noninfectious cause. *Staphylococcus aureus* is usually the organism responsible for infectious blepharitis. The noninfectious variant is known as seborrheic blepharitis and is related to seborrheic dermatitis. Patients have itching, burning, and tearing with crusting of the eyelid margins on awakening. On slit-lamp examination, these patients often have crusted deposits on the eyelashes (traditionally referred to as scurf on the eyelashes in seborrheic blepharitis and collarettes at the base of the eyelashes in staphylococcal blepharitis) with erythematous and thickened eyelid margins (Fig. 1-119). Other signs include eyelash loss or whitening (poliosis) and eyelid margin ulceration (Fig. 1-120). There may be accompanying conjunctival and corneal signs and associated conjunctivitis/keratitis. Multiple chalazia may also occur (Fig. 1-121). Angular blepharitis involves an ulceration at the lateral junction of the upper and lower eyelids (Fig. 1-122). Treatment involves local hygiene therapy consisting of warm compresses, eyelid scrubs (with baby shampoo applied on a wet washcloth or cotton-tip applicator), artificial tears four to six times a day, and antibiotic ointment (e.g., bacitracin, erythromycin) to the eyelid margins at bedtime. More severe cases may benefit from the addition of a short course of topical antibiotic-corticosteroid preparations to the eyelid margins. Proper instruction, patience, and importance of compliance should all be emphasized to the patient. Frequently, patients abandon therapy out of frustration and inconvenience and suffer from persistent disease. When unilateral, asymmetric, or persistent blepharitis or chalazia are noted, sebaceous gland carcinoma should be suspected.

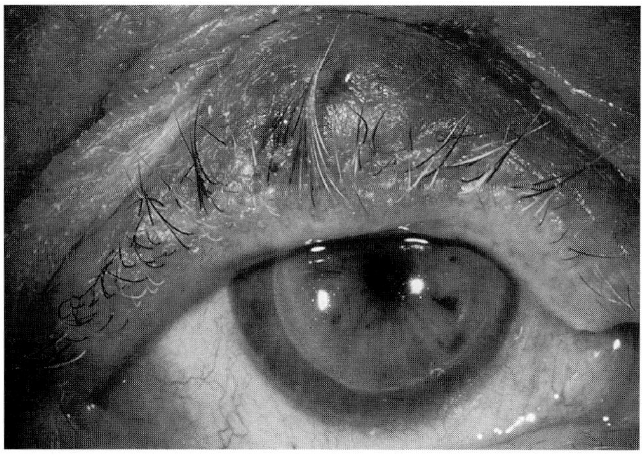

Fig. 1-121 Blepharitis. A large chalazion has formed superiorly in this patient with significant eyelid crusting and inflammation from blepharitis.

Meibomianitis

As mentioned earlier, meibomianitis refers to posterior eyelid margin inflammation and is manifested with similar symptoms but different signs. Patients often have inspissated meibomian gland orifices, evident on squeezing the eyelid margins with a cotton-tip applicator (Figs.

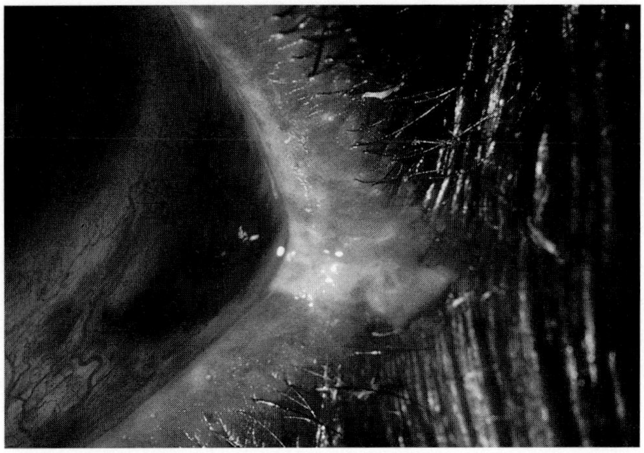

Fig. 1-122 Angular blepharitis. Ulceration at the lateral junction of the upper and lower eyelids occurs in angular blepharitis.

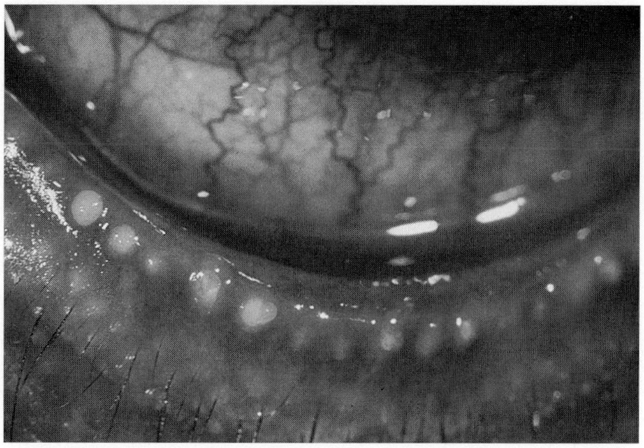

Fig. 1-124 Meibomianitis. Multiple inspissated meibomian glands are apparent in the lower eyelid of this patient with severe meibomian gland disease.

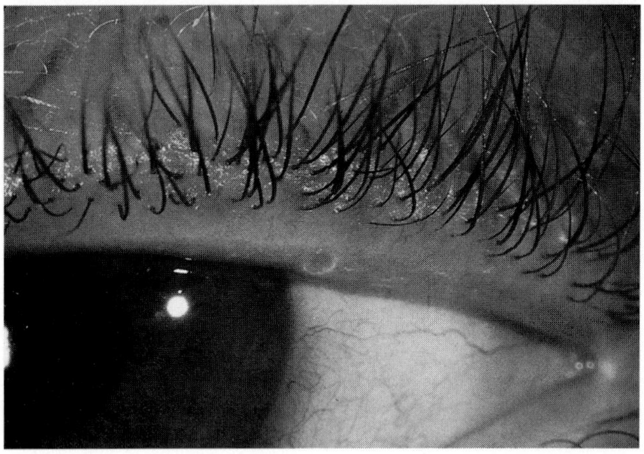

Fig. 1-123 Meibomianitis. An inspissated meibomian gland can be seen in the upper eyelid margin.

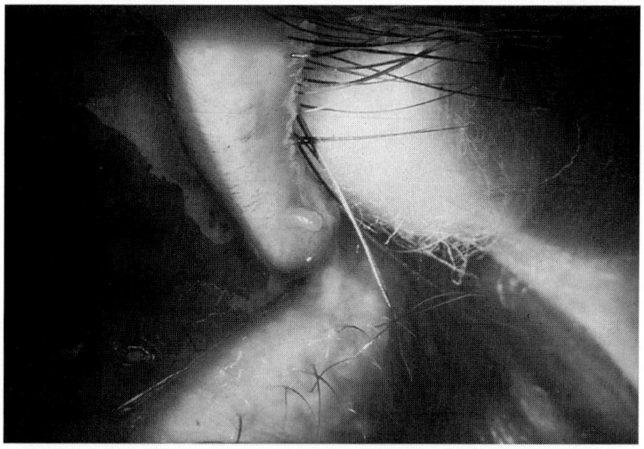

Fig. 1-125 Meibomianitis. Gentle pressure with a cotton-tip applicator expressed a thick secretion from this patient with meibomianitis. This type of secretion is called the "toothpaste sign."

1-123 and 1-124). In patients with severe cases, whitish coagulated secretions may ooze out of meibomian orifices (known as the toothpaste sign) (Fig. 1-125). These patients typically have erythematous, thickened eyelid margins. Treatment is the same as delineated above with the addition of oral antibiotics (e.g., 100 mg doxycycline PO bid for 2 weeks, then 100 mg daily; 250 mg erythromycin PO qid for 2 weeks, bid for 2 weeks, then daily). Recent reports have included some encouraging results with topical metronidazole gel applied to the eyelid margins two to four times a day.

Ocular Rosacea

Acne rosacea is an idiopathic dermatologic condition typically occurring in middle-aged adults. When it affects the eyes (which is quite common), it is more specifically referred to as ocular rosacea. The condition is characterized by sebaceous gland hypertrophy and dysfunction, resulting in familiar facial features such as midfacial erythema, malar rash, telangiectasia, papules, pustules, and rhinophyma (Fig. 1-126). Exacerbation of these features is often noted after the consumption of coffee, alcohol, and spicy foods. Ocular findings are usually bilateral and include chronic, persistent blepharitis, usually meibomianitis, with recurrent chalazia (Fig. 1-127). Involvement may extend to the ocular surface and lead to chronic conjunctivitis, corneal neovascularization, and marginal keratitis. Advanced disease can result in recurrent episcleritis/iritis and corneal scarring, vascularization, and ulceration with melting, necessitating emergency or elective penetrating keratoplasty. Treatment of this disorder involves systemic and ocular medications. Tetracycline (250 mg) PO qid, 250 mg erythromycin PO qid, or 100 mg doxycycline PO bid for 2 to 8 weeks should be started and eventually tapered to

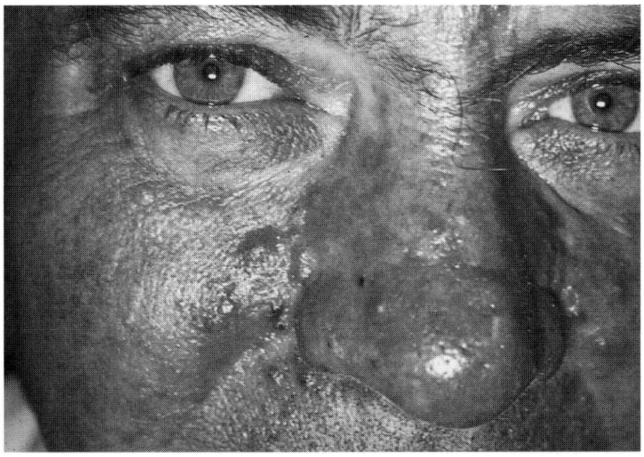

Fig. 1-126 Rosacea. Facial features of rosacea including papules, pustules, telangiectasias, and rhinophyma can be seen in this patient. (Courtesy of Guy F. Webster, M.D., Ph.D.)

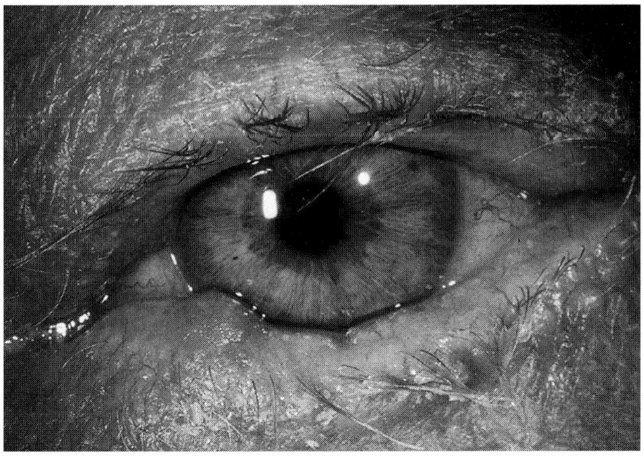

Fig. 1-127 Ocular rosacea. Anterior and posterior blepharitis, as well as eyelid margin telangiectasias and a small chalazion, are seen in this patient with ocular rosacea.

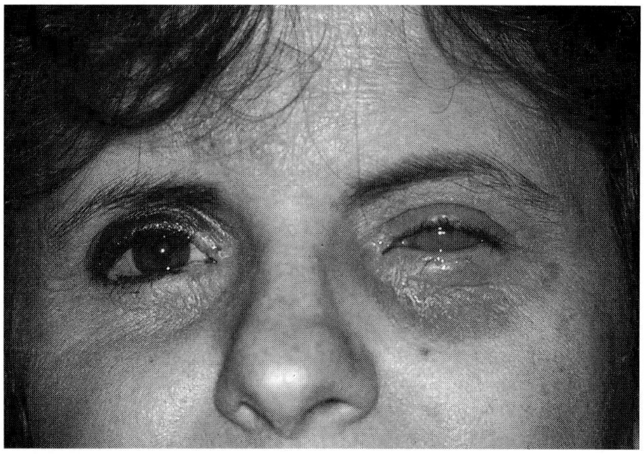

Fig. 1-128 Contact dermatitis. Severe conjunctivitis and dermatitis developed in this patient using unilateral eye drops.

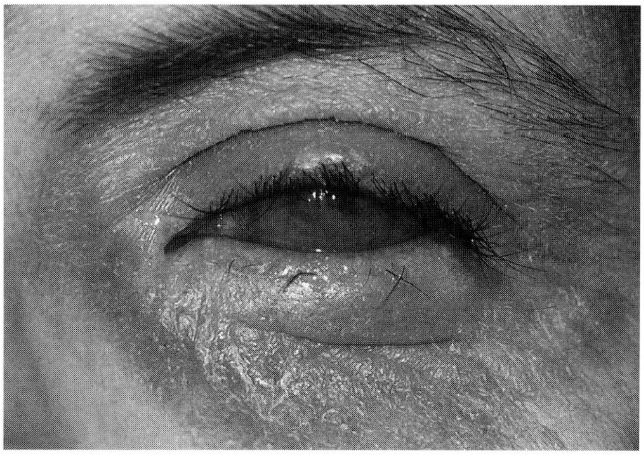

Fig. 1-129 Contact dermatitis. Note the thickening and scaling of the eyelid skin in the patient seen in Fig. 1-128. (See color plate.)

a lower maintenance dose. Patients may also apply a dermatologic cream (e.g., 0.75% to 1.0% metronidazole gel) once or twice a day to the affected skin. When ocular involvement is present, treatment should incorporate the local therapy outlined in the section on meibomianitis. In addition, patients are advised to refrain from possible dietary stimulants. The response to treatment varies, and patients are warned about the chronicity of the disease.

Allergic Disorders of the Eyelids

Contact dermatitis Contact dermatitis is thought to be a type IV mediated delayed hypersensitivity reaction occurring in the periocular skin approximately 24 to 72 hours after the application of topical ophthalmic or dermatologic medications and cosmetics. The condition causes erythema, scaling, and thickening of the periocular skin resembling eczematous dermatitis (Figs. 1-128 and 1-129). Often papillary conjunctivitis and inferior punctate keratitis are present. Unilaterality or bilaterality correlates with the application of the medication or cosmetic. Treatment involves identifying and discontinuing the inciting agent. Patients are then instructed to use cool compresses four to six times a day and, if the condition is severe, mild corticosteroid cream (e.g., 0.05% dexamethasone cream) two to three times a day to the affected areas. Care should be taken not to get corticosteroid cream in the eyes. In addition, a systemic antihistamine (e.g., 25 to 50 mg diphenhydramine PO qid) may be of benefit. The reaction usually resolves in several days without sequelae. Chronic complications such as skin hyperpigmentation and eyelid ectropion may develop in severe cases.

MAJOR POINTS

If a patient has a history of recurrent subconjunctival bleeding, the possibility of a bleeding diathesis either from medication or from a clotting disorder should be suspected, especially if the patient also has easy skin bruising, bleeding from the gums, or nosebleeds.

Ophthalmia neonatorum should be suspected if diffuse conjunctival injection associated with mucopurulent discharge is discovered in one or both eyes of an infant.

Neisseria gonorrhoeae causes the most severe and aggressive form of hyperacute neonatal conjunctivitis, and its suspicion warrants prompt diagnosis and treatment because of the rapid progression to corneal ulceration, perforation, and endophthalmitis.

Treatment of sexual contact(s) should be emphasized to patients with adult inclusion conjunctivitis secondary to *Chlamydia trachomatis* infection. Patients and their sexual contact(s) should be evaluated for other sexually transmitted diseases such as syphilis, gonorrhea, and human immunodeficiency virus.

Blood-tinged debris on the eyelids and eyelashes indicates possible pediculosis.

The diagnosis of superior limbic keratoconjunctivitis is frequently missed simply because the superior conjunctiva (obscured by the upper eyelid) is not carefully inspected or is overlooked on cursory examination. An easy and reliable way to avoid missing this condition is to examine the superior bulbar conjunctiva with the naked eye in a well-lit room while holding up both upper eyelids as the patient looks down.

Floppy eyelid syndrome is also frequently misdiagnosed because the upper eyelid is not everted during ocular examination.

In any patient with chronic conjunctivitis, especially if it is unilateral, examine the eyelids carefully for molluscum contagiosum lesions.

Ocular therapy for the acute phase of Stevens-Johnson syndrome is centered on providing copious lubrication, preventing secondary infection, and decreasing inflammation as needed with topical corticosteroids.

It is important to remember that cicatricial pemphigoid is a systemic disorder that requires systemic treatment, often coordinated with an internist, a dermatologist, or both.

If a patient has severely dry eyes, causes of vitamin A deficiency (e.g., cystic fibrosis, chronic pancreatitis and hepatitis, inflammatory bowel disease, and intestinal bypass surgery for morbid obesity) should be considered.

Hereditary benign intraepithelial dyskeratosis lesions have a distinct appearance but are frequently misdiagnosed as pingueculae/pterygia and squamous cell carcinoma.

Carcinoma in situ is a premalignant lesion that involves full-thickness epithelium of the conjunctiva or cornea but does not extend through the epithelial basement membrane; squamous cell carcinoma is a malignant neoplasm that extends beneath the basement membrane of the conjunctiva and is locally invasive.

Conjunctival nevi, particularly subepithelial and compound nevi, are frequently associated with small epithelial inclusion cysts that help distinguish them from other pigmented conjunctival lesions.

White persons with nevus of Ota lesions are at high risk for malignant transformation of the skin, uvea, conjunctiva, orbit, and brain.

It is important to identify primary acquired melanosis lesions because they have a high (20% to 30%) rate of transformation to malignant melanoma.

Patients with conjunctival lymphoma should undergo complete excisional biopsy for diagnosis, with immediate referral to an oncologist for systemic evaluation.

Kaposi's sarcoma appears clinically as a nodular or diffuse red to purple subepithelial lesion that is frequently mistaken for a subconjunctival hemorrhage. When it is suspected, patients should be questioned about possible symptoms or signs of human immunodeficiency virus infection, because Kaposi's sarcoma can be an early manifestation of acquired immunodeficiency syndrome.

Unilateral, asymmetric, or persistent blepharitis or chalazia may indicate sebaceous gland carcinoma.

CONCLUSION

Disorders of the conjunctiva and eyelids are prevalent. They are among the most common reasons for visits to the ophthalmologist. It is therefore imperative for the diagnostician to have a complete understanding of the many varied pathologic mechanisms that can affect the conjunctiva and the eyelids. Disorders ranging from emergency infectious conjunctivitis to conjunctival tumors to chronic eyelid disease make up this important class of diseases. Thorough patient histories that include such details as chronicity and exposures and results of complete slit-lamp examinations, evaluating the inferior fornices to the superior conjunctiva to the eyelid margins, aid in making the correct diagnosis and in implementing the appropriate treatment.

SUGGESTED READINGS

Journals

Allansmith MR, Korb DR, Greiner JV, et al: Giant papillary conjunctivitis in contact lens wearers, *Am J Ophthalmol* 83: 697-708, 1977.

Browning DJ, Proia AD: Ocular rosacea, *Surv Ophthalmol* 31: 145-158, 1986.

Culbertson WW, Ostler HB: The floppy eyelid syndrome, *Am J Ophthalmol* 92:568-575, 1981.

Driver PJ, Lemp MA: Meibomian gland dysfunction, *Surv Ophthalmol* 40:343-367, 1996.

Foster CS: Cicatricial pemphigoid, *Trans Am Ophthalmol Soc* 84:527-663, 1986.

Friedlaender MH: Conjunctivitis of allergic origin: clinical presentation and differential diagnosis, *Surv Ophthalmol* 38(suppl):105-114, 1993.

Grosskreutz C, Smith LBH: Neonatal conjunctivitis, *Int Ophthalmol Clin* 32:71-79, 1992.

Holland EJ, Chan C, Kuwabara T, et al: Immunohistochemical findings and results of treatment with cyclosporine in ligneous conjunctivitis, *Am J Ophthalmol* 107:160-166, 1989.

Jackson WB: Differentiating conjunctivitis of diverse origins, *Surv Ophthalmol* 38(suppl):91-104, 1993.

Laibson PR: Ocular adenoviral infections, *Int Ophthalmol Clin* 24:49-64, 1984.

Lee GA, Hirst LW: Ocular surface squamous neoplasia, *Surv Ophthalmol* 39:429-450, 1995.

Lemp MA: General measures in the management of the dry eye, *Int Ophthalmol Clin* 27:36-43, 1987.

McCulley JP, Dougherty BS, Deneau DG: Classification of chronic blepharitis, *Ophthalmology* 89:1173-1180, 1982.

McCulley JP, Moore MB, Matoba AY: Mucus fishing syndrome, *Ophthalmology* 92:1262-1265, 1985.

Perkins RE, et al: Bacteriology of normal and infected conjunctiva, *J Clin Microbiol* 1:147-149, 1975.

Schott D, Dempfle CE, Beck P, et al: Therapy with a purified plasminogen concentrate in an infant with ligneous conjunctivitis and homozygous plasminogen deficiency, *N Engl J Med* 339:1679-1686, 1998.

Sendele DD, Kenyon KR, Mobilia EF, et al: Superior limbic keratoconjunctivitis in contact lens wearers, *Ophthalmology* 90:616-622, 1983.

Seregard S: Conjunctival melanoma, *Surv Ophthalmol* 42:321-350, 1998.

Sommer A: Xerophthalmia, keratomalacia, and nutritional blindness, *Int Ophthalmol* 14:195-199, 1990.

Theodore FH, Ferry AP: Superior limbic keratoconjunctivitis-clinical and pathological correlations, *Arch Ophthalmol* 84: 481-484, 1970.

Trocme SD, Aldave AJ: The eye and the eosinophil, *Surv Ophthalmol* 39:241-252, 1994.

Wear DJ, Malaty RH, Zimmerman LE, et al: Cat scratch disease bacilli in the conjunctiva of patients with Parinaud's oculoglandular syndrome, *Ophthalmology* 92:1282-1287, 1985.

Wilson FM II: Adverse external ocular effects of topical ophthalmic medications, *Surv Ophthalmol* 24:57-88, 1979.

CHAPTER 2

Anterior Segment Developmental Anomalies

This chapter is devoted to specific diseases that appear predominantly in early infancy or early childhood as the result of disruption in the normal development of the cornea and the anterior segment. These developmental abnormalities may arise because of one or a combination of genetic, infectious, inflammatory, toxic, metabolic, traumatic, or mechanical processes, and they may occur at any time during tissue induction, differentiation, and maturation. Most of these causative factors are thought to exert their influence either during the period of organogenesis (between the fourth and sixth gestational weeks) or during the period of anterior segment differentiation (between the sixth and sixteenth gestational weeks). Developmental insults of earlier onset result in more severe and extensive injury than do those that take place at a later intrauterine date. Therefore, the nature and the timing of these insults contribute to determining the degree of damage and may aid the clinician in deducing the chronology of embryologic events. Often the exact time points of developmental insult and its pathophysiologic mechanisms and specific causative elements are unknown.

Although they may be encountered rarely in routine ophthalmic practice, it is important for several reasons to recognize these developmental corneal and anterior segment abnormalities in infants and children. The correct diagnosis can provide information regarding the natural history of the condition, indicate the necessary medical or surgical treatment, and determine the appropriate scheduling of follow-up care. Prompt examination can also alert the physician to the various ocular and systemic complications that may accompany the disorder and that warrant additional investigation by other specialists. Finally, accurate identification and analysis of the disease will help parents deal with the realities of the prognosis and guide them in seeking the proper genetic counseling when indicated.

When examining an infant with a cloudy cornea, it helps to remember the STUMPED mnemonic developed by Waring and colleagues: **S** = sclerocornea, **T** = tears in Descemet's membrane from birth trauma (forceps injury) or congenital glaucoma (Haab's striae), **U** = ulceration (infection), **M** = metabolic (e.g., mucopolysaccharidosis), **P** = Peters' anomaly, **E** = edema (e.g., congenital hereditary endothelial dystrophy), and **D** = dermoid. Many of these conditions are discussed in this chapter; others are reviewed elsewhere in this text. It should be emphasized that if a complete examination cannot be conducted in the office, an evaluation under anesthesia should seriously be considered.

DEVELOPMENTAL ANOMALIES OF THE CORNEA

Developmental corneal anomalies make up an interesting collection of conditions caused by a defect in development that results in a departure from normal corneal structure. Such alterations in normal development often involve the neighboring structures of the anterior chamber angle, iris, and lens. Some of the ocular and systemic associations listed for the various corneal anomalies involve the anterior segment and occur because of the close embryologic relationship between these structures and the cornea. However, some of these associations may have no connection with the developmental process and may simply reflect reports of accompanying characteristics.

Absence of the Cornea

True absence of the cornea True absence of the cornea is a rare condition that is always accompanied by the agenesis of other anterior segment structures. It never occurs as an isolated phenomenon because of its close relationship with the embryologic differentiation of other anterior segment structures. Absence of the cornea, iris, lens, and other anterior structures comprises a spectrum of agenesis, with anophthalmos (absence of the entire eye) representing the most extreme example (Table 2-1).

True cryptophthalmos (ablepharon) True cryptophthalmos, otherwise known as ablepharon, is another rare condition that occurs when the eyelids fail to form, leaving the cornea and the conjunctiva unprotected and exposed. Although the cornea and the conjunctiva are present, they undergo metaplastic change (termed dermoid transformation) to form skin. True cryptophthalmos is usually transmitted as an autosomal recessive trait, and it can present unilaterally or bilaterally with equal incidence in males and females. It is accompanied by the absence of lashes and brows and sometimes by the absence of lacrimal glands and canaliculi. The anterior chamber is usually small or absent, and the iris, lens, trabecular meshwork, and Schlemm's canal frequently do not exist or are replaced by connective tissue. The many associated systemic abnormalities that have been cited include craniofacial anomalies (the most common), syndactyly, spina bifida, deformed ears and teeth, cleft lip or palate, laryngeal or anal atresia, ventral hernias, nipple or umbilicus displacement, basal encephalocele, genitourinary anomalies, cardiac anomalies, and mental retardation. The term *cryptophthalmos syndrome* has been used to describe the finding of cryptophthalmos with any extraocular abnormality.

Pseudocryptophthalmos (total ankyloblepharon) Pseudocryptophthalmos, or total ankyloblepharon, is a related condition in which the eyelids form but fail to separate, leaving a normal cornea and conjunctiva that are totally covered by skin. Unlike true cryptophthalmos, in pseudocryptophthalmos both the lashes and brows are present with an otherwise normal eye, and vision is restored by surgical creation of a palpebral fissure.

True absence of the cornea and true cryptophthalmos have dismal visual prognoses and no known treatment. Besides proper education and counseling, the only warranted intervention may be for cosmetic purposes. Although pseudocryptophthalmos is associated with excellent visual potential after surgery, the newly opened eyelids pose a continual challenge because of the need to prevent eyelid reclosure and maintain normal eyelid function.

Anomalies of Corneal Size

The horizontal diameter of a normal newborn cornea measures approximately 10 mm, whereas the horizontal diameter of a normal adult cornea measures approximately 12 mm. The horizontal diameter of the normal cornea virtually always exceeds the vertical diameter by approximately 1 mm because of the prominent scleral encroachment at the superior and inferior limbi. The newborn cornea usually reaches adult size by 2 years of age (Table 2-2).

Table 2-1 Spectrum of conditions involving an absent cornea

Feature	True absence of cornea	True cryptophthalmos (ablepharon)	Pseudocryptophthalmos (total ankyloblepharon)	Anophthalmos
Cause	Unknown	Failure of eyelid formation	Failure of eyelid separation	Unknown
Anatomy	Absent cornea accompanied by agenesis of other anterior segment structures	Abnormal metaplastic cornea	Underlying normal cornea	Absence of the entire eye
Visual prognosis	Poor	Poor	Good	Poor

Table 2-2 Important points of megalocornea and microcornea

Feature	Megalocornea	Microcornea
Horizontal corneal diameter	≥13 mm	≤10 mm
Inheritance	X-linked recessive	Autosomal dominant or recessive
Corneal features	Enlarged but otherwise normal	Smaller and flatter but otherwise normal
Anterior segment features	Enlarged anterior segment and ciliary ring (anterior megalophthalmos)	Crowded anterior segment predisposing to open- and closed-angle glaucoma
Differential diagnosis	Congenital glaucoma	Sclerocornea

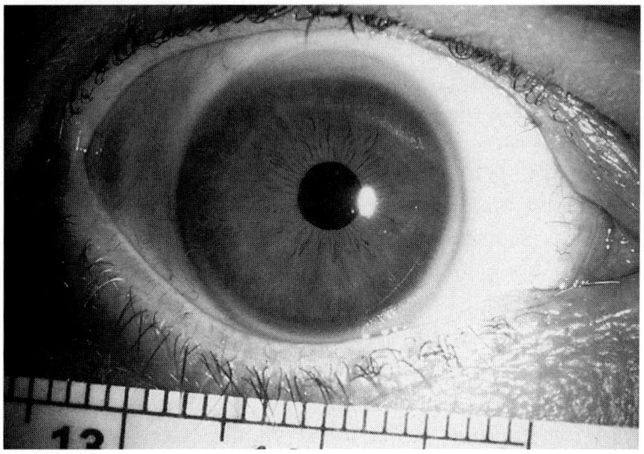

Fig. 2-1 Megalocornea. The horizontal diameter of this eye with megalocornea measures 14 mm. The cornea is essentially clear, and the corneal thickness is normal.

Box 2-1 Major Ocular and Systemic Associations of Megalocornea

OCULAR	SYSTEMIC
Arcus juvenilis	Albinism
Astigmatism (with the rule)	Alport's syndrome
Cataract (usually posterior subcapsular)	Apert's syndrome
Congenital glaucoma	Arachnodactyly
Congenital miosis	Craniosynostosis
Ectopia lentis	Down's syndrome
Ectopia lentis et pupillae	Dwarfism
Iridodonesis	Marfan's syndrome
Iris stromal hypoplasia	Osteogenesis imperfecta
Iris transillumination defects	
Krukenberg's spindle	
Myopia (mild to severe)	
Open-angle glaucoma	
Phacodonesis	
Pigmentation of trabecular meshwork	
Posterior embryotoxon	
Prominent iris processes	
Rieger's anomaly	

Megalocornea Megalocornea, as the name implies, refers to an enlarged cornea defined as having a horizontal diameter greater than or equal to 13 mm. It is a nonprogressive condition that is usually bilateral and symmetric. Because of its predominant transmission as an X-linked recessive trait, 90% of cases are found in males. Autosomal dominant, autosomal recessive, and sporadic cases have also been reported.

Clinical characteristics of megalocornea include an enlarged but clear cornea of normal thickness (Fig. 2-1). At times the cornea may have greater than normal steepness, but keratometry usually reveals that the cornea is of normal curvature. Histologically it is normal in all respects and has normal endothelial cell density. Although megalocornea is frequently an isolated condition, many ocular and systemic associations have been documented (Box 2-1). A steeper cornea usually results in a myopic eye and with the rule astigmatism. Many of the associated ocular findings involving the lens, iris, and anterior chamber angle are thought to occur secondarily to the coexisting anatomic changes of an enlarged anterior segment and ciliary ring, sometimes referred to as a separate condition known as anterior megalophthalmos. The widened ciliary ring presumably causes zonular stretching that results in iridodonesis, phacodonesis, and ectopia lentis (which can make routine cataract extraction challenging!) (Fig. 2-2). The iris also undergoes anatomic stress manifested as stromal hypoplasia and transillumination defects and the subsequent increased pigmentation of trabecular meshwork and formation of Krukenberg's spindles. These changes, coupled with an abnormal angle containing excess mesenchymal tissue and prominent iris processes, predispose the eye to glaucoma.

The differential diagnosis is limited mainly to buphthalmos from congenital glaucoma (Table 2-3). The diagnosis of congenital glaucoma can be easily made if a patient has the classic triad of symptoms (epiphora, photophobia, and blepharospasm) and the obvious signs of elevated intraocular pressure, corneal edema, Haab's striae, and optic disc changes. However, in patients with milder forms of congenital glaucoma, these findings may not be evident. Although difficult, the differentiation may be made by finding a sharply demarcated limbal region, a distinguishing feature of megalocornea not seen in eyes with congenital glaucoma. It may help to measure ocular axial length with A-scan ultrasonography to rule out buphthalmos, a condition in which the entire globe and the cornea are enlarged. Careful examination and use of ancillary studies may help in the crucial distinction between megalocornea and congenital glaucoma, a condition in which early diagnosis and surgical intervention can help prevent severe visual loss.

No definitive treatment other than the correction of significant refractive error is indicated if megalocornea is an isolated anomaly. However, ophthalmologic examination should be performed regularly to detect and monitor the associated findings. Factors that potentially threaten vision (i.e., cataract and glaucoma) should be approached with extreme caution, as medical and laser treatments may be ineffective, and surgery is often complicated.

Microcornea Microcornea is defined as a cornea whose horizontal diameter measures 10 mm or less in a globe of otherwise normal size (Fig. 2-3). Terms that are not to be confused with microcornea are *anterior microphthalmos* (if the entire anterior segment is small), *microphthalmos* (if the entire eye is small and disorganized), and *nanophthalmos* (if the entire eye is small but otherwise normal). Microcornea is nonprogressive and may be unilateral or bilateral. There is no sex predilection, and most cases are inherited in an autosomal dominant or a recessive fashion with very rare sporadic cases.

The small cornea is clear and is of normal thickness, but it is usually flatter than the normal cornea. Histologic specimens have shown the microcornea to be normal in all other respects. Unlike megalocornea, microcornea rarely is an isolated condition; many ocular and systemic anomalies may be associated with it (Box 2-2). The flatter cornea usually gives rise to hyperopia, but any refractive error can exist depending on the axial length of the eye. It is thought that the anatomic changes produced by a smaller cornea contribute to the development of glaucoma, whether narrow or closed-angle glaucoma resulting from a shallow and crowded anterior chamber or

Table 2-3 Differentiating features of megalocornea and congenital glaucoma

Feature	Megalocornea	Congenital glaucoma
Inheritance	X-linked recessive	Sporadic
Time of appearance	Congenital	First year of life
Laterality	Bilateral	Unilateral or bilateral
Natural history	Nonprogressive	Progressive
Symptoms	None or decreased vision	Epiphora, photophobia, blepharospasm
Corneal features	Enlarged diameter but otherwise normal	Diffuse edema, Haab's striae
Anterior segment features	Enlarged anterior segment and ciliary ring (anterior megalophthalmos)	Elevated intraocular pressure, excess mesenchymal tissue on gonioscopy
Other features	Normal globe size	Enlarged globe (buphthalmos), optic disc changes

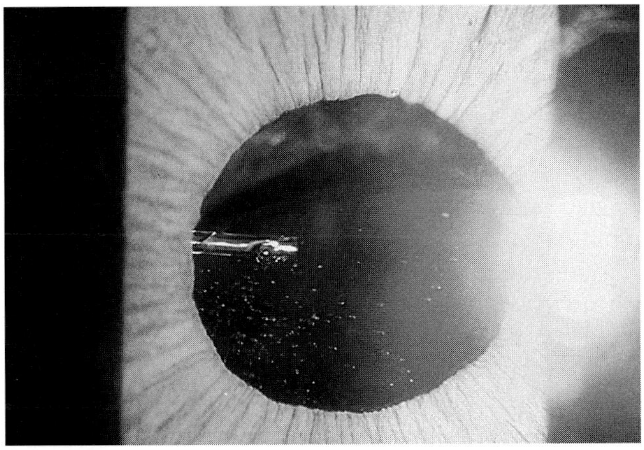

Fig. 2-2 Megalocornea. The widened ciliary ring in megalocornea can cause instability of the natural crystalline lens or of an intraocular implant. The posterior chamber intraocular lens implant in this eye has subluxated inferiorly.

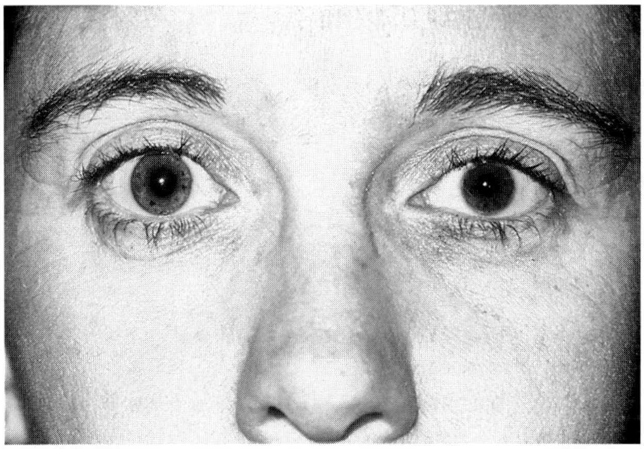

Fig. 2-3 Microcornea. In this patient with unilateral microcornea, the left cornea measures 10 mm. (Courtesy of R. Doyle Stulting, M.D., Ph.D.)

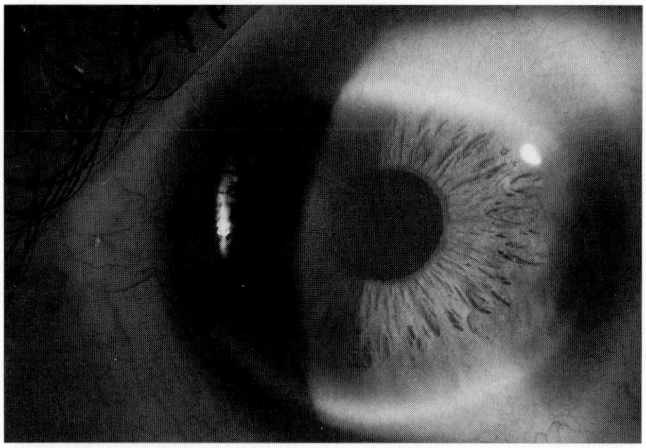

Fig. 2-4 Cornea plana (sclerocornea). Cornea plana refers to the corneal curvature, whereas sclerocornea refers to the corneal anatomy. Cornea plana can be considered a mild form of sclerocornea. In this eye, peripheral scleralization of the cornea is apparent.

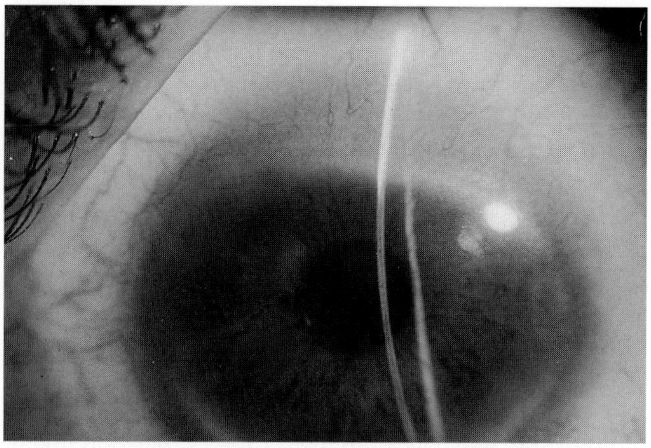

Fig. 2-5 Cornea plana (sclerocornea). The slit beam of the eye seen in Fig. 2-4 demonstrates no change in curvature from the cornea to the sclera, pathognomonic of cornea plana.

Box 2-2 Major Ocular and Systemic Associations of Microcornea

OCULAR	SYSTEMIC
Aniridia	Ehlers-Danlos syndrome
Axenfeld's syndrome	Hallermann-Streiff syndrome
Closed-angle glaucoma	Rubella
Congenital cataract	Trisomy 9, 10, 13-15, 17, 18, 21
Corectopia	Turner's syndrome
Corneal leukoma	Waardenburg's syndrome
Cornea plana	Weill-Marchesani syndrome
Hyperopia	
Infantile glaucoma	
Microphakia	
Narrow-angle glaucoma	
Nystagmus	
Open-angle glaucoma	
Persistent pupillary membrane	
Retinopathy of prematurity	
Rieger's anomaly	
Small orbit	
Uveal coloboma	

open-angle glaucoma caused by angle remnants left during goniodysgenesis.

The differential diagnosis includes sclerocornea and the conditions listed above that may involve a disorganized eye. In addition to careful clinical slit-lamp examination, use of both A- and B-scan ultrasonography and ultrasound biomicroscopy may help differentiate microcornea from these other conditions. When it is an isolated finding, the visual prognosis is excellent, especially with the help of spectacles.

Anomalies of Corneal Shape

Cornea plana (sclerocornea) In cornea plana, the cornea is flat and its curvature is less than 43 D. Although curvature in this condition commonly ranges from 30 to 35 D, patients have been reported to have keratometry readings as low as 20 D. Corneal curvatures that are the same as, or even flatter, than those of the sclera are a pathognomonic finding (Figs. 2-4 and 2-5). The observation that all cases of cornea plana included some degree of peripheral scleralization led to the argument that cornea plana and sclerocornea were the same entity. The similarities in clinical and histopathologic characteristics, inheritance pattern, and ocular and systemic associations between these entities have strengthened this argument. However, some physicians distinguish between the two conditions to emphasize the anomalous flatness of cornea plana versus the anomalous opacification of sclerocornea. This chapter considers cornea plana and sclerocornea as interchangeable, descriptive terms for mild and severe forms of the same condition; it is discussed in more detail later in this chapter.

Congenital anterior staphyloma and keratectasia Congenital anterior staphyloma is defined as an ectatic condition in which an opaque cornea lined posteriorly with uveal tissue protrudes through the palpebral fissure beyond the plane of the normal eyelids (Fig. 2-6). Congenital anterior staphyloma is thought to result from intrauterine keratitis or from some secondary failure in mesenchymal migration of neural crest cells to the developing cornea. The cornea is vulnerable to perforation in

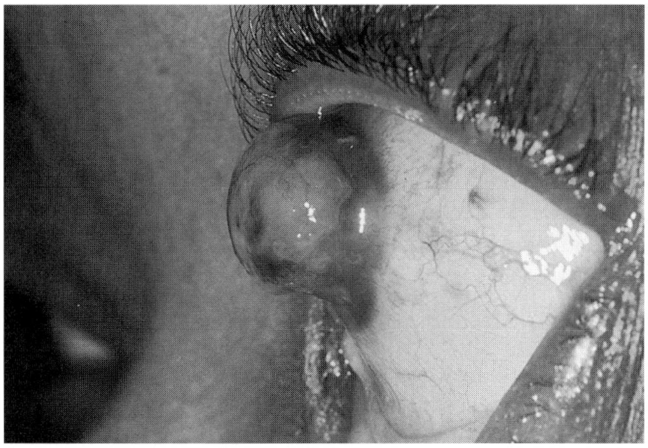

Fig. 2-6 Congenital anterior staphyloma. This severely ectatic cornea protrudes through the palpebral fissure. It is due most commonly to an intrauterine keratitis.

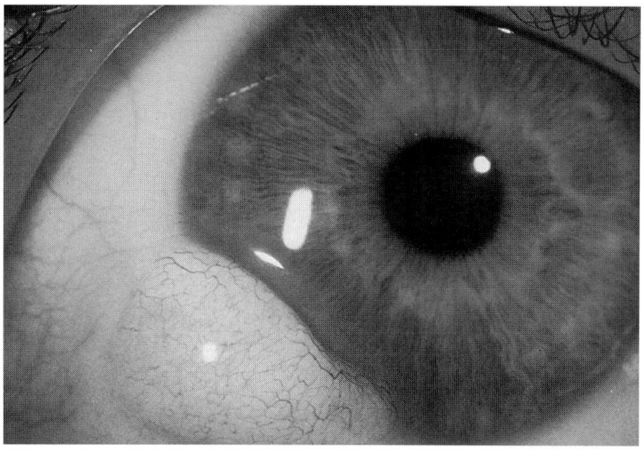

Fig. 2-8 Dermoid. This moderately large dermoid is located inferotemporally. (See color plate.)

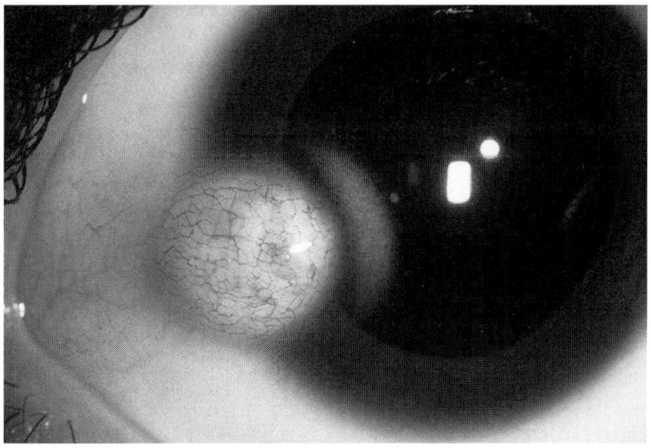

Fig. 2-7 Dermoid. This solid, white, elevated round mass is a classic example of a dermoid. There is a small amount of lipid deposition central to the lesion. Dermoids typically occur inferotemporally.

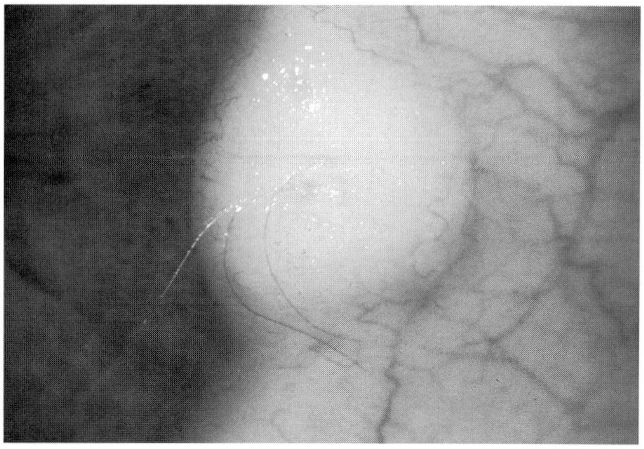

Fig. 2-9 Dermoid. Several hairs protrude from this dermoid.

utero and undergoes dermoid transformation to resemble the stratified squamous epithelium of skin; however, unlike cryptophthalmos, the metaplastic change is limited to the cornea and does not involve the conjunctiva or eyelids. Most reported cases are unilateral and show variable corneal thinning and scarring along with a deep, disorganized anterior segment. The lens may even adhere to the protuberant cornea, mimicking a feature of Peters' anomaly. Characteristic histopathologic findings include an absent Descemet's membrane and endothelium and a posterior uveal lining that represents the remaining pigmented epithelium of an atrophic iris. The visual prognosis is poor because of the severe damage incurred by the anterior segment structures. Although a few patients with milder cases have undergone penetrating keratoplasty of varying degrees of success, enucleation remains the recommended surgical procedure for the blind, glaucomatous, often painful eye.

Keratectasia refers to the same condition of congenital anterior staphyloma without the posterior uveal lining. It is otherwise identical to congenital anterior staphyloma and has the same clinical characteristics and proposed embryologic origins.

Mass Lesions of the Cornea

Dermoid Dermoids are a type of choristoma (normal embryonic tissue in an abnormal location) that commonly affects the cornea. They appear as solid, white, round, elevated mass lesions and are usually found at the inferotemporal limbus (though they may occur anywhere on the globe or in the orbit) (Figs. 2-7 and 2-8). Dermoids are composed of elements not normally found in the cornea/conjunctiva (e.g., sebaceous glands, hair follicles, fat cells) that form fleshy, fibrous tissue (Fig. 2-9). When the fat component of a dermoid predominates, the lesion yellows and is termed a dermolipoma or lipodermoid (Fig. 2-10). Dermolipomas tend to develop superotemporally and may extend posteriorly into the orbit. Other lesions that may look and present similarly include prolapsed orbital fat, prolapsed lacrimal gland, and lymphoma. Careful clinical examination is important in distinguishing these lesions from dermoids and dermolipomas.

Many dermoids are small and cause few, if any, visual or irritative symptoms, but some may cause decreased vision from induced astigmatism or occlusion of visual axis and ocular foreign body sensation. They are, however, usually conspicuous, and patients or parents complain of their cosmetic appearance. They can grow but are considered benign lesions with no potential for malignancy. Although frequently isolated, dermoids may signify associated systemic syndromes such as Goldenhar's syndrome (characterized by upper eyelid colobomas, aural fistulas, preauricular appendages [Fig. 2-11], and vertebral anomalies) and Treacher Collins syndrome (a cranial facial cleft syndrome with lower eyelid colobomas, ear anomalies, antimongoloid slant, microstomia, and malar/mandibular hypoplasia). Therefore, facial and systemic examination should always accompany ocular evaluation of patients with dermoids.

Treatment for symptomatic lesions includes corrective lenses and topical lubrication. When conservative therapy fails, surgical excision may be considered. The indications for surgical excision include decreased vision, prevention of amblyopia, persistent irritation, and cosmesis. Depending on the extent and location of these lesions, various approaches must be considered. Most dermoids involve only the superficial cornea/sclera (usu-

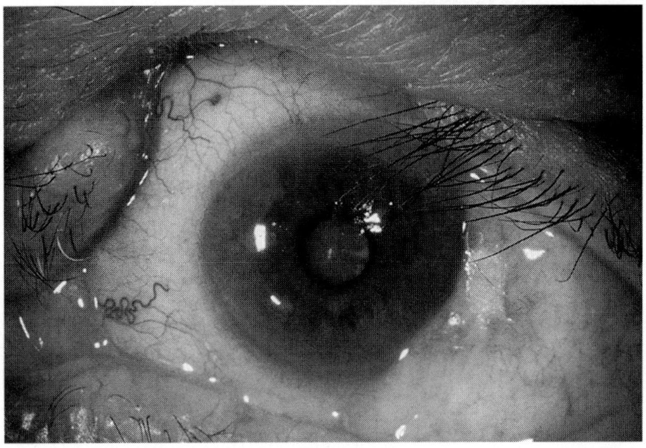

Fig. 2-10 Lipodermoid. This lipodermoid is larger than most dermoids, and it extends superotemporally and posteriorly. Note the upper eyelid coloboma.

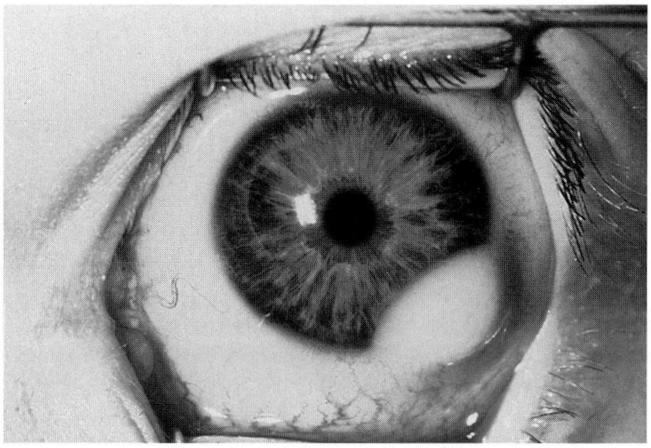

Fig. 2-12 Dermoid. A large inferotemporal dermoid before excision. (Courtesy of R. Doyle Stulting, M.D., Ph.D.)

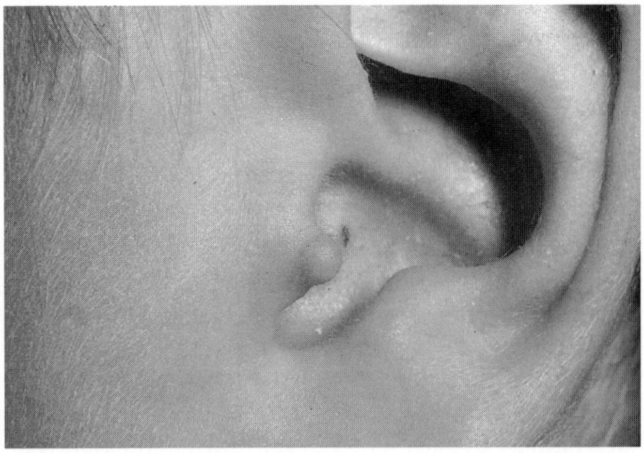

Fig. 2-11 Goldenhar's syndrome. This is a typical preauricular appendage in a patient with a dermoid, an eyelid coloboma, and Goldenhar's syndrome.

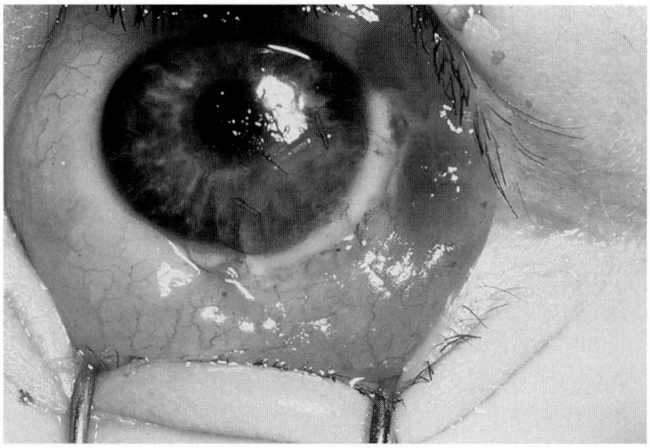

Fig. 2-13 Dermoid. After excision of the dermoid seen in Fig. 2-12. A lamellar corneal graft was performed because of the depth of the pathology. (Courtesy of R. Doyle Stulting, M.D., Ph.D.)

ally the outer third) and require simple lamellar dissection. However, some dermoids can extend more deeply, even into the anterior chamber, necessitating donor corneoscleral tissue for patch grafting (Figs. 2-12 and 2-13). Because it can be difficult to determine the depth of these lesions owing to the opacity of dermoids, donor corneoscleral tissue should be kept available during surgery. Ultrasound biomicroscopy may be helpful before or during surgery to determine the depth of involvement (Fig. 2-14). Central lesions can be treated with penetrating keratoplasty. Generally, dermolipomas extending deeply into the orbit either are observed or are debulked anteriorly because complete excision is difficult and is associated with a high risk for complications.

DEVELOPMENTAL ANOMALIES OF THE ANTERIOR SEGMENT

The terminology describing the various developmental anomalies of the anterior segment has been confusing. Previous terms such as *anterior cleavage syndrome* and *mesodermal dysgenesis syndrome* were used to encompass a spectrum of related disorders thought to arise from an abnormal differentiation of mesodermal tissue. Recent studies have pointed instead to developmental defects in the cranial ectodermal neural crest cells as the unifying origin of these various disorders. The more contemporary terms *anterior segment dysgeneses* and *neurocrestopathies* are used to refer collectively to the group of anomalies consisting of posterior embryotoxon, Axenfeld's anomaly/syndrome, Rieger's anomaly/syndrome, Peters' anomaly types 1 and 2, sclerocornea, and posterior keratoconus.

Peripheral Anomalies

Posterior embryotoxon Posterior embryotoxon refers to a thickened Schwalbe's line that becomes visible on external slit-lamp examination because of its anterior displacement. Schwalbe's line represents the border between Descemet's membrane and the trabecular meshwork and is normally visible on gonioscopy. However, when it becomes prominent and anteriorly displaced, it is visible without gonioscopy as an irregular white ridge along the corneal periphery (notably in the nasal and temporal quadrants but at times extending 360°) (Fig. 2-15).

Posterior embryotoxon can present with no associated ocular abnormalities in approximately 10% of normal eyes. As an isolated condition, it is not associated with an abnormal anterior chamber angle and does not predispose the patient to glaucoma. It is most closely associated with the Axenfeld and Rieger syndromes described below, but it can accompany other anomalies including megalocornea and aniridia. Posterior embryotoxon is thought to be an anatomic variant of the normal Schwalbe's line and is transmitted as an autosomal dominant trait.

Axenfeld's anomaly/syndrome Axenfeld's anomaly describes the finding of posterior embryotoxon coupled with peripheral iris processes extending to or beyond the prominent Schwalbe's line (Fig. 2-16). These iris extensions are actually iridocorneal adhesions that can vary from thin and wispy to broad and ropy. They may involve only parts of the peripheral angle. When they are broad, they are similar to peripheral anterior synechiae and can obstruct visualization of the anterior chamber angle.

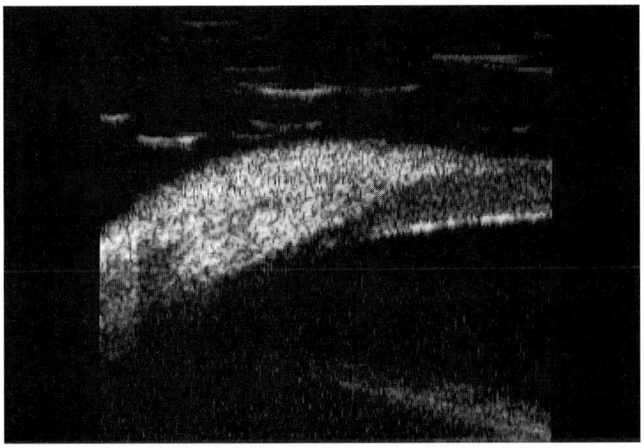

Fig. 2-14 Dermoid. Through ultrasound biomicroscopy, this dermoid was found to reach approximately 90% corneal depth. Whenever excision is to be performed, a corneal graft may be required.

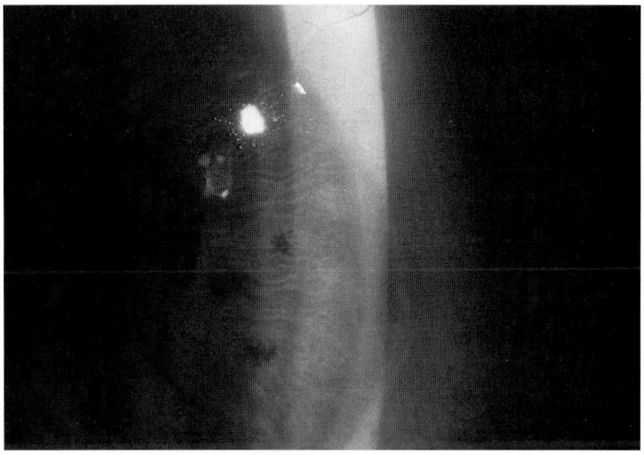

Fig. 2-15 Posterior embryotoxon. Schwalbe's line is seen to be anteriorly displaced in this asymptomatic patient.

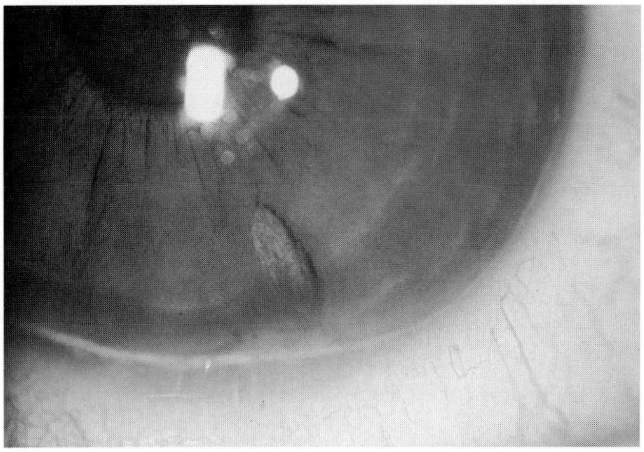

Fig. 2-16 Axenfeld's anomaly. An anteriorly displaced Schwalbe's ring with adherent iris processes is seen.

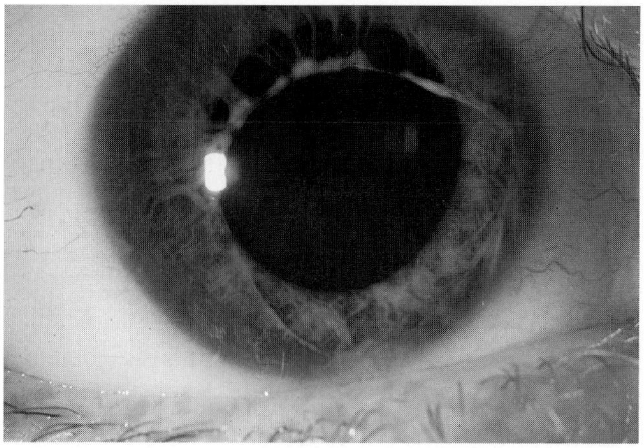

Fig. 2-17 Rieger's anomaly. A small area of prominent Schwalbe's ring with iris processes is seen inferiorly. The most prominent finding is iris stromal atrophy and hypoplasia with polycoria.

The term *Axenfeld's anomaly* simply refers to the structural findings, whereas Axenfeld's syndrome refers to Axenfeld's anomaly when it is accompanied by glaucoma. Abnormal anatomic features are thought to affect the normal function of the angle and to predispose the patient to glaucoma. Glaucoma develops in approximately 50% of patients with Axenfeld's anomaly and must be followed up closely. Some extraocular findings that may accompany Axenfeld's anomaly and syndrome include hypertelorism and hypoplastic shoulder.

Rieger's anomaly/syndrome Rieger's anomaly completes the triad of peripheral angle anomalies and is used when the findings of Axenfeld's anomaly are seen with iris stromal atrophy and hypoplasia (Fig. 2-17). The iris changes of Rieger's anomaly can vary in severity from mild areas of thinning to marked atrophy with subsequent corectopia, polycoria, and ectropion uveae. The angle findings and lack of corneal abnormalities help differentiate this condition from the similar iris appearance seen with the various iridocorneal endothelial syndromes. Glaucoma is associated with Rieger's anomaly in more than 50% of patients. Unlike Axenfeld's syndrome, the term Rieger's syndrome is reserved for patients with associated dental, facial, cranial, and skeletal abnormalities (e.g., microdontia, maxillary hypoplasia, telecanthus, cerebellar hypoplasia, and limb or spinal malformations).

These three conditions represent a continuum of developmental anomalies primarily involving the peripheral anterior segment. Although different hypotheses have been proposed to provide an embryologic explanation, these anomalies probably result from developmental errors occurring sometime during the first to fourth gestational months when the anterior chamber angle is formed. Nevertheless, they include closely related disorders that can be organized according to the extent of maldevelopment. The traditional classification system is useful for the purposes of organization, recollection, and instruction (Box 2-3). All three conditions usually present bilaterally and are transmitted in an autosomal dominant mode with high penetrance.

Box 2-3 Developmental Anomalies of the Peripheral Anterior Segment

- Posterior embryotoxon
  - Centrally displaced and thickened Schwalbe's line
- Axenfeld's anomaly
  - Posterior embryotoxon
  - Iris strands extending to posterior embryotoxon
- Axenfeld's syndrome
  - Posterior embryotoxon
  - Iris strands extending to posterior embryotoxon
  - Glaucoma
- Rieger's anomaly
  - Axenfeld's anomaly
  - Iris atrophy/hypoplasia
- Rieger's syndrome
  - Axenfeld's anomaly
  - Iris atrophy/hypoplasia
  - Extraocular dental, facial, cranial, skeletal abnormalities

Because of the common associations with glaucoma, gonioscopic examination should be performed whenever posterior embryotoxon is seen to rule out the presence of Axenfeld's and Rieger's anomaly and syndrome. When glaucoma is suspected or diagnosed, close monitoring of intraocular pressure, optic disc appearance, and visual field examinations are mandatory. Treatment regimens vary according to the age at which glaucoma appears. Adult patients should receive the same stepwise approach to treatment used for those with open-angle glaucoma. Congenital/infantile glaucoma is more

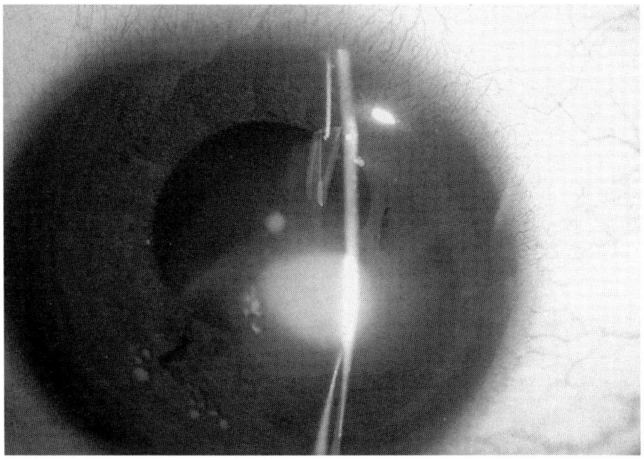

Fig. 2-18 Peters' anomaly. A relatively small central corneal leukoma is seen in this patient with bilateral Peters' anomaly. Note the iris adhesions to the posterior cornea in the area of the scar. (See color plate.)

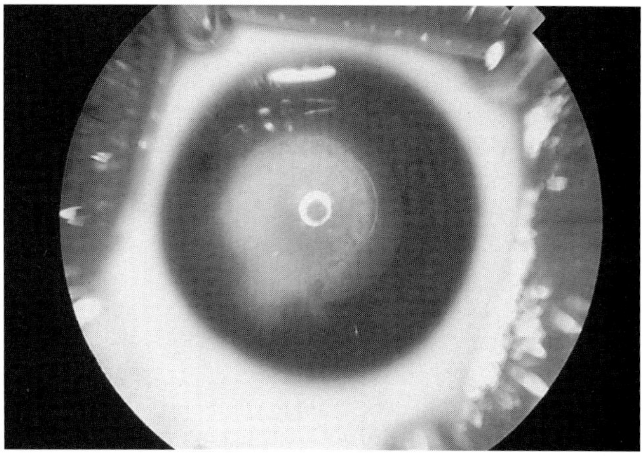

Fig. 2-19 Peters' anomaly. After pupil dilation and before penetrating keratoplasty, a large area of corneal opacity is present in this child with Peters' anomaly.

complex. Trabeculotomy and goniotomy, the conventional surgical procedures, are sometimes contraindicated if there are large, broad iridocorneal adhesions because of the potential for angle damage from trauma and bleeding. Although long-term experience is lacking, the prognosis for filtering surgery in these patients has improved with advances in antimetabolite therapy and seton placement. Cyclodestructive procedures remain an option but are usually reserved for refractory cases because of the associated risks for cataract formation, inflammation, and phthisis.

Central Anomalies

Peters' anomaly Peters' anomaly is a collection of developmental abnormalities involving the central anterior segment. Corneal findings include a central corneal leukoma (scar) with a centrally absent or defective posterior stroma, Descemet's membrane, and endothelium. Associated iris features include strands of iris tissue that extend from the iris collarette and sometimes attach to the central corneal leukoma (Figs. 2-18, 2-19, and 2-20). Additional subclassification of Peters' anomaly denotes type 1 as having no lens involvement and type 2 as having lens involvement. Lens involvement can refer to an associated cataract, an abnormal lens position, or lenticular adherence to the abnormal posterior cornea. Ocular and systemic associations of Peters' anomaly tend to be severe in Peters' anomaly type 2 (the term *Peters' plus syndrome* has been used to signify the presence of these severe anomalies) (Box 2-4). Glaucoma is thought to be a common occurrence in patients with Peters' anomaly; the incidence is as high as 50% to 70%.

The embryologic explanation for this anomaly is thought to lie in the arrest or the incomplete migration of cranial neural crest cells sometime between the tenth

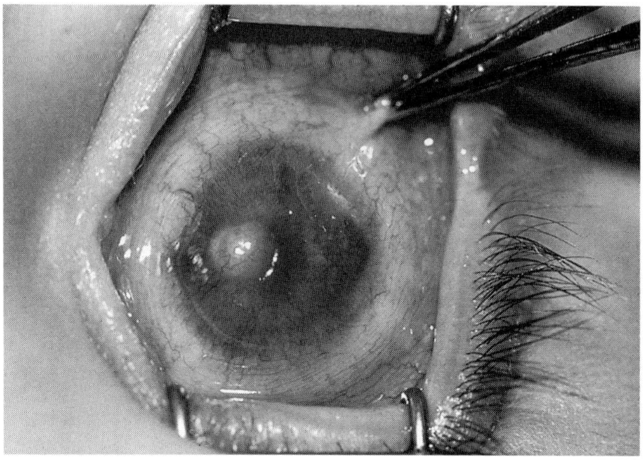

Fig. 2-20 Peters' anomaly. A dense central scar is surrounded by diffuse corneal haze and moderate neovascularization in this child with Peters' anomaly. (Courtesy of R. Doyle Stulting, M.D., Ph.D.)

Box 2-4 Major Ocular and Systemic Associations of Peters' Anomaly

OCULAR	SYSTEMIC
Glaucoma	Cleft palate
Microcornea	Craniofacial dysplasia
Aniridia	Congenital heart defects
Sclerocornea	Skeletal anomalies
Microphthalmia	Genitourinary disorders
Colobomas	Trisomy 13 to 15
	Mosaic trisomy 9
	Partial deletion of 11q

and the sixteenth gestational week (after the full differentiation of the anterior segment and before the complete formation of Descemet's membrane). Peters' anomaly is asymmetrically bilateral with sporadic inheritance (though autosomal dominant and recessive transmission has been reported). Other conditions that are similar to Peters' anomaly and that could represent forms of it include von Hippel's posterior corneal ulcer and posterior keratoconus. These are differentiated from Peters' anomaly by the presence of altered posterior stroma, Descemet's membrane, and endothelium (they are absent in Peters' anomaly).

The diagnosis of Peters' anomaly is essentially a clinical one, but it can be confused with sclerocornea and posterior keratoconus. When visualization of the anterior segment is precluded from corneal scarring, ultrasound biomicroscopy can be a helpful diagnostic tool (Figs. 2-21 and 2-22). Treatment of Peters' anomaly centers around preventing amblyopia (from corneal leukomas and cataracts) and controlling glaucoma. Patients with the type 2 variant have poorer prognoses because of the increased severity of corneal scarring and glaucoma and the need for cataract extraction at the time of corneal transplantation. The success of penetrating keratoplasty has improved with advances in surgical technique and immunosuppressive therapy. Glaucoma management can be difficult and frustrating and should be coordinated with a glaucoma specialist.

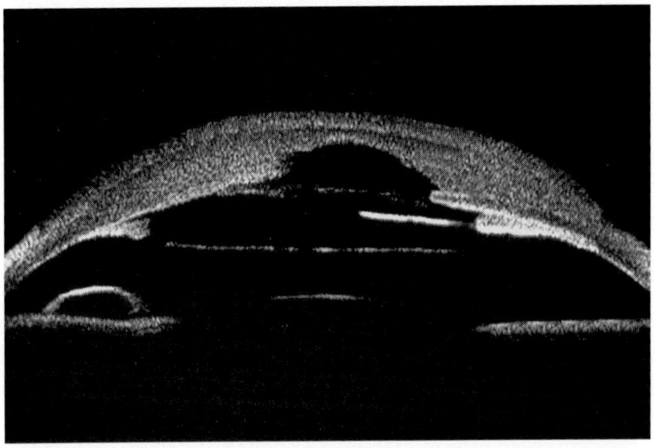

Fig. 2-21 Peters' anomaly. A composite ultrasound biomicroscopy photograph of an eye with Peters' anomaly reveals significant central posterior stromal loss. (Courtesy of Elizabeth L. Affel, M.S.)

Sclerocornea Sclerocornea is a nonprogressive condition that is usually bilateral (and asymmetric) rather than unilateral. Most cases are sporadic; occasionally familial transmission occurs. Pedigrees have demonstrated autosomal dominant and recessive patterns of inheritance. Patients with the autosomal recessive form have a more severe manifestation of total sclerocornea, and those with the autosomal dominant type have a more benign form of peripheral sclerocornea. There is no sex predilection.

Scleralization occurs in varying degrees and progresses from the periphery toward the center. Therefore, only the peripheral cornea (Fig. 2-23) or the entire cornea (Fig. 2-24) is involved. When scleralization is complete (total sclerocornea), the central cornea tends to be somewhat less opaque than the peripheral cornea. The affected cornea appears opaque and vascularized and has no definable limbus. It is as if the sclera and the conjunctiva have extended into the cornea. Histopathologic studies of sclerocornea have revealed morphologic features resembling scleral tissue. The stroma consists of irregularly arranged collagen fibrils of variable and increased diameter present anteriorly and of smaller diameter collagen fibrils present posteriorly (the reverse order is typical for the normal cornea). Because these fibrils lack precise lamellar organization and have accompany-

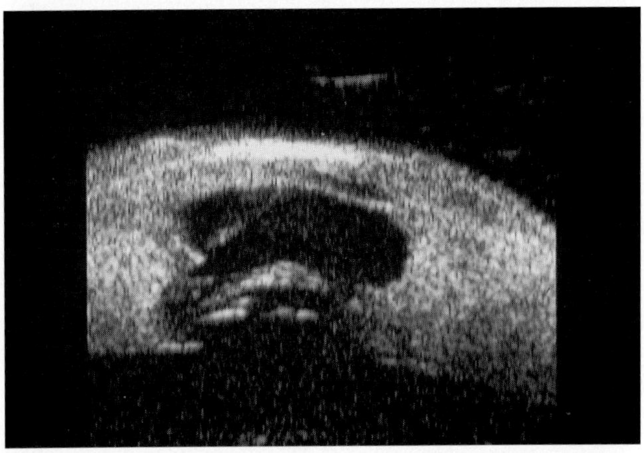

Fig. 2-22 Peters' anomaly. Ultrasound biomicroscopy demonstrates a dense corneal opacity in the anterior cornea centrally. In addition there are significant iridocorneal adhesions and probable anterior lens opacity.

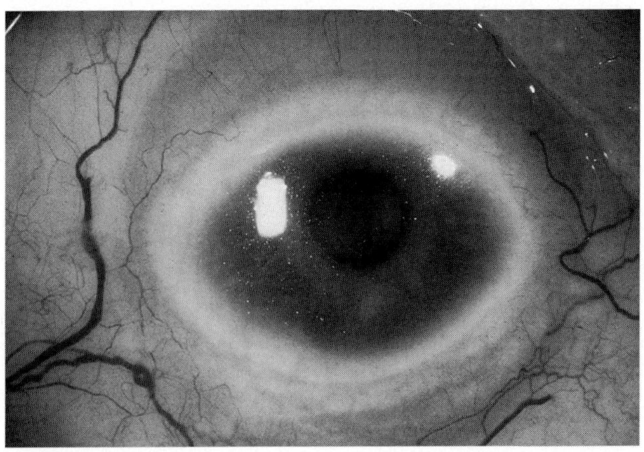

Fig. 2-23 Peripheral sclerocornea. Significant scleralization of the peripheral cornea is evident, whereas the central cornea is spared.

ing blood vessels, optical transparency is lost. When abnormal, Descemet's membrane is generally thin, irregular, and attenuated with focal collagenous deposits. Usually, the anterior chamber angle is difficult to visualize through the opaque cornea, and is frequently abnormal with findings such as peripheral anterior synechiae often leading to the development of glaucoma. Many ocular and systemic conditions are associated with sclerocornea (Box 2-5).

Besides neutralizing any refractive error, treatment is limited to penetrating keratoplasty for cases involving significant central corneal opacification. Because visualization and examination of the anterior segment is often difficult, diagnostic tools such as ultrasound biomicroscopy may be helpful in providing information about associated anterior segment abnormalities and in planning surgery. The visual prognosis after surgery is guarded because of complications related to glaucoma, the frequent association with other severe ocular abnormalities, and the increased risk for allograft rejection. New advances in immunosuppressive therapy (e.g., topical and systemic cyclosporine) have improved the success rates of penetrating keratoplasty for this condition (Figs. 2-25 and 2-26).

Posterior keratoconus Posterior keratoconus is considered a rare developmental condition that bears no relationship to anterior keratoconus and is typically classified as one of the anterior segment dysgeneses.

Box 2-5 Major Ocular and Systemic Associations of Sclerocornea (Cornea Plana)

OCULAR	SYSTEMIC
Aniridia	Cerebellar anomalies
Arcus juvenilis	Cranial dystrophies
Blue sclera	Ear deformities
Cataract	Hallermann-Streiff syndrome
Closed-angle glaucoma	Hurler's syndrome
Ectopia lentis	Maroteaux-Lamy syndrome
Hyperopia	Osteogenesis imperfecta
Microcornea	Polydacyly
Microphthalmos	Trisomy 13, 18
Narrow-angle glaucoma	Unbalanced translocation (17p, 10q)
Open-angle glaucoma	
Peripheral anterior synechiae	
Retinal aplasia	
Retinal coloboma	
Uveal coloboma	

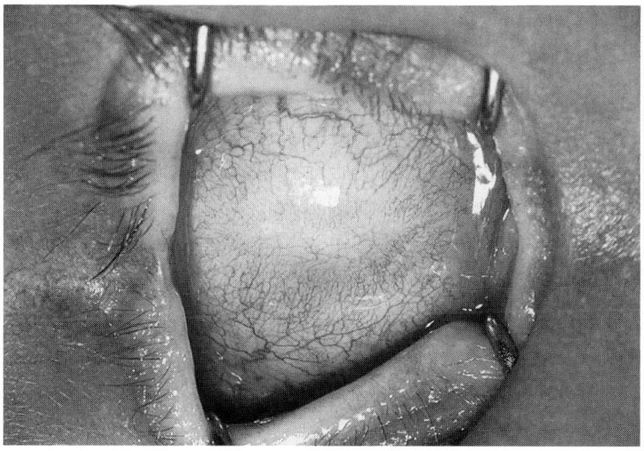

Fig. 2-24 Central sclerocornea. Complete opacification of the cornea is evident in this newborn with sclerocornea. (See color plate.)

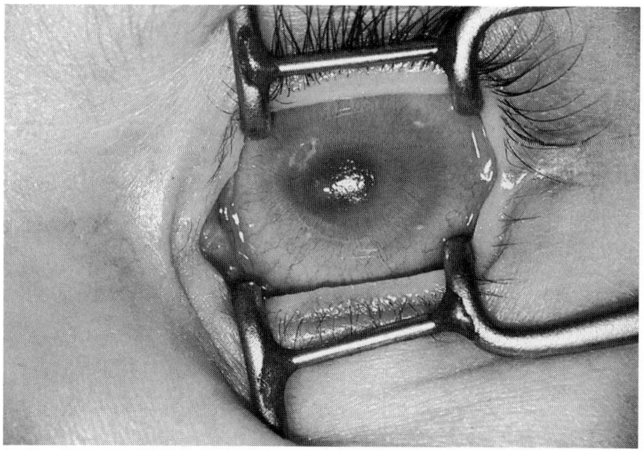

Fig. 2-25 Sclerocornea. This infant with severe bilateral sclerocornea underwent penetrating keratoplasty.

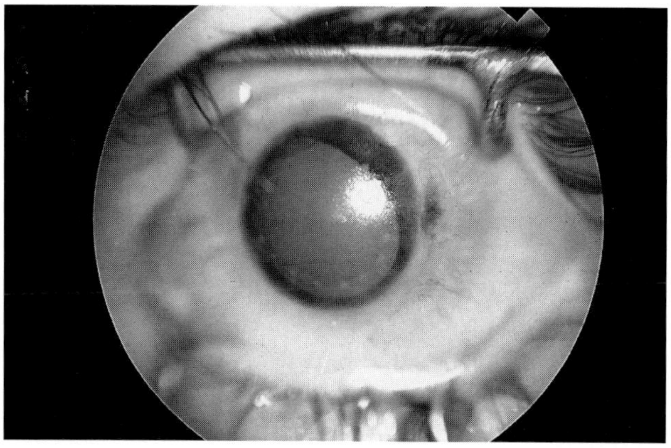

Fig. 2-26 Sclerocornea. A clear graft can be seen after penetrating keratoplasty in the eye seen in Fig. 2-25. Although the prognosis is poor for corneal transplantation in patients with sclerocornea, newer immunosuppressive agents have improved the success rate.

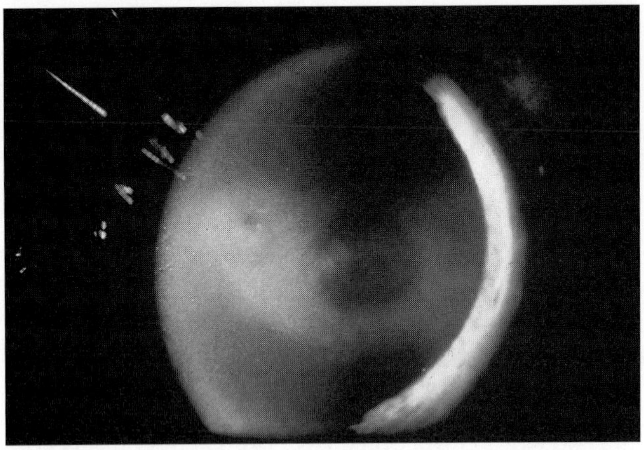

Fig. 2-27 Posterior keratoconus. Note the area of central corneal clarity surrounded by mild haze.

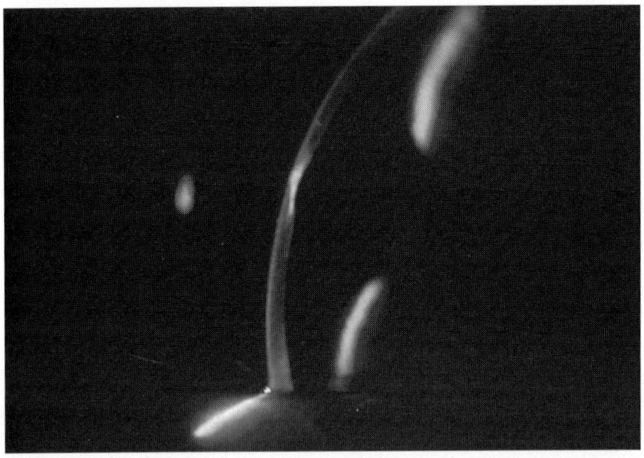

Fig. 2-28 Posterior keratoconus. The slit beam reveals an area of localized central posterior corneal thinning with minimal change in the anterior corneal curvature.

The condition is usually unilateral, nonprogressive, and noninflammatory and is associated with good visual acuity. It may be manifested in a generalized or circumscribed form.

Generalized posterior keratoconus exists when the entire posterior corneal surface has an increased curvature and a normal anterior corneal surface. The more common, though still rare, circumscribed form of posterior keratoconus is characterized by a localized, craterlike lesion in the central posterior cornea (Figs. 2-27 and 2-28). Minimal corneal stromal haze with variable corneal thinning frequently overlies the posterior corneal defect, which is commonly surrounded by endothelial pigment and corneal guttae. This condition may accompany a host of ocular and systemic anomalies (Box 2-6). Although most cases are sporadic, a few familial cases have been cited. It is also thought to represent a mild variant of Peters' anomaly, thereby implying intrauterine inflammation or some other anterior segment dysgenesis as a causative factor. The histopathologic and ultrastructural characteristics of posterior keratoconus include an existent but altered Descemet's membrane and endothelium in the area of the defect. Posterior keratoconus rarely affects visual acuity but may cause a myopic astigmatism that should be corrected with spectacles or contact lenses to prevent amblyopia.

Box 2-6 Major Ocular and Systemic Associations of Circumscribed Posterior Keratoconus

OCULAR	SYSTEMIC
Aniridia	Brachydactyly
Anterior lenticonus	Broad, flat nasal bridge
Anterior polar cataract	Bull/webbed neck
Anterior segment dysgenesis	Cleft lip/palate
Choroidal/retinal sclerosis	Genitourinary anomalies
Ectopia lentis	Growth retardation
Ectropion uveae	Hypertelorism
Glaucoma	Mental retardation
Iris atrophy	
Optic nerve hypoplasia	
Posterior polymorphous dystrophy with iris adhesions	
Ptosis	
Retinal coloboma	
Superior lateral canthus displacement	

Aniridia

Aniridia is a developmental anomaly with striking features involving the cornea and other anterior segment structures. The term *aniridia* does not correctly or adequately describe this condition for two reasons. First of all, despite the clinical appearance of a missing iris, even the most severe cases have been shown, on either gonioscopy or histopathologic analysis, to have some hypoplastic iris tissue. Second, the condition is not limited to the iris but can involve the entire eye (Box 2-7). The diagnosis is commonly made by the dramatic appearance of an absent iris or a large pupil at birth. Gonioscopy can help to visualize a peripheral stump of iris tissue that would normally be invisible by external slit-lamp examination.

Aniridia may be inherited as an autosomal dominant or recessive condition (approximately two thirds of cases) or it may occur sporadically (approximately one third of cases). Sporadic occurrences have important and common systemic associations with Wilms' tumor and the WAGR complex (see Box 2-7). Although other systemic associations develop in familial cases, Wilms' tumor does

Box 2-7 Manifestations of Aniridia

OCULAR	SYSTEMIC
Iris defects (hypoplasia, coloboma)	Wilms' tumor
Corneal pannus and vascularization	WAGR complex
Corneal scarring	Wilms' tumor
Glaucoma (open- and closed-angle)	Aniridia
Cataracts (polar, cortical, subcapsular, lamellar)	Genitourinary malformations
Lens anomalies (microphakia, subluxation)	Retardation
Foveal hypoplasia	
Optic nerve hypoplasia	
Pendular nystagmus	
Strabismus	
Amblyopia	

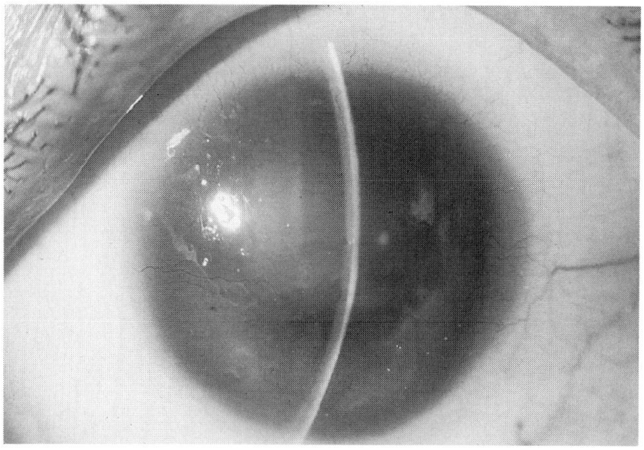

Fig. 2-29 Aniridia. Diffuse corneal haze and irregularity can be seen. There is a small remnant of peripheral iris visible from the 2 to 7 o'clock position.

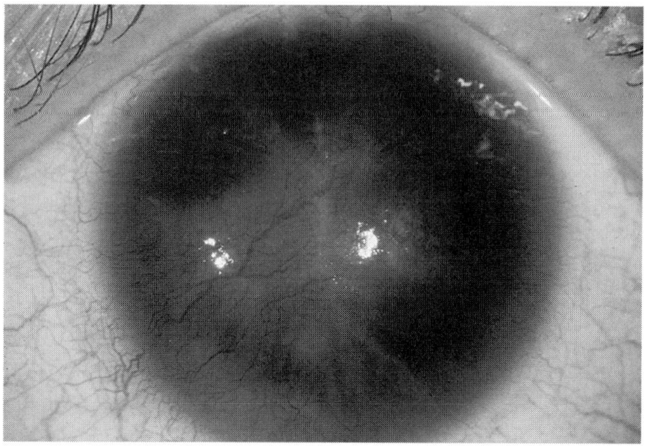

Fig. 2-30 Aniridia. Significant corneal opacity and neovascularization are evident. Diffusely irregular epithelium and mild central fluorescein staining can be seen. (See color plate.)

not. In patients with sporadic aniridia, it is crucial to perform a systemic workup with the help of a pediatrician and to implement regular physical examinations and imaging studies (e.g., renal ultrasonography, brain magnetic resonance imaging). In contrast to anterior segment dysgenesis, aniridia is thought to evolve primarily from a disorder in the neuroectoderm and not in the cranial neural crest cells.

Aniridia is a bilateral condition that can be seen with corneal and other anterior segment findings. Patients often complain of photophobia because of deficient anterior and posterior uveal tissue, but they may also have diminished vision and nystagmus. These patients also generally have symptoms and signs of severe ocular surface disease. Characteristic corneal findings include a superficial grayish haze or opacification with a peripheral pannus that advances centrally (Figs. 2-29 and 2-30). The epithelium is irregular and abnormal and can show whorled patterns with fluorescein staining. Although the pathology primarily involves the superficial corneal layers, secondary stromal scarring that causes significant visual loss may occur. Cataracts may also develop (Figs. 2-31 and 2-32). According to some reports, patients with aniridia have a limbal stem cell deficiency that produces these corneal abnormalities. Histopathologic studies have confirmed the abnormal presence of conjunctival goblet cells on the corneal surface, recurrent inflammatory pannus, and epitheliopathy.

Conservative therapy for the ocular surface disease associated with aniridia is aimed at maintaining a smooth, intact surface and at suppressing inflammation with topical lubricants and corticosteroids. Corneal transplanta-

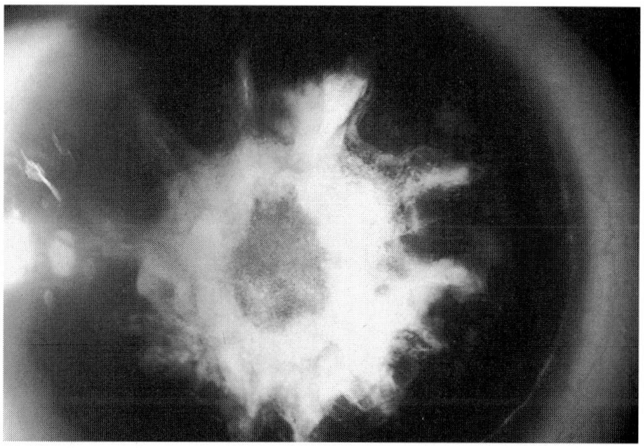

Fig. 2-31 Aniridia. A dense central cataract is apparent in this eye with aniridia. A small amount of peripheral iris can be seen from the 1 to 5 o'clock position. (Courtesy of R. Doyle Stulting, M.D., Ph.D.)

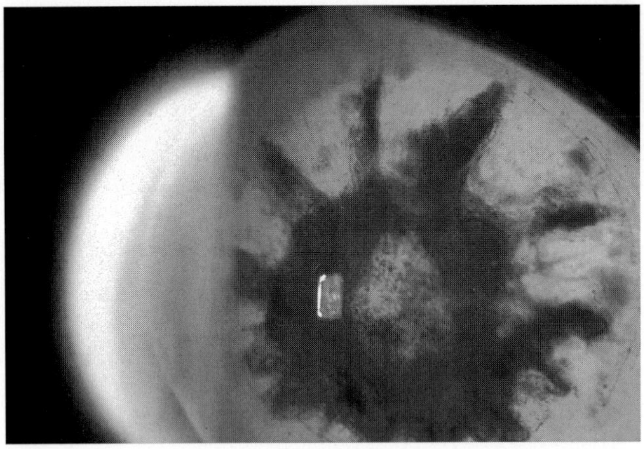

Fig. 2-32 Aniridia. Retroillumination off the iris highlights the cataract seen in Fig. 2-31. The edge of the crystalline lens can be seen from the 7 to 10 o'clock positions because of the lack of iris tissue. (Courtesy of R. Doyle Stulting, M.D., Ph.D.) (See color plate.)

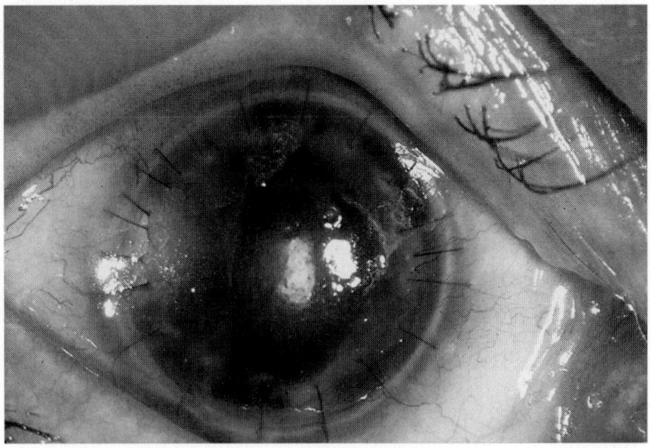

Fig. 2-33 Aniridia. After corneal transplantation in aniridia, problems with epithelial healing often develop because of abnormal limbal stem cells. Note the moderate epithelial irregularity.

tion is indicated when persistent epitheliopathy and inflammation lead to visually significant corneal scarring and vascularization. Unfortunately, the prognosis after corneal transplantation is guarded, with a 64% rate of graft rejection and a 27% rate of graft failure caused by recurrent surface disease and neovascularization (Figs. 2-33 and 2-34). Studies recommending the use of a limbal stem cell transplant procedure before penetrating keratoplasty have shown improved and encouraging results. When deciding whether to proceed with corneal transplantation, the surgeon should anticipate problems with epithelial healing, be prepared to treat the patient with aggressive lubrication and lateral tarsorrhaphy, and consider limbal cell transplantation before the procedure. According to a new classification system, proposed by Holland and colleagues, a conjunctival limbal allograft (from a living relative) or a keratolimbal allograft (from a cadaveric donor) should be considered the procedures of choice. Such procedures require prolonged systemic immunosuppression. Studies have shown no statistically significant difference between the two procedures regarding ocular surface stability and improved visual acuity.

Besides corneal opacification, cataract and glaucoma are the other anterior segment findings associated with aniridia that can compromise visual acuity. Cataracts may be observed at birth as anterior and posterior polar opacities and, in most patients, can progress within the first two decades of life to cortical, subcapsular, and lamellar opacities. Cataract surgery should be approached with caution because of accompanying zonular dehiscence and lens subluxation. Some surgeons have strongly discouraged the use of capsule-supported intraocular lenses during cataract surgery because of the high incidence of intraocular lens decentration and subluxation/dislocation. Open- and closed-angle glaucoma can develop. Open-angle glaucoma arises from a dysfunctional or absent aqueous drainage system, whereas the acute attacks of closed-angle glaucoma occur even with a hypoplastic stump of peripheral iris tissue. Medical therapy usually fails, and filtering surgery and cyclodestructive procedures are frequently necessary.

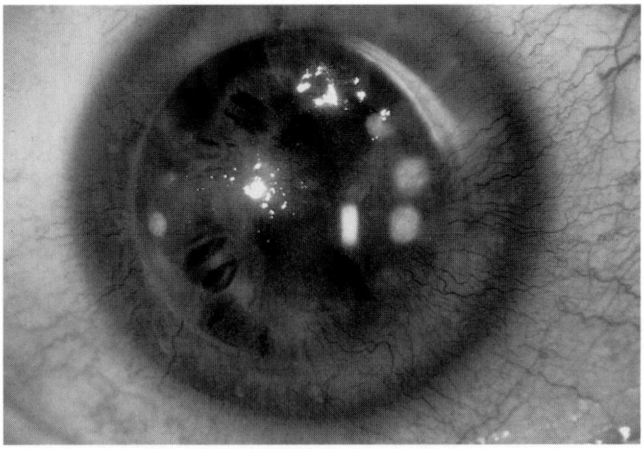

Fig. 2-34 Aniridia. Several years after penetrating keratoplasty for aniridia, progressive corneal neovascularization and chronic epithelial irregularity have developed.

CONCLUSION

A systematic approach, such as that indicated by the STUMPED mnemonic, is extremely important when faced with an infant or a child with an anterior segment abnormality. Acute infections must be ruled out promptly, and congenital glaucoma, if it is present, must be diagnosed immediately. Other metabolic, dystrophic, and developmental conditions must be diagnosed accurately for proper treatment of the entire patient, not only of the eye. In addition, a precise diagnosis is important so that parents may be informed of the long-term systemic and visual prognosis and the heritability of the condition.

MAJOR POINTS

The STUMPED mnemonic is often helpful for remembering the primary causes of a congenital cloudy cornea: S = sclerocornea, T = tears in Descemet's membrane, U = ulceration, M = metabolic, P = Peters' anomaly, E = edema, and D = dermoid.

When an adequate examination cannot be conducted in the office, an evaluation under anesthesia should be considered.

True absence of the cornea, true cryptophthalmos, and anophthalmos have dismal visual prognoses; there are no known treatments.

The widened ciliary ring associated with megalocornea presumably causes zonular stretching and results in phacodonesis, iridodonesis, and ectopia lentis (which can make routine cataract extraction challenging!).

Careful examination skills and use of ancillary studies can help in the crucial distinction between megalocornea and congenital glaucoma, a condition in which early diagnosis and surgical intervention can help prevent severe visual loss and other complications.

In sclerocornea, the anterior segment is typically difficult to visualize through the opaque cornea and is frequently associated with other abnormal ocular findings. Diagnostic tools such as ultrasound biomicroscopy are helpful in anticipating complications and in planning surgery.

Because the depth of dermoid lesions can be difficult to determine, donor corneoscleral tissue should always be ordered in advance and be readily available if surgical excision is considered.

The sporadic cases of aniridia have important and common systemic associations with Wilms' tumor and the WAGR complex, whereas the familial cases are not associated with Wilms' tumor.

When deciding whether to proceed with corneal transplantation for aniridia, the surgeon should anticipate problems with epithelial healing, be prepared to treat the patient with aggressive lubrication and lateral tarsorrhaphy, and should consider limbal cell transplantation before proceeding with the corneal transplantation.

SUGGESTED READINGS

Books

Kim T, Palay DA: Developmental corneal anomalies of size and shape. In Krachmer JH, Mannis MJ, Holland EJ, editors: *Cornea,* St Louis, 1997, Mosby.

Journals

Dana MR, Schaumberg DA, Moyes AL, Gomes JAP: Corneal transplantation in children with Peters anomaly and mesenchymal dysgeneses, *Ophthalmology* 104:1580-1586, 1997.

Goldstein JE, Cogan DG: Sclerocornea and associated congenital anomalies, *Arch Ophthalmol* 67:761-768, 1962.

Gupta SK, De Becker I, Tremblay F, et al: Genotype/phenotype correlations in aniridia, *Am J Ophthalmol* 126:203-210, 1998.

Holland EJ, Schwartz GS: The evolution of epithelial transplantation for severe ocular surface disease and a proposed classification system, *Cornea* 15:549-556, 1996.

Kenyon KR: Mesenchymal dysgenesis in Peters' anomaly, sclerocornea and congenital endothelial dystrophy, *Exp Eye Res* 21:125-142, 1975.

Mansour AM, Barber JC, Reinecke RD, Wang FM: Ocular choristomas, *Surv Ophthalmol* 33:339-358, 1989.

Meire FM: Megalocornea: clinical and genetic aspects, *Doc Ophthalmol* 87:1-121, 1994.

Nelson LB, Spaeth GL, Nowinski TS, et al: Aniridia: a review, *Surv Ophthalmol* 28:621-642, 1984.

Nishida K, Kinoshita S, Ohashi Y, et al: Ocular surface abnormalities in aniridia, *Am J Ophthalmol* 120:368-375, 1995.

Shields MB, Buckley E, Klintworth GK, Thresher R: Axenfeld-Rieger syndrome: a spectrum of developmental disorders, *Surv Ophthalmol* 29:387-409, 1985.

Waring GO, Rodrigues MM, Laibson PR: Anterior chamber cleavage syndrome: a stepladder classification, *Surv Ophthalmol* 20:3-27, 1975.

CHAPTER 3

Corneal Dystrophies, Degenerations, and Ectatic Conditions

Corneal dystrophies include a wide variety of conditions affecting all levels of the cornea. They are, as a rule, hereditary, bilateral, and relatively symmetric (Box 3-1). Generally, they are evident only in the cornea and there are no associated systemic findings, though there are exceptions. Corneal dystrophies may be apparent at birth but usually become evident later in life. Often they are visible when patients are young but are not clinically significant until many years later. These dystrophies typically cause two difficulties: painful, recurrent epithelial erosions and decreased vision. Treatment of corneal dystrophies varies, depending on the specific dystrophy, clinical problem, and severity of the condition. Recurrent erosion can be treated with conservative medical therapy or minor corneal surgery to induce better adherence of the epithelium to the underlying stroma. The usual treatment of diminished vision from the anterior corneal dystrophy is removal of the anterior corneal opacities with a blade or a laser. Visual problems from deeper stromal or endothelial dystrophies are generally treated by partial-thickness or full-thickness corneal transplantation.

Corneal degenerations are often age-related phenomena. Unlike corneal dystrophies, they are not inherited. Corneal degenerations can be unilateral or bilateral, symmetric or asymmetric. Depending on the exact degeneration and the location of the pathology, vision may or may not be affected. Deposition of material found naturally in the body but not normally in the cornea, such as

Box 3-1 Genetic Association of Corneal Dystrophies

AUTOSOMAL DOMINANT

Anterior basement membrane dystrophy
Meesmann's dystrophy
Reis-Bücklers' dystrophy (CDB-1)
Thiel-Behnke dystrophy (CDB-2)
Granular dystrophy
Lattice dystrophy, types 1 and 2
Avellino dystrophy
Schnyder's crystalline dystrophy
Fleck dystrophy
Central cloudy dystrophy of François
Posterior amorphous stromal dystrophy
Congenital hereditary stromal dystrophy
Fuchs' dystrophy
Posterior polymorphous dystrophy
Congenital hereditary endothelial dystrophy (less common)

AUTOSOMAL RECESSIVE

Macular dystrophy
Lattice dystrophy, type 3
Congenital hereditary endothelial dystrophy (more common)

calcium or lipid, is usually secondary to other eye abnormalities, such as chronic inflammation or new blood vessel invasion into the cornea. Many of these conditions require no therapy, whereas others should be managed by treating the underlying cause. Occasionally, actual removal of the corneal lesion is required to improve visual function.

Ectatic corneal conditions include a family of disorders. Keratoconus is, by far, the most common of these abnormalities, but pellucid marginal degeneration and keratoglobus share many characteristics. These conditions all involve areas of pathologic corneal thinning and protrusion, resulting in corneal irregularity and decreased vision. Depending on the severity of the disease, vision can often be improved with glasses, contact lenses, or corneal surgery.

ANTERIOR CORNEAL DYSTROPHIES (Table 3-1)

Anterior Basement Membrane Dystrophy

The most common anterior corneal dystrophy is epithelial basement membrane dystrophy, also called anterior basement membrane (ABM) dystrophy and map-dot-fingerprint dystrophy. It has also been termed Cogan's microcystic dystrophy, emphasizing the less common creamy white microcysts seen in this condition.

Histopathologically, ABM dystrophy is caused by an abnormality of epithelial cell production, maturation, and turnover, creating a basement membrane with poorly functioning adhesion complexes, hemidesmosomes, and anchoring fibrils. It can lead to reduplication of epithelial cells with superimposed basement membrane layers (Fig. 3-1). This condition tends to be autosomal dominant. It is generally bilateral but may be asymmetric.

The presenting symptoms of all corneal conditions relate to the level of corneal involvement. As the pathology in ABM dystrophy is in and just below the epithelium, it can cause decreased vision from epithelial irregularity and pain from epithelial defects. The onset of symptoms tends to be in early to middle adulthood.

Painful symptoms generally arise during sleep or on awakening, and they vary from mild foreign body sensation to severe pain. Mild symptoms typically resolve rapidly, over minutes, but they can last hours. Severe pain can last for hours to days, depending on the extent of epithelial damage. The abnormal adhesion complexes lead to a relatively weak attachment of the epithelial layer to Bowman's membrane. There is less tear production overnight, which allows the undersurface of the eyelids to stick to the epithelium, causing problems ranging from a slight dislodgment of the epithelial layer inducing mild discomfort to a frank epithelial defect inducing severe pain. When these uncomfortable or painful symptoms occur repeatedly, it is termed recurrent erosion syndrome. Minor corneal trauma, which would not affect a normal cornea, can cause an epithelial defect in an eye with ABM dystrophy. These eyes are at the greatest risk for the development of recurrent erosion syndrome after trauma, especially from sharp objects such as fingernails, paper, and tree branches.

Although visual acuity is poor when the epithelium is dislodged or absent centrally, vision can also be affected without any ocular discomfort. Because the air-tear interface is the most important refractive surface of the eye, any small epithelial irregularity can lead to distorted and decreased vision. These visual problems can be transient or constant and can occur even without painful erosions.

The clinical findings of ABM dystrophy include map lines, fingerprint lines, and dots or microcysts anywhere in the epithelium (Figs. 3-2, 3-3, and 3-4). Map lines are often associated with fine, gray patchy opacities. Fingerprint lines are thin and often concentric refractile ridges, whereas microcysts are dot sized, pearly white, and generally circular or ovoid. Microcysts occasionally coalesce to form broad lines or even shapes resembling Chinese characters. Many of the changes are best seen with a wide slit-lamp beam shone from the side (Fig. 3-5). With topical fluorescein and cobalt blue light, a rapid tear

Table 3-1 Characteristics of the three major anterior dystrophies

Feature	Anterior basement membrane dystrophy	Meesmann's dystrophy	Corneal dystrophies of Bowman's membrane
Also known as	Map-dot-fingerprint dystrophy	Hereditary juvenile epithelial dystrophy	Reis-Bücker's dystrophy, Thiel-Behnke dystrophy
Age of onset	15-50 years	Infancy	5-10 years
Laterality	Bilateral, often asymmetric	Bilateral	Bilateral
Visual symptoms	Decreased vision, halos, monocular diplopia	Glare, photophobia	Decreased vision
Recurrent erosions	Common, especially after corneal trauma	Occasional	Common, begin early
Inheritance	Autosomal dominant	Autosomal dominant	Autosomal dominant
Corneal appearance	Map lines with gray patchy opacities Fingerprint lines with refractile ridges Pearly-white microcysts	Multiple tiny dotlike cysts in interpalpebral fissure	Bowman's membrane and superficial stromal opacities Honeycomb pattern
Pathologic abnormality	Abnormal epithelial basement membrane Reduplication of basement membrane	Accumulation of periodic acid-Schiff–positive "peculiar substance"	Electron microscopy rodlike bodies and curly filaments
Treatment	Lubrication Bandage soft contact lens Epithelial debridement Superficial keratectomy with diamond burr or excimer laser PTK	Sunglasses Lubrication Bandage soft contact lens	Lubrication Superficial keratectomy with excimer laser PTK

PTK, Phototherapeutic keratectomy.

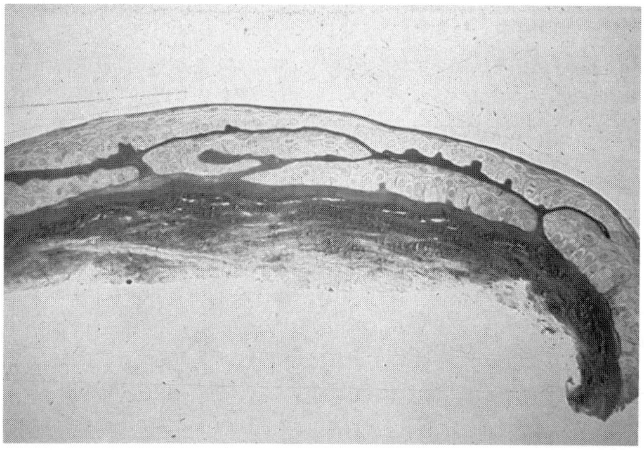

Fig. 3-1 Anterior basement membrane dystrophy. Histopathology (periodic acid-Schiff stain) of an anterior corneal specimen reveals multiple layers of epithelial cells with reduplicated epithelial basement membrane.

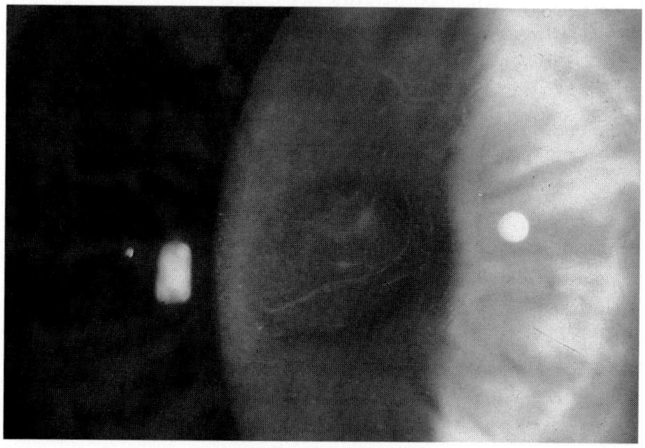

Fig. 3-2 Anterior basement membrane dystrophy. Central corneal map changes. Gray areas of corneal epithelium indicate where the basement membrane is reduplicated.

break-up time and negative staining may be noted over areas of elevated irregular epithelium (Fig. 3-6). Additionally, retroillumination through a dilated pupil can highlight subtle ABM dystrophy findings (Fig. 3-7).

The treatment of ABM dystrophy takes a stepwise approach and depends on the type, severity, and duration of symptoms. Painful symptoms are initially treated with topical lubrication such as an artificial tear or sodium chloride ointment at night, unless an epithelial defect is present in which case an antibiotic ointment is used until the defect is healed. If the patient has daytime dry eye symptoms, artificial tear supplements can be used.

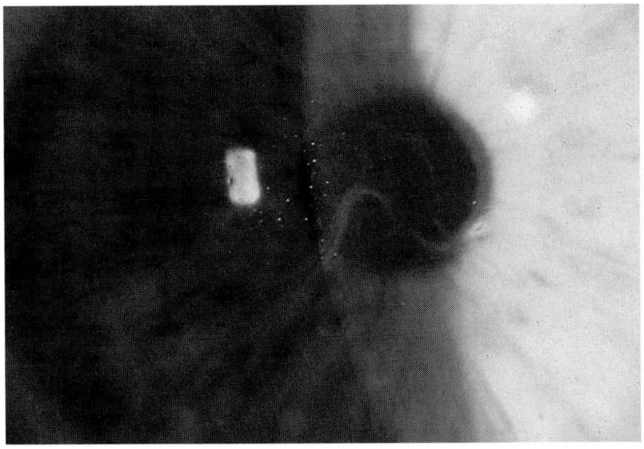

Fig. 3-3 Anterior basement membrane dystrophy. Corneal map changes with a mare's tail pattern approaching the 7 o'clock position.

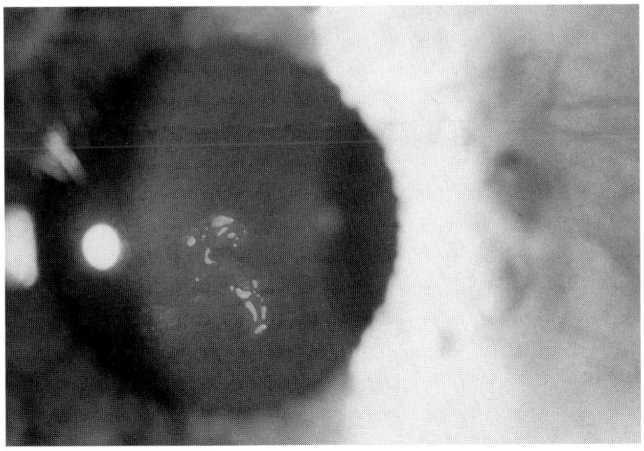

Fig. 3-4 Anterior basement membrane dystrophy. Central corneal dot changes. These Cogan's microcysts are intraepithelial. They are surrounded by a gray halo of abnormal epithelial basement membrane.

Nighttime ointments must be continued for at least 3 to 6 months after resolution of the symptoms to allow for permanent adhesion of the epithelium to Bowman's membrane. Some patients find that placing a drop of artificial tears in the affected eye before opening the eye (but allowing the drop to seep in) each morning helps prevent erosions from recurring. If the painful symptoms continue despite medical treatment, a bandage soft contact lens, which places a protective layer between the cornea and the eyelid, can be tried. Bandage soft contact lenses are effective at improving painful, and occasionally visual, symptoms while the lens is in place. However, the lenses must be used for at least 3 months and often closer to 6 or 12 months for permanent pain relief; even then, there is no guarantee of success.

Surgical treatments for painful symptoms include anterior stromal micropuncture, epithelial debridement

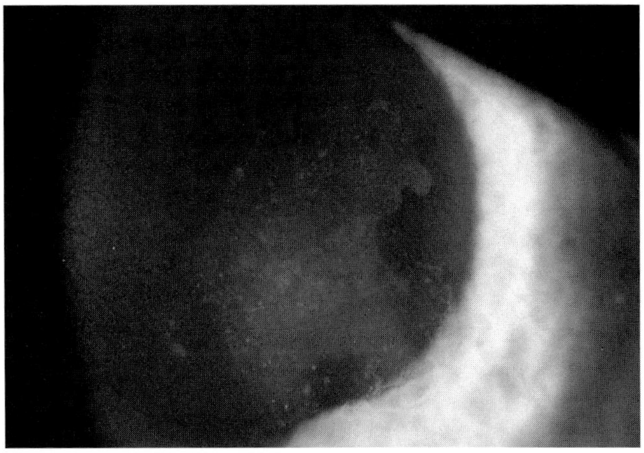

Fig. 3-5 Recurrent corneal erosion. Irregular epithelium the morning after an episode of recurrent corneal erosion. There is no frank epithelial defect, but the epithelial surface is irregular and picks up fluorescein dye over several minutes.

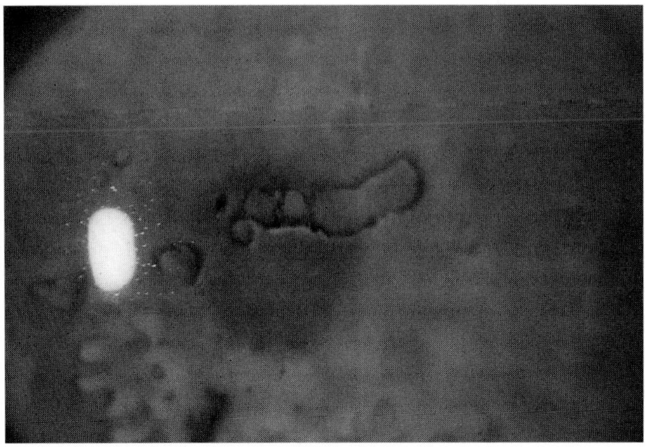

Fig. 3-6 Anterior basement membrane dystrophy. Negative staining of elevated epithelium in an eye with moderate anterior basement dystrophy. It is best noted with fluorescein dye.

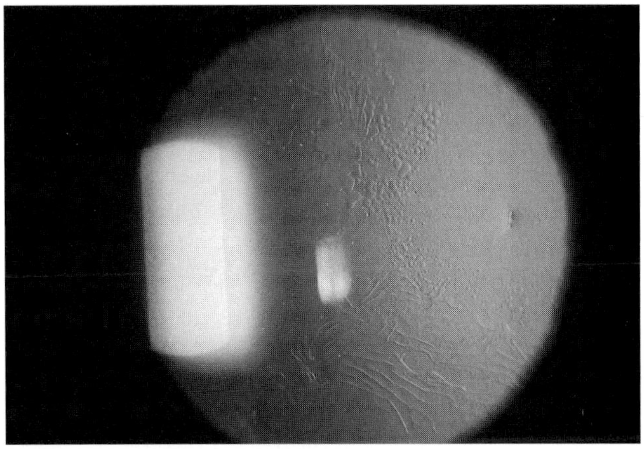

Fig. 3-7 Anterior basement membrane dystrophy. Fingerprint lines, primarily seen superiorly and inferiorly, are highlighted in retroillumination, whereas bleblike changes are seen toward the 1 o'clock position.

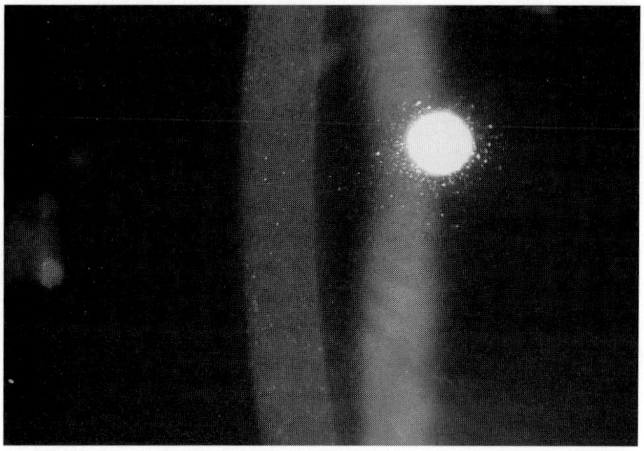

Fig. 3-8 Meesmann's dystrophy. Tiny intraepithelial gray-white dots are noted on direct illumination and illumination off the iris.

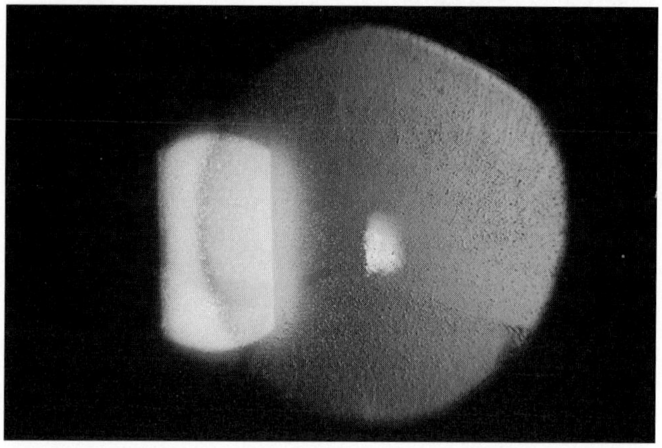

Fig. 3-9 Meesmann's dystrophy. Pinpoint dots are often best noted in retroillumination.

Box 3-2 Surgical Treatment Options for Anterior Basement Membrane Dystrophy

FOR PAINFUL RECURRENT EROSIONS

Anterior stromal micropuncture
Epithelial debridement alone
Epithelial debridement with diamond burr polishing of Bowman' s membrane
Excimer laser phototherapeutic keratectomy

FOR IMPROVED VISION

Epithelial debridement alone
Epithelial debridement with diamond burr polishing of Bowman's membrane
Excimer laser phototherapeutic keratectomy

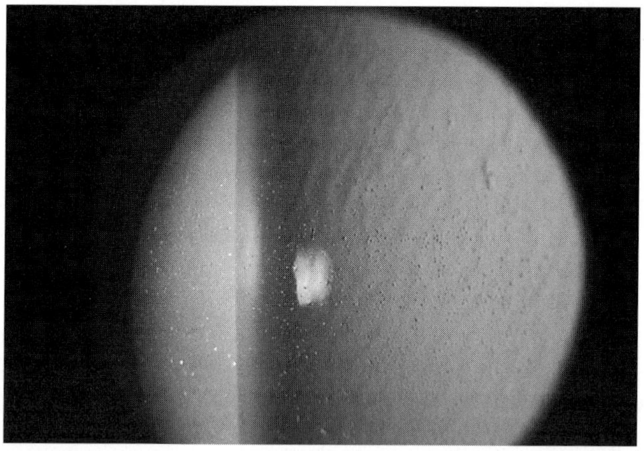

Fig. 3-10 Meesmann's dystrophy. High-magnification retroillumination demonstrates that the microcysts are most concentrated in the interpalpebral zone.

alone or in combination with diamond burr polishing of Bowman's membrane, and excimer laser phototherapeutic keratectomy (PTK). Anterior stromal micropuncture is best used for localized, noncentral ABM dystrophy changes, usually caused by traumatic corneal abrasion. Visual symptoms result from an irregular epithelium that often does not respond, or responds only momentarily, to topical lubricants. For these patients all treatments (Box 3-2) except anterior stromal micropuncture can be curative. The idea is that the new epithelium will be smoother, yielding better visual acuity.

Epithelial debridement to remove all areas of abnormal loose epithelium can be successful at promoting better adherence to the stroma. Diamond burr polishing of Bowman's membrane to remove adherent abnormal basement membrane complexes has a better success rate than epithelial debridement alone. Excimer laser PTK, which removes a fraction of Bowman's membrane after mechanical epithelial debridement, is another effective method to treat recurrent erosions that do not respond to more conventional therapies.

Meesmann's Dystrophy

Meesmann's dystrophy, a rare autosomal dominant condition affecting the epithelium, becomes apparent early in life, often within the first few months; consequently, it is also called hereditary juvenile epithelial dystrophy. Primary symptoms include glare, diminished vision, and mild foreign body sensation, but occasionally painful recurrent erosions develop. Meesmann's dystrophy tends to be bilateral and symmetric.

On slit-lamp examination, tiny intraepithelial dotlike cysts are visible (Fig. 3-8). They are best appreciated in retroillumination through a dilated pupil, where they appear translucent (Figs. 3-9 and 3-10). The cysts, which

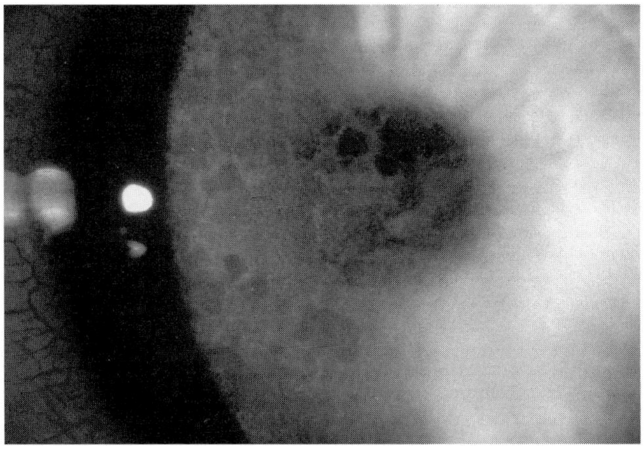

Fig. 3-11 Corneal dystrophy of Bowman's membrane, type 1 (Reis-Bücklers' dystrophy). The gray-white honeycomb pattern is evident throughout the anterior cornea.

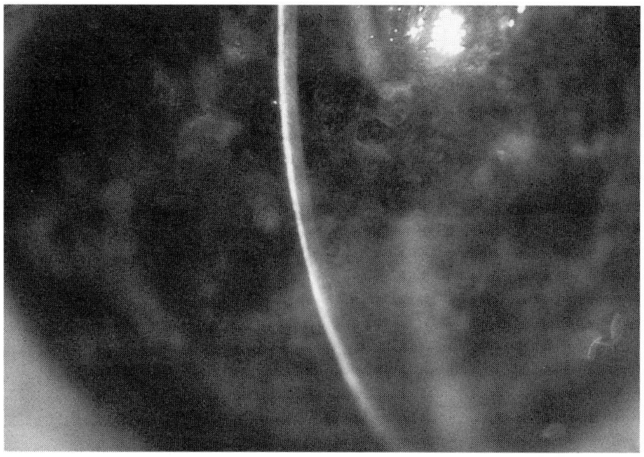

Fig. 3-12 Corneal dystrophy of Bowman's membrane, type 1 (Reis-Bücklers' dystrophy). The slit beam demonstrates the anterior nature of this condition. The opacity also involves the corneal periphery.

look gray-white on direct illumination, often concentrate in the interpalpebral zone, and they can extend from limbus to limbus. Histopathologically, the epithelium is thickened with a multilayered basement membrane. The epithelial cells contain a periodic acid-Schiff (PAS)-positive substance of unknown composition known as peculiar substance.

The treatment of Meesmann's dystrophy depends on the symptoms. Often sunglasses improve glare and visual symptoms. Lubricating drops and ointments can alleviate foreign body symptoms. Patients with painful recurrent erosions can be treated with bandage soft contact lenses or superficial corneal surgery as described for ABM dystrophy. Occasionally, patients have been treated with excimer laser PTK with initial success, but Meesmann's dystrophy tends to recur.

Corneal Dystrophies of Bowman's Membrane

Because of confusion in the literature, the terminology for the specific dystrophies of Bowman's membrane is evolving. Reis-Bücklers' dystrophy is the most common term used for these conditions. Because of histopathologic similarities, Reis-Bücklers' dystrophy is also known as a superficial variant of granular dystrophy. There is another dystrophy involving Bowman's membrane that is similar, though not identical, to Reis-Bücklers' dystrophy known as Thiel-Behnke dystrophy or honeycomb dystrophy. Some investigators have split these entities into corneal dystrophy of Bowman's membrane type 1 (CDB-1, Reis-Bücklers' dystrophy) and type 2 (CDB-2, Thiel-Behnke dystrophy).

Both dystrophies of Bowman's membrane are bilateral, relatively symmetric, and autosomal dominant.

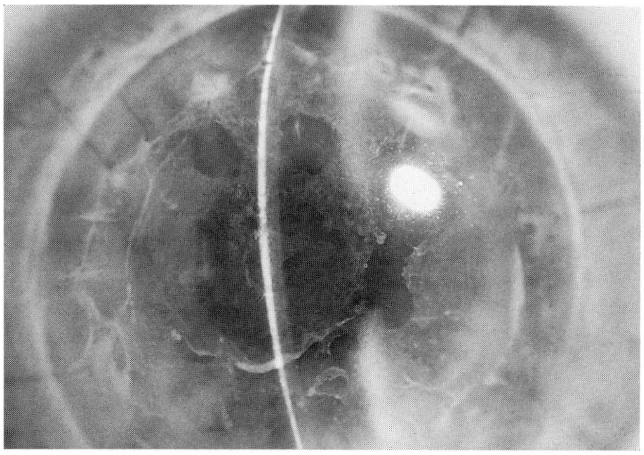

Fig. 3-13 Corneal dystrophy of Bowman's membrane, type 1 (Reis-Bücklers' dystrophy). Recurrent Reis-Bücklers' dystrophy in a corneal graft. As with most recurrent dystrophies, it primarily affects the superficial cornea and thus is amenable to excimer laser phototherapeutic keratectomy.

They usually present in the first decade of life with symptoms of painful corneal erosion. Early in life, slit-lamp examination reveals a gray-white, reticular, honeycomb-shaped opacity involving Bowman's membrane and anterior stroma (Figs. 3-11, 3-12, and 3-13). Whereas it is most dense centrally and anteriorly, the condition can involve the deeper stroma and the corneal periphery as it progresses. The pathology creates a rough, irregular surface, resulting in decreased vision because of corneal opacity and irregular astigmatism. Decreased vision typically begins in the second to fourth decades but can occur earlier. After multiple recurrent erosions, subepithelial fibrosis develops; it tends to ameliorate the pain of erosion but further diminishes vision.

Clinically, CDB-1 and CDB-2 are difficult to distinguish from each other. CDB-2 tends to have a smoother corneal surface and decreases vision later in life than CDB-1. Histopathologically, transmission electron microscopy differentiates these two variants. CDB-1 demonstrates rod-like bodies, similar to those found in granular dystrophy, whereas in CDB-2 curly filaments are found.

Therapy for these two dystrophies is identical. Recurrent erosion is treated medically, as described for ABM dystrophy. When medical management fails or visual acuity is significantly compromised, surgical treatment should be considered. Superficial keratectomy with a blade or with excimer laser PTK works well to clear the central cornea, to decrease recurrent erosions, and to improve vision. The dystrophies do recur over a few years and occasionally even more rapidly. Retreatment with excimer laser PTK can yield good results. In advanced cases with deeper pathologic abnormalities, lamellar or penetrating keratoplasty may be indicated. Recurrence of the dystrophy also occurs after corneal grafts, but generally not as rapidly as after superficial keratectomy.

STROMAL CORNEAL DYSTROPHIES (Table 3-2)

Granular Dystrophy

Granular dystrophy is one of the three classic corneal stromal dystrophies. Granular dystrophy and lattice dystrophy are much more prevalent than the third classic stromal dystrophy, macular dystrophy (Box 3-3). Granular dystrophy is autosomally dominantly inherited. It becomes apparent in childhood, but it does not become symptomatic until adulthood. The primary symptom is diminished vision, but painful recurrent erosions may develop in patients with especially superficial disease.

Slit-lamp examination reveals multiple focal, distinct, white opacities in the anterior stroma. The opacities resemble crushed bread crumbs and can also be found in the middle or even the deep stroma. The intervening spaces between opacities are clear, at least early in life (Figs. 3-14, 3-15, 3-16, and 3-17). With time these clear spaces also become involved, but much more superficially than the early opacities (Fig. 3-18). The lesions involve the central cornea, spare the periphery, and do not extend to the limbus.

In general visual acuity is minimally affected in the first two decades of life, when the spaces between the opacities are clear. With increasing age, as patients reach their 20s to 30s, the pathology slowly becomes confluent and vision declines. Occasionally the lesions can extend anteriorly, through Bowman's membrane, and result in painful symptoms that are managed as recurrent erosions. Histopathologically, the granular material is hyaline. It stains bright red with Masson trichrome (Fig. 3-19). The superficial variant of granular dystrophy, which shares some histopathologic characteristics with granular dystrophy, is really a dystrophy of Bowman's layer and was discussed earlier.

Decreased vision is treated by removal of the pathology. Because the abnormality causing most of the visual decrease is the superficial confluent opacity, removing this outermost layer dramatically improves vision. Lamellar keratectomy can be performed with a blade in a freehand fashion, with a microkeratome, or with excimer laser PTK (the usual method). If the pathology is especially deep, lamellar or penetrating keratoplasty may be indicated. The dystrophy will recur after any of these treatments, but the time it takes depends on the amount of tissue removed. Vision may remain excellent for several years after superficial keratectomy, whereas a corneal transplant may remain clear for many years or even decades before central recurrence affects vision. Often a superficial keratectomy, such as with PTK, can be repeated or can be used to treat recurrence in a corneal transplant.

Lattice Dystrophy

Lattice dystrophy is typically autosomal dominant, though there is more variable clinical expression. Signs can often be seen on slit-lamp examination within the first two decades of life. Painful recurrent erosions are generally the earliest symptoms of the condition, initially occurring in the teens and 20s. Here, as in granular dystrophy, the disease begins as discrete lesions with relatively clear intervening spaces that do not dramatically affect vision. As the condition progresses, and especially after numerous recurrent erosions, confluent scarring develops and severely affects vision.

The classic slit-lamp appearance of lattice dystrophy is branching grayish refractile linear opacities in the anterior and mid-stroma (Figs. 3-20, 3-21, 3-22, and 3-23). The lines are best appreciated on retroillumination off the iris or against the red reflex (Fig. 3-24). Early in life, central subepithelial white dots and haze are seen. Later in life, superficial scarring and irregularity often develop (Fig. 3-25). With time the stroma can acquire a ground-glass appearance. The opacities generally remain central and midperipheral and spare the limbus.

Histopathologically, the deposits in lattice dystrophy are amyloid. In addition the amyloid accumulates subepithelially, disrupting normal epithelial adhesions and predisposing the cornea to erosions. Amyloid deposits stain reddish-orange with congo red dye, stain positively with PAS and Masson trichrome, and stain metachromatically with crystal violet (Fig. 3-26). Apple-green birefringence and red-green dichroism are noted when a polarizing filter is used (Fig. 3-27).

Table 3-2 Characteristics of the four major stromal dystrophies

Feature	Granular dystrophy	Lattice dystrophy (type 1)	Macular dystrophy	Schnyder's crystalline dystrophy
Age of onset				
Deposits	<10 years	<10 years	<10 years	15-20 years
Painful symptoms	20-30 years	10-20 years	<10 years	None
Visual loss	20-30 years	20-40 years	10-20 years	>50 years
Inheritance	Autosomal dominant	Autosomal dominant	Autosomal recessive	Autosomal dominant
Erosions	Uncommon	Frequent	Infrequent	None
Corneal appearance	Gray-white bread crumb opacities Intervening spaces clear early, hazy late Periphery spared	Multiple fine refractile lines Subepithelial dots Subepithelial fibrosis late Periphery clear, except in severe cases	Gray-white opacities, with hazy margins Central lesions anterior stroma Peripheral lesions posterior stroma Limbus to limbus Cornea guttata often present	Central superficial crystalline pattern Early arcus senilis Central and diffuse stromal haze late
Corneal thickness	Normal	Normal	Thinned	Normal
Histochemical stains	Masson trichome	Congo red Periodic acid-Schiff Crystal violet	Colloidal iron Alcian blue Periodic acid-Schiff	Oil red O
Abnormal material	Hyaline	Amyloid	Glycosaminoglycans	Cholesterol, neutral fats

Box 3-3 Key Distinguishing Features of the Three Major Stromal Dystrophies

GRANULAR DYSTROPHY

Early clear spaces between dense opacities
Periphery remains clear

LATTICE DYSTROPHY

Refractile dots and lines

MACULAR DYSTROPHY

Autosomal recessive
Limbus-to-limbus involvement
Opacities superficial centrally, deep peripherally
No clear intervening spaces
Cornea thinned

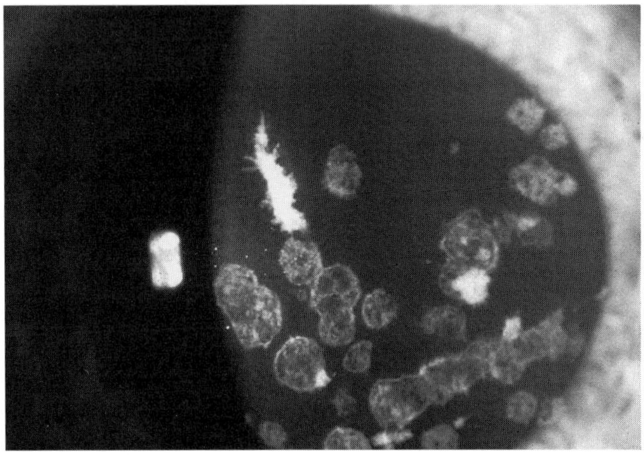

Fig. 3-14 Granular dystrophy. Multiple, distinct, crushed bread crumb white opacities involve the central cornea. Early in the course of the dystrophy, the intervening spaces are clear and vision is good.

Three main types of lattice dystrophy have been identified (Table 3-3). Type 1, classic lattice dystrophy, is by far the most common. It is autosomal dominant. Type 1 has the earliest clinical onset, usually in the first decade or two of life, the earliest painful symptoms, usually in the teens or 20s, and earliest vision loss, typically in the 30s or 40s. The lattice lines are numerous, relatively fine, and spare the limbus. There is no systemic involvement clinically.

Type 2 lattice dystrophy is Meretoja syndrome, or systemic amyloidosis. It is also autosomal dominant. Symptoms generally include diminished vision and occasionally recurrent erosions, but they are rare in patients younger than 50 years. In the cornea the amyloid lines are much fewer but significantly thicker than they are in type 1 lattice dystrophy. The lines extend to the limbus, are densest in the corneal midperiphery, and tend to spare the visual axis. Systemic amyloidosis can involve

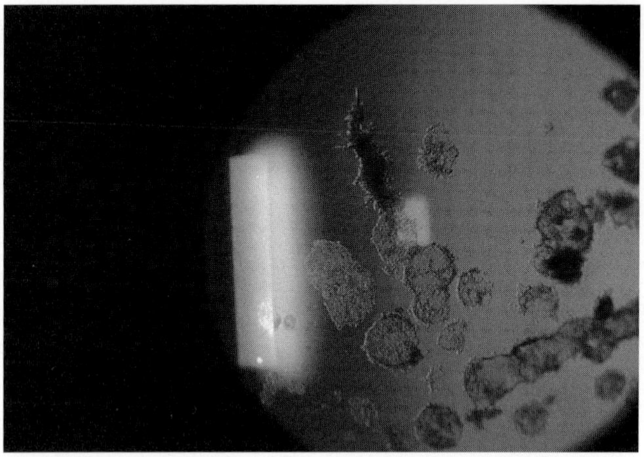

Fig. 3-15 Granular dystrophy. The same cornea seen in Fig. 3-14, now in retroillumination. Clear intervening spaces are apparent.

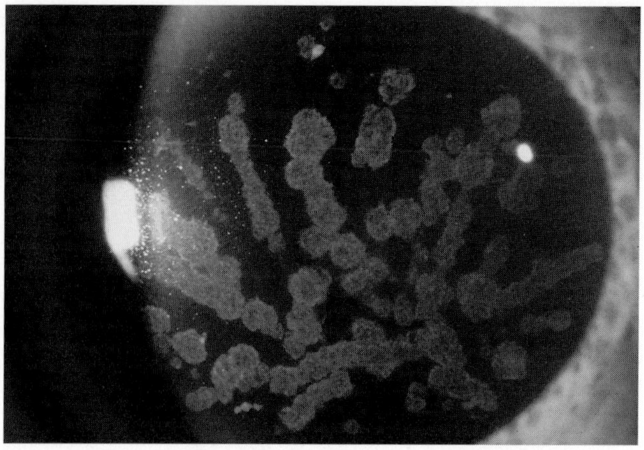

Fig. 3-16 Granular dystrophy. Gray-white opacities primarily involve the central cornea. Intervening spaces are clear. (See color plate.)

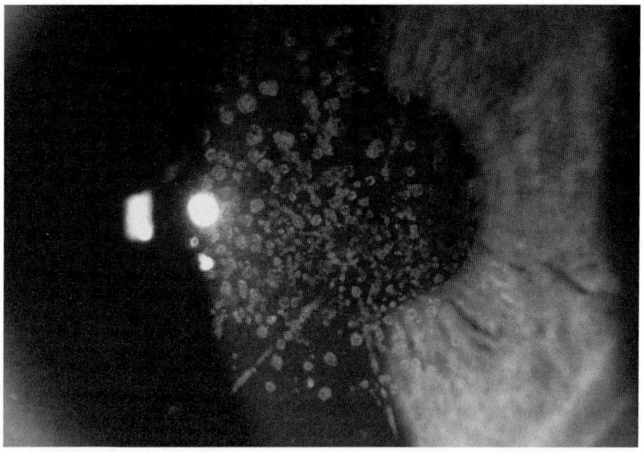

Fig. 3-17 Granular dystrophy. Opacities are densely packed centrally. Intervening spaces are becoming involved with the dystrophy. At this point vision begins to decline significantly.

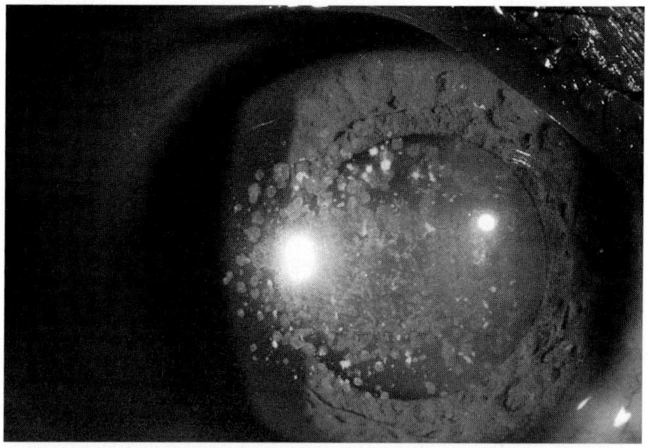

Fig. 3-18 Granular dystrophy. The central cornea is almost completely involved, and there are essentially no clear intervening spaces. Vision is poor. Dull gray, moderately large opacities are superficial, whereas small, densely white opacities are in the middle to deep stroma.

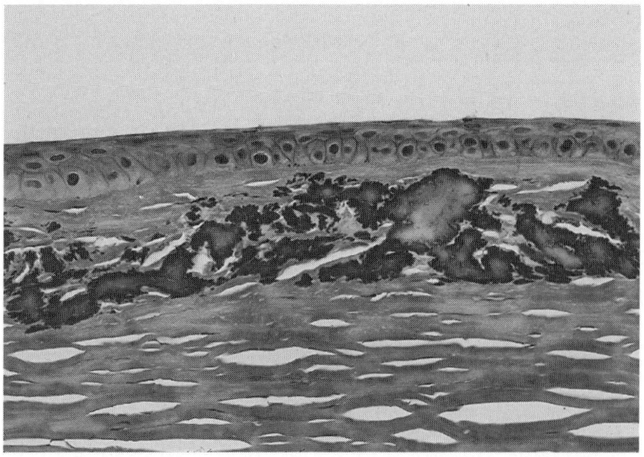

Fig. 3-19 Granular dystrophy. Masson trichrome stain revealing the hyaline deposits in the anterior stroma. (Courtesy of Ralph C. Eagle, Jr., M.D.) (See color plate.)

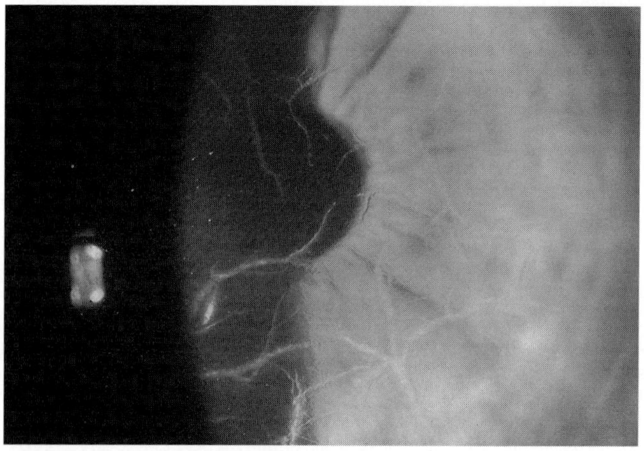

Fig. 3-20 Lattice dystrophy. Multiple white branching lines of amyloid are seen. (See color plate.)

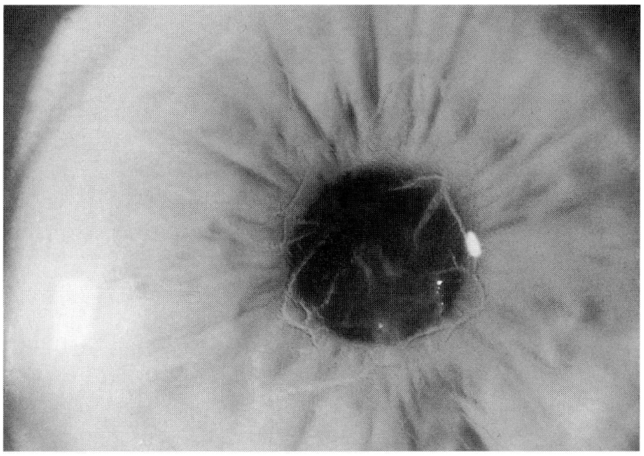

Fig. 3-21 Lattice dystrophy. Numerous branching refractile lines are observed, primarily in the central cornea. Note the mild elevated corneal scar at the inferior aspect of the pupil.

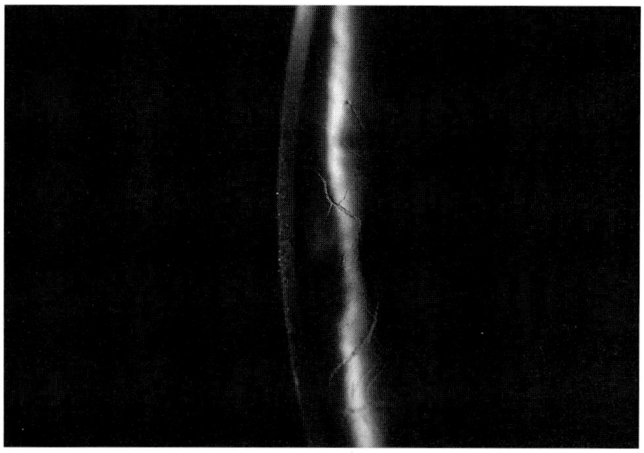

Fig. 3-22 Lattice dystrophy. The refractile nature of the amyloid deposits is highlighted using the slit beam to retroilluminate the cornea off the iris.

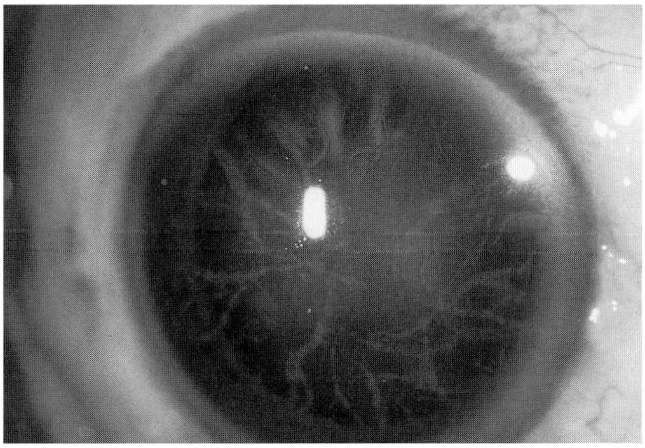

Fig. 3-23 Lattice dystrophy. Multiple refractile amyloid lines can be seen encompassing most of the central cornea but not involving the periphery.

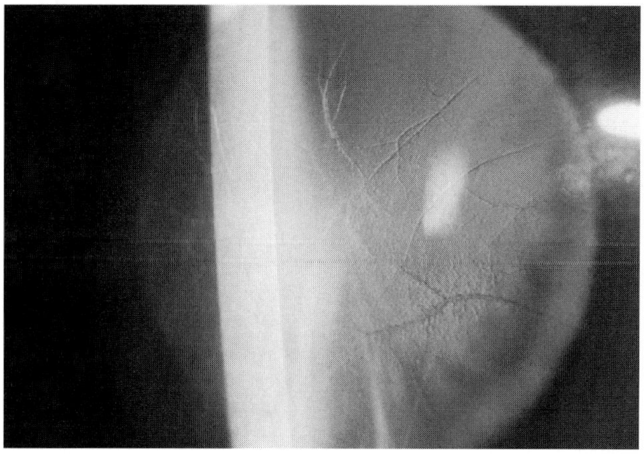

Fig. 3-24 Lattice dystrophy. Retroillumination off the retina demonstrates the refractile amyloid lines well.

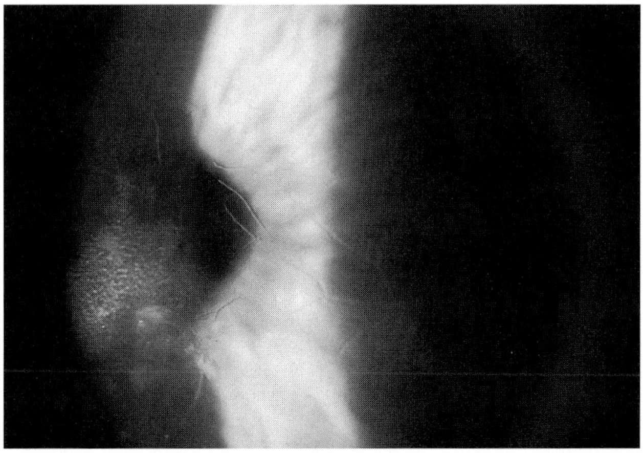

Fig. 3-25 Lattice dystrophy. After many recurrent erosions, the anterior stroma develops a diffuse haze as seen in the central cornea. This superficial corneal opacity causes significantly diminished vision. Because it is superficial, it is often amenable to treatment with excimer laser phototherapeutic keratectomy.

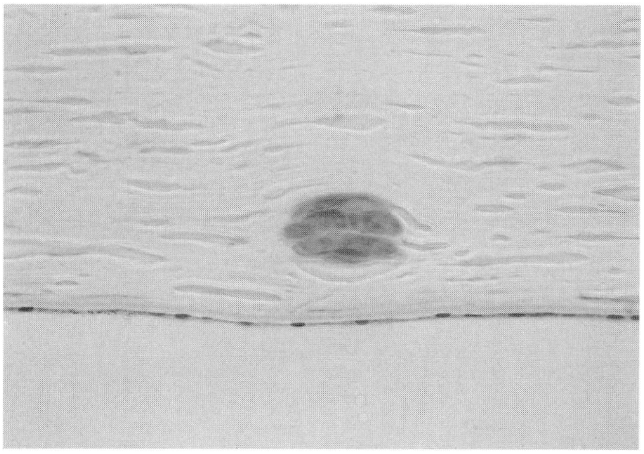

Fig. 3-26 Lattice dystrophy. Congo red stain demonstrates deep corneal amyloid deposits. (Courtesy of Ralph C. Eagle, Jr., M.D.) (See color plate.)

the skin, causing blepharochalasis and the characteristic bloodhound facies. It can also affect the arteries and nerves, producing cranial and peripheral neuropathies (Box 3-4).

Lattice type 3 is autosomal recessive. It is associated with thick lattice lines that usually do not affect vision until late in life. They are not associated with recurrent erosions, and there is no systemic involvement.

The treatment of lattice dystrophy is similar to that for granular dystrophy. Painful symptoms, which occur more often than they do in granular dystrophy, are treated as recurrent erosions. Because vision is relatively unaffected until the central superficial scarring becomes significant, lamellar keratectomy either with a free-hand blade, microkeratome, or excimer laser PTK is typically a first-line treatment. Lamellar or penetrating keratoplasty may be necessary for deep lesions. Eventually the dystrophy will recur in the graft. Interestingly, recurrent lattice dystrophy tends not to exhibit the classic branching lattice lines, but rather diffuse anterior corneal haze and subepithelial opacities and is consequently often amenable to treatment with excimer laser PTK. Frequently, the recurrences are first seen near the suture scars in the donor button. Lattice dystrophy recurs somewhat more rapidly than granular dystrophy after similar treatments.

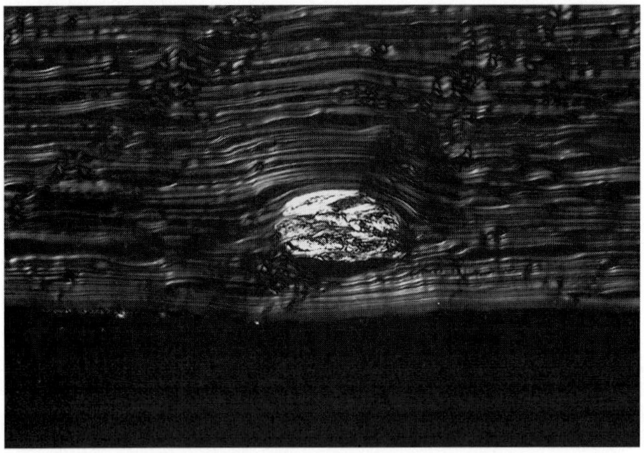

Fig. 3-27 Lattice dystrophy. Apple-green birefringence of the amyloid material is apparent using a polarizing filter. (Courtesy of Ralph C. Eagle, Jr., M.D.) (See color plate.)

Avellino Dystrophy

Avellino dystrophy, originally described in families whose ancestry could be traced to the Italian province of Avellino, is a variant of granular dystrophy in which lattice deposits are also found. The discrete gray-white bread crumb granular dystrophy opacities appear first, and later in life the refractile amyloid deposits of lattice dystrophy appear (Fig. 3-28). Amyloid deposits collect more posteriorly than they do in classic lattice dystrophy. Patients with Avellino dystrophy experience more recurrent erosion symptoms than do those with granular dystrophy. The treatment is the same as it is for granular and lattice dystrophies.

Macular Dystrophy

Macular dystrophy is the third of the classic stromal dystrophies, but that is where the similarities end. Macular dystrophy is autosomal recessive (compared to autosomal dominant for the other two) and much rarer. It involves the entire cornea to the periphery, and it causes decreased vision at a younger age than do granular and lattice dystrophies.

Slit-lamp examination reveals focal gray-white opacities that are circular and that have ill-defined edges (Figs. 3-29 and 3-30). They are located in the superficial stroma in the central cornea and in the deep stroma in the periphery (Fig. 3-31 and 3-32). The peripheral lesions are more distinct than the central lesions. Although

Table 3-3 Different types of lattice dystrophy

Feature	Type 1	Type 2 (Meretoja syndrome)	Type 3
Inheritance	Autosomal dominant	Autosomal dominant	Autosomal recessive
Age of onset	<10 years	25-40 years	>40 years
Age of visual loss	10-30 years	>60 years in severe cases	>60 years
Recurrent erosions	Frequent, begin at a young age	Infrequent	None
Corneal appearance	Multiple fine lattice lines Subepithelial dots Late subepithelial fibrosis	Few thick lines Few subepithelial dots	Multiple thick lines Diffuse subepithelial dots
Location of lattice lines	Central early, periphery late	Periphery early, central late	Limbus to limbus
Systemic involvement	None	Amyloidosis of skin, especially face Cranial and peripheral neuropathies Arterial, kidney, other organ involvement	None

the opacities are quite apparent, the intervening stroma is not clear but is diffusely grayish-white. With time the focal opacities become larger and can coalesce, and the entire full-thickness cornea becomes diffusely cloudy. Descemet's membrane can become gray, and significant corneal guttae may be seen. Unlike granular and lattice dystrophies in which the corneal thickness is normal, in macular dystrophy the central cornea tends to be thin. Corneal thicknesses of 400 to 450 μm are common.

Visual loss occurs early in patients with macular dystrophy because the intervening spaces between the macules are unclear. Patients note significantly diminished vision and glare symptoms in the second and third decades. Recurrent erosions may occur but are unusual.

The abnormal deposits in macular dystrophy are glycosaminoglycan (acid mucopolysaccharide). Histopathologically, they stain positively with colloidal iron (Fig. 3-33), Alcian blue, and PAS stains. There are two subtypes of macular dystrophy that are clinically similar. In type 1, the more common form, there is no keratan sulfate in the cornea or serum. In type 2, keratan sulfate is present, but the levels are approximately 30% below normal. An enzyme-linked immunosorbent assay serum test can help diagnose type 1 macular dystrophy even before it is clinically apparent.

Therapy for macular dystrophy, as for all dystrophies, depends on the symptoms. The rare patient with recurrent erosions should be treated appropriately. Occasionally glare is the chief symptom, and sunglasses or tinted contact lenses may be helpful. Significantly decreased vision must be treated with penetrating keratoplasty. Excimer laser PTK and lamellar keratoplasty are generally not good options because of the depth of the pathology. Macular dystrophy, as with all the dystrophies, recurs after corneal transplantation, but it takes many years for the recurrence to become clinically significant.

Box 3-4 Systemic Associations of Corneal Dystrophies

LATTICE DYSTROPHY, TYPE 2 (MERETOJA SYNDROME)

Systemic amyloidosis

SCHNYDER'S CRYSTALLINE DYSTROPHY

Hypercholesterolemia, with or without hypertriglyceridemia
Genu valgum
Xanthelasma

Schnyder's Crystalline Dystrophy

Schnyder's crystalline dystrophy, also called central crystalline dystrophy, though not one of the classic stromal dystrophies, is more prevalent than macular dystro-

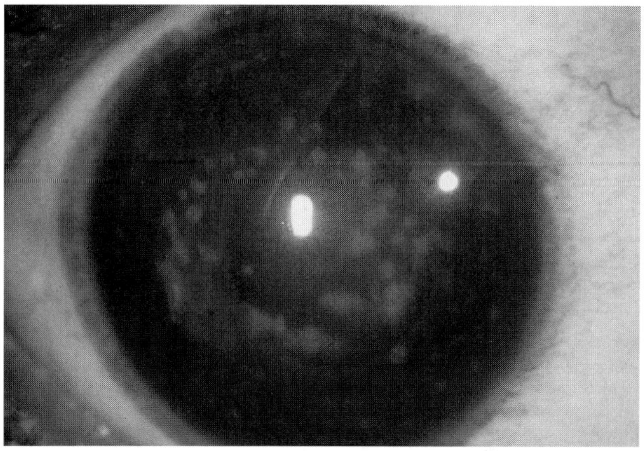

Fig. 3-29 Macular dystrophy. Diffuse central and peripheral corneal deposits are seen.

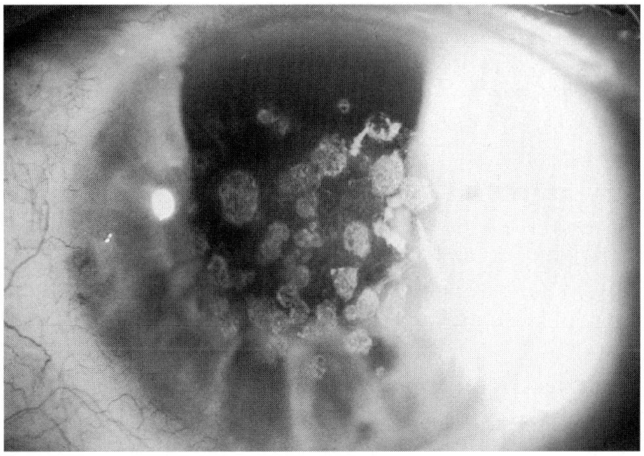

Fig. 3-28 Avellino dystrophy. Lattice lines are seen among the more numerous granular dystrophy deposits.

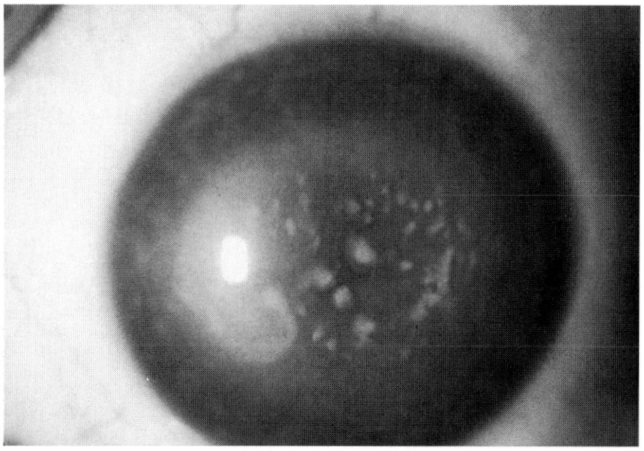

Fig. 3-30 Macular dystrophy. Dense deposits are seen along with diffuse central corneal opacification. Here, too, the disease involves the corneal periphery.

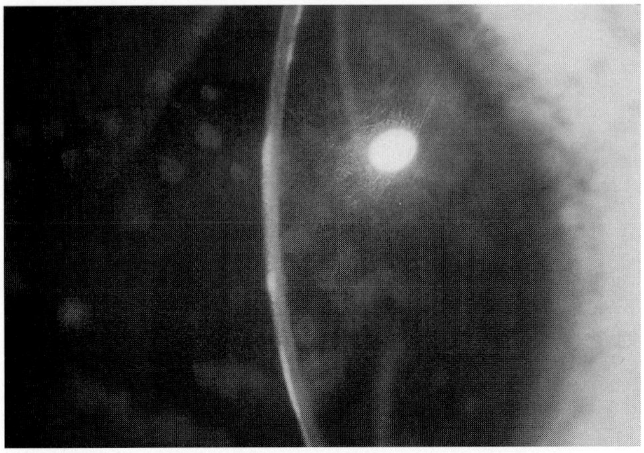

Fig. 3-31 Macular dystrophy. Central deposits involve the anterior cornea, whereas peripheral deposits involve the deep stroma and Descemet's membrane.

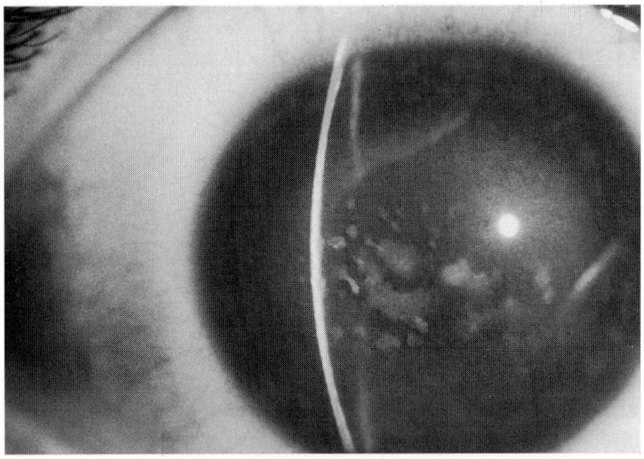

Fig. 3-32 Macular dystrophy. Central macules are anterior and are surrounded by diffuse corneal haze, whereas the peripheral deposits are in the deep cornea. (See color plate.)

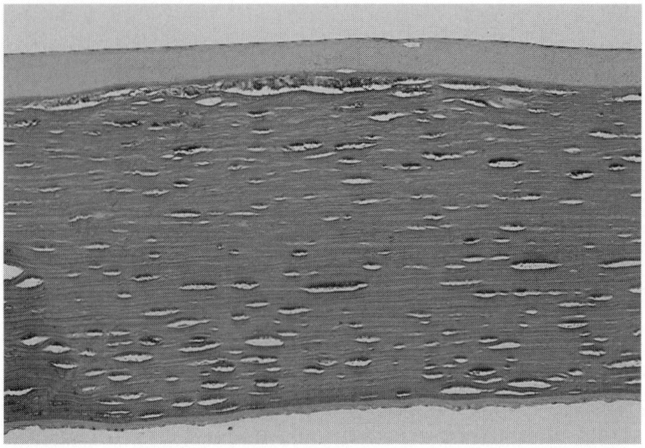

Fig. 3-33 Macular dystrophy. The colloidal iron stain demonstrates the glycosaminoglycan (acid mucopolysaccharide) as blue deposits concentrated in the anterior cornea but evident throughout the stroma. (Courtesy of Ralph C. Eagle, Jr., M.D.) (See color plate.)

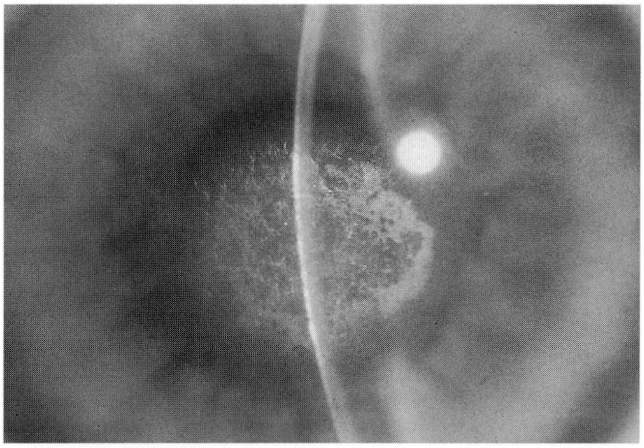

Fig. 3-34 Schnyder's crystalline dystrophy. White crystalline deposits in the superficial stroma are generally noted first in this dystrophy. The deposits, lipid, neutral fats, and cholesterol, may have a feathery pattern.

phy in the United States. It is similar to granular and lattice dystrophies in that it is autosomal dominant, appears early in life, is slowly progressive, and tends not to cause symptoms until years later. It is different from many of the other dystrophies, however, because it has several systemic associations.

The clinical course begins with tiny yellow-white refractile crystals in the superficial central stroma, often within the first decade of life (Fig. 3-34). After the age of 23 years, a prominent arcus lipoides or arcus senilis has often developed. After the age of 40 years, a full-thickness central corneal haze has developed (Figs. 3-35, 3-36, and 3-37). Numerous patterns of Schnyder's crystalline dystrophy have been described, including a central discoid opacity without crystals (sine crystals) (Fig. 3-38) and a relatively clear central area within a surrounding dense, ring-shaped opacity.

Histopathologic evaluation reveals that the crystals are lipid, neutral fat, and cholesterol. This dystrophy is associated with hypercholesterolemia, with or without hypertriglyceridemia. However, the serum lipid levels do not necessarily correlate with the density of the corneal opacities. Schnyder's crystalline dystrophy is also associated with genu valgum and xanthelasma. Fasting serum cholesterol and triglyceride levels should be checked (see Box 3-4).

Patients are generally asymptomatic. Sometimes they have glare symptoms or, in severe cases, decreased vision. Excimer laser PTK has been successful in some patients at removing the superficial opacities, which may

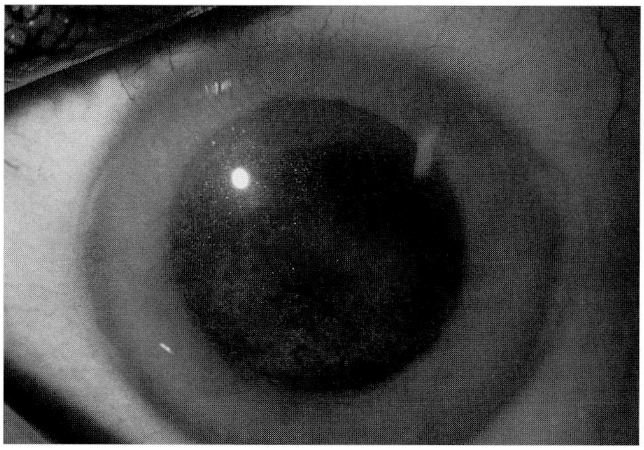

Fig. 3-35 Schnyder's crystalline dystrophy. The central crystals may be diffuse. In this patient a dense central area of opacity is surrounded by a less dense halo and then by a ring of denser material.

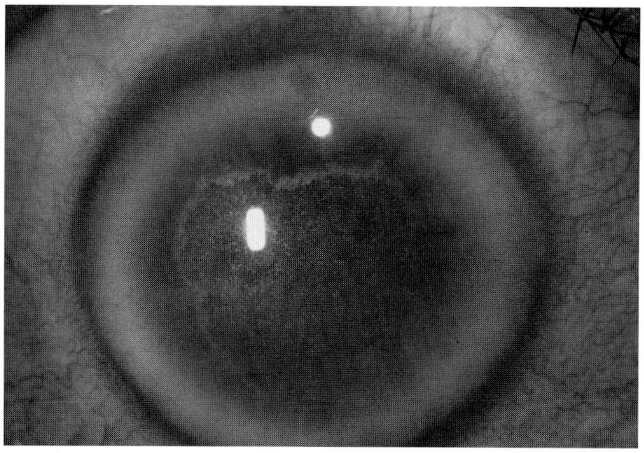

Fig. 3-37 Schnyder's crystalline dystrophy. Central crystalline deposits with a prominent outer crystalline ring are seen. The dense arcus lipoides is also obvious. (See color plate.)

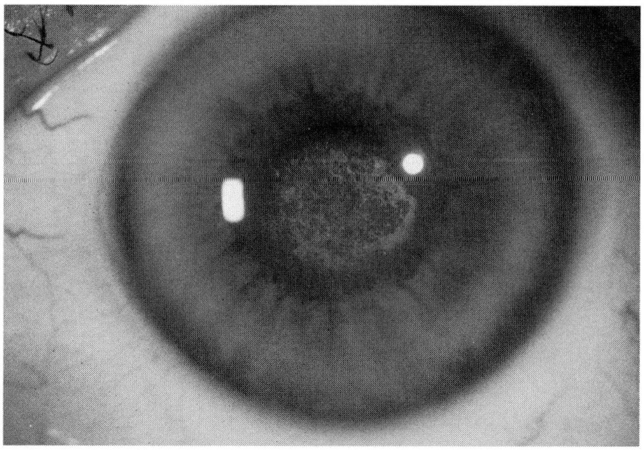

Fig. 3-36 Schnyder's crystalline dystrophy. The central circle of crystalline deposition is evident. As patients age, a dense arcus lipoides becomes apparent.

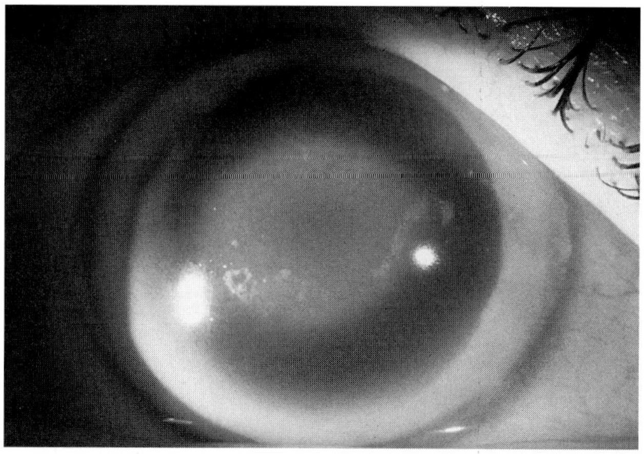

Fig. 3-38 Schnyder's crystalline dystrophy. In this patient the full-thickness central corneal opacity is prominent, whereas the crystals are difficult to observe (sine crystals).

improve glare symptoms, but the deep central stromal opacities remain. Penetrating keratoplasty is necessary when vision is significantly diminished. The dystrophy can recur, but it does so extremely slowly.

Fleck Dystrophy

Fleck dystrophy is a rare autosomal dominant condition. It is seen in the first decade of life and may be congenital. Slit-lamp examination reveals small, discrete, flat gray-white opacities in all layers of the stroma (Fig. 3-39). They have distinct margins, though they can vary in shape and size and can involve the central and peripheral cornea. The condition is nonprogressive. Histopathologically, certain stromal keratocytes contain excess glycosaminoglycan and lipid.

Fleck dystrophy causes no visual or painful symptoms and is typically found on routine examination. No treatment is necessary.

Central Cloudy Dystrophy of François

The central cloudy dystrophy of François is autosomal dominant. It is bilateral, relatively symmetric, and nonprogressive. It consists of multiple gray-white polygonal opacities without distinct margins, separated by lines of clearer cornea. The opacities primarily involve the central three quarters of the cornea and taper off in the periphery (Fig. 3-40). They are densest in the posterior stroma. Clinically, central cloudy dystrophy of François is identical to the corneal degeneration known as posterior crocodile shagreen. The diagnosis of the dystrophy is

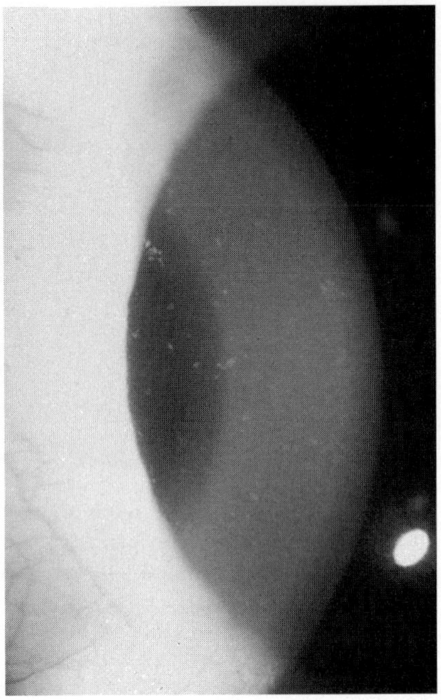

Fig. 3-39 Fleck dystrophy. Multiple small, discrete, gray-white opacities are seen throughout the stroma. There are no associated visual symptoms.

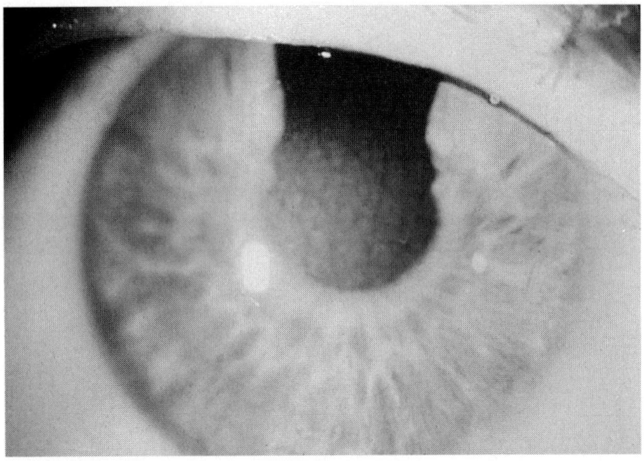

Fig. 3-40 Central cloudy dystrophy of François. Multiple central corneal polygonal opacities are found in the posterior stroma. They appear identical to posterior crocodile shagreen but are considered a dystrophy when they are found in multiple members of a family.

made when the condition is found in multiple family members of different generations and an autosomal dominant inheritance pattern is present. It may also develop earlier in life in those patients with the dystrophy.

Central cloudy dystrophy of François does not cause painful recurrent erosions or decreased visual acuity, and it is usually diagnosed on routine examination. No treatment is needed.

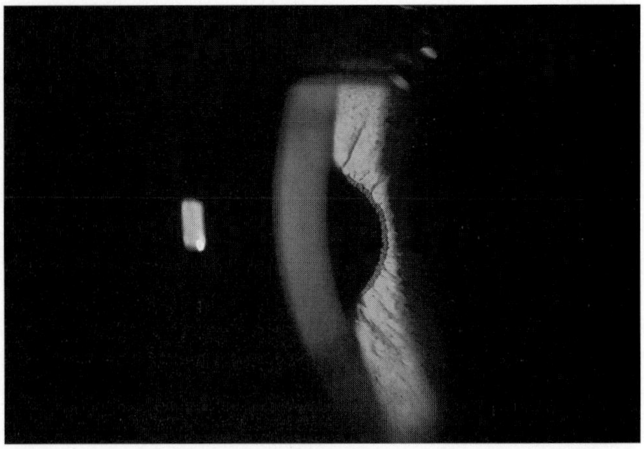

Fig. 3-41 Posterior amorphous stromal dystrophy. Large sheet-like gray-white opacities are noted in the deep stroma. The opacity may reach the periphery. There is often significant corneal thinning and flattening.

Posterior Amorphous Stromal Dystrophy

Posterior amorphous stromal dystrophy is a rare autosomal dominant entity that is bilateral and symmetric. It appears in the first decade of life and can be slowly progressive. Slit-lamp examination demonstrates large sheet-like, gray-white opacities in the deep stroma (Fig. 3-41). It can involve Descemet's membrane and reach the corneal periphery. It is associated with significant corneal thinning (as low as 300 μm), corneal flattening (as low as keratometry readings in the mid-30 D range) and hyperopia. Iris abnormalities, including fine iris processes, have been seen with posterior amorphous stromal dystrophy.

Vision is generally not affected. No treatment is indicated once any refractive error has been corrected.

Congenital Hereditary Stromal Dystrophy

Congenital hereditary stromal dystrophy is another rare bilateral, symmetric, autosomal dominant condition. It is apparent at birth and is nonprogressive. The central cornea is diffusely hazy with feathery, white opacities in the superficial stroma. The corneal periphery is relatively clear, and the endothelium and corneal thickness are normal. Histopathologically, the stroma is made up of abnormal collagen lamellae that cause the opacity.

Congenital hereditary stromal dystrophy can be dense enough to lead to poor vision, nystagmus, and esotropia. However, tearing and photophobia generally do not develop. If it is severe, treatment involves penetrating keratoplasty when patients are young to prevent dense amblyopia.

Table 3-4 Characteristics of the three major posterior corneal dystrophies

Feature	Fuchs' dystrophy	PPMD	CHED
Age of onset	40-60 years	10-30 years, rarely in infancy	Birth or infancy
Inheritance	Autosomal dominant	Autosomal dominant	Autosomal recessive (more common) Autosomal dominant (less common)
Corneal appearance	Cornea guttata, often pigmented Beaten metal appearance of Descemet's membrane Stromal edema early ABM dystrophy changes Epithelial edema later Subepithelial fibrosis latest	Endothelial vesicles, bands Diffuse endothelial gray areas Corneal stromal and epithelial edema	Severe corneal edema
Other ocular findings	Narrow angles	Fine peripheral anterior synechiae Broad iridocorneal adhesions Glaucoma	None
Specular microscopy	Polymorphism Polymegethism Decreased endothelial cell count Variably sized dark holes in endothelial mosaic	Areas of normal and abnormal endothelial cells Vesicles and bands visible	Not visible
Corneal graft required	Uncommonly	Rarely	Commonly
Prognosis for graft	Very good	Good to very good Best if no glaucoma or iridocorneal adhesions	Fair for infants, better if older

PPMD, Posterior polymorphous dystrophy; *CHED,* congenital hereditary endothelial dystrophy; *ABM,* anterior basement membrane.

POSTERIOR CORNEAL DYSTROPHIES (Table 3-4)

Endothelial Dystrophy

The terminology used for the conditions cornea guttata, endothelial dystrophy, and Fuchs' dystrophy is not standardized. For this text, corneal guttae are lesions on the central endothelial surface in endothelial and Fuchs' dystrophies. Endothelial dystrophy is the presence of central cornea guttata *without* clinically apparent corneal edema, whereas Fuchs' dystrophy is central cornea guttata *with* corneal edema. Cornea guttata is often autosomal dominant. Note that peripheral corneal guttae constitute a common degenerative finding called Hassall-Henle bodies.

Cornea guttata appears in the central cornea bilaterally as dark spots on the endothelial surface, best seen with specular reflection. On retroillumination they resemble multiple tiny water droplets on the endothelium. There is often a dusting of fine pigment overlying the cornea guttata (Figs. 3-42 and 3-43). As the condition progresses, Descemet's membrane thickens and begins to opacify. At that point the Descemet's membrane/endothelium complex takes on an orange peel or beaten metal pattern (Fig. 3-44). Patients with endothelial dystrophy are asymptomatic, but it may be observed on routine examination. There is no treatment for this dystrophy. Patients are warned that they are at increased risk for corneal edema as a result of aging or of any trauma to

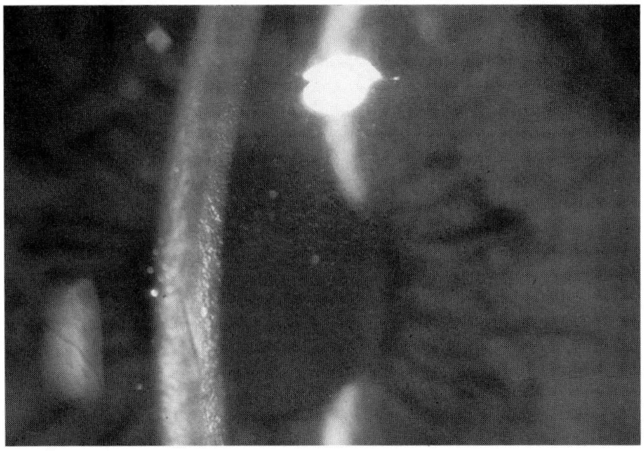

Fig. 3-42 Endothelial dystrophy. Cornea guttata creates a beaten metal pattern in Descemet's membrane and the endothelium. This pattern is evident in the slit beam, demonstrating the corrugated surface to the posterior cornea. Brown endothelial pigment can also be seen.

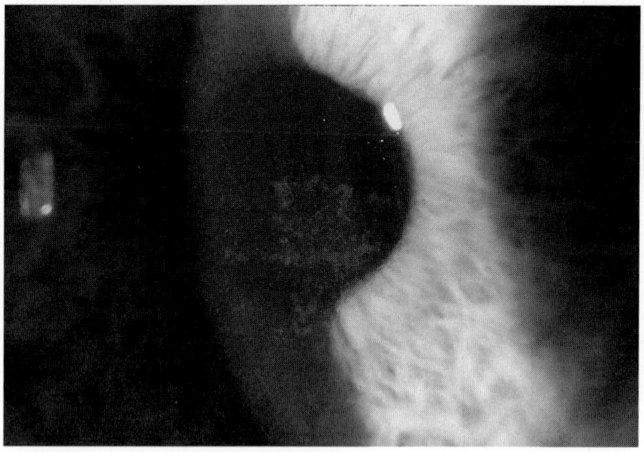

Fig. 3-43 Endothelial dystrophy. The pigment dusting is apparent on the endothelial surface.

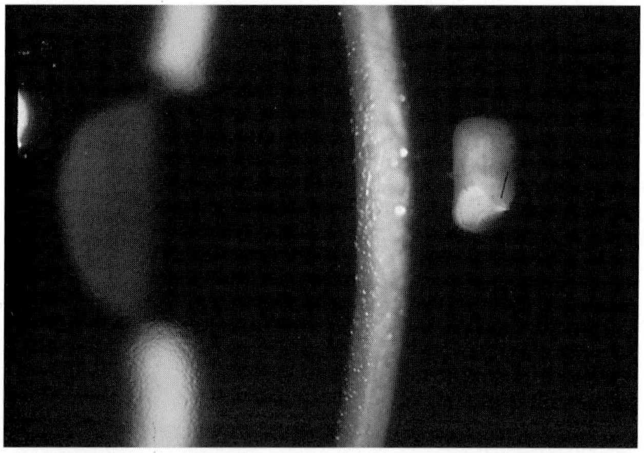

Fig. 3-44 Endothelial dystrophy. The beaten metal appearance in the posterior cornea can be seen with retroillumination off the iris and at the posterior corneal edge of the slit beam.

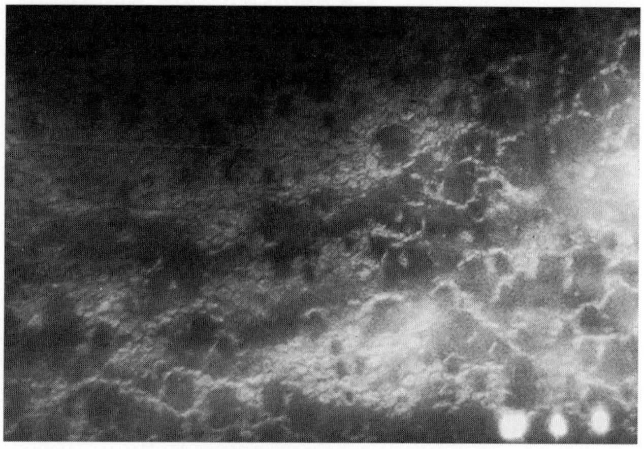

Fig. 3-45 Endothelial dystrophy. Specular microscopy reveals numerous irregular dark areas devoid of endothelial cells. Cells that can be seen are often larger and more varied in size (polymegethism) and shape (polymorphism).

the corneal endothelial cells, such as from intraocular surgery or inflammation. Symptomatic corneal edema develops in only a small percentage of patients with endothelial dystrophy.

Histopathologically, the endothelial cells in endothelial and Fuchs' dystrophies lay down new collagenous tissue over Descemet's membrane, leading to an abnormally thickened Descemet's layer. Descemet's membrane can become two to three times its normal thickness. Usually this new tissue appears as discrete excrescences that protrude into the anterior chamber (corneal guttae). It can also appear as buried excrescences in an abnormally thickened Descemet's membrane or sometimes as a thickened Descemet's membrane without excrescences. The excrescences and the thickened Descemet's membrane affect the overlying endothelial cells and their function. They cause the cells to thin and lose their characteristic hexagonal shape. Specular microscopy reveals small to large dark areas devoid of cells, demonstrating the guttate excrescences, and adjacent endothelial cells. The cells are more varied in size (polymegethism) and shape (polymorphism), and many cells have more than six sides (Fig. 3-45). Endothelial cell density tends to be decreased. The endothelial cells lose their Na^+, K^+-ATPase pump function, increase their permeability, or both to allow the cornea eventually to swell. At that point, it becomes Fuchs' dystrophy.

Fuchs' Dystrophy

Fuchs' dystrophy demonstrates an autosomal dominant inheritance pattern. It is rare for symptoms to develop before age 50, although cornea guttata/endothelial dystrophy can be seen decades earlier. It is found bilaterally, but it may be markedly asymmetric. Women have endothelial and Fuchs' dystrophies three to four times more often than men. There may be an association between Fuchs' dystrophy and axial hypermetropia, shallow anterior chambers, and angle-closure glaucoma.

Endothelial dystrophy is the precursor of Fuchs' dystrophy, but, because it is asymptomatic, patients generally do not know they have that condition. As the endothelial cells lose more and more of their pump and barrier functions, fluid starts to accumulate in the cornea, leading to the diagnosis of Fuchs' dystrophy. The edema typically begins in the posterior stroma and progresses to the anterior stroma with time (Fig. 3-46). Mild to severe folds may develop in Descemet's membrane. Corneal thickness, as measured by pachymetry, can increase from a normal of approximately 520 μm centrally to 600 to 1000 μm. With increasing fluid accumulation, epithelial edema develops. It begins as intracellular microcystic edema, appearing as a stippled epithelial pattern (bedewing). Using topical fluorescein dye,

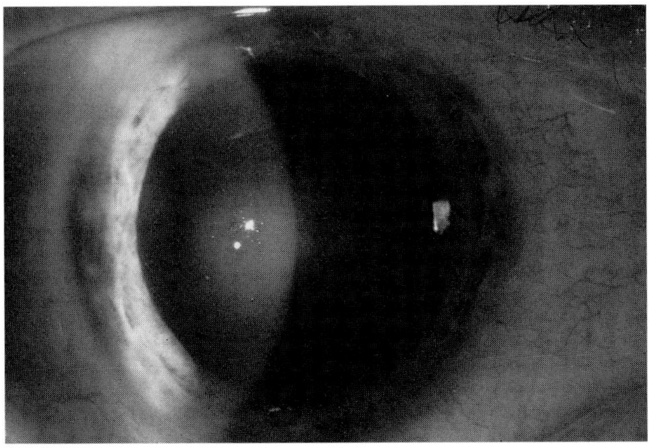

Fig. 3-46 Fuchs' dystrophy. As the endothelial cells continue to lose their ability to keep the cornea in a state of deturgescence, edema develops. Posterior stromal edema occurs first, followed by anterior stromal edema and haze. When epithelial edema occurs, vision diminishes dramatically.

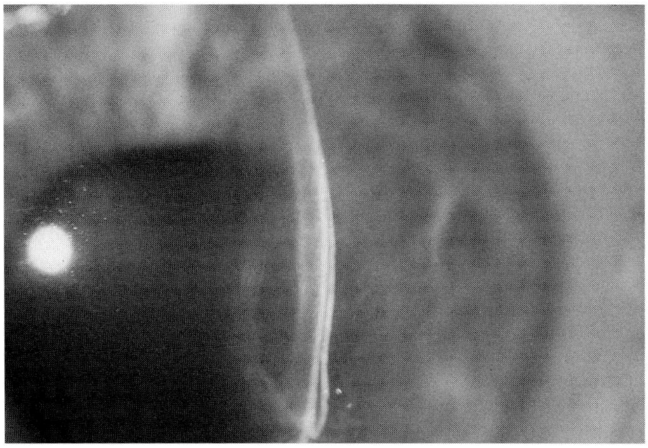

Fig. 3-47 Fuchs' dystrophy. A large epithelial bulla is obvious on slit-beam examination. At this point the vision is poor, and there are often severe painful erosion symptoms.

severe disruption of the tear film can be seen. Once epithelial edema occurs, the vision becomes significantly affected. Epithelial edema can be associated with fingerprint lines and recurrent erosion symptoms. The intracellular edema can progress to intercellular edema, causing the microcysts to coalesce and form epithelial bullae. This thickened, irregular epithelium causes severe loss of vision. These bullae cause a foreign body sensation and extreme pain when they burst (Fig. 3-47). Chronic epithelial edema leads to anterior stromal haze and permanent stromal and subepithelial scarring. Interestingly, as the subepithelial scarring worsens, the epithelial edema decreases and the painful symptoms improve. The vision, however, continues to decline.

The treatment of Fuchs' dystrophy follows a step-wise approach dependent on the severity of the condition. Generally, mild stromal edema causes minimal symptoms and requires no treatment. Vision begins to become significantly affected when epithelial edema develops. The earliest symptom patients note is blurred vision in the morning that clears in the next several hours. A classic history is that the patient cannot read the newspaper at 7 AM but can by 10 AM. This transient decreased vision results from overnight corneal edema caused by a lack of evaporation from the corneal surface during sleep. This type of mild edema can be treated with hypertonic drops (5% sodium chloride) during the day and, more importantly, hypertonic ointment (5% sodium chloride) at bedtime. These preparations can act to dehydrate the cornea slightly. Another method to improve vision is to use a hair dryer held at arm's length to blow warm, dry air across the corneas for 5 to 10 minutes each morning to dehydrate them. It works only for mild epithelial edema and consequently is the best way to clear early morning swelling in the beginning stages of Fuchs' dystrophy.

Because of the hydrostatic forces in the aqueous and cornea, an elevated intraocular pressure tends to promote epithelial edema. When the intraocular pressure is even moderately elevated, it is occasionally helpful to reduce it medically. Painful symptoms from severe corneal edema can be treated with a bandage soft contact lens. This treatment does not generally improve visual acuity and may make it worse. A bandage soft contact lens is only used when the visual potential is poor or the painful symptoms outweigh the decrease in vision. It is generally a temporary solution because it is associated with an increased risk for corneal infection.

For patients with painful symptoms or with little or no visual potential, or for those who are unable to undergo corneal transplantation, several treatment options exist. One method is to scar the corneal surface to prevent epithelial bullae from forming. Controlled scarring of the corneal surface can be achieved through cautery of Bowman's membrane (Salleras cautery), anterior stromal micropuncture, and excimer laser PTK. Another option to eliminate painful symptoms is a conjunctival flap. Although more surgically complex than the scarring techniques, it offers excellent long-term pain relief.

The standard treatment to improve vision and ameliorate painful symptoms for patients with Fuchs' dystrophy is penetrating keratoplasty. Here the abnormal cornea and the poorly functioning endothelial cells are replaced with a donor cornea with healthier endothelial cells, allowing the new cornea to remain clear. The short- and long-term success of corneal transplantation for Fuchs' dystrophy is very good. Because many patients requiring corneal transplantation for Fuchs' dystrophy are elderly, they often have concomitant significant lens opacities. For these patients, combined keratoplasty, cataract ex-

Box 3-5 Differential Diagnosis of Congenital Corneal Edema

Birth trauma, especially forceps injury
Congenital glaucoma
Posterior polymorphous dystrophy
Congenital hereditary endothelial dystrophy

traction, and intraocular lens implantation can be performed.

Whether to perform combined corneal transplantation and cataract surgery is an extremely important clinical question. Certain patients will present with significant corneal edema requiring corneal transplantation but only a moderate cataract. The density of the cataract and the patient's age help determine the need for combined surgery. The denser the cataract and the older the patient, especially if the patient is older than 60 to 65 years, lead toward combined surgery. Of course, cataract surgery can be performed after corneal transplantation (with the added benefit of stable keratometry readings on which to base intraocular lens calculations), but additional surgical risk and delayed visual rehabilitation are consequences of a second intraocular procedure. In addition, second surgery increases the risk for graft rejection and graft failure.

Other patients will present with visually significant cataracts, requiring cataract surgery, with mild Fuchs' dystrophy. The severity of the corneal edema determines the need for combined surgery. If the patient has decreased vision in the mornings or on humid days, indicating clinically significant epithelial edema, it is doubtful that the cornea will survive even the gentlest cataract surgery, and a combined technique is indicated. In general, corneal thickness measurements of 650 to 700 μm or greater are associated with corneal decompensation after cataract surgery. However, endothelial dystrophy in and of itself is not a reason to perform a penetrating keratoplasty with cataract surgery if there is no corneal edema. Even with significant cornea guttata, the cornea may survive for many years after cataract surgery, often delaying or averting the need for corneal transplantation. Additionally, corneal transplantation in a patient with a posterior chamber intraocular lens implant is a less complicated procedure than combined corneal transplantation, cataract extraction, and lens implantation.

Posterior Polymorphous Dystrophy

Posterior polymorphous dystrophy (PPMD) is an uncommon autosomal dominant corneal dystrophy. It generally presents early in life and can be congenital, so it should be included in the differential diagnosis of the cloudy cornea at birth (Box 3-5). It is bilateral but may be asymmetric, and it has been associated with Alport's syndrome (hereditary hemorrhagic nephritis and sensorineural hearing loss).

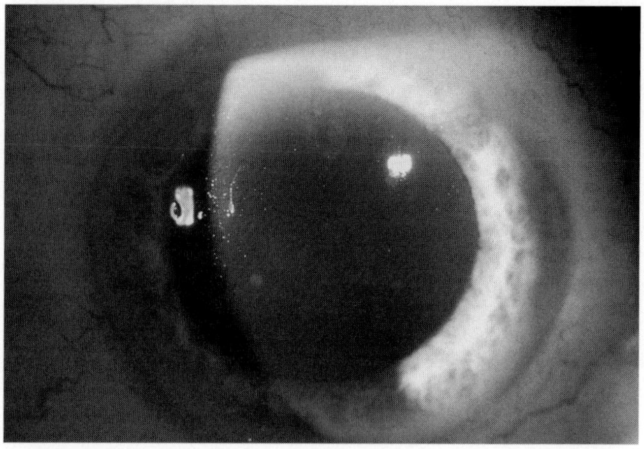

Fig. 3-48 Posterior polymorphous dystrophy. A patch of geographic gray endothelial opacities is noted superiorly, whereas a band with scalloped edges is seen in the inferocentral cornea.

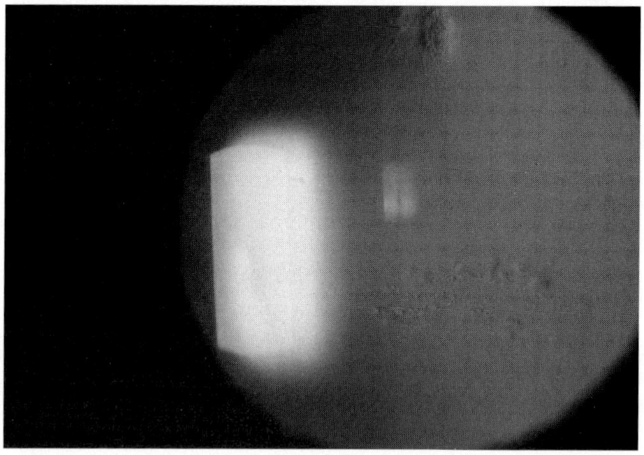

Fig. 3-49 Posterior polymorphous dystrophy. The same eye as in Fig. 3-48 is examined in retroillumination. The superior irregularities and inferocentral band are evident.

Clinically, there are three main features of the posterior corneal surfaces in eyes with PPMD: grouped vesicles, discrete geographic gray lesions, and broad bands with scalloped edges. Vesicles are small, round lesions that may appear singly but typically occur in groups of 3 to 20. Grouped vesicles are surrounded by a gray halo. Geographic lesions are dense gray regions with distinct borders. Bands are broad, often 1 mm wide, and are curvilinear, with prominent scalloped edges (Figs. 3-48, 3-49, 3-50, and 3-51). Bands can be several millimeters long. These abnormalities of the endothelium can be serious enough to cause corneal edema. In severe cases, the entire endothelium can have the appearance of beaten metal (Table 3-5).

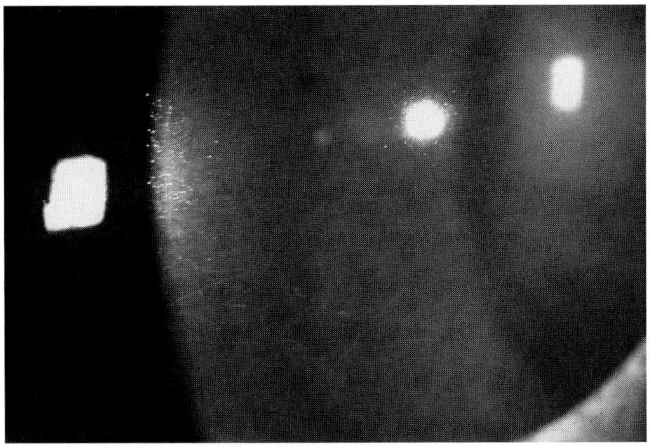

Fig. 3-50 Posterior polymorphous dystrophy. A scalloped edge band is seen in the inferior cornea.

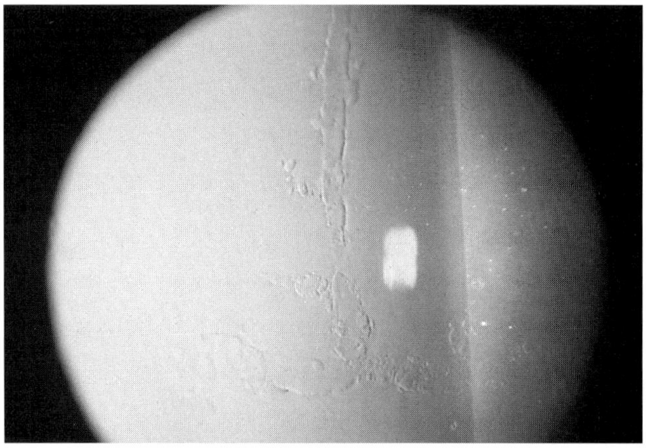

Fig. 3-51 Posterior polymorphous dystrophy. Retroillumination using the red reflex easily demonstrates a central corneal scalloped band.

Table 3-5 Characteristics of posterior polymorphous dystrophy and iridocorneal endothelial syndrome

Feature	PPMD	ICE syndrome
Age of onset	10-30 years, rarely in infancy	20-40 years
Inheritance	Autosomal dominant	None
Laterality	Bilateral	Unilateral
Corneal appearance	Endothelial vesicles, bands, gray areas May develop corneal edema	Diffuse hammered silver appearance May develop corneal edema
Specular microscopy	Focal dots and bands of abnormal cells	More diffuse patches of abnormal cells Abnormal cells large, with white peripheries, dark bodies, and a white central dot
Pathology	Epithelialization of endothelium	Endothelialization of the angle and iris
Glaucoma	Uncommon (15%)	Very common (90%)
Iris abnormalities	Fine peripheral anterior synechiae Broad iridocorneal adhesions	Broad-based peripheral anterior synechiae Iris atrophy and holes Multiple small iris nodules, heterochromia
Progression	Minimal	Severe

PPMD, Posterior polymorphous dystrophy; *ICE,* iridocorneal endothelial.

In addition to the corneal findings, iris abnormalities can be seen. Abnormal iris processes, broad peripheral iridocorneal adhesions, and corectopia are associated with PPMD. Elevated intraocular pressure is found in 15% of patients with PPMD. There is significant variability in the severity of PPMD manifestations; in fact, members of the same family may exhibit different ends of the severity spectrum.

A condition called posterior corneal vesicle syndrome describes corneal changes similar to those seen in PPMD, but the abnormalities are unilateral, usually mild, and develop without a family history of PPMD. These lesions are nonprogressive, are not associated with iris abnormalities, and do not cause corneal edema.

Specular microscopy in PPMD reveals findings similar to those seen on slit-lamp examination. The vesicles, gray areas, and bands correspond to dark, abnormal-appearing areas, whereas adjacent areas have relatively normal-appearing endothelial cells. Histopathologically, the endothelial cells in PPMD resemble epithelial cells. They have microvilli, stain positively for epidermal keratin, have intercellular desmosomes, and grow easily in cell culture.

Most patients with PPMD never have clinical problems. Occasionally, corneal edema or glaucoma develops and must be treated. Corneal edema is managed similarly to Fuchs' dystrophy. The principal treatment to improve visual acuity is penetrating keratoplasty, which has a reasonably good prognosis. Risk factors indicating the need for corneal transplantation include iridocorneal adhesions and increased intraocular pressure. Unfortunately, these same two conditions are also risk factors for a poor outcome of penetrating keratoplasty.

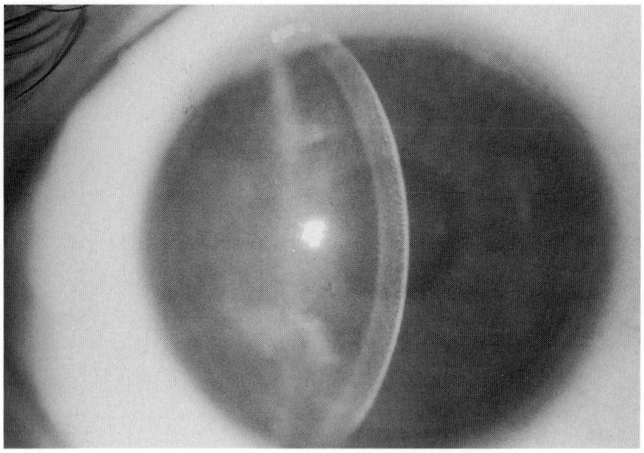

Fig. 3-52 Congenital hereditary endothelial dystrophy. The cornea is diffusely cloudy and thickened with a ground-glass appearance.

Box 3-6 Critical Features of Congenital Hereditary Endothelial Dystrophy

AUTOSOMAL RECESSIVE FORM

Present at birth
Nonprogressive
Associated with nystagmus

AUTOSOMAL DOMINANT FORM

Appears within first 2 years of life but can be congenital
Slowly progressive
Associated with pain, tearing, and photophobia
Wider spectrum of involvement
Relatives may have corneal changes of PPMD
Typically not associated with nystagmus

Congenital Hereditary Endothelial Dystrophy

Congenital hereditary endothelial dystrophy has two separate forms. One is autosomal recessive, appears at birth, is nonprogressive, and is associated with nystagmus. The other is autosomal dominant, appears within the first 2 years of life, but may be congenital. The autosomal dominant form is slowly progressive and is associated with pain, tearing, and photophobia, but typically not with nystagmus. This form has a wider spectrum of involvement, from minimal to severe, both in affected patients and in family members. Interestingly, relatives of patients with the autosomal dominant form often have the corneal changes associated with PPMD (Box 3-6).

Box 3-7 Corneal Dystrophies Requiring Penetrating Keratoplasty

REQUIRE AT BIRTH OR SOON THEREAFTER

Congenital hereditary endothelial dystrophy
Posterior polymorphous dystrophy (rarely)
Congenital hereditary stromal dystrophy

REQUIRE DURING THE SECOND TO FOURTH DECADES

Reis-Bücklers' dystrophy (CDB-1)
Macular dystrophy
Lattice dystrophy, type 1

REQUIRE DURING THE THIRD TO FIFTH DECADES

Granular dystrophy
Thiel-Behnke dystrophy (CDB-2)

REQUIRE AT ADVANCED AGE OR NEVER

Schnyder's crystalline dystrophy
Fuchs' dystrophy
Posterior polymorphous dystrophy
Lattice dystrophy, types 2 and 3

Box 3-8 Recurrence of Corneal Dystrophies after Penetrating Keratoplasty

RECUR FASTEST (WITHIN A FEW YEARS)

Reis-Bücklers' dystrophy (CDB-1)
Thiel-Behnke dystrophy (CDB-2)

RECUR THE NEXT FASTEST (WITHIN 4 TO 8 YEARS)

Lattice dystrophy, type 1

RECUR THE NEXT FASTEST (WITHIN 5 TO 10 YEARS)

Granular dystrophy

RECUR THE SLOWEST (OVER 10 YEARS)

Schnyder's crystalline dystrophy
Macular dystrophy
Lattice dystrophy, types 2 and 3

TEND NOT TO RECUR

Fuchs' dystrophy
Posterior polymorphous dystrophy
Congenital hereditary endothelial dystrophy
Congenital hereditary stromal dystrophy

Both forms demonstrate severe limbus-to-limbus corneal edema involving primarily the stroma. The cornea is diffusely blue-gray with a ground-glass appearance (Fig. 3-52). Descemet's membrane is generally thickened. The endothelial cells are abnormal or, more typically, absent. The stroma can be two to three times the normal thickness.

Congenital hereditary endothelial dystrophy is usually a diagnosis of exclusion. Other causes of congenital cloudy corneas must be ruled out, such as infantile glaucoma, forceps injury, infectious ulceration, metabolic disorders, and other dystrophies including congenital hereditary stromal dystrophy and early-onset PPMD.

Treatment depends on the severity of the corneal edema and clarity. Patients with the autosomal recessive form tend to have severe corneal edema at birth, and often bilateral penetrating keratoplasty is necessary early in life to give them the best chance for good vision. The autosomal dominant form tends to develop after birth, and the need is often less urgent for early keratoplasty (Boxes 3-7 and 3-8).

CORNEAL DEGENERATIONS

Degenerations Related to the Aging Process

Arcus senilis Arcus senilis (corneal arcus) refers to bilateral white-yellow lipid deposition in the peripheral corneal stroma. It begins inferiorly, then superiorly, and later progresses nasally and temporally. The lipid deposition is denser in the anterior and posterior stroma, resembling an hourglass pattern. The border of the deposition is sharper peripherally and less distinct centrally. There is a clear zone between the limbus and the lipid deposition (Fig. 3-53). Occasionally, mild to moderate corneal thinning develops in this clear zone and is termed furrow degeneration. However, furrow degeneration is not associated with decreased vision, inflammation, vascularization, or perforation. Patients with arcus senilis and furrow degeneration are asymptomatic.

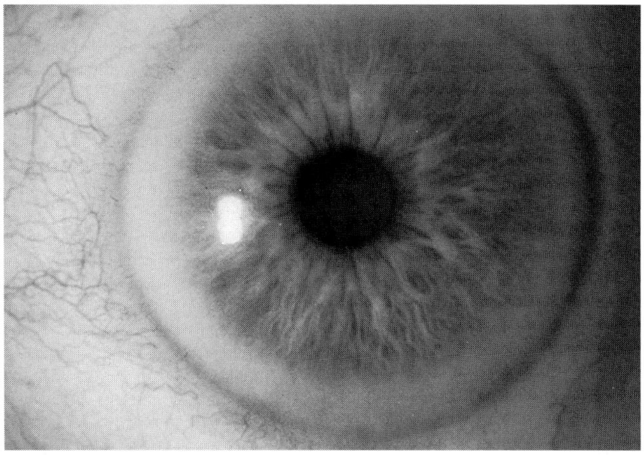

Fig. 3-53 Arcus senilis. A peripheral white-yellow lipid deposition is seen in the peripheral cornea. The clear zone between the limbus and the arcus is evident.

Arcus senilis is common. It is found in 60% of men between the ages of 40 and 60 years and in almost 100% of men older than 80. It occurs later in women and earlier in blacks. Although generally age related, it can be indicative of a lipid abnormality (hyperlipoproteinemia and hypercholesterolemia), especially if it is found in patients younger than 35 to 40 years. If it develops in a young person, a lipid/cholesterol workup is indicated. Unilateral arcus senilis is associated with carotid artery disease that is more severe on the side without the arcus senilis. These patients should undergo carotid studies.

Hassall-Henle bodies Hassall-Henle bodies are small, localized, peripheral excrescences in Descemet's membrane. These protrusions, also called Descemet's warts, are a normal change associated with aging. They are caused by an overproduction of basement membrane by the peripheral endothelial cells. They are rare in patients younger than 25 years but increase with age until they are common in patients older than 65 years. Histopathologically, they are identical to central cornea guttata of endothelial dystrophy, but they do not cause progressive endothelial damage.

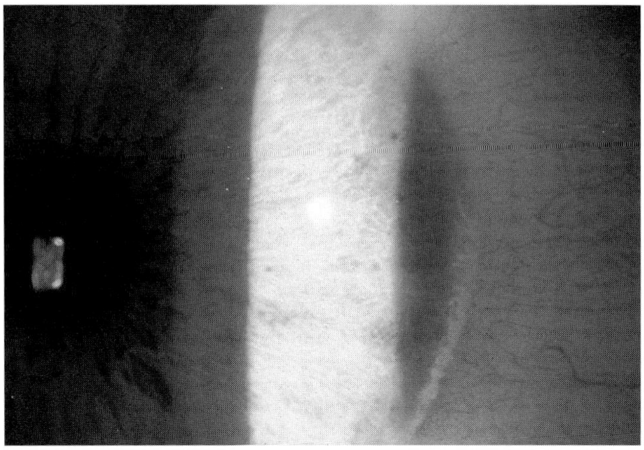

Fig. 3-54 Limbal girdle of Vogt. A narrow, moderately dense white line of elastotic degeneration is found at the limbus nasally and temporally. It often has tiny irregular linear extensions toward the central cornea.

Limbal girdle of Vogt The limbal girdle of Vogt is a superficial, narrow, white peripheral opacity adjacent to the limbus nasally and temporally (Fig. 3-54). There is no clear zone between the limbal girdle and the limbus. At its central edge, it can have tiny irregular linear extensions. It is typically bilateral and symmetric. This lesion is composed of elastotic degeneration, similar to that seen in pingueculae and pterygia. It is age related and is seen as frequently as arcus senilis. Its finding is incidental, it does not cause symptoms, and no treatment is required. Vogt originally described another form of the limbal girdle that is now thought to be early calcific degeneration.

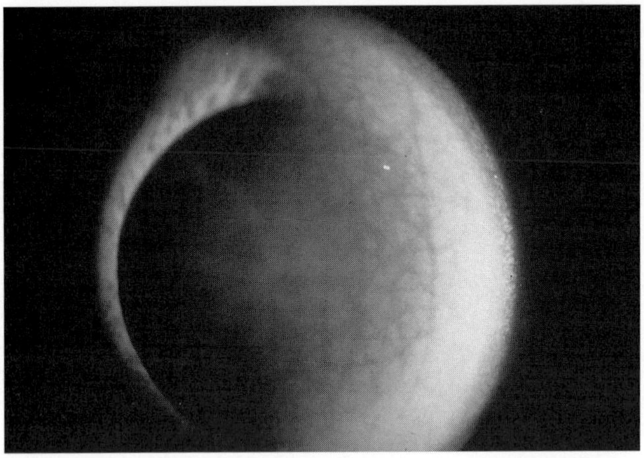

Fig. 3-55 Crocodile shagreen. A common degeneration consisting of a mosaic of multiple gray-white polygonal opacities. They may be concentrated anteriorly or posteriorly. There are no associated visual symptoms.

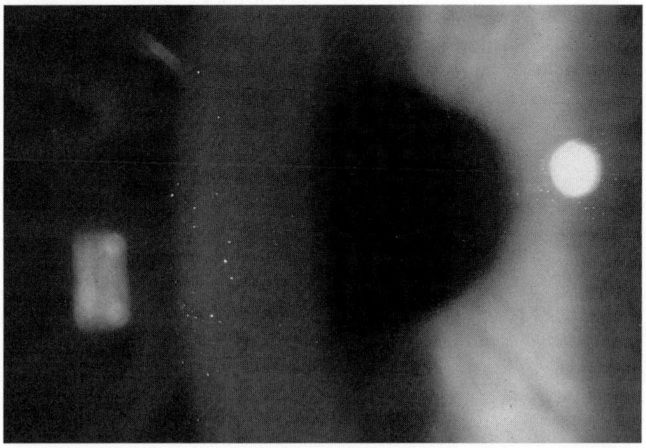

Fig. 3-56 Cornea farinata. Thousands of dustlike dots are found in the posterior stroma. They can be observed in the slit beam but are best seen in retroillumination off the iris and at the edge of the pupil.

Crocodile shagreen Anterior and posterior forms of crocodile shagreen have been observed. Both are characterized by a mosaic pattern of polygonal gray-white opacities separated by relatively clear spaces. Both develop centrally, and their incidence increases with age. The anterior form occurs at the level of Bowman's membrane and superficial stroma, whereas the posterior form is found in the deep stroma and Descemet's membrane (Fig. 3-55). Histologically, there are irregularities in the collagen lamellae centrally. The posterior form may be related to central cloudy dystrophy of François, as discussed earlier. Corneal thickness is normal, vision is unaffected, and no treatment is necessary.

Cornea farinata Cornea farinata is an age-related phenomenon of bilateral fine, pinpoint opacities in the posterior stroma. They resemble flour in color and size, hence the name farinata, which means flour in Latin. They are best seen as dustlike dots on retroillumination off the iris (Fig. 3-56). Histopathologically, they are composed of a lipofuscin-like substance. They do not affect vision, and they require no treatment.

Polymorphic amyloid degeneration Polymorphic amyloid degeneration is a primary localized degenerative form of amyloid deposition in the cornea. It is generally seen in patients older than 50 years, and it is typically bilateral but may be asymmetric. The amyloid deposits are found throughout the cornea but are mostly posterior, and they develop more frequently in the center than in the periphery. The deposits appear gray-white on direct illumination (Figs. 3-57 and 3-58), but are best seen with retroillumination off the iris or retina, where they appear refractile (Fig. 3-59). The shapes of the opacities range from dots, to commas, to single lines, to branching lines reminiscent of lattice corneal dystrophy. They are an incidental finding, do not cause recurrent erosions or decreased vision, and do not necessitate treatment.

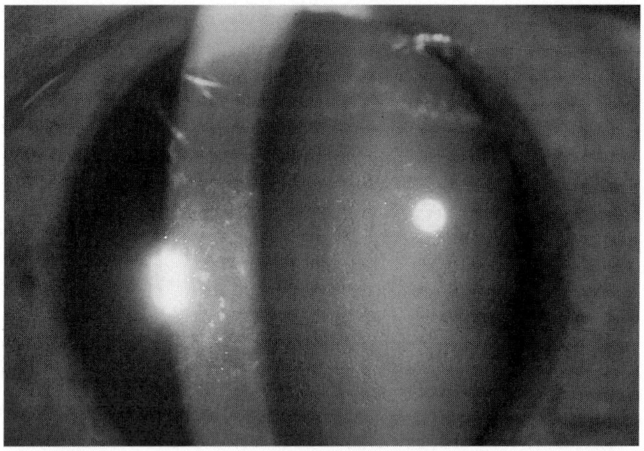

Fig. 3-57 Polymorphic amyloid degeneration. Multiple small refractile opacities in the middle and posterior stroma can be seen in retroillumination off the lens.

Degenerations Not Related to the Aging Process

Terrien's marginal degeneration Terrien's marginal degeneration is a peripheral corneal thinning disorder considered an inflammatory and a degenerative condition. It affects men more than women, and it develops at any age but most commonly between the ages of 20 and 40 years. It is bilateral but it may be asymmetric, and it is slowly progressive. Its cause is unknown (Box 3-9).

Clinically, there is peripheral corneal thinning, which usually begins superiorly but can begin inferiorly. It starts with peripheral white opacities that coalesce to create an arc of corneal thinning (Fig. 3-60). The involved area can progress to severe corneal thinning that may even bulge, but it rarely perforates. The thinned cornea is vascularized and has radial vessels from the limbus (Fig. 3-61).

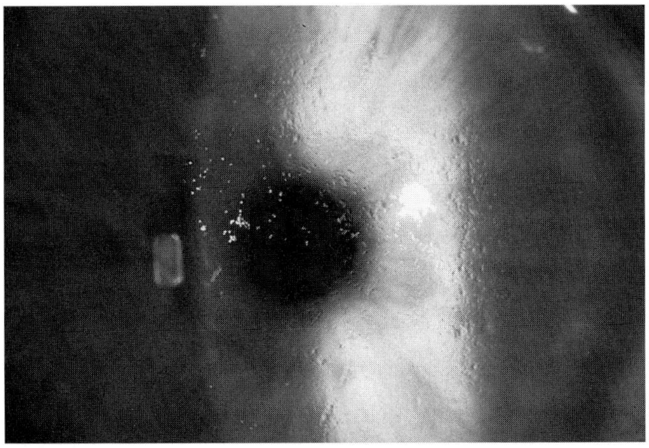

Fig. 3-58 Polymorphic amyloid degeneration. Hundreds of globular and comma-shaped dots are highlighted in retroillumination off the iris.

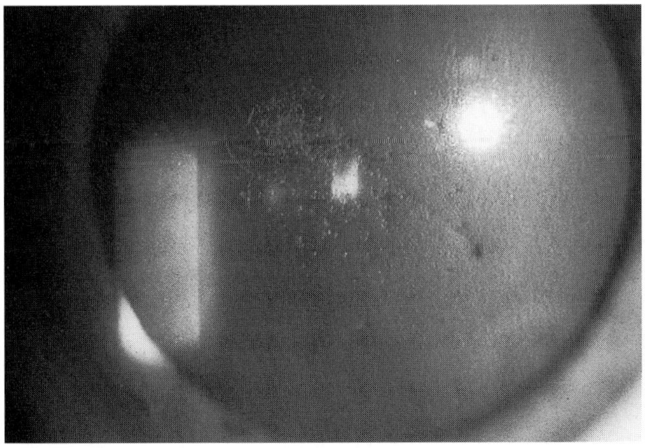

Fig. 3-59 Polymorphic amyloid degeneration. The refractile nature of the amyloid opacities is evident using the red reflex. They are typically dotlike but may be linear (nasally in this left cornea), resembling lattice corneal dystrophy.

There is a relatively abrupt transition from the involved area to the normal thickness cornea (Figs. 3-62 and 3-63). At the central extension of the thinning is a line of yellow-white lipid deposition. The epithelium remains intact throughout this process. It generally progresses circumferentially, but it can progress centrally. In most patients the eyes are white and quiet, and there is little to no active clinical inflammation. However, some patients have recurrent episodic bouts of peripheral keratitis with which associated episcleritis may develop. The active inflammatory process tends to respond to topical corticosteroids, but these medications should be used judiciously.

Terrien's marginal degeneration can create significant irregular astigmatism. When the thinning is primarily superior or inferior, against-the-rule astigmatism develops. Patients' symptoms are generally related to the induced irregular astigmatism that causes decreased vision. In patients with severe corneal thinning, the bulging may cause symptoms of foreign body sensation. With minor or even no trauma, corneal hydrops or perforation can rarely occur. For irregular astigmatism, a rigid or hybrid contact lens can significantly improve vision. Surgical treatment with an inlay crescentic, lamellar, or full-thickness corneal graft may stabilize severe corneal thinning or perforation.

Calcific band keratopathy Calcific band keratopathy, or simply band keratopathy, is a slowly progressive degenerative condition involving calcium deposition across the cornea at the level of Bowman's membrane. It occurs in the interpalpebral zone, typically beginning as a gray-white opacity nasally and temporally (Fig. 3-64), and progressing centrally in a band-shaped pattern (Fig.

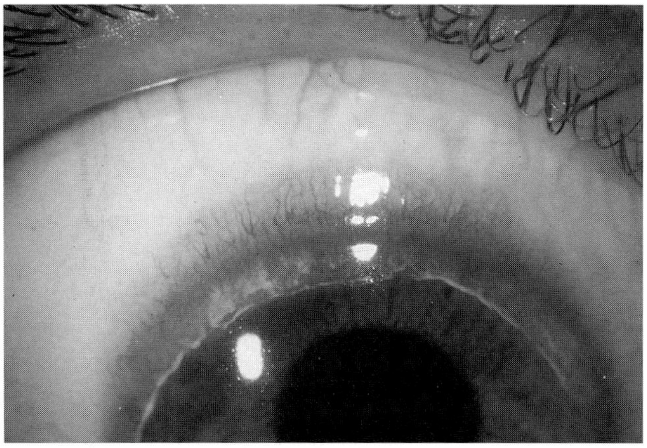

Fig. 3-60 Terrien's marginal degeneration. The superior peripheral cornea is thinned with creamy white infiltrates. The central edge has a dense white line of confluent lipid opacity.

Box 3-9 Critical Features of Terrien's Marginal Degeneration

- Peripheral thinning disorder, usually begins superiorly
- Bilateral but may be asymmetric
- Thinned cornea is vascularized with radial vessels from the limbus
- Lipid deposition at the central extension of the thinning
- Abrupt transition from the involved area to the normal cornea
- Causes significant irregular astigmatism, typically against-the-rule
- Can cause severe corneal thinning and rarely perforation
- Considered inflammatory and degenerative
- Affects men more than women
- Most common between the ages of 20 and 40 years
- Slowly progressive
- Cause unknown

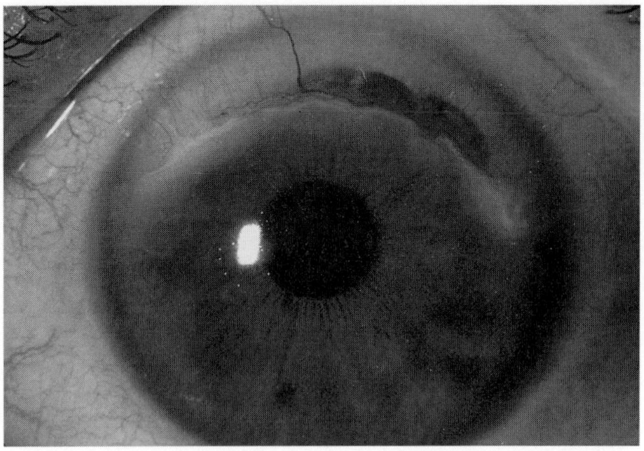

Fig. 3-61 Terrien's marginal degeneration. The thinned area is often vascularized. The vessels typically run radially from the limbus to the leading edge and then track circumferentially.

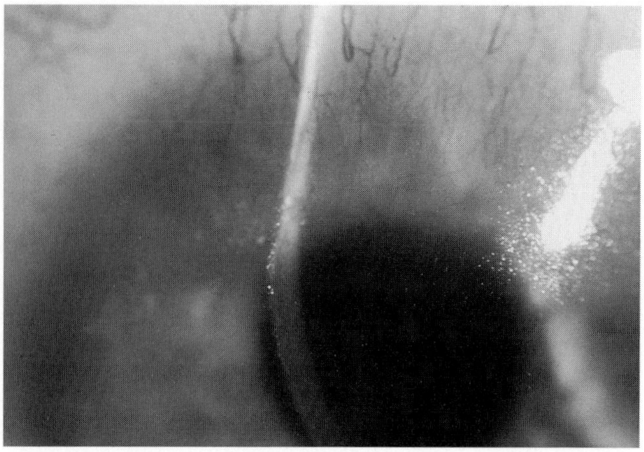

Fig. 3-63 Terrien's marginal degeneration. The slit beam reveals moderate thinning between the limbus and the leading lipid edge.

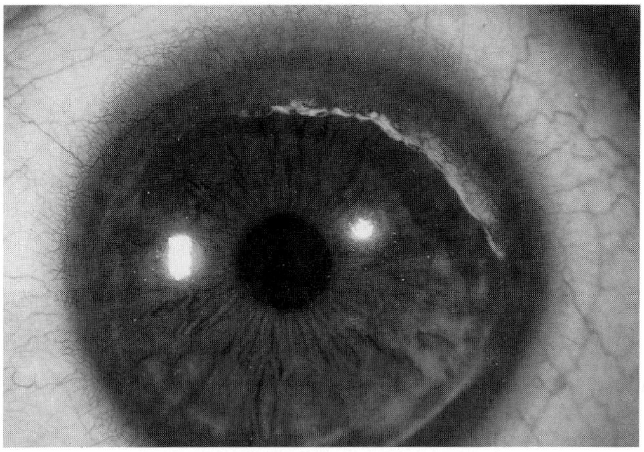

Fig. 3-62 Terrien's marginal degeneration. The thinning and lipid infiltration can involve a few to many clock hours of the peripheral cornea.

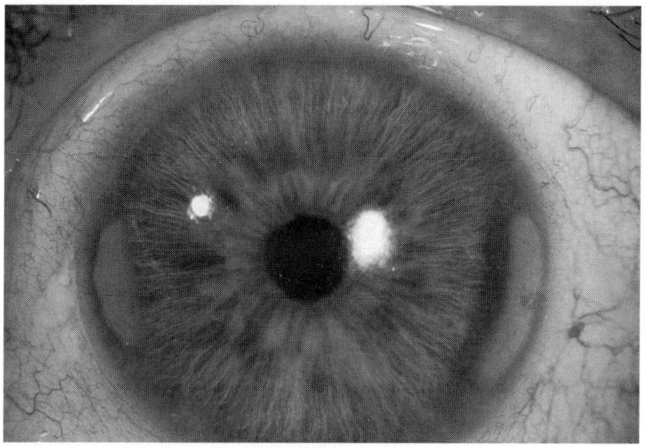

Fig. 3-64 Calcific band keratopathy. In early band keratopathy, the calcium deposition often begins adjacent to the limbus nasally and temporally.

3-65). Occasionally, it can begin centrally. It has a distinct peripheral edge where it is separated from the limbus by a small clear zone. The central border is less well demarcated (Fig. 3-66). There are typically multiple small holes in the band, where corneal nerves penetrate the Bowman's membrane. The calcium deposits can be in a thin, diffuse, relatively uniform strip across the cornea, or they can be in thick discrete plaques. The plaques can flake off, leaving painful epithelial defects at risk for infection. There may be underlying corneal scarring.

Calcific band keratopathy has numerous causes (Box 3-10). The most common is chronic ocular disease that encompasses any chronic inflammatory process, specifically uveitis, especially juvenile rheumatoid arthritis, interstitial keratitis, and phthisis. Other causes include hypercalcemia (associated with renal failure), hyperphosphatemia without hypercalcemia, chronic mercury exposure in the form of vapors or preservatives in ophthalmic preparations, silicone oil in an aphakic eye, and primary hereditary band keratopathy. Noncalcific band keratopathy consisting of yellow urate deposits in the epithelium may develop in patients with gout.

Patients are generally asymptomatic in the early stages of band keratopathy because it involves the peripheral cornea. As the condition progresses, the calcium deposits can cross into the visual axis and affect visual acuity or flake off and cause painful, recurrent, erosive symptoms. In patients with poor visual potential in whom pain does not develop, the cosmetic appearance may be the chief symptom.

The first step in the management of calcific band keratopathy is to determine the underlying cause and to treat it if possible. If discomfort is the primary symptom and visual potential is poor, lubricating ointments may bring significant improvement. However, the best treatment for band keratopathy is calcium chelation or chem-

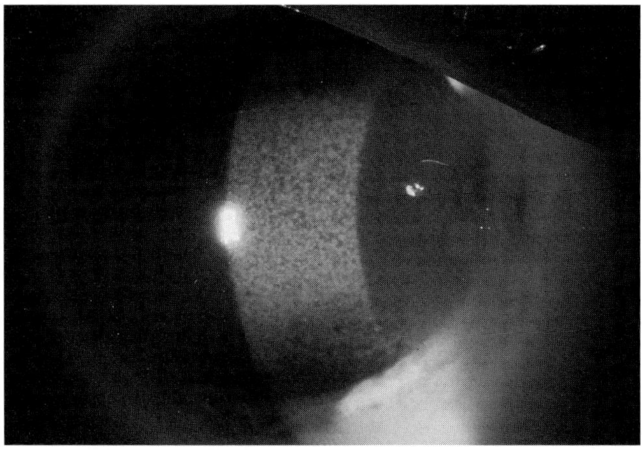

Fig. 3-65 Calcific band keratopathy. In advanced band keratopathy, calcium is deposited from the nasal limbus to the temporal limbus. A Swiss-cheese pattern forms, with tiny clear areas where corneal nerves penetrate Bowman's membrane.

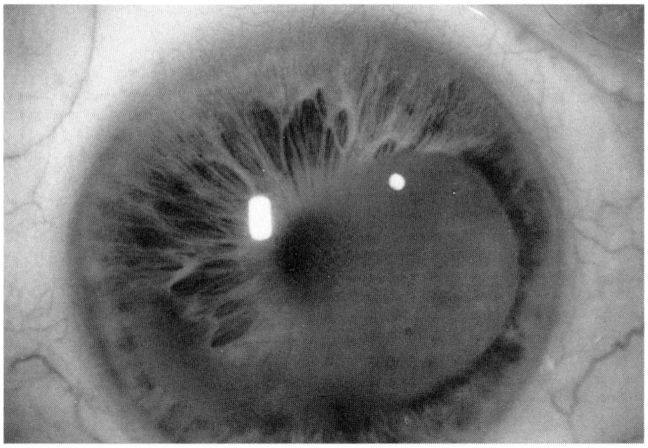

Fig. 3-66 Calcific band keratopathy. There is typically a well-defined clear zone between the limbus and the calcium deposition, whereas the central edge is less distinct. In this eye the opacity is severe enough to almost completely obscure the iris.

ical removal of the calcium. This in-office procedure can be performed using the slit-lamp biomicroscope or the operating microscope. After topical anesthesia is applied and an eyelid speculum is placed, the epithelium overlying the entire area of calcium deposition is removed with a blunt spatula or sharp blade (e.g., no. 15 Bard Parker blade). A cellulose sponge is soaked with diluted disodium ethylenediaminetetraacetic acid (EDTA; Endrate 150 mg/ml). [Note: do not use sodium EDTA.] The EDTA is diluted 1:4 with normal saline. The cellulose sponge is then rubbed against the calcium deposits until they are completely dissolved. Superficial calcium is readily removed, leaving Bowman's membrane intact. The time it takes to achieve complete calcium removal depends on the severity of the band keratopathy, but it

Box 3-10 Causes of Calcific Band Keratopathy

MORE COMMON CAUSES

Chronic ocular disease
- Chronic uveitis (e.g., juvenile rheumatoid arthritis)
- Interstitial keratitis
- Long-standing corneal edema or keratitis
- Phthisis

Silicone oil in an aphakic eye
Idiopathic

LESS COMMON CAUSES

Hypercalcemia (associated with renal failure)
Hyperphosphatemia without hypercalcemia
Chronic mercury exposure (vapors from preservatives in ophthalmic preparations)
Primary hereditary band keratopathy

ranges from 5 to 45 minutes. If thick calcium plaques have formed, it may be possible to scrape them away before the EDTA is applied. Superficial corneal scarring may be present under the calcium and will not respond to chelation. Excimer laser PTK may be used to treat this residual corneal scarring. PTK has been used to treat band keratopathy, but, given the difficulty of treating inhomogeneous pathology, EDTA chelation is the treatment of choice. After surgery the eye is treated for a large corneal abrasion. Band keratopathy can recur after treatment, but it may take years to become symptomatic, and repeat chelation may be necessary in the future.

Spheroidal degeneration Spheroidal degeneration, also called climatic droplet keratopathy, has a variety of other names, including Labrador keratopathy, hyaline degeneration, and chronic actinic keratopathy. Although climatic droplet keratopathy and chronic actinic keratopathy accurately describe its relationship to sun exposure, the condition also involves the conjunctiva so the term spheroidal degeneration will be used.

Clinically this condition begins with clumps of small, clear droplets under the corneal or conjunctival epithelium, and sometimes under both. The droplets generally begin peripherally and advance centrally. With progression of the disorder, the droplets can become gray, white, yellow, and eventually gold or even brown. Small droplets can coalesce, enlarge, and even become elevated. It is found in exposed areas of cornea and conjunctiva, typically interpalpebrally (Fig. 3-67). When the conjunctiva is involved, the spherules are usually smaller and fewer in number. The condition is usually bilateral. It does not generally cause symptoms until the opacities reach the pupillary axis and diminish vision.

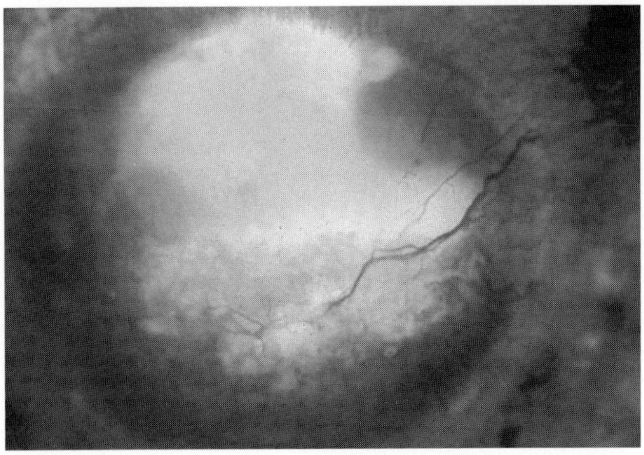

Fig. 3-67 Spheroidal degeneration. Elevated yellow-white globular deposits have become confluent to cover the inferocentral cornea.

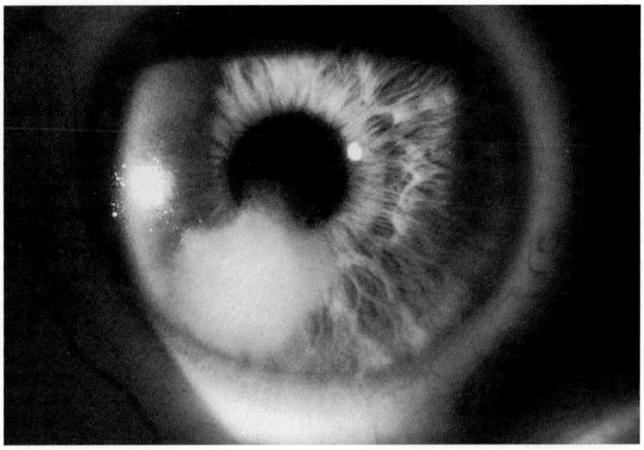

Fig. 3-68 Salzmann's nodular degeneration. A white elevated mass is seen inferiorly. The lesion becomes thinner with fine fingerlike projections at its central edge.

The exact cause of spheroidal degeneration is unclear, but it appears to be related to sun or ultraviolet light exposure, ocular dryness, and exposure to wind, sand, and ice (reflected ultraviolet exposure). It is more prevalent in older patients. It may also be related to chronic corneal inflammation. Although spheroidal degeneration is usually bilateral, if one eye has experienced less actinic exposure, for example from congenital ptosis, or one eye has had more chronic inflammation, the condition may be asymmetric or even unilateral. Histologically, the droplets are composed of hyaline material. Spheroidal degeneration tends to be slowly progressive as long as the causative factors remain.

Treatment is considered when the opacities become symptomatic, which typically means they affect the vision. However, large lesions can cause foreign body sensation or even cosmetic problems. Surgical removal is generally successful. Conjunctival lesions can be excised directly. Elevated and anterior corneal lesions can be removed by superficial keratectomy with a blade or by excimer laser PTK. Deeper lesions may require lamellar or penetrating keratoplasty.

Salzmann's nodular degeneration Salzmann's nodular degeneration usually develops in corneas with a history of a chronic inflammatory condition, such as interstitial keratitis, vernal keratoconjunctivitis, and keratoconjunctivitis sicca, but it may appear in eyes with no known history of keratitis. It is often, but not always, bilateral. Salzmann's nodules are more prevalent in women than in men and develop more frequently as patients age.

Clinically, single or multiple white or gray-white elevated lesions are found in the corneal periphery, midperiphery, or central cornea (Figs. 3-68 and 3-69). Size and elevation of the nodules vary greatly. Between the nodules the cornea is relatively unaffected. The underlying cornea may be scarred, vascularized, edematous, or normal, depending on the patient. Long-standing Salzmann's nodules may demonstrate iron pigment deposition surrounding the base of the lesions.

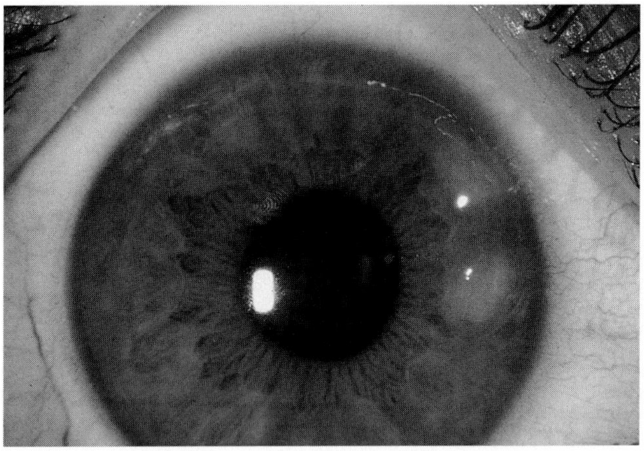

Fig. 3-69 Salzmann's nodular degeneration. Two large lesions are present at the 2 and 3 o'clock positions of the peripheral cornea. They are moderately elevated. A faint early lesion can be seen in the periphery at the 9 o'clock position.

Histopathologically, the nodules are composed of hyalinized collagen material between the epithelium and the stroma. Bowman's membrane may be intact or absent under the lesion.

Patients are usually asymptomatic unless the lesions involve the visual axis. Occasionally, elevated lesions can affect contact lens wear or cause epithelial erosions. Symptomatic patients can typically be successfully treated with superficial keratectomy with a blade. Under topical or local anesthesia, the nodules are generally easily removed by peeling them from the cornea, leaving Bowman's membrane intact. Occasionally, a smooth plane between Bowman's membrane and the lesion

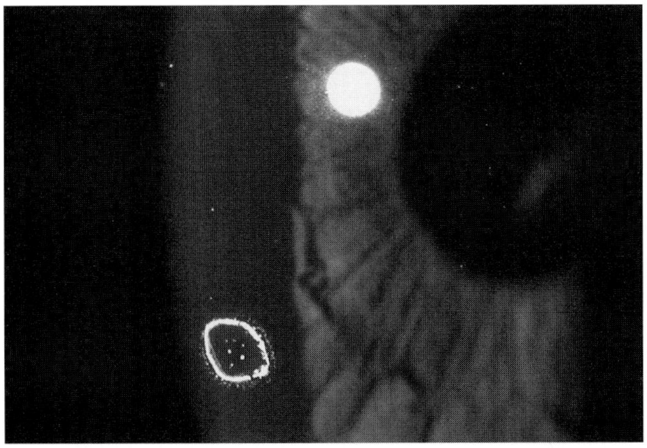

Fig. 3-70 Coats' white ring. A small, dense, white oval ring is present after the removal of an iron foreign body.

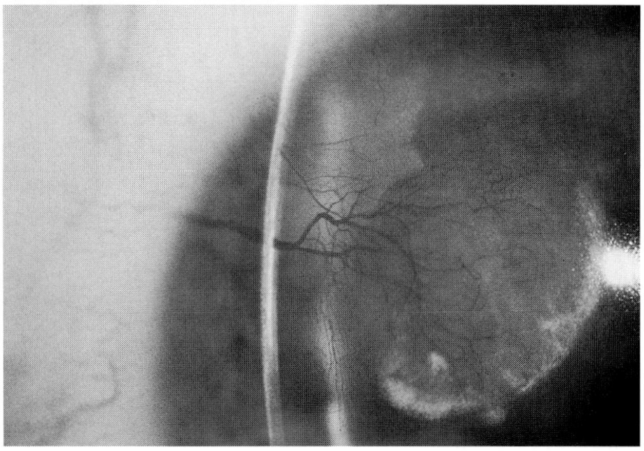

Fig. 3-72 Lipid keratopathy. A lipid fan develops at the terminus of a large area of corneal neovascularization in the eye of a patient with herpes simplex keratitis.

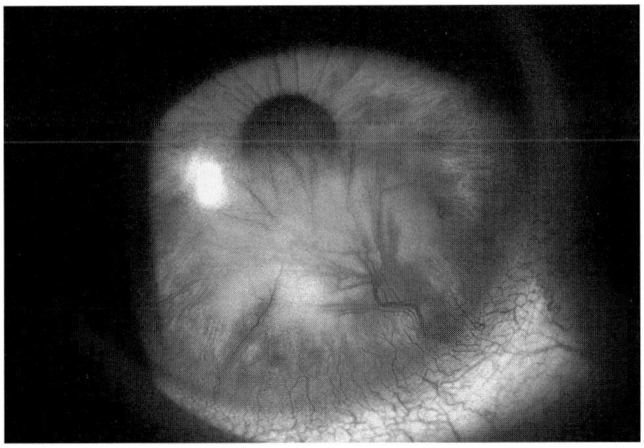

Fig. 3-71 Lipid keratopathy. Long-standing deep corneal neovascularization, secondary to contact lens abuse, causes a severe lipid deposition around the blood vessels.

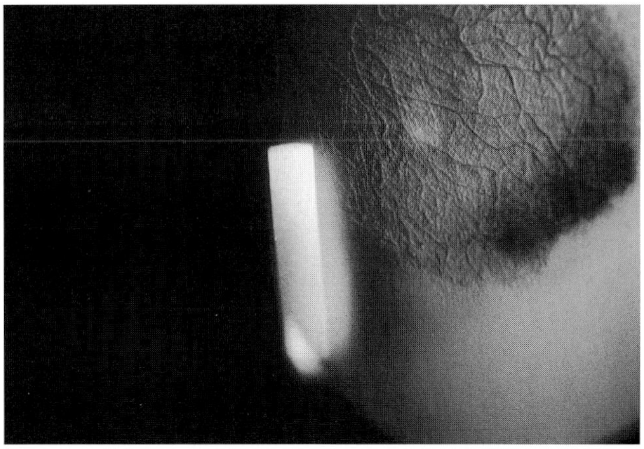

Fig. 3-73 Lipid keratopathy. The neovascularization is well seen in the red reflex. The blurred terminus is the lipid deposition.

cannot be created, and excimer laser PTK may be the best treatment option. Even more rarely is lamellar or penetrating keratoplasty indicated for deep stromal disease beneath the degenerative changes.

Coats' white ring Coats' white ring rarely causes any symptoms and is typically an incidental finding. It consists of a small white ring, generally 1 mm or smaller in diameter, in the superficial cornea, usually in Bowman's membrane or the anterior stroma (Fig. 3-70). It may be a partial or complete oval or circle. The overlying epithelium is normal. The lesion is composed of iron and is caused by previous trauma from a metallic foreign body.

Lipid keratopathy Primary lipid keratopathy is rare; secondary lipid keratopathy is more common. In the primary form lipids are deposited in both eyes, usually centrally, in a nonvascularized cornea without a history of corneal trauma or inflammation. Secondary lipid keratopathy, or lipid degeneration, is related to the presence of corneal blood vessels or, less often, to previous corneal necrosis. It can be found in any eye with corneal stromal neovascularization but is seen most typically after corneal trauma or ulceration and in eyes with interstitial keratitis or herpetic (simplex or zoster) keratitis. Severe corneal neovascularization related to hypoxia from contact lens abuse, though rare, can also cause lipid keratopathy.

In secondary lipid keratopathy, dense yellow-white lipid deposits appear in the stroma around the area of vascularization (Fig. 3-71). It typically has a feathery appearance at the edge away from the blood vessels. A fanlike pattern can develop at the ends of the blood vessels (Figs. 3-72 and 3-73). There may be refractile crystalline deposits in the stroma alone or in addition to denser opacities. It usually takes months to years for them to develop, but they may arise quickly.

Clinical management consists of treating the underlying condition. Any therapy, such as topical corticosteroids, to reduce or eliminate the corneal neovascularization may lead to improvement in the lipid deposition or may control disease progression. Laser treatment of the corneal neovascularization usually does not permanently close the blood vessels or bring about resolution of the lipid deposition. Corneal transplantation can be attempted for severe vision-threatening lipid keratopathy, but the prognosis for grafts in vascularized corneas is guarded because of the increased risk for graft rejection and the nature of the underlying disease. Additionally, if the neovascularization remains, lipid deposits may recur (Box 3-11).

Box 3-11 Dystrophies and Degenerations That Do and Do Not Affect Vision

GENERALLY AFFECT VISION

- Meesmann's dystrophy
- Reis-Bücklers' dystrophy (CDB-1)
- Thiel-Behnke dystrophy (CDB-2)
- Granular dystrophy
- Lattice dystrophy, type 1
- Avellino dystrophy
- Fuchs' dystrophy
- Congenital hereditary endothelial dystrophy
- Macular dystrophy
- Terrien's marginal degeneration
- Calcific band keratopathy
- Spheroidal degeneration
- Salzmann's nodular degeneration
- Lipid keratopathy

MAY AFFECT VISION

- Anterior basement membrane dystrophy
- Schnyder's crystalline dystrophy
- Posterior amorphous stromal dystrophy
- Congenital hereditary stromal dystrophy
- Posterior polymorphous dystrophy
- Lattice dystrophy, types 2 and 3

GENERALLY DO NOT AFFECT VISION

- Fleck dystrophy
- Central cloudy dystrophy of François
- Arcus senilis
- Hassall-Henle bodies
- Limbal girdle of Vogt
- Crocodile shagreen
- Cornea farinata
- Polymorphic amyloid degeneration
- Coats' white ring

CORNEAL PIGMENTATIONS

Iron

Iron is a common source of pigment deposition in the cornea. Needless to say, an iron foreign body can enter the cornea and a portion may remain at any level. Coats' white ring, a small circle of residual iron deposition in the anterior stroma that forms after the entry of a superficial corneal foreign body, was discussed previously. Otherwise, most corneal iron deposition occurs in the epithelial cells.

Numerous iron lines have been identified (Fig. 3-74). A Hudson-Stähli line, a wavy horizontal line of iron deposition at the inferior third of the cornea where the lower eyelid meets the cornea, is associated with aging. Many iron lines develop at the base of corneal topographic abnormalities. A Fleischer ring is iron deposition at the base of the cone in keratoconus. Depending on the severity of the keratoconus, the ring may be small or large, complete or incomplete. A Ferry line is iron deposition at the anterior edge of a filtering bleb. A Stocker line is iron deposition at the head of a pterygium. Iron lines can be seen at the base of other corneal irregularities, such as Salzmann's nodules. Stellate iron patterns are also found after refractive surgery for myopia, such as radial keratot-

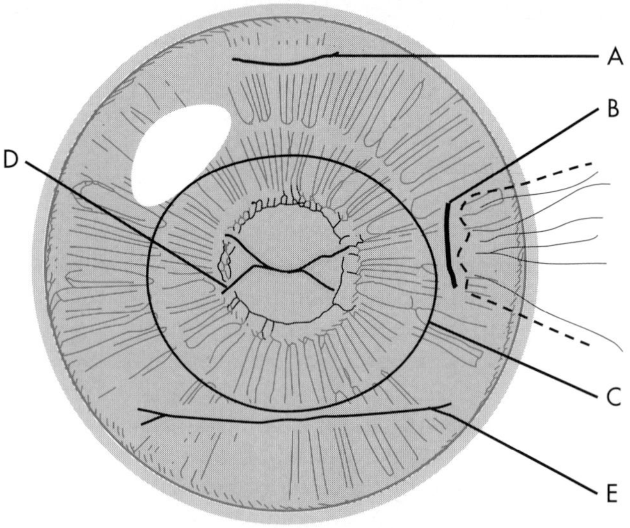

Fig. 3-74 Corneal iron lines. A Ferry line (**A**) is located central to a filtering bleb. A Stocker line (**B**) is found central to a pterygium. A Fleischer ring (**C**) is located at the base of the cone in keratoconus. It may be partial or complete and may be found centrally or inferiorly, depending on the severity and location of the cone. After myopic refractive surgery, an iron line, often stellate (**D**), can be seen centrally. A Hudson-Stähli line (**E**) is a horizontal iron line found at the level of the lower eyelid tear meniscus, approximately one third the way up the cornea.

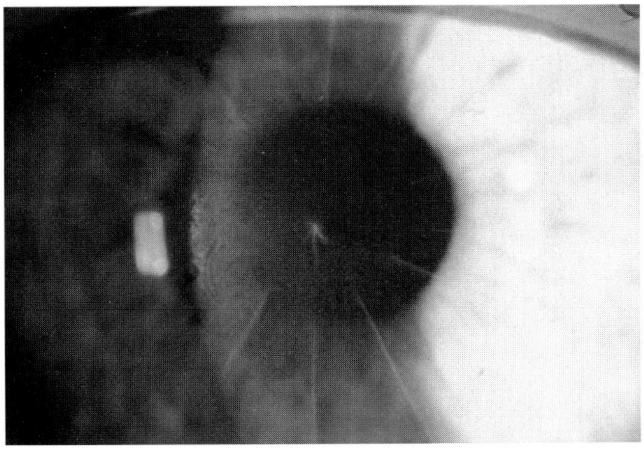

Fig. 3-75 An iron line after refractive surgery. A stellate iron pattern forms in the central cornea many years after 16-incision radial keratotomy.

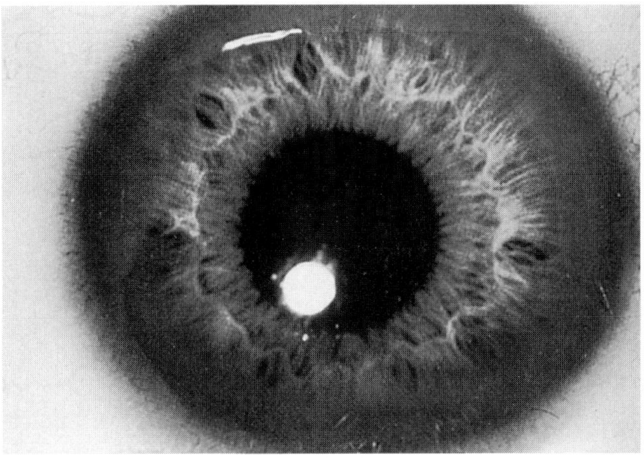

Fig. 3-76 Kayser-Fleischer ring. A brown peripheral corneal ring is seen in the deep cornea and Descemet's membrane, primarily in Wilson's disease. In early stages, it may be visible only on gonioscopy.

Box 3-12 Epithelial Iron Lines

Hudson-Stähli line—inferior third of the cornea, associated with aging
Fleischer ring—base of the cone in keratoconus
Ferry line—anterior edge of a filtering bleb
Stocker line—head of a pterygium
Base of other corneal irregularities, such as Salzmann's nodules
Central stellate patterns after refractive surgery

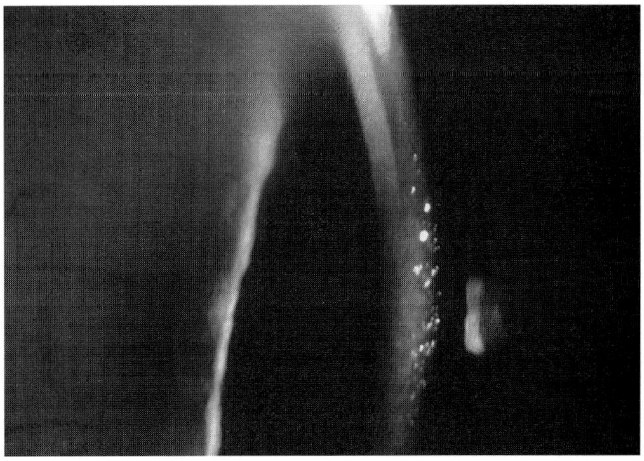

Fig. 3-77 Kayser-Fleischer ring. The brown copper pigment can be seen in the deep peripheral cornea using the slit beam.

omy (Fig. 3-75), excimer laser photorefractive keratectomy, and laser in situ keratomileusis (Box 3-12).

Siderosis is iron deposition within the eye. It generally occurs from an intraocular foreign body, but it can also result from systemic iron overload such as may occur in hemochromatosis. In the anterior segment the iron can be deposited in the iris to cause heterochromia and mydriasis or may be deposited in the lens to cause a cataract. Yellow-brown iron pigment may develop in the posterior stroma, especially if the metal foreign body is in the anterior chamber. Irreversible retinal degeneration can also occur.

Melanin

Striate melanokeratosis refers to the epithelial pigment lines that run centrally from the limbus. It usually occurs in dark-skinned persons or after ocular trauma or inflammation. Rarely, corneal melanin results from conjunctival melanoma that may or may not appear significantly pigmented.

Copper

Ocular chalcosis is copper deposition in the eye. It usually occurs secondary to an intraocular copper foreign body. In the cornea, it causes a gray-green discoloration of Descemet's membrane. If the copper content of the foreign body is greater than 85%, it can cause severe suppurative endophthalmitis.

A Kayser-Fleischer ring is a yellow-brown or gray-green discoloration at the level of Descemet's membrane in the corneal periphery (Figs. 3-76 and 3-77). It is seen earliest with the use of gonioscopy in the superior cornea. It is found in Wilson's disease (hepatolenticular degeneration), an autosomal recessive disorder resulting in the accumulation of copper in the body. It is sometimes seen in patients with primary biliary cirrhosis, chronic

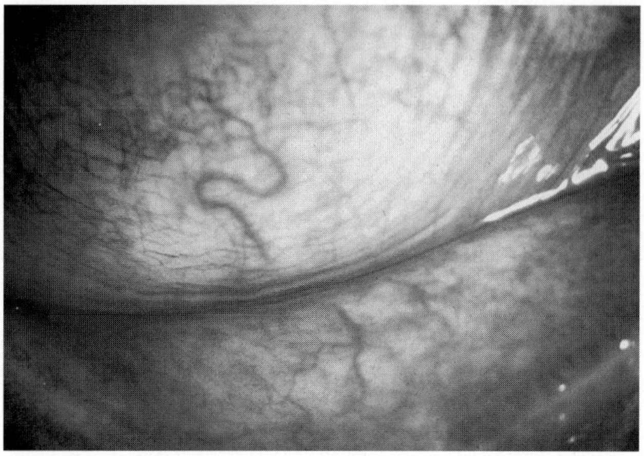

Fig. 3-78 Argyrosis. Long-term use of silver-containing medications (e.g., Argyrol) can lead to a gold-gray deposition of silver in the bulbar and palpebral conjunctiva.

active hepatitis, progressive intrahepatic cholestasis, and, even more rarely, multiple myeloma. Treatment to remove copper from the patient's body, such as with D-penicillamine, can be monitored by following the disappearance of the Kayser-Fleischer ring.

Gold

Gold deposition in the cornea, termed corneal chrysiasis, results from systemic gold treatment, typically for rheumatoid arthritis. The gold deposits are yellow-brown and generally occur in the deep stroma and Descemet's membrane. Although the deposits do not cause ocular symptoms and do not necessitate the discontinuation of therapy, the deposits may be reversible if the gold treatments cease.

Silver

Argyrosis is the term for silver deposition in the eye. While it occurred commonly in the past with the widespread use of silver-containing topical medications such as Argyrol, argyrosis is rarely seen today. The deposits cause a diffuse gray discoloration of the conjunctiva (Fig. 3-78) and eyelid skin. Descemet's membrane becomes gold-gray in the periphery, but this discoloration does not affect vision.

IRIDOCORNEAL ENDOTHELIAL SYNDROME

The term iridocorneal endothelial (ICE) syndrome comprises three related entities, Chandler's syndrome, essential iris atrophy, and iris nevus syndrome. The primary abnormality involves the corneal endothelium. This entity shares many characteristics with posterior polymorphous dystrophy. However, PPMD is hereditary, bilateral, and slowly progressive, whereas the ICE syndrome is sporadic, usually unilateral, and more rapidly progressive (see Table 3-5). Additionally, in the ICE syndrome, there are often glaucoma and iris abnormalities, including peripheral anterior synechiae, iris atrophy, iris holes, and iris nodules. The three components of the ICE syndrome vary in their degree of corneal and iris abnormality (Box 3-13 and Table 3-6).

Box 3-13 Characteristics of Iridocorneal Endothelial Syndrome

Sporadic
Usually unilateral
Relatively rapidly progressive
Often difficult to control glaucoma
Abnormal corneal endothelial cells with epithelial cell properties
Three components
- Chandler's syndrome
- Essential iris atrophy (progressive iris atrophy)
- Iris nevus syndrome (Cogan-Reese syndrome)

In Chandler's syndrome the corneal endothelial abnormalities are the most prominent. Here, the posterior corneal surface has a hammered silver appearance. There is a variable degree of corneal edema, from none to bullous keratopathy. Specular microscopic evaluation demonstrates patches of normal endothelial cells adjacent to patches of abnormal cells. The pathologic cells are larger than normal and have white peripheries, dark bodies, and a white central dot. There may be related iris abnormalities.

Iris changes are most notable in essential (or progressive) iris atrophy and iris nevus syndrome. In essential iris atrophy there are broad-based peripheral anterior synechiae. The central iris is pulled toward the synechiae, leading to ectropion uveae, corectopia, and iris atrophy (Figs. 3-79 and 3-80), and eventually hole formation on the opposite side (Figs. 3-81, 3-82, 3-83, and 3-84). Gonioscopic examination reveals endothelialization of the anterior chamber angle, occasionally severe enough to cause angle-closure glaucoma.

Iris nevus syndrome, also called Cogan-Reese syndrome, is really a misnomer. Small iris nodules result from endothelialization of the iris, causing flattening of the normal iris crypt architecture, but small knuckles of iris stroma protrude anteriorly through holes in the membrane, simulating nevi. It can also appear as a diffuse flat, pigmented area, resembling a large iris nevus and causing iris heterochromia.

The clinical presentation of ICE syndrome depends on the particular variant. Chandler's syndrome typically presents with decreased vision, and occasionally painful

Table 3-6 Iridocorneal endothelial syndrome: three clinical variations

Feature	Chandler's syndrome	Essential (progressive) iris atrophy	Iris nevus (Cogan-Reese) syndrome
Primary symptom	Corneal edema	Iris atrophy, holes, corectopia	Iris nodules or areas of increased pigment
Corneal edema	Early	Possible	Possible
Iris abnormalities	Minimal	Severe	Severe
		Broad-based peripheral anterior synechiae	Multiple small pigmented iris nodules
		Iris atrophy and holes on opposite side of synechiae	Large iris nevi
			Iris heterochromia

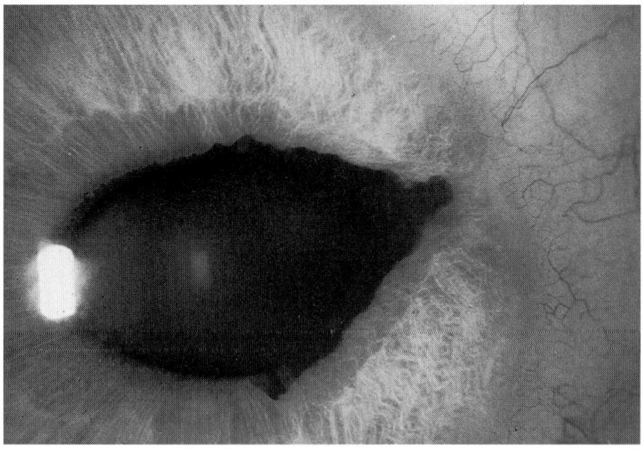

Fig. 3-79 Iridocorneal endothelial syndrome. Ectropion uveae and corectopia are evident in this eye with essential iris atrophy.

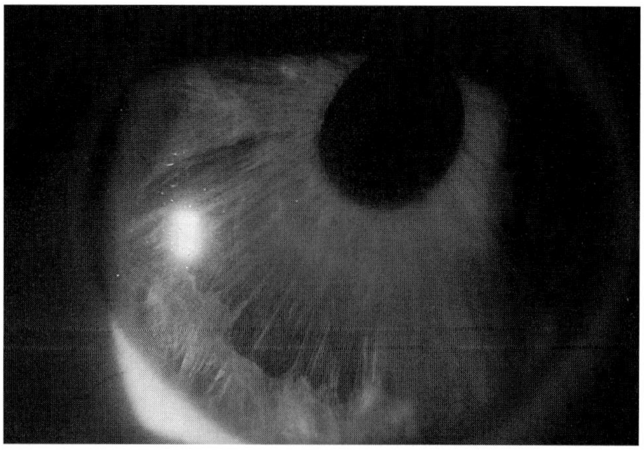

Fig. 3-81 Iridocorneal endothelial syndrome. In this eye with essential iris atrophy, the iris is pulled toward the 1 o'clock position, and there is notable stretching and thinning of the iris from the 5 to 10 o'clock positions.

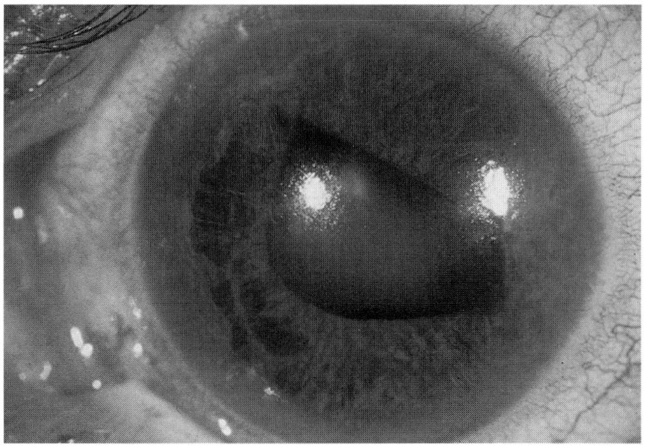

Fig. 3-80 Iridocorneal endothelial syndrome. Extensive iris abnormalities are present in this patient with essential iris atrophy. Ectropion uveae is noted at the 4 and 11 o'clock positions. Broad peripheral anterior synechiae can be seen from the 6 to 12 o'clock positions.

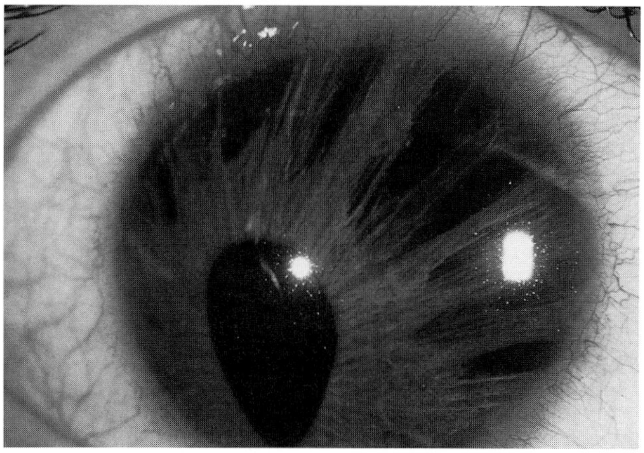

Fig. 3-82 Iridocorneal endothelial syndrome. Multiple iris holes are evident superiorly in this patient with severe essential iris atrophy.

symptoms, from bullous keratopathy. Patients with essential iris atrophy and iris nevus syndrome generally have good vision unless glaucoma develops. Often the diagnosis is made on routine evaluation or when the patient seeks care for an iris irregularity.

Histopathologic evaluation of ICE syndrome has found endothelial overgrowth in the anterior chamber. The corneal endothelial cells can migrate over the angle to cover the trabecular meshwork (pulling the iris and causing the PAS and iris holes in essential iris atrophy) leading to the restriction of outflow and causing glaucoma. In patients with iris nevus syndrome, the endothelium can grow

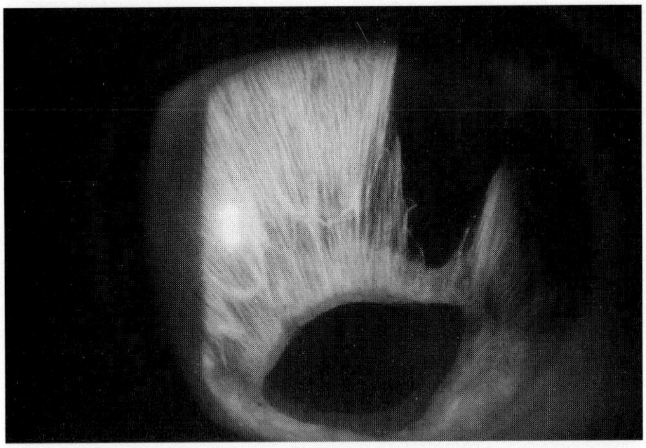

Fig. 3-83 Iridocorneal endothelial syndrome. Ectropion uveae is present inferiorly and a large hole in the iris is present superiorly in this eye with essential iris atrophy.

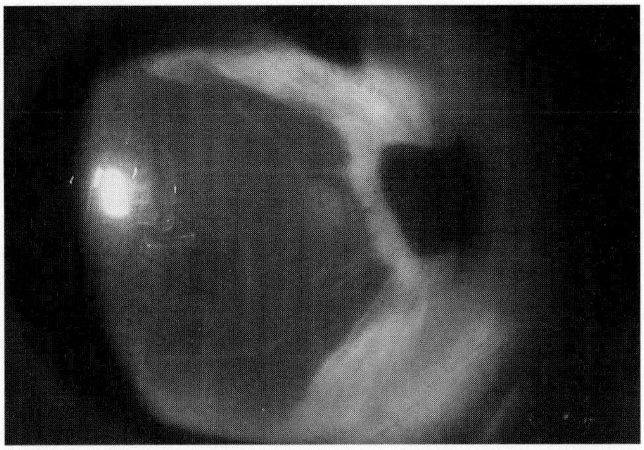

Fig. 3-84 Iridocorneal endothelial syndrome. Severe essential iris atrophy is present, with large-hole formation from the 7 to 10 o'clock positions and only a small pupil present at the 3 o'clock position. There is moderate corneal edema with Descemet's folds.

over large sections of the iris, leaving small holes through which the iris stroma pokes out. Normal and abnormal populations of corneal endothelial cells are seen. Abnormal endothelial cells often have characteristics of epithelial cells, such as surface microvilli. These epithelial characteristics include loss of contact inhibition, allowing endothelialization of the anterior segment to occur. Interestingly, though ICE syndrome is clinically unilateral, specular microscopic changes of pleomorphism and polymegethism have been noted in contralateral eyes. The cause of ICE syndrome is unknown, but a herpes simplex viral etiology is suspected based on polymerase chain reaction studies.

The management of ICE syndrome depends on the symptoms and the clinical problem. In Chandler's syndrome, corneal edema predominates. Mild corneal edema can be treated with topical hyperosmotics and intraocular pressure-lowering medications, even when the intraocular pressure is only mildly elevated. Severe corneal edema, affecting vision or causing painful symptoms, can be treated with penetrating keratoplasty. In all three variants, glaucoma is a common problem that is difficult to treat. Medical management is often successful temporarily, but surgical treatment is frequently required. Although trabeculectomy is frequently successful, these blebs are subject to failure from endothelialization. Control of the glaucoma in ICE syndrome is extremely important for maintaining good vision and a clear graft.

ECTATIC CONDITIONS

Keratoconus, pellucid marginal degeneration, and keratoglobus are all disorders of corneal ectasia without evidence of active corneal inflammation (Table 3-7 and Fig. 3-85).

Keratoconus

Keratoconus is by far the most prevalent ectatic corneal condition. Typically, the pathologic process in keratoconus is central or inferocentral corneal thinning and steepening. The thinnest area of the cornea is at the apex of the cone. Keratoconus may begin earlier, but it is generally first noted during puberty to late adolescence. It starts off mild, progresses for years, and then stabilizes. It is found in males and females. Keratoconus is usually bilateral, though frequently asymmetric. It presents most commonly with decreased vision that is not fully correctable with spectacles. Often patients try multiple prescriptions for spectacles within a short period of time, none of which are satisfactory. The sine qua non of keratoconus is irregular astigmatism, which explains why spectacles do not adequately correct the vision (Box 3-14).

Early signs of keratoconus include central or inferocentral corneal thinning and steepening that may be seen on careful slit-lamp examination (Fig. 3-86). Multiple fine vertical or oblique stress lines (Vogt's striae) are often seen in the posterior stroma at the apex of the cone. These lines may change direction or may disappear when gentle pressure is placed at the limbus. An iron line (Fleischer ring) may be visible around the base of the cone (Fig. 3-87). It may be a complete ring, especially in central cones, or a partial ring, seen in inferior cones. The Fleischer ring is brown and is best seen using a broad slit beam from the side. A cobalt blue filter may aid in visualizing faint Fleischer rings. Even in mild keratoconus, the retinoscopic reflex is distorted, yielding a scissors pattern on streak retinoscopy. With keratometry, the mires are irregular, and the central readings steep, which become even steeper as the patient looks up and the inferior cornea is measured. Placido disc evaluation demonstrates ovoid rings shaped like water droplets.

Table 3-7 Characteristics of the three ectatic conditions of the cornea

Feature	Keratoconus	Pellucid marginal degeneration	Keratoglobus
Frequency	Uncommon	Very uncommon	Rare
Age of onset	12-25 years	20-40 years	Birth
Laterality	Bilateral, often asymmetric	Bilateral, often asymmetric	Bilateral
Area of greatest thinning	Inferocentral and central	Inferior periphery, 1-2 mm wide, from 4-8 o'clock positions	Entire cornea, especially peripherally
Area of greatest protrusion	At apex of thinnest area	Just above band of thinning	Entire central cornea
Iron line	Partially or entirely surrounds cone Fleischer ring	Occasional	None
Scarring	Common at apex of cone	Uncommon	Uncommon
Corneal stress lines	Common Vogt's striae	Uncommon	Uncommon
Hydrops	Uncommon	Very uncommon	Rare
Perforation	Rare	Rare	Not uncommon, with little or no trauma
Contact lenses	Usually successful	Often successful	Often contraindicated to decrease trauma to cornea
Surgical treatment	Penetrating keratoplasty	Large eccentric penetrating keratoplasty	Large tectonic lamellar graft May require secondary small central penetrating graft

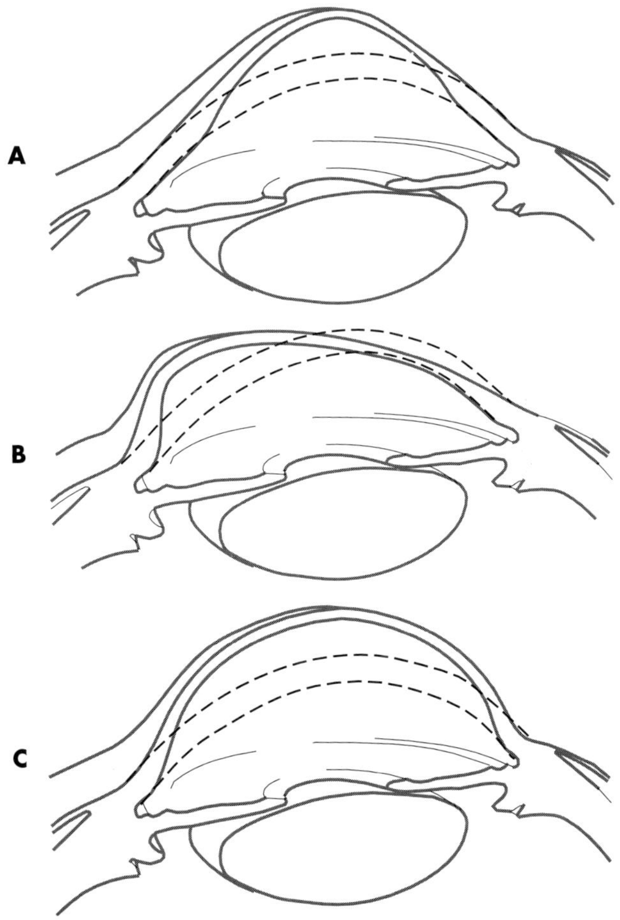

Fig. 3-85 Ectatic corneal conditions. (**A**) Keratoconus. The thinning is central or inferocentral. The thinnest and most protruded portions of the cornea are in the same location. (**B**) Pellucid marginal degeneration. The thinning occurs 1 to 2 mm from the inferior corneal periphery. The most protruded area of the cornea is slightly more central than the thinnest area of cornea. (**C**) Keratoglobus. The entire cornea is thinned to the periphery.

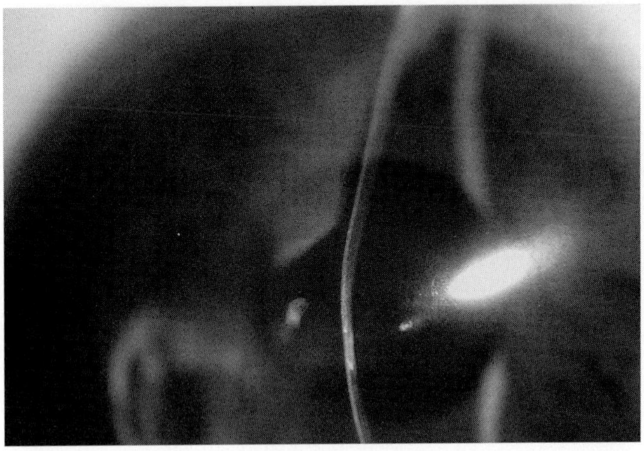

Fig. 3-86 Keratoconus. Central corneal thinning and irregularity are present. The superior cornea appears abnormally flat, whereas the inferior cornea appears steep.

Fig. 3-87 Keratoconus. A prominent Fleischer ring, iron deposition in the epithelial cells at the base of the cone, can be seen in this well-dilated eye.

Box 3-14 Early and Late Signs of Keratoconus

EARLIEST SIGNS

Inferior steepening and irregular astigmatism on computed corneal topography
Inferior steepening on keratometric examination
Irregular scissors reflex on retinoscopic examination

EARLY SIGNS

Mild central or inferocentral corneal thinning
Mild central or inferocentral corneal steepening
Fleischer ring
Vogt's stria

LATER SIGNS

Superficial corneal scarring
Breaks in Bowman's membrane
Visible corneal nerves
Munson's sign
Apical corneal nodule

LATEST SIGNS

Acute corneal hydrops
Dense central corneal scarring
Severe apical corneal thinning

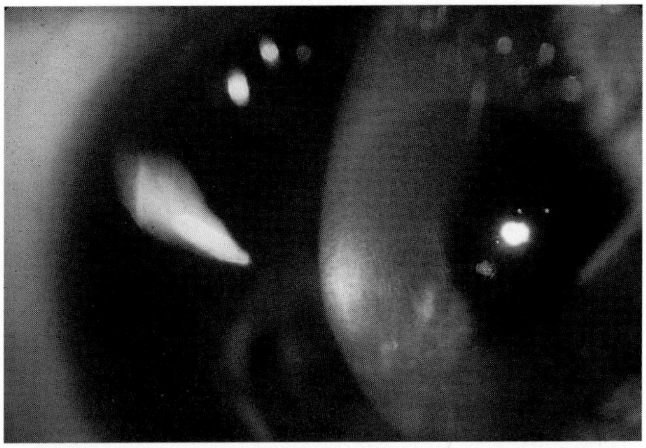

Fig. 3-88 Keratoconus. Corneal scarring is apparent at the inferior aspect of the pupil. A segment of a Fleischer ring is present at the superior edge of the pupil. Faint Vogt's striae, vertical stress lines in the posterior stroma, can be seen in the 6 to 7 o'clock portion of the pupil.

Later signs include superficial corneal scarring, typically at the protrusion of the cone (Fig. 3-88). Breaks in Bowman's membrane may become visible. Corneal nerves may also become more apparent. In some patients a nodule develops at the apex of the cone, typically related to a contact lens, and may interfere with comfortable contact lens wear or even vision. Munson's sign is apparent in advanced keratoconus. It can be seen by noting the V-shaped pattern the cone forms in the lower eyelid as the patient gazes downward and the upper eyelid is raised.

Acute corneal hydrops develops when Descemet's membrane is stretched so much that it tears. This acute opening in Descemet's membrane allows aqueous fluid to rush into the cornea, causing immediate pain, corneal edema, and diminished vision (Figs. 3-89 and 3-90). Acute hydrops rarely leads to corneal perforation, and it is not an indication for emergency corneal transplantation. The edema is observed or treated medically with hypertonic drops and aqueous suppressants and generally resolves within 3 to 6 months. Corneal scarring remains, but the cornea may be flatter than before (Fig. 3-91). If the scar is outside the visual axis, the flatter cornea may improve vision and contact lens tolerance.

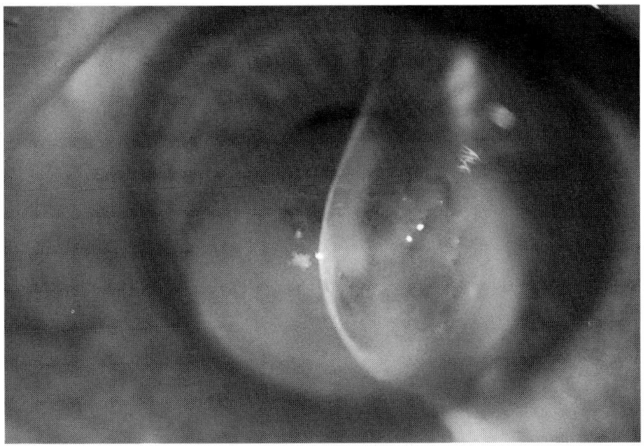

Fig. 3-89 Keratoconus. Acute corneal hydrops occurs when a break develops in Descemet's membrane, suddenly allowing aqueous fluid into the corneal stroma. The slit beam demonstrates the dramatic corneal thickening, perhaps five times the normal corneal thickness. The clear space at the inferior aspect of the hydrops is an intracorneal cleft filled with aqueous.

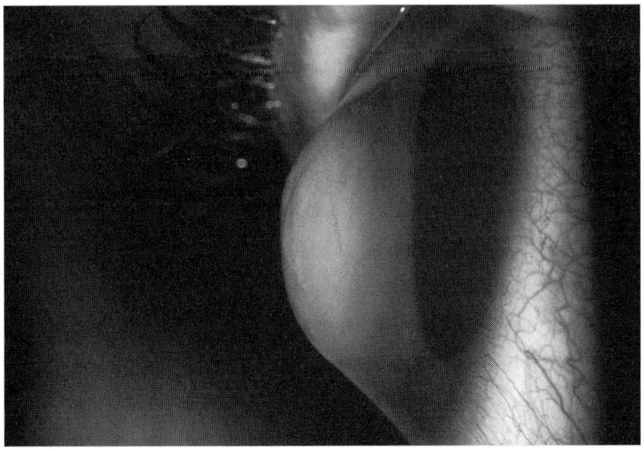

Fig. 3-90 Keratoconus. Side view of the severe corneal thickening in acute corneal hydrops.

However, more typically, the vision is decreased after acute hydrops, eventually necessitating corneal transplantation for better vision.

In moderate and severe keratoconus, it is not difficult to make the diagnosis. However, in milder cases, it is not always apparent. The most sensitive method for evaluating corneal curvature and detecting mild irregularities is computerized videokeratography or corneal topography. This evolving technology, reviewed in detail in Chapter 9, can demonstrate very mild changes in corneal curvature that are not readily visible on slit-lamp or keratometric examination. Mild irregular astigmatism or inferior or central corneal steepening may indicate subclinical or early keratoconus (Fig. 3-92). Whereas most ophthalmologists require some slit-lamp changes consistent with keratoconus to make the diagnosis, early signs of keratoconus on corneal topography can be helpful in

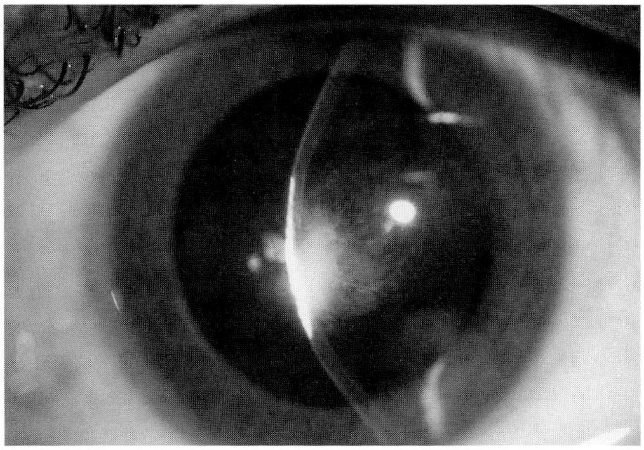

Fig. 3-91 Keratoconus. Significant central corneal scarring remains after an episode of acute corneal hydrops. A faint Fleischer ring can be seen superiorly.

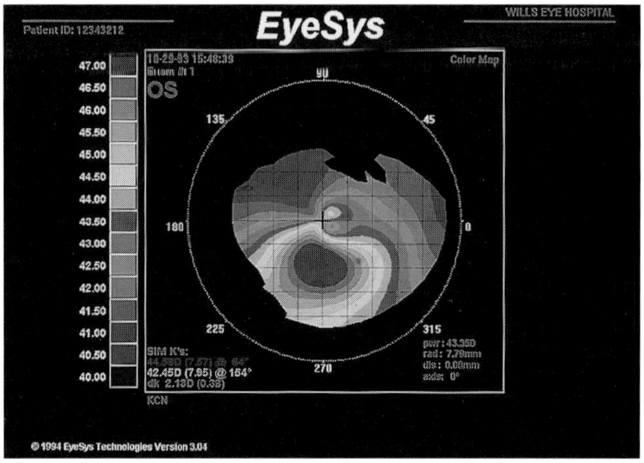

Fig. 3-92 Keratoconus. Computerized corneal topographic analysis of an eye with keratoconus. The scale on the left side indicates the dioptric power of each color. The red area in the inferior aspect of the cornea, in conjunction with the blue area superiorly, indicates significant inferior corneal steepening consistent with keratoconus. The diagnosis must be confirmed by careful slit-lamp examination. (See color plate.)

making the correct diagnosis. When no slit-lamp findings are noted, the terms subclinical keratoconus or forme fruste keratoconus have been used. These terms, though not ideal, attempt to differentiate keratoconus suspected solely on topographic evidence from those in which physical corneal changes are found. Topographic data suggest that keratoconus is usually bilateral yet asymmetric.

Keratoconus does not appear to be hereditary in most cases, but it runs in families 5% to 20% of the time. Interestingly, when corneal topographic analyses are performed on family members of patients with keratoconus,

Box 3-15 Keratoconus Associations

OCULAR DISORDERS

Floppy eyelid syndrome
Leber's congenital amaurosis
Eye rubbing
Contact lens wear (?)

SYSTEMIC DISEASES

Down's syndrome
Atopic disease
Collagen vascular diseases (e.g., Ehlers-Danlos syndrome)

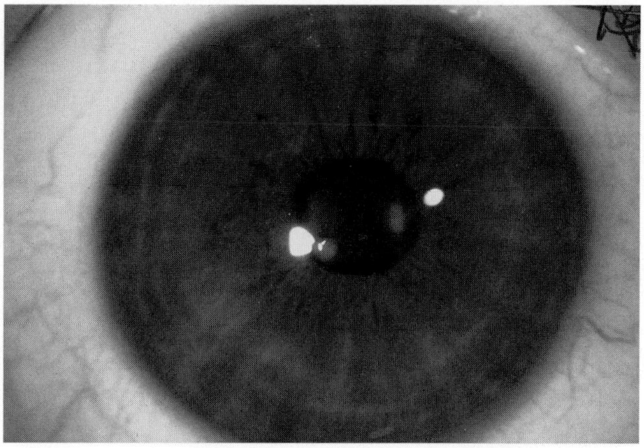

Fig. 3-93 Keratoconus. A small, superficial corneal nodule can develop on the apex of the cone and interfere with contact lens wear and vision. It is evident at the 7 o'clock aspect of the pupil.

approximately half demonstrate topographic analyses consistent with subclinical keratoconus. It may be that keratoconus has a genetic basis with incomplete penetrance and variable expressivity.

Numerous conditions are associated with keratoconus, including ocular disorders such as floppy eyelid syndrome and Leber's congenital amaurosis, as well as systemic diseases such as Down's syndrome, atopic disease, and certain collagen vascular diseases such as Ehlers-Danlos syndrome. Many of the associated conditions have the common link of eye rubbing, and many investigators believe that eye rubbing plays an important role in the development and the progression of keratoconus. Whether contact lenses, especially the polymethylmethacrylate hard lens but occasionally soft lenses, also have a role in causing or aggravating keratoconus is more controversial, but it may in some patients (Box 3-15).

On histopathologic examination, corneas with keratoconus demonstrate disruptions in Bowman's layer. There is corneal thinning and scarring, occasionally severe, at the apex of the cone. The cornea can be thinned to half the normal corneal thickness or less, with overlying epithelial hypertrophy. Epithelial iron deposition, the Fleischer ring, can also be found. After episodes of acute hydrops, Descemet's membrane is noted to be split with the retracted edges in scrolls.

Management of keratoconus begins with an attempt at spectacle correction in mild cases. Usually, the irregular astigmatism prevents good vision with glasses (or soft lenses), and rigid contact lenses are required. Most patients with keratoconus can be comfortably fit with rigid gas-permeable lenses, yielding good vision. As the severity of the keratoconus progresses, with increased apical protrusion, the lens fit becomes more problematic. Superficial corneal scarring can also seriously impede good vision. As visual acuity and contact lens tolerance decline, surgical alternatives are considered.

Infrequently, a superficial nodular lesion develops on the vertex of the cone, usually related to chronic apical touch of the rigid contact lens, which impedes contact lens wear (Fig. 3-93). In these cases, lamellar keratectomy with a blade or excimer laser PTK, can be extremely helpful in removing the nodule and reestablishing comfortable contact lens wear.

Thermokeratoplasty, the use of mild heat to scar and flatten the cone, was used in the past to treat keratoconus. The results were variable and there were significant complications, including severe corneal neovascularization. Recently, it has been used on occasion to flatten severely ectatic corneas in patients for whom intraocular surgery is not suitable. For example, some patients with Down's syndrome have severe corneal ectasia, and penetrating keratoplasty is contraindicated because of the high risk for traumatic wound dehiscence. Such flattening can occasionally improve comfort and vision without the risk inherent in intraocular surgery. Additionally, it can be used to treat severe hydrops that does not improve after several months.

The standard treatment for patients who cannot tolerate contact lenses is penetrating keratoplasty. In fact, globally keratoconus is one of the leading indications for penetrating keratoplasty. There are several important points regarding corneal transplantation for keratoconus. Surgically, the size and placement of the graft should encompass the entire cone, often best approximated by the Fleischer ring. It is most effective to identify the area of thinning and to determine the size and location of the planned graft at the slit-lamp before surgery. This goal of excising the entire cone tends to lead to larger and more inferiorly placed corneal transplants than for most other diagnoses, possibly increasing the risk for graft rejection. Many patients with keratoconus are highly myopic because of longer than average axial lengths. Some surgeons have advocated transplanting a graft slightly smaller than the recipient opening to flatten the corneal

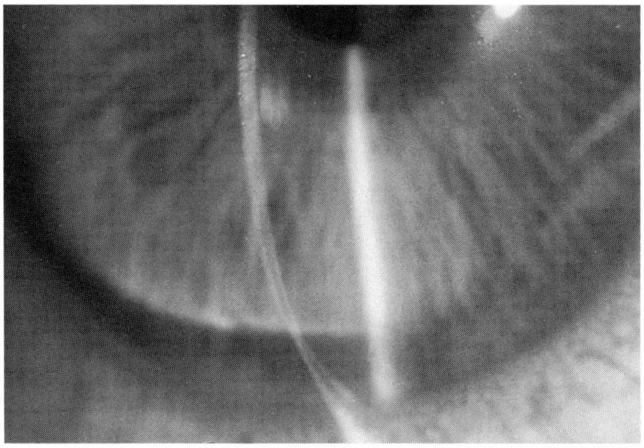

Fig. 3-94 Pellucid marginal degeneration. The slit beam depicts corneal thinning 1 to 2 mm from the inferior limbus.

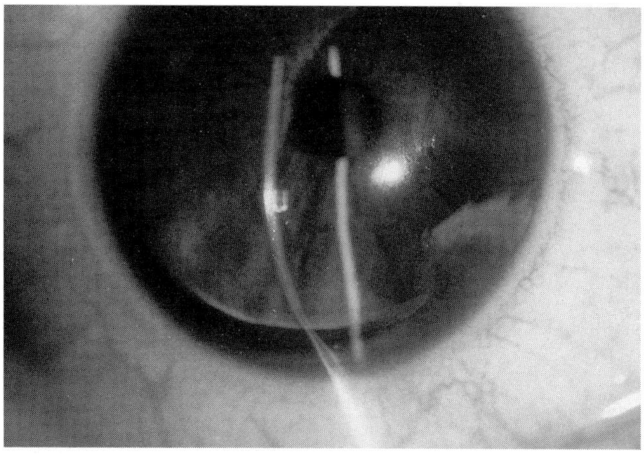

Fig. 3-95 Pellucid marginal degeneration. The most protruded aspect of the cornea is just above the area of thinning.

curvature and to decrease the myopia. However, this technique can lead to remarkably flat corneal grafts, which may be impossible to fit with a contact lens if it becomes necessary. Urrets-Zavalia syndrome is a permanently dilated pupil after corneal transplantation for keratoconus. Some surgeons think it is caused by the use of strong mydriatic agents after surgery and advocate against them. Many others think it is caused by iris trauma during surgery, either from the trephination or from posterior pressure pushing the iris against the corneal opening after removal of the corneal button. Whatever the reason, this problem is less prevalent than when it was first reported in the 1960s.

Corneal grafts for keratoconus have some of the best graft clarity and visual acuity results of all the indications for transplantation. More than 90% of patients can be expected to achieve 20/30 or better best-corrected visual acuity after surgery. Although as many as one quarter to one third of keratoconus transplants will undergo episodes of graft rejection, few grafts fail because of it. Rarely, keratoconus has been reported to recur in grafts, but this is probably the result of incomplete excision at the time of the graft.

Pellucid Marginal Degeneration

Pellucid marginal degeneration is similar to keratoconus in that it is a noninflammatory ectatic condition of the cornea. It is also bilateral, often asymmetric, slowly progressive, and occurs in men and women. It is different from keratoconus, however, in that the area of corneal thinning is 1 to 2 mm wide and occurs 1 to 2 mm from the limbus from the 4 to 8 o'clock positions in the inferior corneal periphery (Figs. 3-94 and 3-95). The most ectatic area of cornea is just above the area of thinning. This is also in contrast to keratoconus in which the thinnest area and the most protruded area are the same

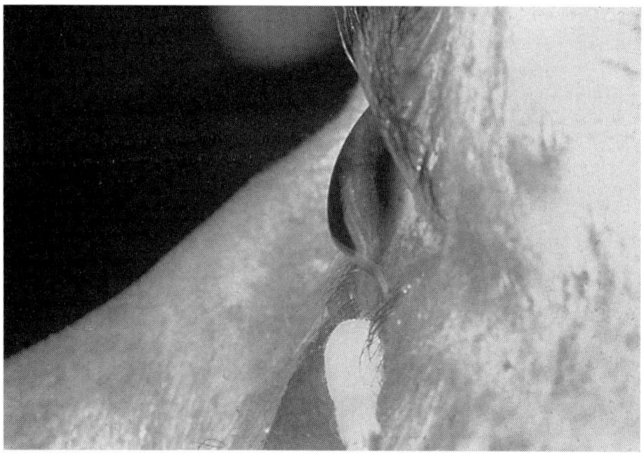

Fig. 3-96 Pellucid marginal degeneration. Side view demonstrates the sagging nature of the cornea. The most protruded part of the cornea is just above the area of severe thinning.

(Fig. 3-96). Like keratoconus, pellucid marginal degeneration causes irregular astigmatism. Unlike keratoconus, it typically causes a recognizable against the rule pattern that tends to be flatter than normal on corneal topography (Fig. 3-97 and Box 3-16).

Pellucid marginal degeneration is much less prevalent than keratoconus and is usually diagnosed at an older age, typically when patients are between the ages of 20 and 50 years. Rarely, keratoconus and pellucid marginal degeneration are found in the same patient and even in the same eye.

Symptoms are similar to those of keratoconus, with decreased vision not fully corrected by spectacles the most common. Acute corneal hydrops can also occur, but less often than it does in keratoconus. Treatment depends on the severity of the symptoms. In mild cases, spectacles may correct the vision adequately. If not, a

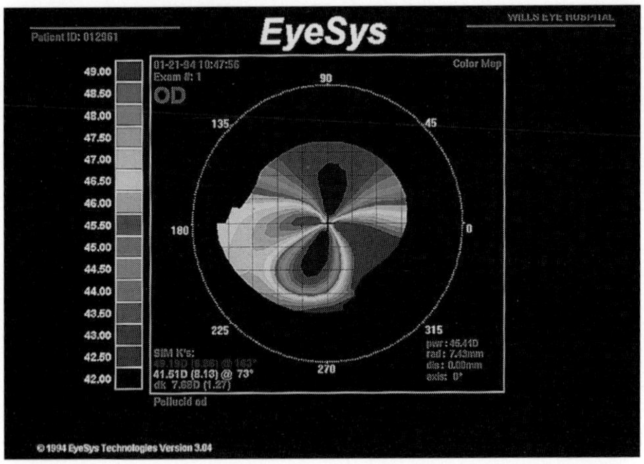

Fig. 3-97 Pellucid marginal degeneration. Computerized corneal topographic analysis of an eye with pellucid marginal degeneration. The scale on the left side indicates the dioptric power of each color. The red area of corneal steepening nasally and temporally is seen to arc inferiorly. This irregular color pattern of against-the-rule astigmatism is classic for pellucid marginal degeneration. The diagnosis must be confirmed by careful slit-lamp examination. (See color plate.)

Box 3-16 Critical Features of Pellucid Marginal Degeneration

- Noninflammatory ectatic condition of the cornea
- Less common than keratoconus
- Bilateral but often asymmetric
- Most ectatic area of cornea is just above the area of thinning
- Area of corneal thinning is 1 to 2 mm in width, occurs 1 to 2 mm from the limbus from 4 to 8 o'clock positions
- Causes irregular astigmatism, typically against-the-rule
- Slowly progressive
- Occurs in men and women
- Typically diagnosed between the ages of 20 and 50 years

rigid contact lens can often be comfortably fit to give excellent vision. Contact lenses are more difficult to fit than in keratoconus because of the inferior corneal protrusion and the flat central cornea.

When contact lenses no longer provide satisfactory vision and comfort, surgical treatment may be attempted. Large inferiorly placed penetrating keratoplasties are often successful, but they are at increased risk for graft vascularization and rejection due to their proximity to the limbus. Careful preoperative slit-lamp planning is necessary to ensure that the graft wound is peripheral to the thin area of cornea. Other surgical options, such as crescentic lamellar resections in the area of thinning or lamellar keratoplasties, have been performed with variable results.

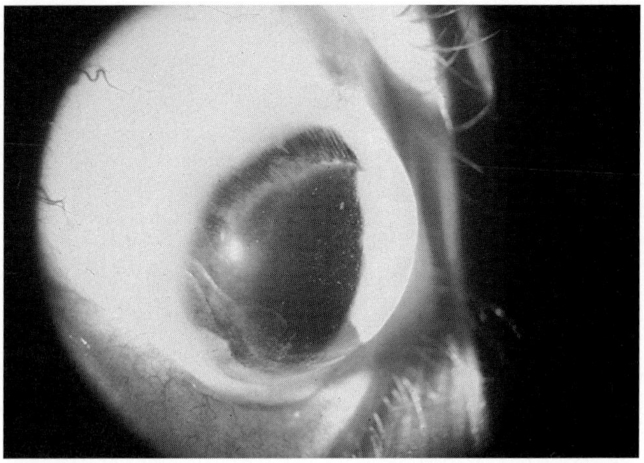

Fig. 3-98 Keratoglobus. The entire cornea is protruded in keratoglobus. The peripheral cornea is thinned.

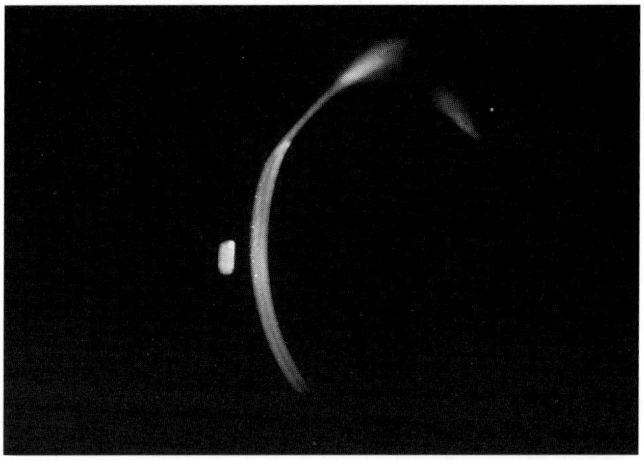

Fig. 3-99 Keratoglobus. This slit beam illustrates the peripheral corneal thinning.

Keratoglobus

Keratoglobus is an extremely rare ectatic disorder characterized by generalized corneal thinning greatest in the mid-periphery and the periphery (Figs. 3-98 and 3-99). The cornea can be as thin as 20% its normal thickness. It results in a globoid protrusion of the cornea causing increased corneal curvature, astigmatism, and decreased vision (Fig. 3-100). It is bilateral, found in men and women, and stationary or slowly progressive. Acute hydrops can occur in keratoglobus, but not as commonly as in keratoconus. Corneal perforation is not uncommon

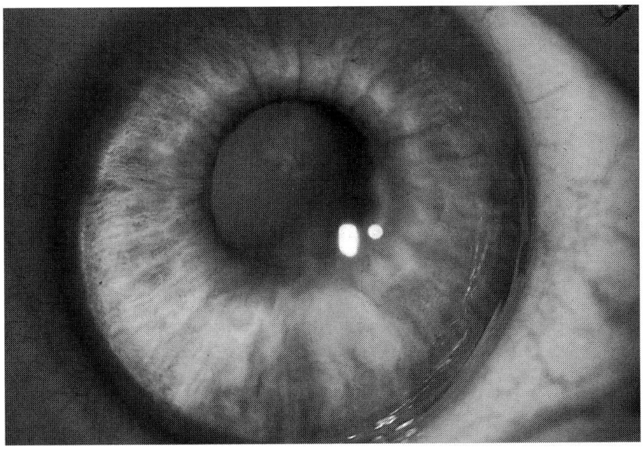

Fig. 3-100 Keratoglobus. The peripheral cornea, especially inferiorly, is noted to protrude anteriorly away from the limbus. Mild corneal scarring can be seen.

Box 3-17 Critical Features of Keratoglobus

- Rare ectatic corneal disorder
- Bilateral
- Generalized corneal thinning, greatest in the periphery
- Globoid protrusion of the entire cornea
- Causes increased corneal curvature, myopia, and astigmatism
- Stationary or slowly progressive
- Found in men and women
- Corneal perforation can occur because of the severe corneal thinning
- Surgical treatment is extremely difficult

MAJOR POINTS

- Anterior basement membrane dystrophy can cause decreased vision as well as painful recurrent erosions.
- Granular dystrophy spares the periphery, whereas macular dystrophy does not.
- In granular and lattice dystrophies, the vision dramatically decreases when the central clear spaces become opacified.
- Macular dystrophy causes decreased vision early in life because the stroma between the dense opacities is not clear.
- Granular, lattice, and Schnyder's crystalline dystrophies are autosomal dominant whereas macular dystrophy is autosomal recessive.
- Patients with Schnyder's crystalline dystrophy should undergo a workup for hypercholesterolemia and hypertriglyceridemia.
- Cornea guttata without corneal edema is called endothelial dystrophy whereas cornea guttata with corneal edema is termed Fuchs' dystrophy.
- In patients with corneal edema, the vision decreases significantly with the development of epithelial edema.
- Small refractile amyloid deposits in the mid to deep stroma in an older patient without a long history of decreased vision or painful erosions and with no family history of lattice dystrophy most likely signify polymorphic amyloid degeneration.
- Patients with Terrien's marginal degeneration typically present with decreased vision due to regular and irregular astigmatism and can usually be managed with glasses or rigid contact lenses.
- Band keratopathy is most effectively treated with EDTA chelation.
- Most Salzmann's nodular degeneration lesions can be readily excised with superficial keratectomy with a blade.
- ICE is different from PPMD in that it is sporadic, unilateral, and more rapidly progressive, whereas PPMD is autosomal dominant, bilateral, and more slowly progressive.
- In keratoconus the thinnest and most protruded area of cornea are one and the same whereas in pellucid marginal degeneration the protrusion occurs above the area of greatest thinning.

because of the severe corneal thinning. Perforation can occur with minimal trauma and even with no history of trauma. Keratoglobus has been associated with Leber's congenital amaurosis and a condition similar to Ehlers-Danlos syndrome type 6 (Box 3-17).

Treatment is extremely problematic. Spectacles can occasionally give reasonable vision and do provide a measure of protection against trauma. Contact lenses are difficult to fit and are relatively contraindicated because of the risk for trauma with insertion and removal. Patients may do well with scleral lenses. Surgical treatment is difficult at best and should be delayed whenever possible. Penetrating keratoplasty requires a limbus-to-limbus graft with a high risk for postoperative complications, including graft vascularization, rejection, and glaucoma. Most surgeons think the best surgical option is a tectonic lamellar graft, which goes across the limbus for 360° to flatten the entire cornea. Although it is occasionally successful alone, usually a subsequent smaller, central penetrating graft is required to achieve good vision.

CONCLUSION

Although ectatic disorders, corneal dystrophies, and corneal degenerations are generally not emergency situations, they are important conditions to recognize and to manage appropriately. They tend to be slowly progressive, and a step-wise approach to treatment generally works well. Because many of these disorders are inherited, it is important that they be correctly identified and that genetic counseling be offered when necessary.

SUGGESTED READINGS

Bron AJ: The corneal dystrophies, *Curr Opin Ophthalmol* 1:333-346, 1990.

Holland EJ, Daya SM, Stone EM, et al: Avellino corneal dystrophy: clinical manifestations and natural history, *Ophthalmology* 99:1564-1568, 1992.

Krachmer JH, Feder RS, Belin MW: Keratoconus and related noninflammatory corneal thinning disorders, *Surv Ophthalmol* 28:293-322, 1984.

Kuchle M, Green WR, Volcker HE, Barraquer J: Reevaluation of corneal dystrophies of Bowman's layer and the anterior stroma (Reis-Bücklers' and Thiel-Behnke types): a light and electron microscopy study of eight corneas and a review of the literature, *Cornea* 14:333-354, 1995.

Rabinowitz YS: Keratoconus, *Surv Ophthalmol* 42:297-319, 1998.

Waring GO, Rodrigues MM, Laibson PR: Corneal dystrophies: I. Endothelial dystrophies, *Surv Ophthalmol* 23:71-122, 1978.

Waring GO, Rodrigues MM, Laibson PR: Corneal dystrophies: II. Dystrophies of the epithelium, Bowman layer and stroma, *Surv Ophthalmol* 23:147-168, 1978.

Weiss JS: Schnyder's dystrophy of the cornea, *Cornea* 1:93-101, 1992.

Wilson SE, Bourne WM: Fuchs' dystrophy, *Cornea* 7:2-18, 1988.

CHAPTER 4

Corneal Infections, Inflammations, and Surface Disorders

Infectious, inflammatory, and surface diseases of the cornea are major causes of ocular morbidity and visual loss throughout the world. Many of the diseases included in this chapter are commonly encountered in everyday practice and account for a significant proportion of emergency visits to an ophthalmologist's office. This chapter discusses the important aspects of the history, clinical presentation, pathophysiology, diagnosis, and treatment of each condition.

Infectious and inflammatory corneal diseases include bacterial, fungal, viral, parasitic, and inflammatory keratitis. Bacterial keratitis and viral keratitis are the most frequently encountered conditions in this category. Bacterial keratitis develops most often in patients with compromised corneal surfaces and in contact lens users; therefore a significant population is at risk. Rapid diagnosis and treatment significantly improves the visual prognosis in affected patients. It is essential that the ophthalmologist understand the risk factors for infection and the various clinical presentations of bacterial keratitis. Viral keratitis in the form of herpes simplex or herpes zoster keratitis remains a significant cause of ocular disease in the United States and around the world. Diagnosing and treating these conditions can be difficult and frustrating because of their numerous clinical manifestations, their high rate of recurrence, and their chronic nature. Progressive corneal scarring and visual loss cannot always be avoided, despite appropriate therapy, and corneal transplantation remains an option for many of these patients.

Corneal surface disorders are a group of frequently overlooked or misdiagnosed conditions that can produce significant discomfort or visual limitation in affected patients. Many of these conditions are related to contact lens wear. Tight contact lenses and solution toxicity are common causes of discomfort and contact lens intolerance, and the symptoms may be similar. However, patients are often examined after having discontinued contact lens wear for several days, and consequently have few objective findings. A heightened clinical suspicion of a corneal surface disorder and a complete contact lens history aid in diagnosis and treatment, thereby helping these patients safely and successfully continue contact lens wear.

In addition to contact lens–related disorders, many surface diseases such as dry eye syndrome, superficial punctate keratopathy (SPK), exposure keratopathy, and recurrent erosions may present with minimal findings on initial examination. Although nonspecific ocular discomfort may be the most common symptom of these conditions, severe or vision-threatening complications occasionally develop because chronic surface diseases predispose the cornea to infection and scarring. Early recognition and treatment of the underlying causes of these conditions may provide significant symptomatic relief and help preserve vision.

INFECTIOUS AND INFLAMMATORY KERATITIS

Bacterial Keratitis

Bacterial keratitis is the most common form of infectious keratitis, and it is an ocular emergency. Prompt recognition and initiation of appropriate antimicrobial therapy are crucial to limit the amount of tissue destruction and to improve the patient's visual prognosis, particularly if the ulcer involves the central cornea.

Normal flora The eye is constantly bathed in a variety of microorganisms that constitute the normal flora of the eyelids and the conjunctivae (Box 4-1). Gram-positive bacteria predominate; however, with increasing age more gram-negative organisms may be found. Fungi are occasionally present. The exact composition of the normal flora varies among populations and geographic regions.

Ocular defense mechanisms The eye has several defense mechanisms that limit the growth of microorganisms and prevent their penetration into the cornea. These methods of protection can be divided into two categories: chemical defenses and mechanical defenses. The major chemical defenses include lysozyme, lactoferrin, and immunoglobulins located in the aqueous portion of the tear film. Lysozyme is an enzyme that aids in the breakdown of the bacterial cell wall and that is active against many gram-positive bacteria, but it is less effective against gram-negative bacteria. Lactoferrin is a metal-chelating protein that may interfere with the uptake of iron by bacteria and thereby reduce their virulence. Secretory immunoglobulin-A, the most predominant immunoglobulin in tears, helps prevent bacterial adherence to epithelial cells.

Box 4-1 Predominant Normal Flora of the External Ocular Surface

GRAM POSITIVE

Staphylococcus aureus (more common)
Staphylococcus epidermidis (more common)
Diphtheroids
Propionibacterium acnes
Streptococcus pneumoniae
Streptococcus viridans

GRAM NEGATIVE (LESS COMMON)

Escherichia coli
Klebsiella spp
Proteus spp
Moraxella spp

FUNGI (LESS COMMON)

Candida spp

Mechanical defenses include the blink response and the anatomic barrier effect of the corneal epithelium. The sweeping action of the blink response helps to reduce bacterial colonization by washing bacteria suspended in the tears toward the lacrimal puncta, where they are then pumped into the lacrimal sac. However, the most important mechanical defense against the development of infectious keratitis is the surface epithelium of the cornea. A smooth, intact corneal epithelium provides a significant anatomic barrier to the adherence of microorganisms to the corneal stroma and their penetration into it. As a result, the major risk factors for the development of infectious keratitis involve the compromise of this protective layer.

Risk factors for infection Trauma and contact lens wear are the most common risk factors for microbial keratitis. Direct trauma to the cornea may damage or even remove the epithelium, rendering the underlying stroma more susceptible to microbial colonization and infection. Penetrating trauma may directly inoculate the stroma. Once organisms reach the stroma, they may adhere, replicate, and begin to liberate enzymes and toxins that destroy tissue and incite an inflammatory reaction.

Contact lens use is the most common risk factor for microbial keratitis in otherwise healthy eyes. All contact lens wearers, whether they use soft, rigid, gas-permeable, daily wear, extended wear, or disposable lenses, are at risk. However, overnight contact lens wear is associated with a 10 times greater risk for ulcerative keratitis than daily wear, and each additional night of overnight lens wear further increases the risk for infection. Bacterial contamination of contact lens storage cases and solutions is common. Bacteria (especially *Pseudomonas*) have been shown to adhere to contact lenses, and they may be transferred directly to the corneal surface when the lens is placed on the eye. Contact lenses may produce microscopic or macroscopic trauma to the corneal epithelium, providing those organisms with easier access to the stroma. Meticulous hygiene and contact lens care can help reduce the risk for infection.

Previous ocular surgery is another risk factor for bacterial keratitis, particularly if a patient has loose sutures. Exposed sutures provide a surface on which microorganisms may adhere and proliferate. They also provide a ready-made tract deep inside ocular tissues for the easy initiation of infection. All loose, exposed sutures should be removed.

Additional risk factors for infection include ocular adnexal and primary corneal disorders that may result in external infection, decreased corneal sensation, or corneal epithelial damage. Ocular adnexal conditions such as ectropion, entropion, and trichiasis produce chronic corneal exposure or mechanical epithelial trauma that predispose the cornea to infection. Similarly, chronic surface diseases of the cornea such as keratoconjunctivitis sicca, recurrent erosions, bullous keratopathy, and neurotrophic keratopathy also compromise the integrity of the corneal epithelium, removing the primary mechanical barrier to corneal infection (Box 4-2).

Evaluation and workup The evaluation of infectious keratitis begins with a careful patient history. Understanding the patient's risk factors for infection is often crucial for determining the likely underlying pathogens. It is therefore necessary to get a comprehensive medical, social, and contact lens history. Knowing a patient's occupation, hobbies, and exposures may help pinpoint the cause of the infection.

A complete ophthalmic examination should be performed to the extent possible, given the patient's symptoms and ability to cooperate. Evaluation should include careful slit-lamp examination of the eyelids and conjunctiva for evidence of eyelash and eyelid abnormalities, infection, inflammation, ulceration, or foreign bodies. The sclera should be examined for signs of inflammation, thinning, or ischemia.

The corneal ulcer is the hallmark of bacterial keratitis. An infiltrate is defined as a focal collection of inflammatory cells within the corneal stroma (Fig. 4-1), whereas an ulcer clinically appears as a dense, white, inflammatory infiltrate in the cornea (Fig. 4-2) accompanied by an overlying epithelial defect and tissue loss (Fig. 4-3).

Box 4-2 Risk Factors for Microbial Keratitis

CONTACT LENS WEAR

TRAUMA

TOPICAL CORTICOSTEROIDS

CHRONIC CORNEAL SURFACE DISEASE

Viral keratitis
Bullous keratopathy
Exposure keratopathy
Keratoconjunctivitis sicca
Neurotrophic keratopathy
Stevens-Johnson syndrome
Ocular cicatricial pemphigoid

OCULAR SURGERY

Cataract extraction
Keratoplasty
Pterygium excision
Loose corneal sutures
Refractive surgery

OCULAR ADNEXAL CONDITIONS

Entropion
Ectropion
Trichiasis
Blepharitis/rosacea

SYSTEMIC DISEASE

Immunosuppression
Systemic infection
Diabetes mellitus
Collagen vascular disease
Substance abuse
Poor general health/malnutrition

There may be mild to severe tissue destruction. The epithelial defect may be the same size as the underlying infiltrate or it may be smaller or larger. Usually the infiltrate is sufficiently dense to obscure the examiner's view of the iris while looking through the infiltrate. In eyes with sterile corneal melts, there may be little to no infiltrate, but there may be extensive tissue loss. It is important to describe the location, shape, size, border morphology, and color of the infiltrate because sometimes these characteristics suggest a particular pathogen. For example, feathery edges or satellite lesions may suggest fungus, whereas a ring infiltrate may suggest *Pseudomonas* or *Acanthamoeba* spp (Box 4-3). The slit beam should be used to determine the depth of the infiltrate and the amount of tissue loss and to measure the size of the epithelial defect and the infiltrate. These measurements are helpful in assessing the progress of the

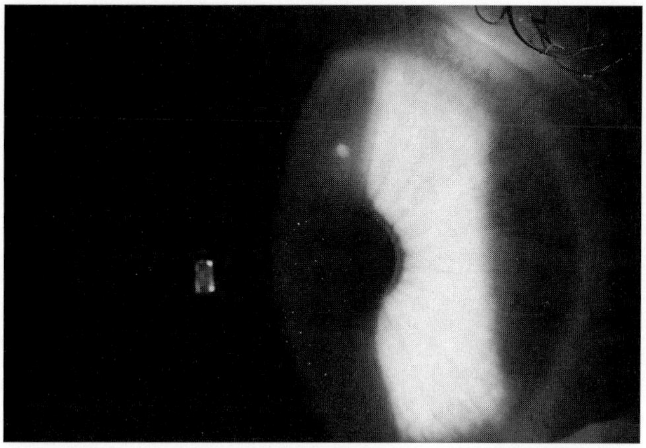

Fig. 4-1 Corneal infiltrate. A small, gray-white corneal infiltrate is seen in this wearer of soft contact lenses. Mild surrounding corneal edema but no anterior chamber reaction is present.

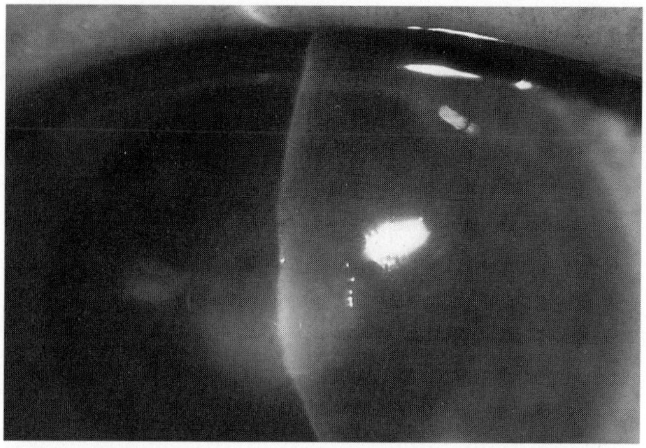

Fig. 4-3 Corneal ulcer. A slit-beam view of this central corneal ulcer reveals moderate corneal tissue loss and thinning.

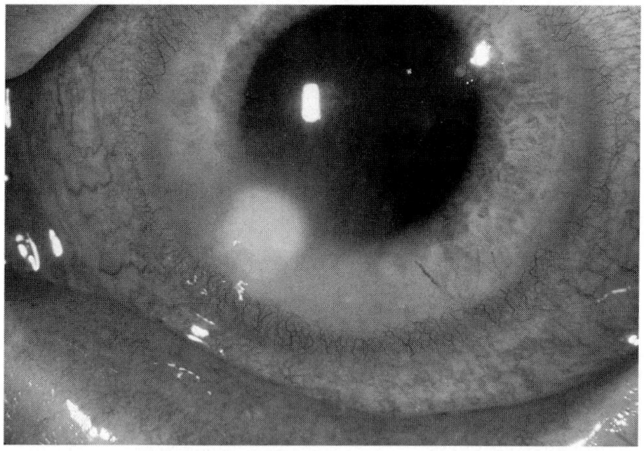

Fig. 4-2 Corneal ulcer. A moderately large, dense, white corneal ulcer is present inferonasally. Note the significant surrounding corneal edema. The ulcer blocks the view of the iris.

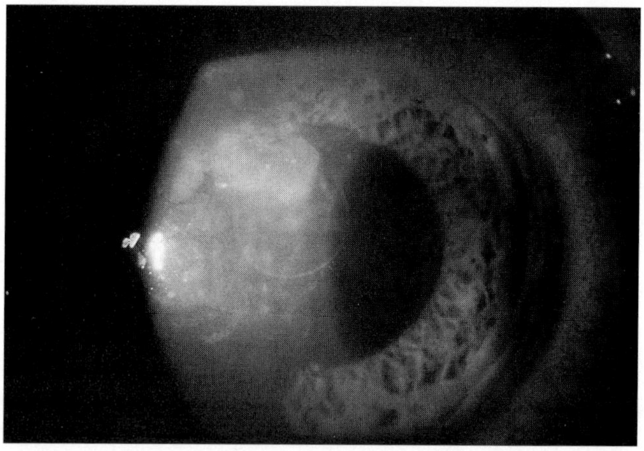

Fig. 4-4 Corneal ulcer with an immune ring. One focus of this corneal ulcer is associated with an immune ring, a circular stromal inflammatory reaction.

infection and the response to therapy. A circular immune ring may be noted surrounding an infiltrate (Fig. 4-4). The cornea should also be evaluated for evidence of vascularization, foreign bodies, and keratic precipitates. The anterior chamber should be examined for evidence of cell, flare, and hypopyon (Fig. 4-5). Anterior chamber depth should be assessed. Seidel's testing should be performed, particularly in patients with ulcers and extensive tissue loss, to look for occult or frank perforation (Fig. 4-6). Bloody pigment in the ulcer, protrusion of the infiltrate, or radiating folds in Descemet's membrane may be an indication of perforation. Sudden loss of a hypopyon may also signal perforation. Infections in a trabeculectomy bleb should be treated aggressively because of the thin barrier separating the organisms from the inside of the eye (Fig. 4-7).

Once bacterial keratitis is suspected, corneal scrapings for staining and culture may be obtained to identify the underlying pathogen. Cultures often allow the clinician to guide or modify therapy if the clinical response is poor and to eliminate the administration of unnecessary and potentially toxic medications. However, if the infiltrate is small (1 to 2 mm or smaller in diameter) and peripheral and if unusual organisms are not suspected after a thorough history and examination, initial cultures

Box 4-3 Differential Diagnosis of a Ring Infiltrate

Pseudomonas (acute onset, suppurative)
Acanthamoeba (delayed 3 to 6 weeks)
Fungus (uncommon)
Herpes simplex virus (immune ring)
Herpes zoster virus (immune ring)
Anesthetic abuse
Central corneal infiltrate in a contact lens wearer

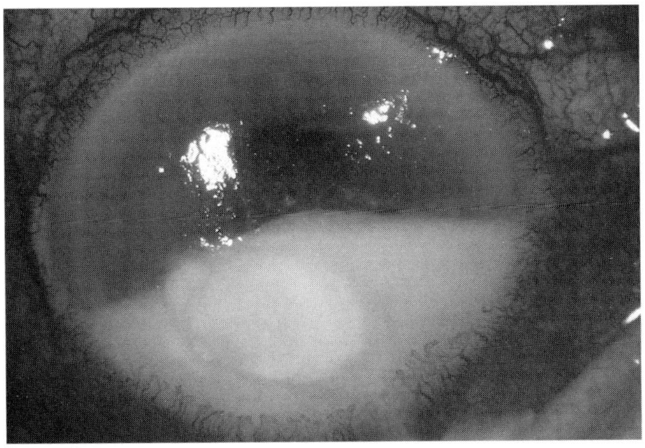

Fig. 4-5 Corneal ulcer with a hypopyon. An extremely large hypopyon can be seen related to this corneal ulcer.

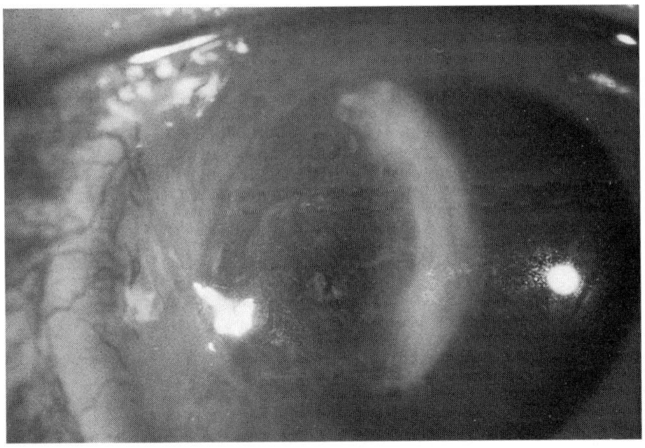

Fig. 4-6 Corneal ulcer with thinning. The central aspect of this large corneal ulcer is densely infiltrated. The lateral aspect appears clearer because of significant corneal thinning. Such severe corneal ulceration should prompt a Seidel test to evaluate for frank or occult perforation.

may be deferred (Box 4-4). Intensive broad-spectrum antibiotic therapy should be started, and the patient should be observed closely. If a prompt clinical response to therapy does not take place, cultures should be obtained.

In general large or central infiltrates, infiltrates associated with hypopyons, or unusual infiltrates should be cultured. If in doubt as to the diagnosis, then culture. Cultures should be performed with a heat-sterilized metal spatula used to scrape the corneal infiltrate after topical anesthesia has been applied. Be sure to allow sufficient time for the spatula to cool before applying it to the cornea! If a sizzling sound occurs as the spatula touches the cornea, the spatula was too hot. Once a scraping is obtained, the spatula should directly inoculate the culture media. The initial culture media should include blood agar, chocolate agar, Sabouraud's dextrose agar (without cyclohexamide), and thioglycolate broth. The spatula should be heat sterilized and cooled between scrapings. Alternatively, a no. 15 Beaver blade or a calcium alginate swab may be used to obtain scrapings. Scrapings should also be smeared on two or more glass slides and sent for Gram stain and either Giemsa or calcofluor white stain. Other stains and cultures may be obtained if the clinical situation warrants (Table 4-1). Cultures of the conjunctiva and eyelid margins may also be performed if they appear to be infected, though the results may not necessarily establish which bacteria are responsible for the corneal infection.

If the infectious process progresses despite repeat negative cultures, a corneal biopsy specimen may be taken (Fig. 4-8) either at the slit lamp on a cooperative patient or under the operating microscope. Using a blade or a small trephine, a small piece of tissue is excised from the clinically affected area of the cornea. This piece is then sectioned under sterile conditions, and the portions are sent to the pathologist for examination and to the microbiology laboratory for culture.

Specific organisms The most common bacterial organisms cultured from corneal ulcers are *Staphylococcus aureus,* coagulase-negative *Staphylococcus, Streptococcus, Pseudomonas,* and *Moraxella.* Although it is not

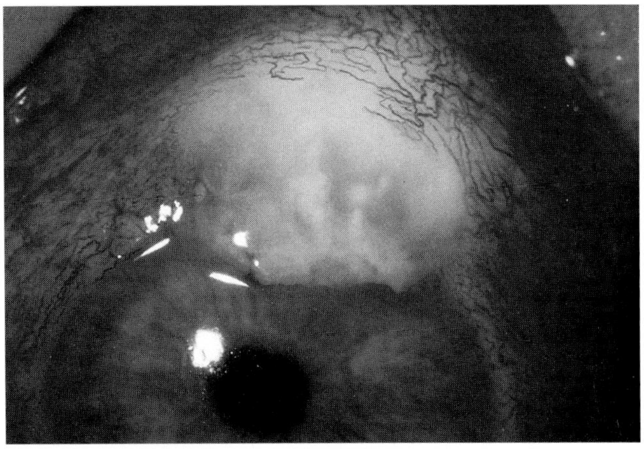

Fig. 4-7 Blebitis. This trabeculectomy bleb has become acutely inflamed and infiltrated. Small accumulations of white blood cells can be seen loculated in the bleb. Such infections must be treated aggressively.

Box 4-4 When to Culture Suspected Infectious Corneal Ulcers

- Infiltrate larger than 1 to 2 mm with an epithelial defect
- Central or paracentral ulcers
- Significant tissue loss
- Presence of hypopyon
- Unusual organisms suspected by history or examination
- Lack of response to empiric therapy
- Postoperative eye

Table 4-1 Diagnostic stains and culture media in infectious keratitis

Stain or culture media	Predominant organisms cultured or visualized
STAINS	
Gram stain	Bacteria, fungi
Giemsa stain	Fungi, bacteria, *Chlamydia* Details of the inflammatory cellular response
GMS stain	Fungi
Calcofluor white stain	Fungi, *Acanthamoeba*
Acid fast stain	Mycobacteria, filamentous bacteria *(Nocardia)*
Acridine orange stain	*Acanthamoeba,* fungi, bacteria
CULTURE MEDIA	
Blood agar	Aerobic and facultatively aerobic bacteria, fungi
Sabouraud's agar	Fungi
Chocolate agar	*Neisseria, Haemophilus*
Thioglycolate broth	Aerobic and anaerobic bacteria, fungi
Löwenstein-Jensen agar	Mycobacteria
Nonnutrient agar with *Escherichia coli* overlay	*Acanthamoeba*
Anaerobic culture media	*Propionibacterium acnes*

GMS, Gomori's methenamine silver.

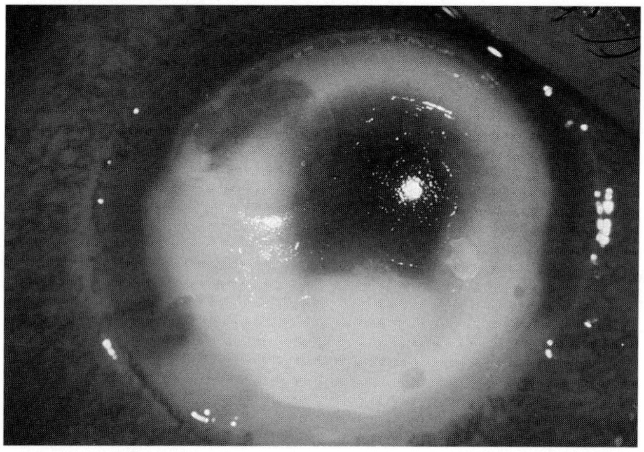

Fig. 4-8 Corneal biopsy. A corneal biopsy specimen was taken from this large, chronic, corneal ulcer with a significant hypopyon that was not responding to treatment to determine the cause of the infection. The 3-mm circular biopsy site can be seen at the 10 o'clock position.

possible to distinguish reliably between gram-positive and gram-negative infections based on their clinical appearance, some generalizations may be made (Table 4-2).

Pseudomonas is a gram-negative rod that may be isolated in a significant proportion of patients with bacterial keratitis associated with contact lens wear. It may cause rapidly progressive and destructive keratitis that perforates the cornea if appropriate treatment is delayed. Infiltrates near the corneal periphery can spread to involve the contiguous sclera. The resultant infectious scleritis may be devastating and result in loss of the eye. The intense destructive capacity of this organism stems from its production of exotoxins, which rapidly digest corneal

Table 4-2 General clinical features of gram-positive and gram-negative keratitis

Feature	Gram positive	Gram negative
Appearance	Mild to dense infiltrate	Dense infiltrate, necrosis
Borders	Distinct infiltrate borders	Indistinct borders
Surrounding cornea	Generally clear	Often hazy
Hypopyon	Less common	More common

glycosaminoglycans. Additionally, its cell wall contains endotoxin, which serves to potentiate the corneal inflammatory response. Once the organism gains access to the corneal stroma, a rapidly progressive suppurative keratitis ensues. Within 18 to 24 hours, an extensive infiltrate with a marked mucopurulent exudate and anterior chamber reaction or hypopyon may be present (Fig. 4-9). The surrounding epithelium may appear diffusely gray because of inflammatory epithelial edema. The infiltrate may continue to spread concentrically, forming a dense, circular pattern. Profound tissue loss at the center of the infiltrate may give it the appearance of a ring infiltrate. Untreated infection leads to rapid corneal melting, descemetocele formation, and perforation. *Pseudomonas* spp are usually sensitive to aminoglycosides, antipseudomonal penicillins, and fluoroquinolones.

It is also important to note that *Pseudomonas* infection of the cornea related to contact lens wear may rarely present in a superficial form that initially resembles SPK. Additionally, small infiltrates in contact lens wearers may

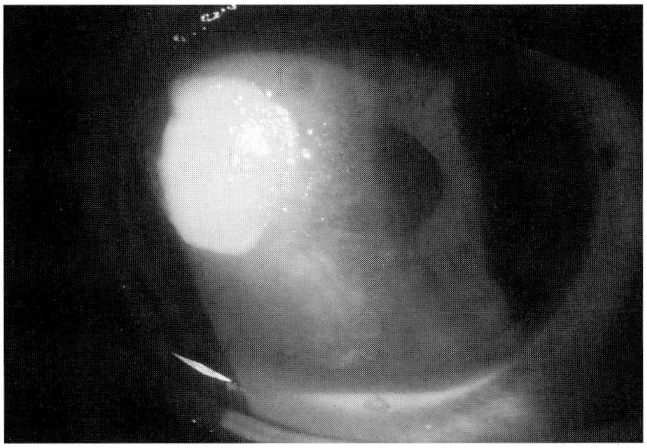

Fig. 4-9 *Pseudomonas* corneal ulcer. A dense, white corneal ulcer with moderate surrounding corneal edema and a small hypopyon caused by *Pseudomonas* is present.

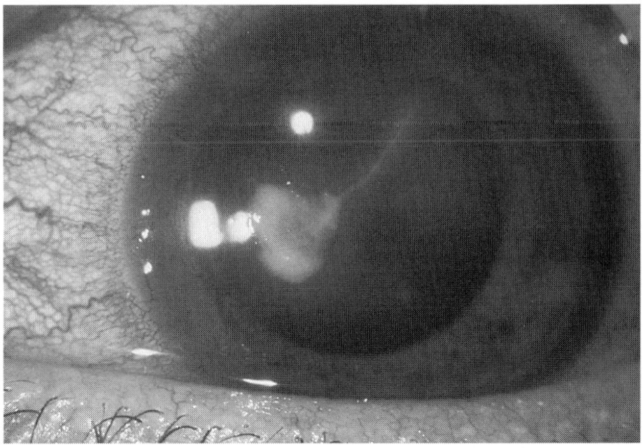

Fig. 4-10 *Pseudomonas* corneal ulcer. Spread of infection along a corneal nerve can be caused by bacteria, such as in this *Pseudomonas* ulcer, but can also be caused by other organisms, including *Acanthamoeba*.

be caused by *Pseudomonas*. The organism may spread along the corneal nerves (Fig. 4-10). If left untreated, this infection progresses to suppurative keratitis as described above.

Staphylococcus is a gram-positive coccus that causes infectious keratitis, usually in patients with underlying chronic corneal surface diseases such as bullous keratopathy, dry eyes, persistent epithelial defects, rosacea keratitis, or chronic herpetic keratitis. *Staphylococcus aureus* may be distinguished from *Staphylococcus epidermidis* in the laboratory in that *S. aureus* is coagulase positive and ferments mannitol. Clinically, they both often present with a well-defined, white or creamy infiltrate. Untreated, these infiltrates gradually invade the deeper stroma, though they may also take a rapidly progressive course. The anterior chamber reaction is variable. Staphylococcal organisms are generally sensitive to many antibiotics, including cephalosporins, bacitracin, erythromycin, neomycin, and vancomycin. Coagulase-negative *Staphylococcus* is less virulent than *S. aureus*, but it is more variable with regard to antibiotic sensitivity. Vancomycin is the drug of choice for methicillin-resistant staphylococcal infection, though its use should be limited to resistant cases or to patients with allergies to penicillin or cephalosporin to help limit the emergence of resistant strains.

Streptococcus pneumoniae is another gram-positive coccus that frequently infects compromised eyes. It typically presents with a dense, suppurative stromal infiltrate, which may advance superficially before producing deeper necrosis. Often the leading edge of the infiltrate has a serpiginous shape. A significant anterior chamber reaction or hypopyon usually results, and there may be adherent fibrin or an endothelial inflammatory plaque underlying the infiltrate. Other β-hemolytic streptococci may present with a similar clinical picture, whereas viridans streptococci usually present with more localized and chronic infections. Severe streptococcal infections can present similarly to *Pseudomonas* ulcers. Streptococci are usually sensitive to penicillin, cephalosporins, vancomycin, bacitracin, erythromycin, and trimethoprim. Fluoroquinolones are less effective against streptococcal infections.

A special form of streptococcal infection is infectious crystalline keratopathy. This unusual infection is usually due to *Streptococcus viridans* that proliferates between the lamellae of the corneal stroma. It produces a minimal inflammatory response and sometimes leaves an intact epithelium. Discrete needlelike opacities with minimal surrounding inflammation, much like a true crystalline deposit within the corneal stroma, may be seen (Fig. 4-11). Infectious crystalline keratopathy usually occurs in eyes with suppressed or impaired inflammatory responses. Risk factors include topical corticosteroid use, previous surgery (especially penetrating keratoplasty), remaining corneal sutures, contact lens wear, corneal edema, neurotrophic cornea, and topical anesthetic abuse. Although *Streptococcus* spp account for most cases of infectious crystalline keratopathy, other bacterial and fungal organisms have been reported. In these unusual cases, it is important to determine the causative organism by culture or biopsy.

Neisseria gonorrhoeae, a type of gram-negative bacteria consisting of diplococci, is an important cause of hyperacute conjunctivitis in the adult, ophthalmia neonatorum, and severe keratitis. It may be distinguished in the laboratory from *Neisseria meningitidis* through its sugar fermentation pattern. *N. gonorrhoeae* ferments glucose, whereas *N. meningitidis* ferments glucose and maltose. Clinically, it presents with a rapid, hyperacute onset of marked conjunctival chemosis associated with a massive purulent discharge and preauricular adenopathy (Fig. 4-12). Untreated gonococci may penetrate an intact

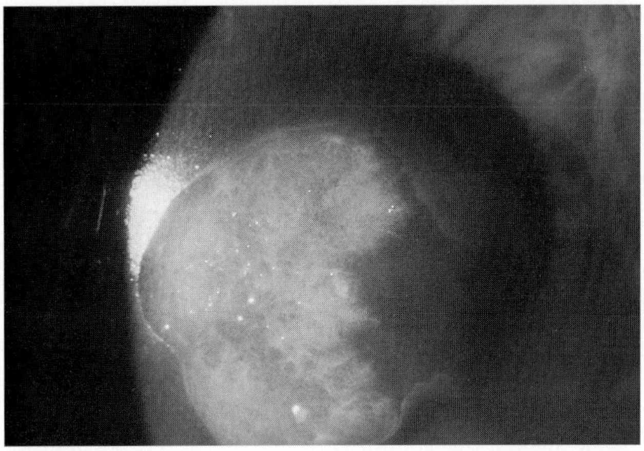

Fig. 4-11 Infectious crystalline keratopathy. Crystalline, needlelike projections in the anterior stroma are evident in this eye with a *Streptococcus viridans* infection. This eye was neurotrophic after a herpes zoster infection.

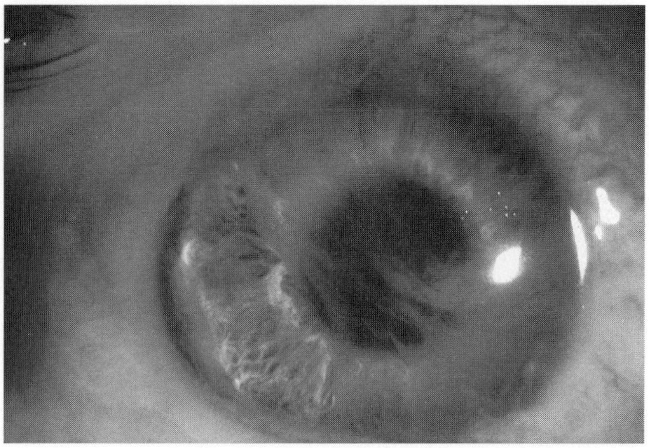

Fig. 4-13 *Neisseria gonorrhoeae* conjunctivitis. This cornea is coated with a purulent discharge from *Neisseria gonorrhoeae*.

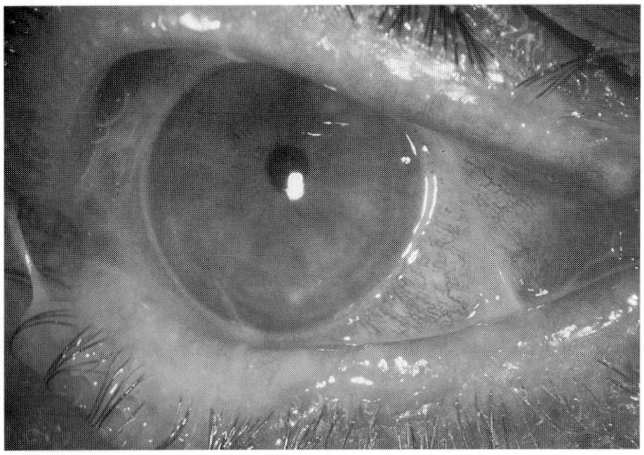

Fig. 4-12 *Neisseria gonorrhoeae* conjunctivitis. A copious purulent discharge can be seen in this eye with hyperacute conjunctivitis.

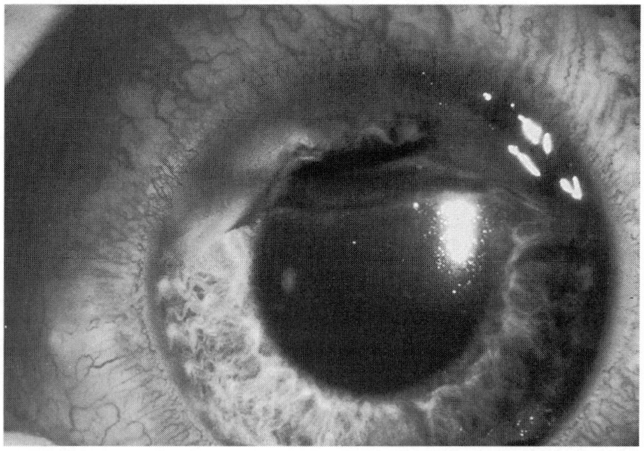

Fig. 4-14 *Neisseria gonorrhoeae* corneal ulcer. A superior corneal ulcer developed in the eye seen in Fig. 4-13. The entire cornea must be evaluated in all eyes with hyperacute conjunctivitis because corneal ulceration often occurs under the upper eyelid.

corneal epithelium (Box 4-5), producing rapid stromal ulceration, necrosis, and perforation as early as 24 to 48 hours after infection (Figs. 4-13, 4-14, and 4-15). Rapid diagnosis by Gram stain (gram-negative intracellular diplococci) and treatment with systemic antibiotics are required. The organism must be cultured on chocolate agar maintained in a 10% carbon dioxide environment. The current treatment of choice is 1 g ceftriaxone intramuscularly once for conjunctivitis and 1 g intramuscularly or intravenously every 12 hours for 3 to 5 days for corneal involvement. Ciprofloxacin and spectinomycin are alternatives for patients allergic to penicillin or cephalosporin. Topical treatment alone with ciprofloxacin is insufficient for these patients, though it may be a helpful adjunct. Frequent irrigation may be required because of the copious amount of purulent discharge produced. Patients should be tested for other sexually transmitted diseases, including syphilis and human immunodeficiency virus, and concurrent treatment with oral tetracycline, doxycycline, or erythromycin should be considered for possible chlamydial infection. Sexual partners should be evaluated and treated for sexually transmitted diseases.

Box 4-5 Organisms That Can Penetrate an Intact Epithelium

Neisseria gonorrhoeae
Haemophilus aegyptius
Corynebacterium
Listeria

Moraxella spp are gram-negative coccobacilli that may produce infectious keratitis, usually in debilitated

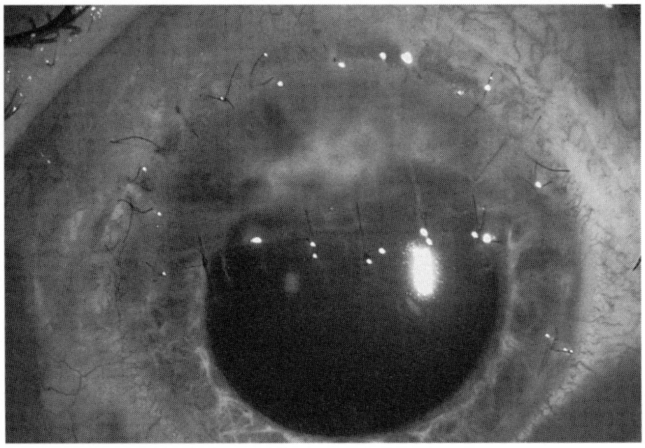

Fig. 4-15 *Neisseria gonorrhoeae* corneal ulcer repair. The corneal ulcer seen in Fig. 4-14 perforated and required a large corneal patch graft.

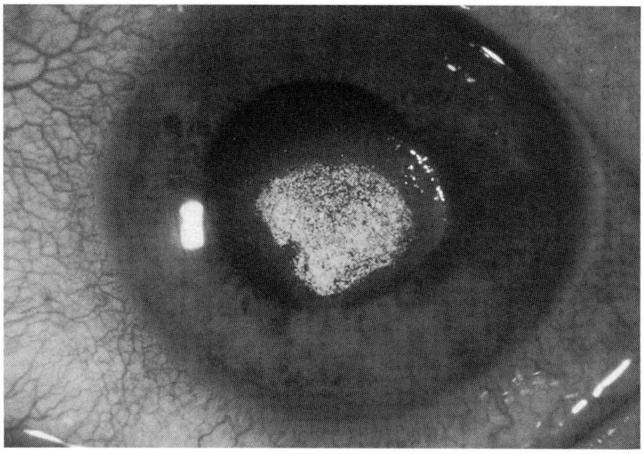

Fig. 4-16 Ciprofloxacin corneal deposits. Frequent topical ciprofloxacin use with an epithelial defect can result in medication deposits in the superficial cornea.

patients and chronically sick eyes. It often presents with a superficial infiltrate that progresses with a slow, indolent course. It tends to respond gradually to antibiotics and has a relatively high perforation rate compared with other bacteria. Surprisingly, these organisms tend to be sensitive to antibiotics such as cefazolin and vancomycin that are generally more effective against gram-positive organisms. Ciprofloxacin is also effective, but the response to aminoglycosides is variable.

Treatment The initial treatment of bacterial keratitis is usually empirical and involves frequent instillation of broad-spectrum antibiotics. Traditionally, a fortified cephalosporin such as cefazolin (50 mg/ml) and a fortified aminoglycoside such as tobramycin (15 mg/ml) or gentamicin (15 mg/ml) are used in combination as initial therapy. These agents are usually started every 15 or 30 minutes to 60 minutes around the clock after an initial loading dose (5 drops over 5 minutes), depending on the patient's condition. This combination provides excellent gram-positive and gram-negative coverage, and it may be modified based on clinical progress and culture results. The use of a fluoroquinolone alone every 15 to 30 minutes as a single-agent therapy may be considered for small peripheral ulcers because it provides relatively broad-spectrum activity against gram-positive and gram-negative organisms, including *Pseudomonas*. However, the fluoroquinolone antibiotics are relatively weak against some gram-positive organisms, especially *Streptococcus*, and anaerobes, and resistance to fluoroquinolones appears to be increasing. The combination of a fluoroquinolone and fortified cefazolin may be as effective as the traditional combination of fortified cefazolin and a fortified aminoglycoside. Topical corticosteroids should not be used in the initial treatment of infected corneal ulcers. Frequent use of topical ciprofloxacin in an eye with a large epithelial defect may cause ciprofloxacin deposits to adhere to the superficial corneal stroma (Fig. 4-16). Although the deposits do not appear to impede reepithelialization, they may limit visualization of the deep cornea and the anterior chamber.

Once antibiotic therapy has been initiated, the patient should be followed up daily until a significant clinical response to treatment is noted. Dramatic improvement in severe infections is not expected for a few days. Improved patient comfort within the first 24 to 48 hours is a good indication that the infection is improving. Clinical signs of improvement include decrease in size and density of the infiltrate, consolidation of the infiltrate and the development of well-defined borders, loss of adherent mucopurulent discharge, reduction in hypopyon or anterior chamber reaction, reduction in surrounding stromal edema, and progressive reepithelialization (Box 4-6). Once improvement has begun, the frequency of antibiotic administration may be slowly tapered according to the patient's condition. Overnight dosing may be reduced or eliminated first to allow the patient to get more sleep. Antibiotic ointment at bedtime should then be added. Daytime administration may be reduced gradually, again according to the patient's response, and fortified antibiotics may be converted to commercially available antibiotics. Culture results may allow the elimination of less effective medications that contribute to toxicity.

Modification of the initial antibiotic therapy is based on the culture results and on the clinical response. Resistance to the initial antibiotics and worsening or lack of improvement in the patient's condition should prompt a change in therapy. Similarly, if the patient's condition worsens significantly before culture results and sensitivity information are available, a change in therapy should be considered. If the cultured organism is sensitive to more than one agent used, the less effective one should be reduced or eliminated to reduce toxicity. The dura-

Box 4-6 Clinical Signs of Resolution of Bacterial Corneal Ulcers

Improved patient comfort
Progressive reepithelialization over the infiltrate
Decreasing size and density of the infiltrate
Loss of adherent mucopurulent discharge
Reduction in hypopyon or anterior chamber reaction
Reduction of stromal edema surrounding the infiltrate
Development of well-defined infiltrate borders

tion of treatment depends on the severity of the infection and the specific organism. Small infiltrates may only require 5 to 7 days of antibiotics, whereas large ulcers may require treatment for several weeks (Figs. 4-17 and 4-18). Gram-negative ulcers generally require longer treatment than gram-positive ulcers, and they often recrudesce if the antibiotics are tapered too rapidly.

An ulcer that continues to worsen after intensive broad-spectrum therapy has begun is worrisome. Resistance to antibiotics or an inadequate choice of initial agents may be responsible, and a change in therapy should be considered. Culture and sensitivity results may be helpful, but if the cultures are negative or the sensitivity data are unavailable, an empiric change may be necessary. For gram-positive organisms, vancomycin may be a useful alternative. For gram-negative organisms, an antipseudomonal penicillin (such as mezlocillin or piperacillin) may be added, or ceftazidime or amikacin may be used instead of gentamicin or tobramycin. If cultures are negative and the patient's condition worsens or does not improve with broad-spectrum therapy, repeat corneal scrapings or corneal biopsy may be required. Nonbacterial causes of infectious keratitis should also be considered, and additional scrapings for cultures on special media should also be obtained. Lack of improvement after therapy has begun may be related to poor patient compliance with the intensive medication schedule. It is important to ascertain exactly how often the patient is actually using the medications. Ask patients to demonstrate how they instill their drops. The results may be surprising. If doubt exists as to a patient's ability to administer the required medication at the required frequency, recommend hospital admission. The reliable administration of medication by the hospital staff may be all that is required to turn a worsening ulcer into a resolving one.

Ulcers that continue to progress despite aggressive, maximal medical therapy and that threaten to (or actually do) perforate the cornea or spread to the sclera may require patch grafting or penetrating keratoplasty. Surgical intervention should be deferred, if possible, until initial antibiotic therapy has been given for 1 to 2 days, depending on whether the anterior chamber is formed. Systemic antibiotics occasionally are helpful.

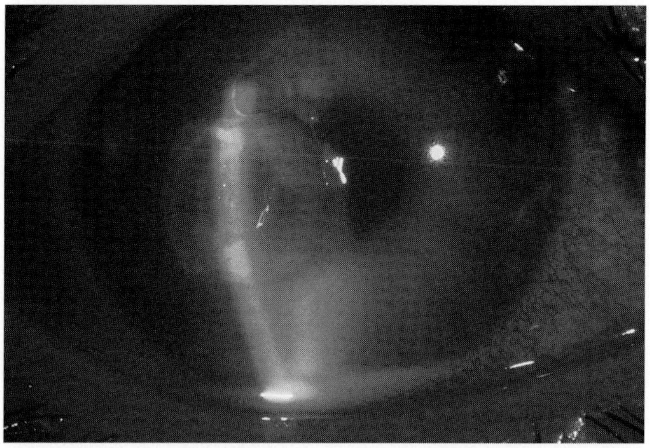

Fig. 4-17 Corneal ulcer. A moderately large *Pseudomonas* corneal ulcer and a hypopyon resulting from contact lens wear are treated aggressively with topical antibiotics.

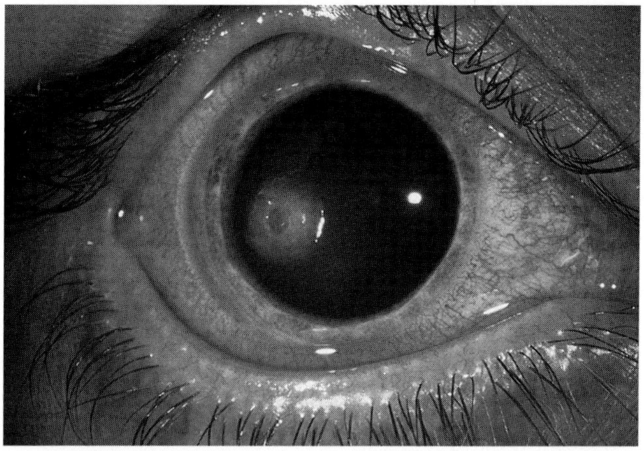

Fig. 4-18 Corneal ulcer. After 10 days of aggressive treatment with topical antibiotics, the corneal ulcer seen in Fig. 4-17 is responding well.

The use of topical corticosteroids in the management of bacterial keratitis is controversial. Corticosteroids may help reduce the stromal inflammatory reaction, thus limiting the tissue damage produced by neutrophils, the degree of neovascularization, and the amount of postinflammatory scar formation. However, suppression of the host's inflammatory response to infection, particularly if current antibiotic therapy is incomplete or inadequate, may allow the bacteria to survive. Corticosteroids have been implicated in the late recrudescence of *Pseudomonas* keratitis once antibiotics are tapered. In general corticosteroids should be avoided if the causative organism and the efficacy of bactericidal agents are not known for sure. Cautious use of corticosteroids may be considered for patients who have mild to moderate disease, who are threatened by scarring of the visual axis, and for whom the causative organism, positive response to antibiotic therapy, and patient compliance have been established (this usually requires at least 72 hours of treatment).

Corticosteroid therapy should be tapered along with the antibiotic tapering regimen, and it should be discontinued before the antibiotic is discontinued.

The treatment of contact lens-related erosions and infiltrates deserves special attention. Because of the significant risk for infection, particularly with *Pseudomonas*, all contact lens-related epithelial erosions should be treated with frequent antibiotic therapy, which includes coverage for *Pseudomonas.* Patching is contraindicated for these patients, and the patient should be reexamined in 24 hours. Contact lens-related corneal infiltrates larger than 1 to 2 mm that include an overlying epithelial defect should be scraped for culture, and hourly antibiotic therapy with adequate coverage for *Pseudomonas* should be started. If possible, the contact lens and the lens case should also be cultured.

Not all contact lens-related infiltrates result from bacterial infection. Corneal hypoxia from a tight contact lens or a hypersensitivity reaction to lens cleaning and disinfection solutions may produce inflammatory infiltrates in the cornea. However, these infiltrates tend to be peripheral and do not usually include an overlying epithelial defect, surrounding edema, or an anterior chamber reaction. Therefore if a patient has a contact lens-related corneal infiltrate without an epithelial defect, cultures may be deferred, but contact lens use should be discontinued, and prophylactic antibiotics with adequate *Pseudomonas* coverage should be started. Topical corticosteroids should be avoided, and frequent observation is warranted.

Fungal Keratitis

Keratomycosis was once rare. Recently, however, there has been an increase in the prevalence of these infections. This increased prevalence may be related to better recognition because of improved diagnostic capabilities and heightened clinical awareness, though the widespread use of broad-spectrum antibiotics and topical corticosteroids has also been implicated. Fungal keratitis, relatively uncommon in temperate climates, is a significant cause of ocular morbidity in tropical regions.

Fungal organisms that cause corneal infections may be divided into three categories: yeasts (unicellular fungi), filamentous fungi (molds), and dimorphic fungi. The typical yeast form is *Candida*. Yeasts generally are round or oval, and they reproduce by budding. Filamentous fungi produce long, branching structures called hyphae. Hyphae are categorized as septate if they contain distinct inner divisions between elements; the alternative form is nonseptate. The filamentous fungi most frequently isolated from corneal ulcers are all septate varieties and include *Fusarium, Aspergillus, Penicillium, Alternaria,* and *Curvularia*. Nonseptate filamentous fungi rarely cause corneal disease, though the most notorious of this group, *Mucor,* is an important cause of ocular morbidity in the forms of orbital cellulitis and cavernous sinus syndrome in patients with diabetes and in immunocompromised hosts. Dimorphic fungi exist in either a yeast form or a filamentous form, depending on temperature and local conditions. Dimorphic fungi such as *Histoplasma* are rare causes of keratomycosis.

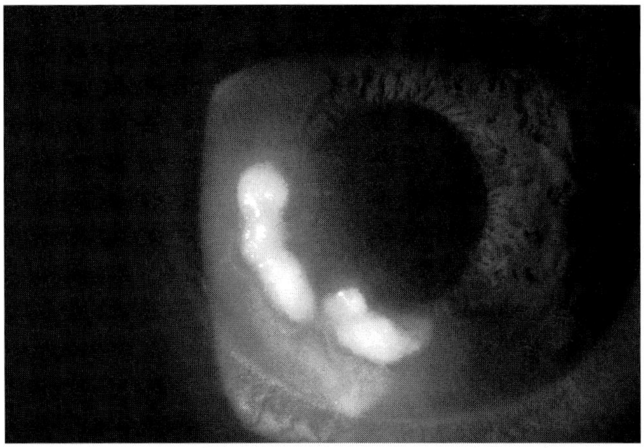

Fig. 4-19 Fungal keratitis. A multicentric dense corneal infiltrate is seen. Fungal cultures were positive for *Candida* spp.

Major risk factors for keratomycosis are trauma, especially when caused by vegetable matter (typically filamentous fungi), chronic ocular disease, and an immunocompromised cornea (typically caused by *Candida*). The trauma may seem trivial, but it could be significant (e.g., trauma involving vegetable matter to a farmer, a gardener, or a stable worker). A corneal ulcer in an otherwise healthy eye without any apparent risk factors for infection should prompt an in-depth review of medical, occupational, and social factors that may be contributory. Chronic ocular disease such as a severe dry eye or ocular cicatricial pemphigoid and topical corticosteroid use (particularly in patients with chronic underlying corneal disease) may also predispose to fungal infection.

The clinical onset of keratomycosis is often insidious because fungal infections are typically slow growing. The predisposing event may have occurred days to weeks before the patient seeks treatment. The patient may report irritation that was followed by an asymptomatic period; it was during this time that a smoldering infiltrate formed. The classic clinical appearance of fungal keratitis is a patchy white or grayish-white infiltrate with feathery edges (Figs. 4-19 and 4-20), satellite lesions (Fig. 4-21), and a variable epithelial defect. An immune ring may be present surrounding the infiltrate, and there may be an anterior chamber reaction, an inflammatory endothelial plaque, or even a hypopyon (Fig. 4-22). Although this clinical appearance is highly suggestive of a fungal process, it should be noted that several of these features may be present in other infectious processes, such as *Acanthamoeba* infection, herpes simplex keratitis, and atypical mycobacteria keratitis. It is important

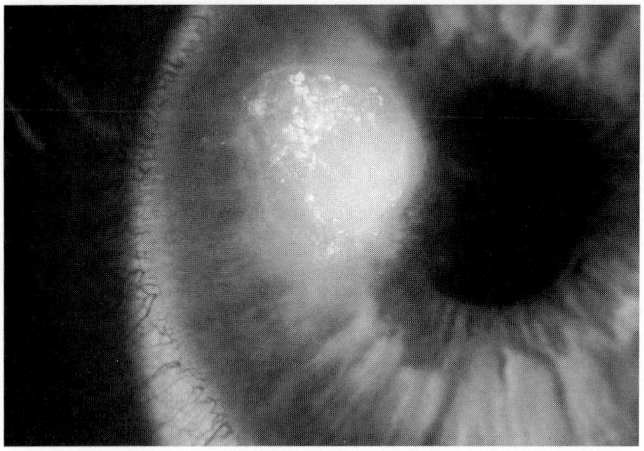

Fig. 4-20 Fungal keratitis. This dense corneal ulcer with feathery edges was caused by *Fusarium* infection.

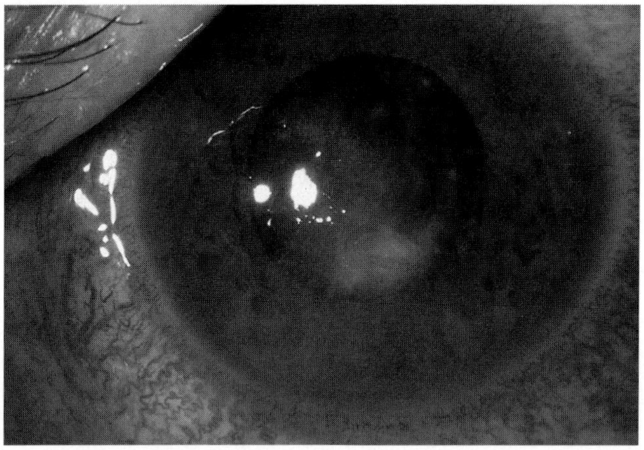

Fig. 4-21 Fungal keratitis. A patchy corneal infiltrate with satellite lesions is commonly seen in fungal keratitis.

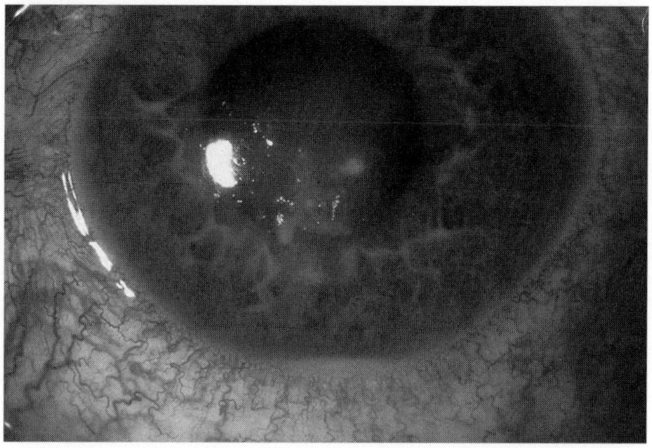

Fig. 4-22 Fungal keratitis. A small, patchy, fungal corneal infiltrate has an associated hypopyon.

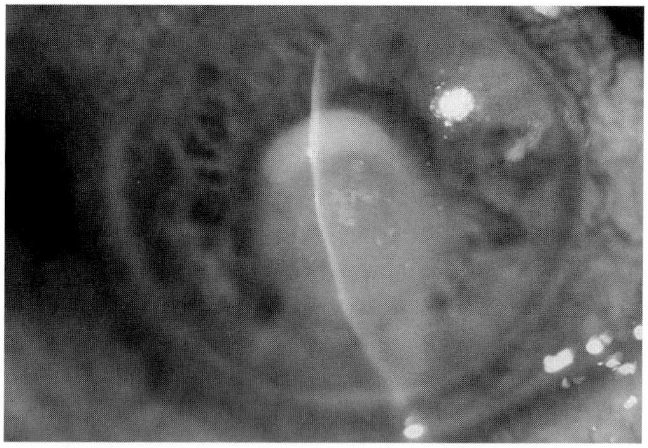

Fig. 4-23 Fungal keratitis. This dense ulcer and small hypopyon did not respond to intensive topical, fortified antibiotics. Smears and cultures were negative. It advanced rapidly and required emergency corneal transplantation.

to remember that fungal infiltrates are sometimes clinically indistinguishable from bacterial infiltrates or may coexist with them. Thus it is critical to establish a differential diagnosis based on the patient's history and clinical findings and to obtain the necessary smears and cultures. Fungal cultures should be included in the laboratory workup of any suspected infectious corneal infiltrate.

If left untreated, fungal organisms can penetrate deep into the stroma (Fig. 4-23). This deep infection may be accompanied by progressive thinning, descemetocele formation, and perforation. Fungal infiltrates may penetrate deeply without significant thinning, often with resolution of the epithelial defect and the superficial areas of infiltration. These deep foci permit fungal elements to find refuge from poorly penetrating topical antifungal medication, to proliferate, and to allow penetration of Descemet's membrane and entry to the anterior chamber *without* corneal perforation (which bacteria generally cannot do).

The diagnosis of a suspected fungal corneal ulcer is confirmed by corneal scraping for stain and culture. Deep infections, which may not be accessible by superficial scraping, may require that a corneal biopsy specimen be taken for diagnosis. Stains for fungi include Gram, Giemsa, Gomori's methenamine silver (Fig. 4-24), periodic acid-Schiff, acridine orange, and calcofluor white. Note that the calcofluor white stain requires a fluorescent microscope. Fungus grows on Sabouraud's agar without cycloheximide and on blood agar and chocolate agar at room temperature. Growth also occurs in thioglycolate broth and in brain-heart infusion media. Most species grow within 3 to 5 days; however, cultures should be held for 3 weeks to allow for late growth. In

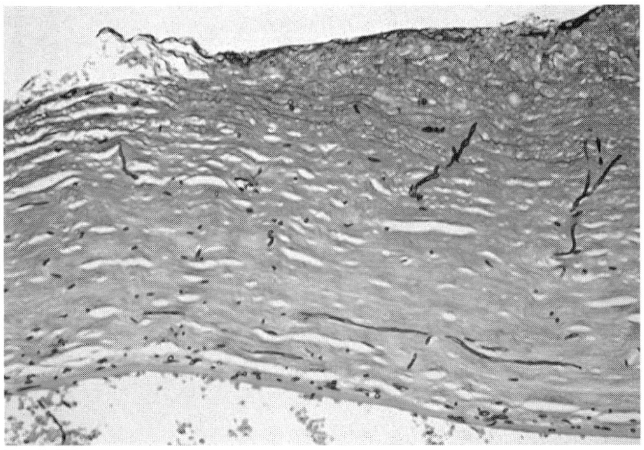

Fig. 4-24 Fungal keratitis. The histopathology of the cornea seen in Fig. 4-23, stained with Gomori's methenamine silver, revealed numerous fungal elements throughout the stroma. (Courtesy of Ralph C. Eagle, Jr., M.D.)

vitro susceptibility testing is available for fungal isolates, but little evidence correlates in vitro susceptibility data with clinical results.

Two main categories of antifungal medications are available: polyenes and imidazoles (Box 4-7). Polyenes are agents that bind preferentially to ergosterol in the fungal cell membrane, thereby altering membrane permeability. Natamycin, a polyene, is the only commercially available topical antifungal, and it is the initial agent of choice for filamentous fungal infections. However, it penetrates the cornea poorly, largely because of extremely limited penetration through the corneal epithelium. Epithelial debridement significantly increases the drug's penetration and efficacy. This is especially important if the epithelium has healed over a deep stromal infection that may still be active. Amphotericin B, another polyene, is the treatment of choice for yeast infections, particularly those caused by *Candida,* but it is less effective against filamentous fungi. It may be formulated into a drop, usually at a 0.15% concentration, from the intravenous preparation. It may be administered intravitreally, if necessary, to treat fungal endophthalmitis. As with natamycin, epithelial debridement enhances the corneal penetration and efficacy of amphotericin B.

The imidazoles (see Box 4-7) are another class of antifungal agents that may inhibit fungal ergosterol synthesis and damage fungal cell walls. These agents are effective against yeasts and filamentous fungi and vary in efficacy by individual drug. All these medications are commercially available for systemic antifungal therapy, and topical preparations can be compounded. Several of these agents, most notably fluconazole and itraconazole, penetrate the aqueous reasonably well after oral administration and have been used in conjunction with the topical administration of other antifungal agents.

Box 4-7 Currently Available Antifungal Agents

POLYENES

Natamycin (better for filamentous fungi)
Amphotericin B (better for yeasts)
Mycostatin

IMIDAZOLES

Ketoconazole
Miconazole
Clotrimazole
Fluconazole
Itraconazole

Initial management of suspected fungal corneal ulcers should include smears for fungal identification and morphology and scrapings for culture. If the smear reveals hyphae, natamycin is the initial drug of choice, whereas if yeast forms are present, 0.15% amphotericin B may be considered initially. Typically, these drops are used every hour around the clock initially and are tapered extremely slowly. If cultures and smears are negative and fungus is still suspected, corneal biopsy should be considered. The response to antifungal therapy is usually slow, with resolution taking weeks to months. Signs of improvement are reduced pain, reduced infiltrate size, and loss of satellite lesions. Antifungal agents are continued as long as a patient has active corneal infiltration. Beware of infiltrates that continue to penetrate deeper into the stroma. If the keratitis progresses despite aggressive therapy, consider adding systemic therapy, changing the topical therapy, or both. Culture results may be helpful in this situation. Corticosteroids may potentiate fungal proliferation and should be avoided. If the infection continues to progress deeply into the cornea or toward the limbus despite maximal medical therapy, therapeutic penetrating keratoplasty may be necessary.

Acanthamoeba Keratitis

Acanthamoeba spp are free-living protozoans found in tap water, ponds and lakes, swimming pools, hot tubs, sea water, and soil. They are a relatively uncommon, though important, cause of ocular infection; they may produce painful, relentlessly progressive, and potentially blinding keratitis. *Acanthamoeba* organisms exist in two forms: an active trophozoite and a dormant cyst. It is the resistant cyst form that contributes to the difficulty in eradicating this serious infection.

Contact lens use, trauma, and exposure to contaminated soil or water are the major risk factors for infection. Most forms of *Acanthamoeba* keratitis are related to con-

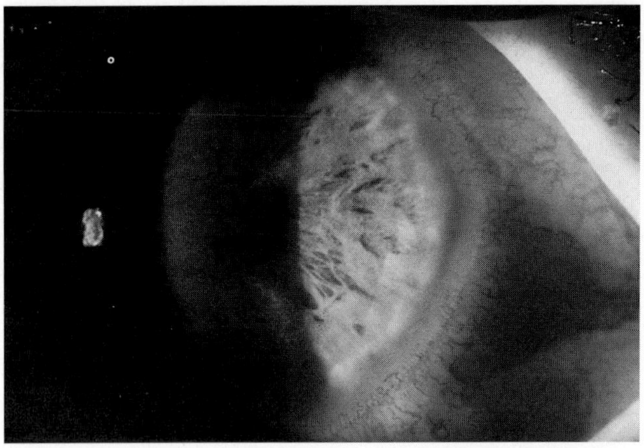

Fig. 4-25 *Acanthamoeba* keratitis. Mildly elevated gray-white epithelial opacities in a dendritiform pattern are seen in the early stages of *Acanthamoeba* keratitis.

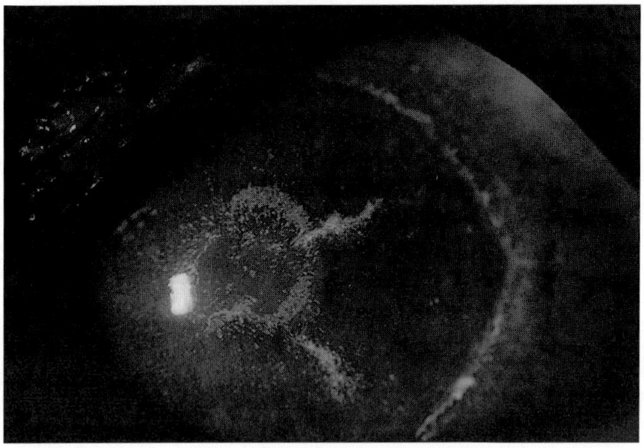

Fig. 4-26 *Acanthamoeba* keratitis. Fluorescein dye staining of the cornea seen in Fig. 4-25 reveals a dendritiform staining pattern. Early *Acanthamoeba* keratitis is consequently often misdiagnosed as herpes simplex keratitis. (See color plate.)

tact lens use. All contact lens types, whether soft or hard—but especially daily wear soft contact lenses—have been associated with *Acanthamoeba* infection. Swimming with contact lenses, poor contact lens cleaning and disinfection, and using ineffective disinfecting systems are the most frequent contact lens–related risk factors for *Acanthamoeba* infection. In the past, tap water and homemade saline made from distilled water and salt tablets were significant risk factors. Trophozoites have been shown to adhere more readily to soft contact lenses, particularly those of higher water content, than to rigid lenses. Proper lens cleaning procedures successfully remove adherent cysts and trophozoites from lenses.

Corneal infection may begin with an epithelial irregularity and infiltrate, often in a dendritiform pattern resembling a herpes infection (Figs. 4-25 and 4-26). This

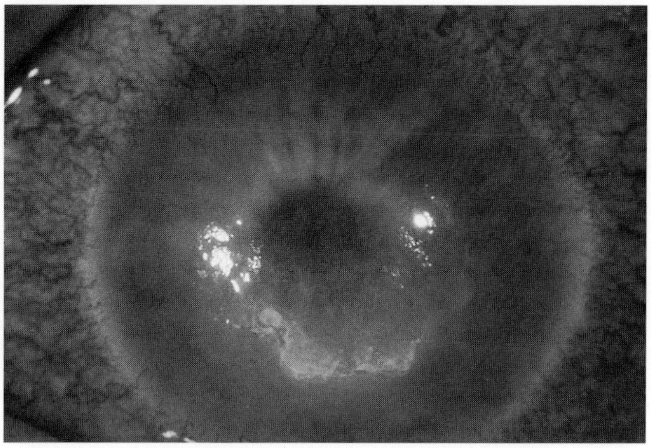

Fig. 4-27 *Acanthamoeba* keratitis. A large, patchy, stromal infiltrate is seen in this eye with chronic keratitis. Corneal scrapings revealed *Acanthamoeba* cysts.

unfortunate similarity often contributes to a delay in diagnosis. However, patients with *Acanthamoeba* infection are characteristically in intense pain, out of proportion to the clinical findings, because of the organism's affinity for corneal nerves. Patients with herpes keratitis generally have less pain than expected because of the relative neurotrophic state of their corneas. If left untreated, the *Acanthamoeba* infection may progress more deeply into the stroma, producing patchy anterior stromal infiltrates (Fig. 4-27) that coalesce into a ring infiltrate in 3 to 6 weeks (Fig. 4-28). Radial infiltrates surrounding corneal nerves may also be found (Fig. 4-29). Corneal neovascularization is relatively absent early in the infection. Although not pathognomonic, a ring infiltrate and radial keratoneuritis are highly suggestive of *Acanthamoeba* infection. Untreated stromal infection may progress to suppurative, necrotizing deep stromal keratitis with thinning and perforation.

A heightened degree of clinical suspicion is essential for the early diagnosis of *Acanthamoeba* keratitis. This infection is often misdiagnosed as herpes simplex keratitis, though bacterial and fungal infections and anesthetic abuse may present with similar findings. The diagnosis of *Acanthamoeba* infection is confirmed by the observation of *Acanthamoeba* organisms in smears of corneal scrapings. Gram stain, Giemsa stain (Fig. 4-30), and acridine orange stain may identify both forms of the organism, but calcofluor white only stains the cysts. The calcofluor white stain requires a fluorescent microscope. Confocal microscopy may help make an early diagnosis. Cultures are obtained by directly inoculating corneal scrapings onto nonnutrient agar with an overlay of a gram-negative rod such as *Escherichia coli* or *Klebsiella.* These plates are then examined for surface trails left by the motile trophozoites. Corneal biopsy may be required for deeper infections. Contact lenses and cases can also be cultured.

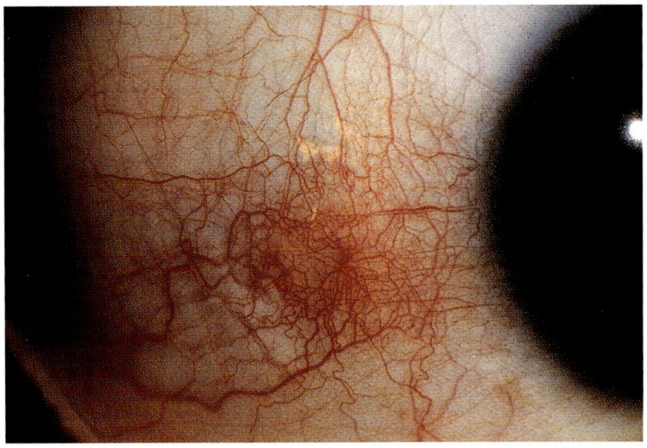
Plate 1-3

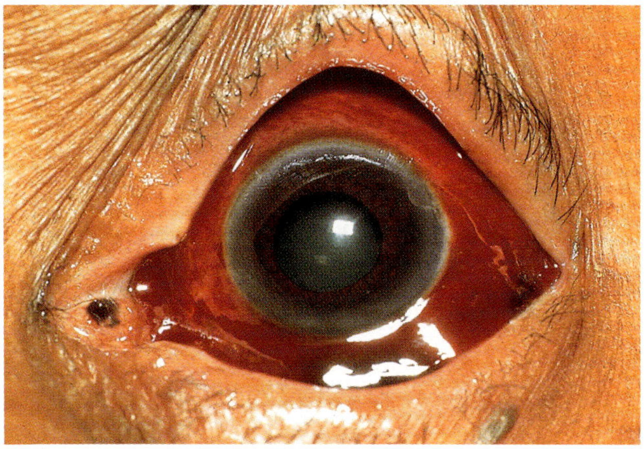
Plate 1-5

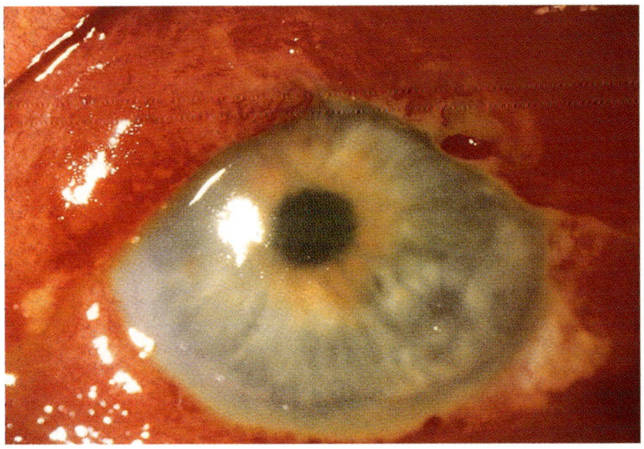
Plate 1-19

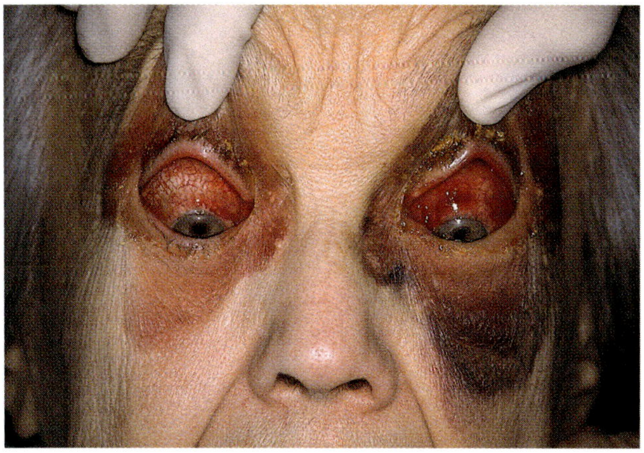
Plate 1-24

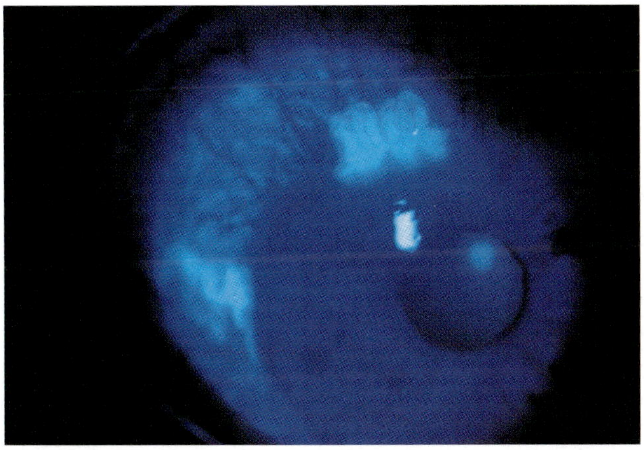
Plate 1-25

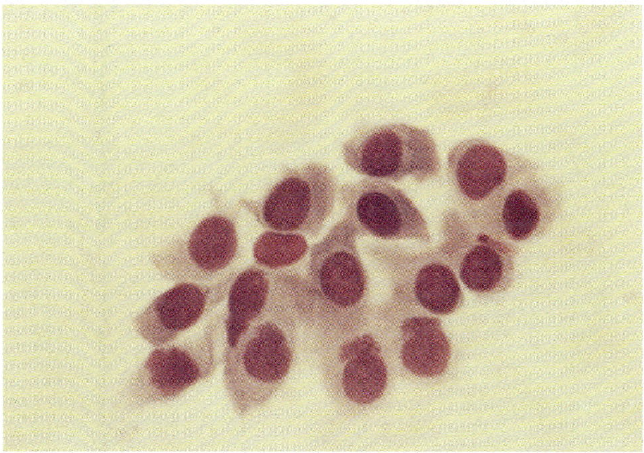
Plate 1-34

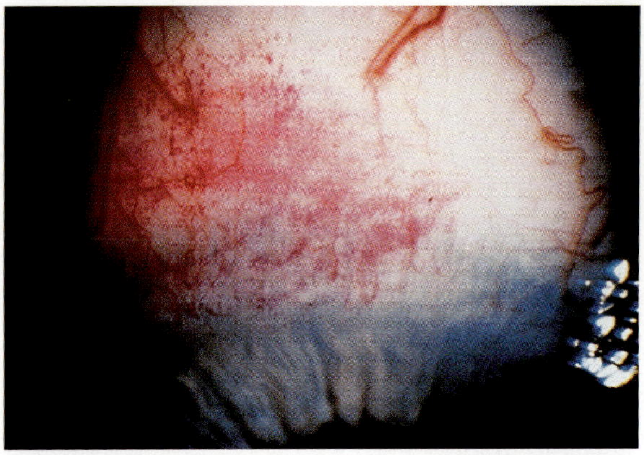

Plate 1-50

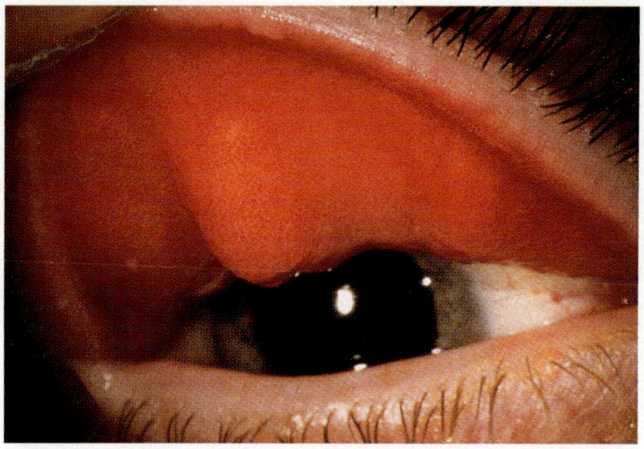

Plate 1-53

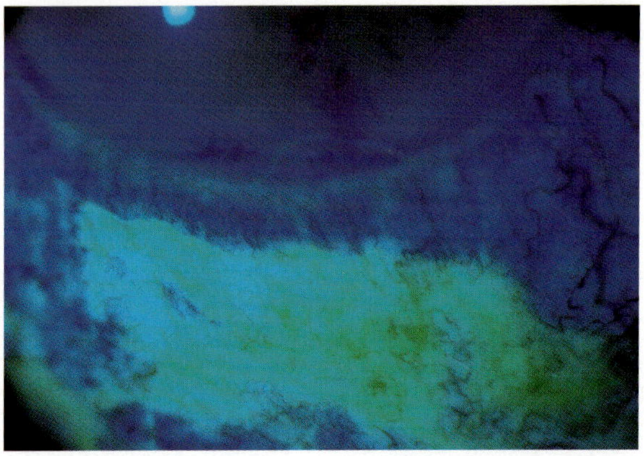

Plate 1-58

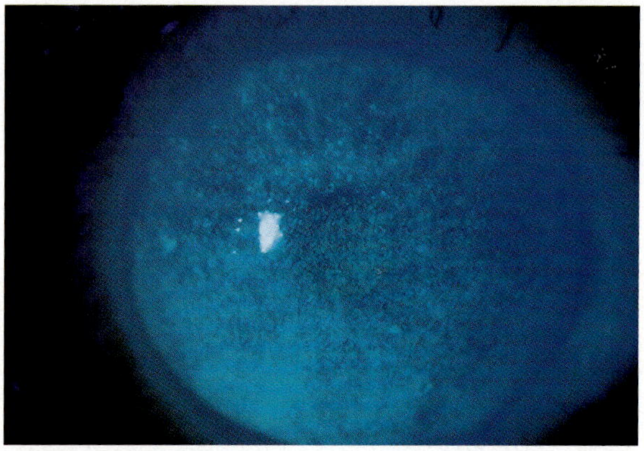

Plate 1-60

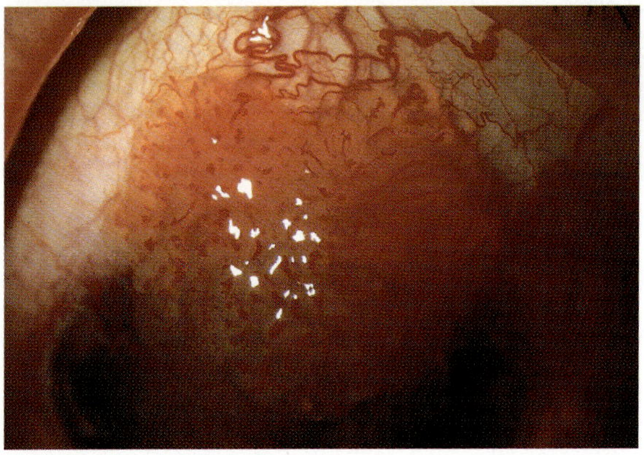

Plate 1-95

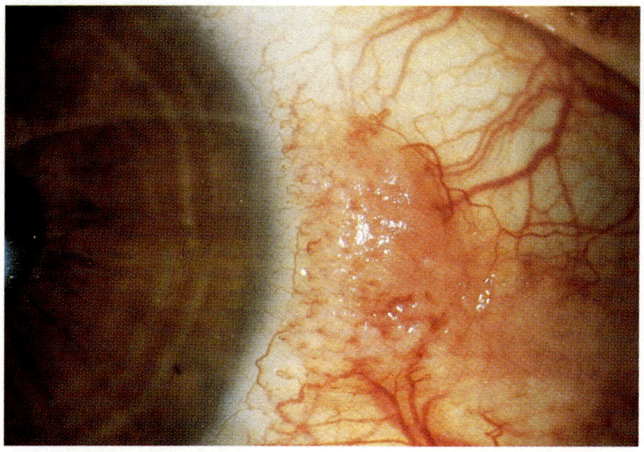

Plate 1-96

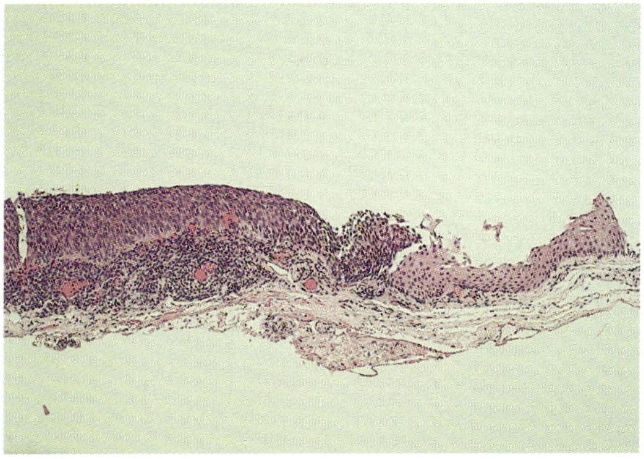

Plate 1-98

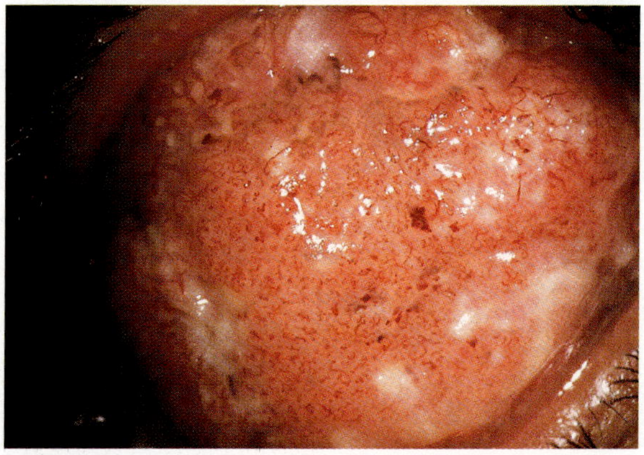

Plate 1-102

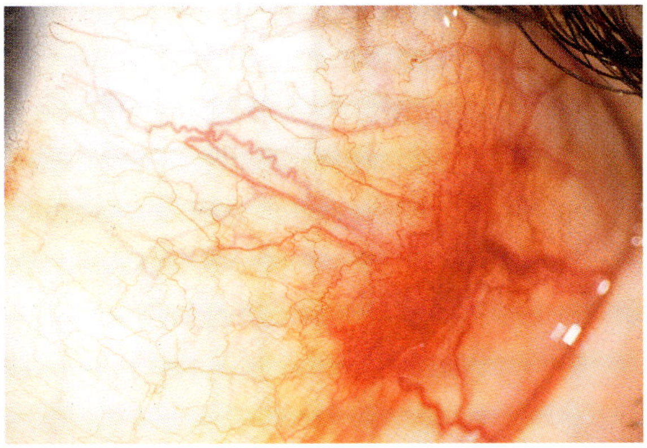
Plate 1-116

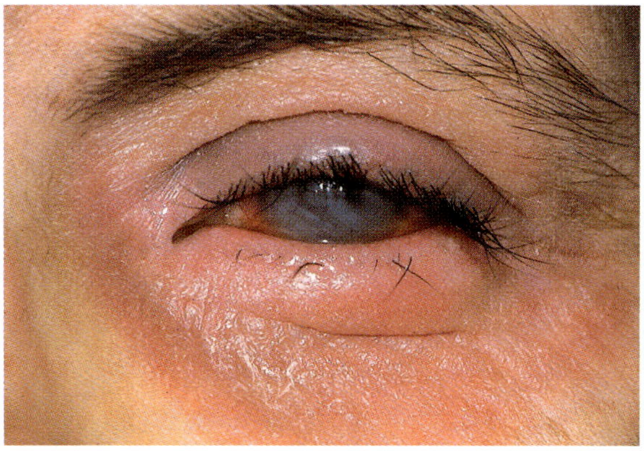
Plate 1-129

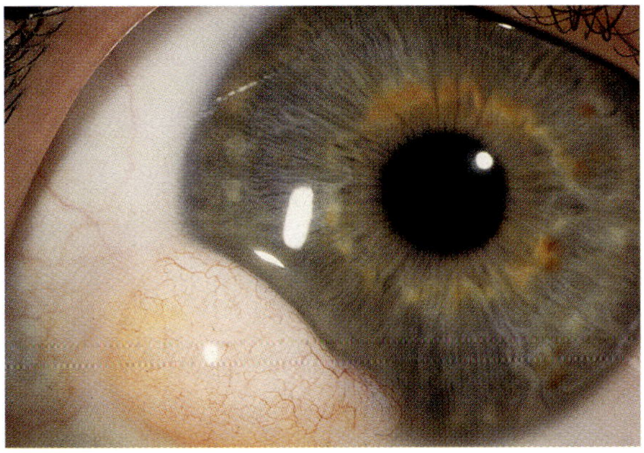
Plate 2-8

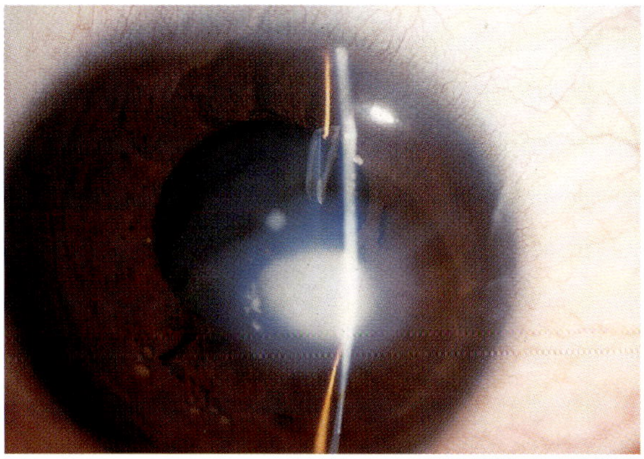
Plate 2-18

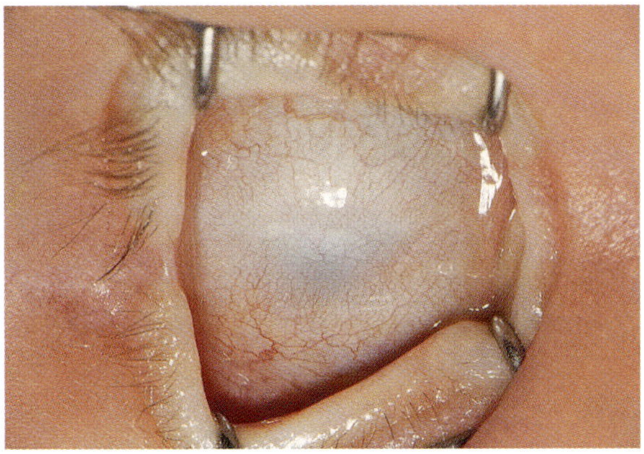
Plate 2-24

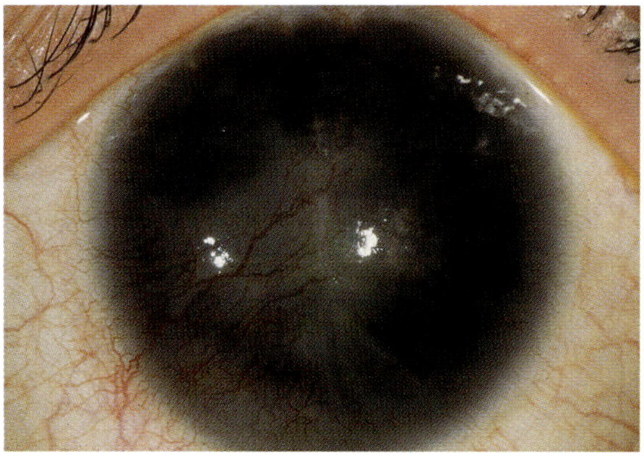
Plate 2-30

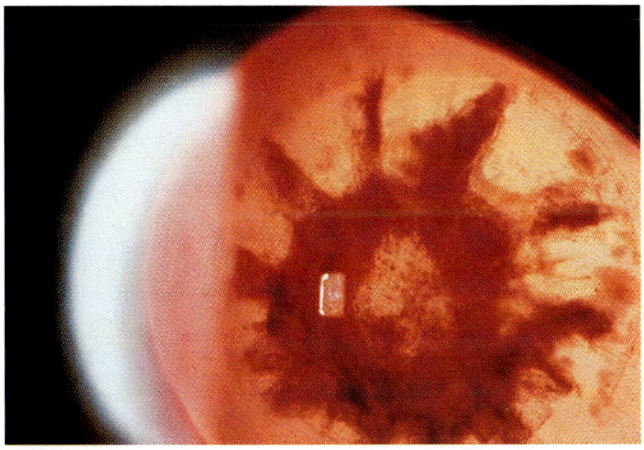
Plate 2-32

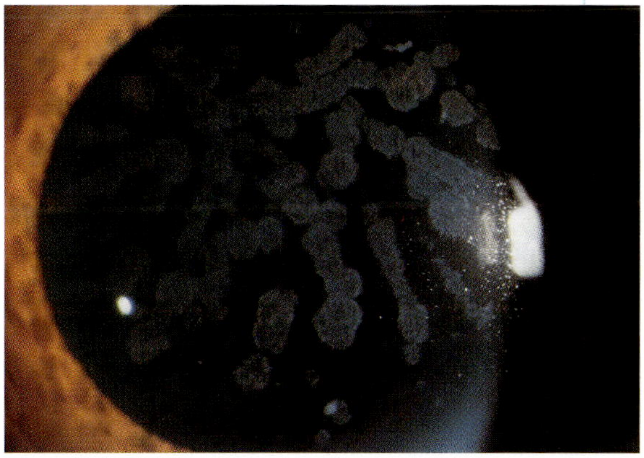
Plate 3-16

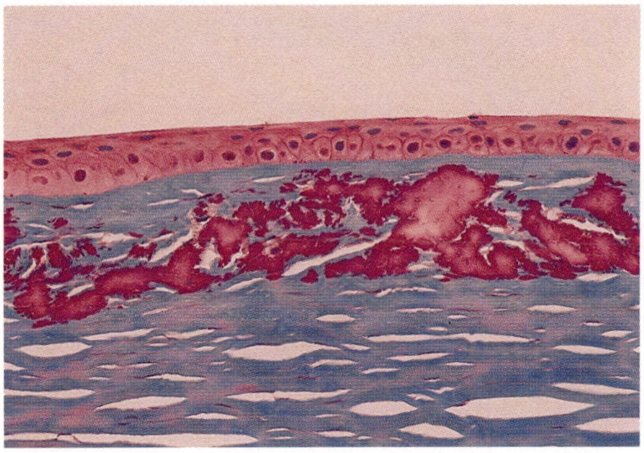

Plate 3-19

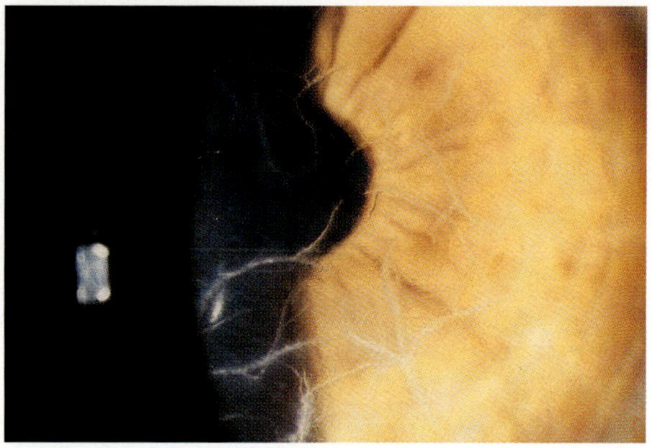

Plate 3-20

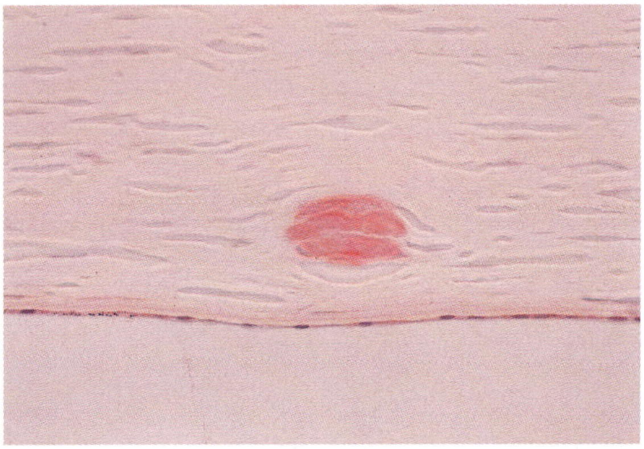

Plate 3-26

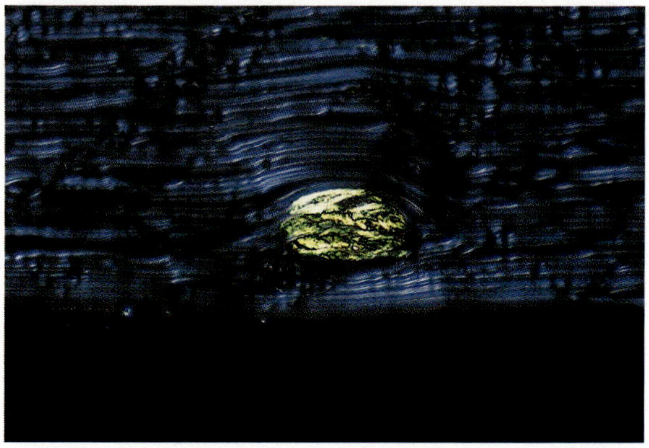

Plate 3-27

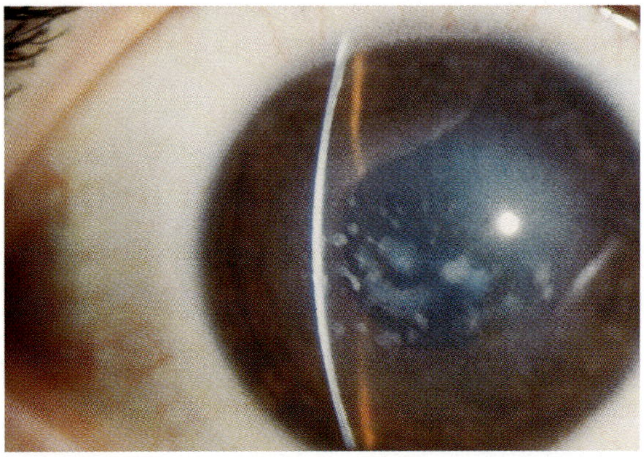

Plate 3-32

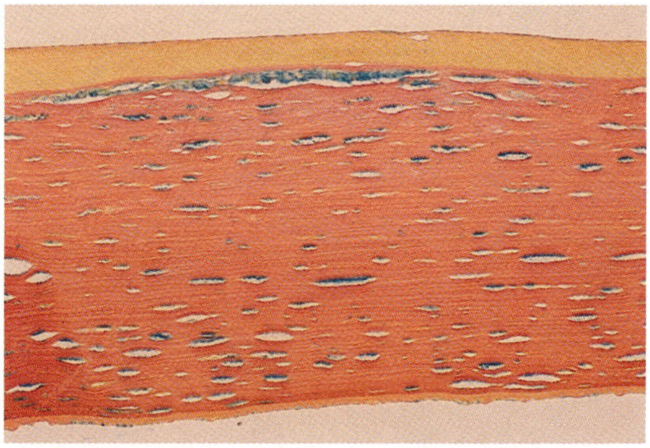

Plate 3-33

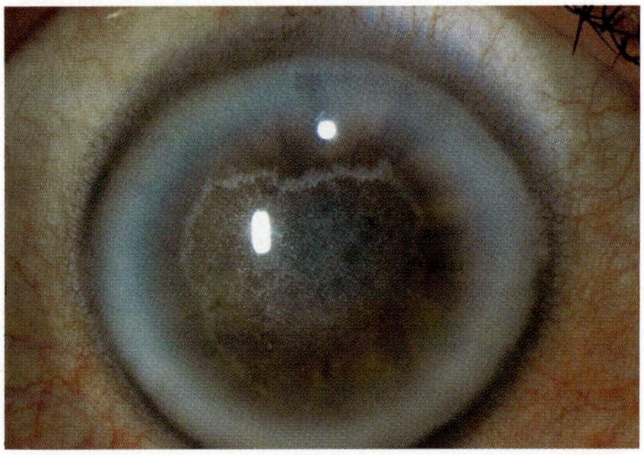

Plate 3-37

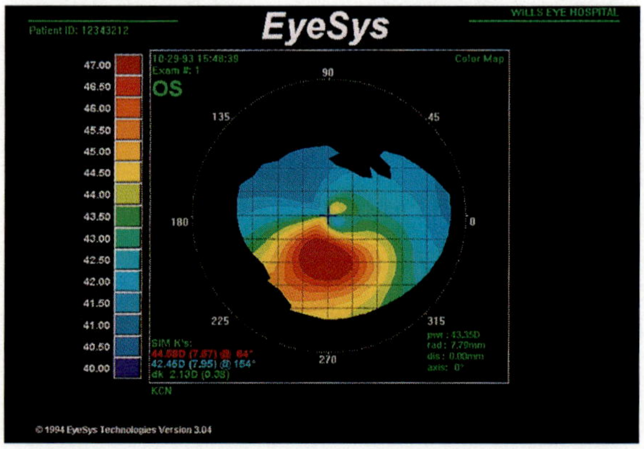

Plate 3-92

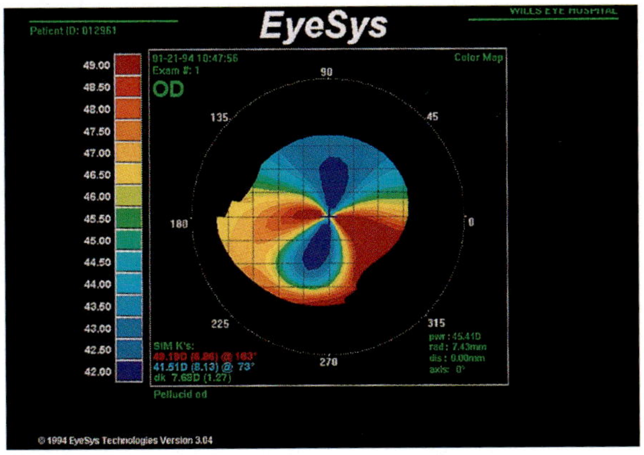

Plate 3-97

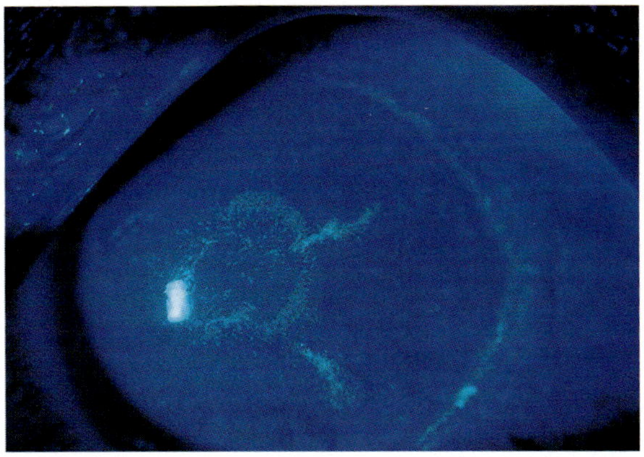

Plate 4-26

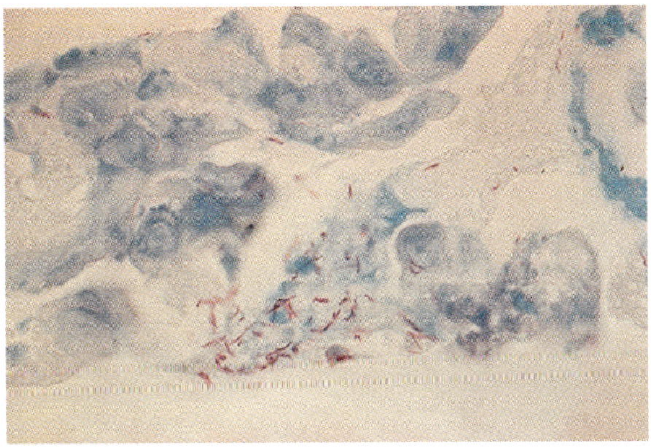

Plate 4-32

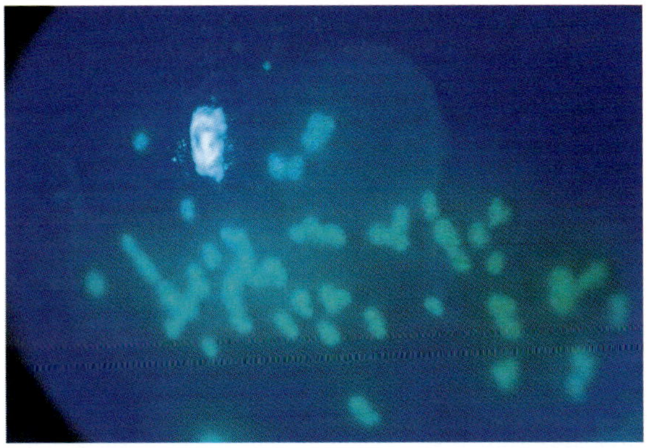

Plate 4-35

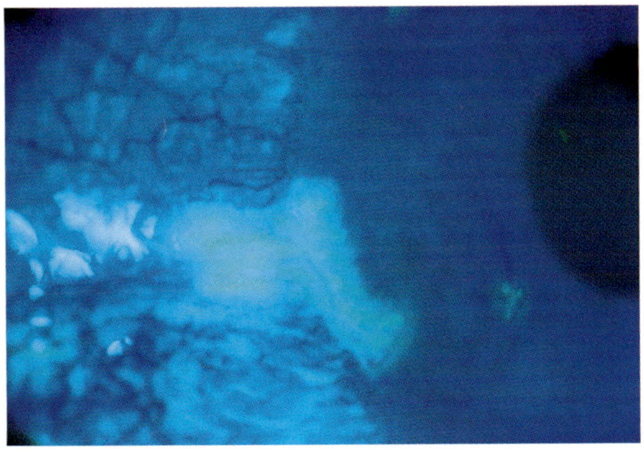

Plate 4-39

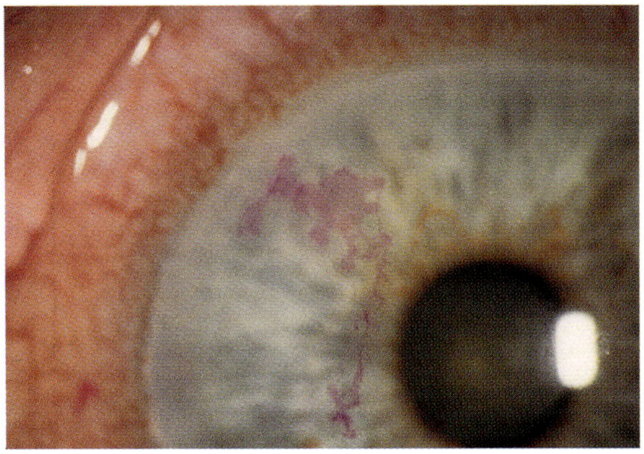

Plate 4-41

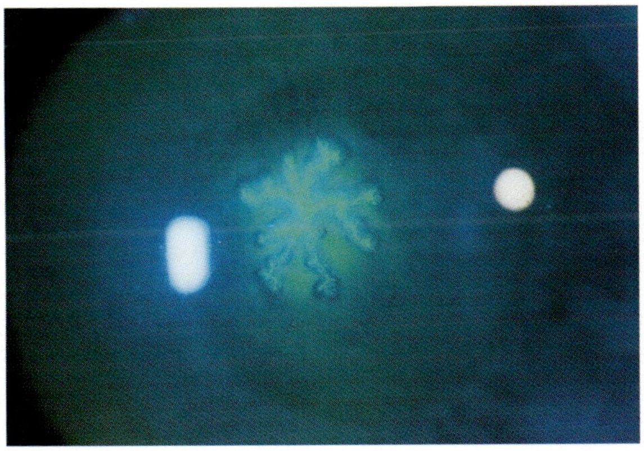

Plate 4-43

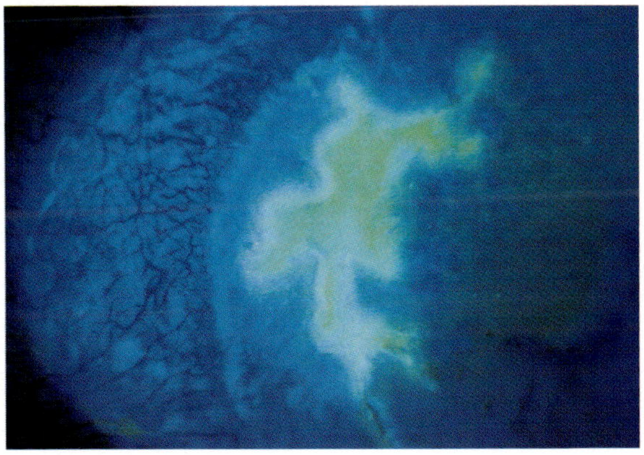

Plate 4-44

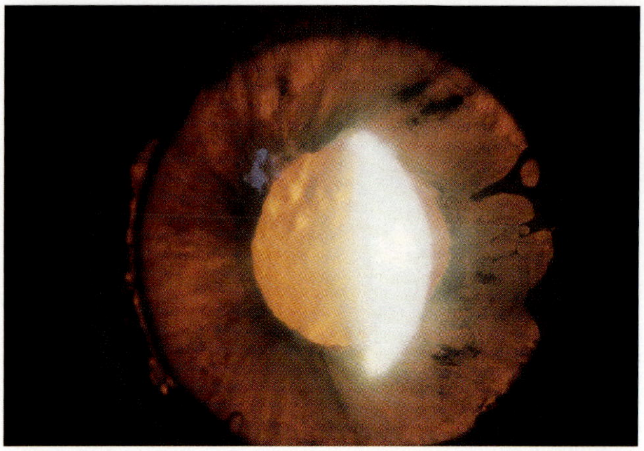
Plate 4-54

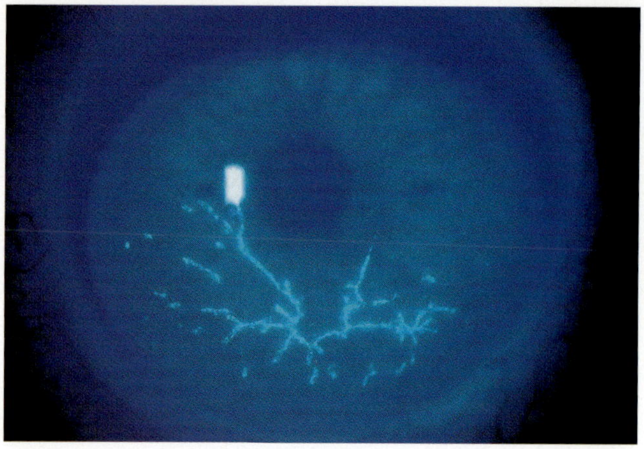
Plate 4-63

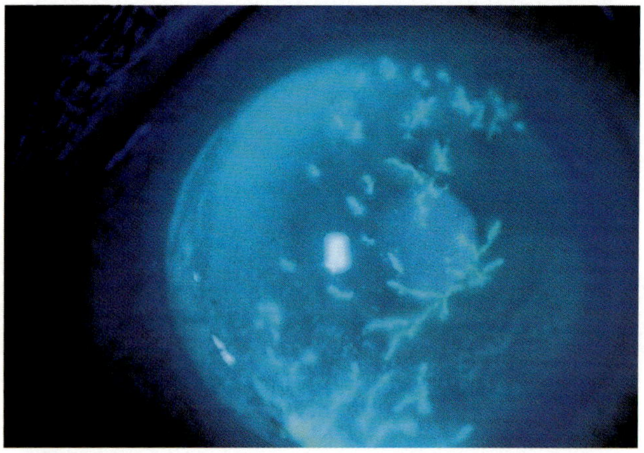
Plate 4-65

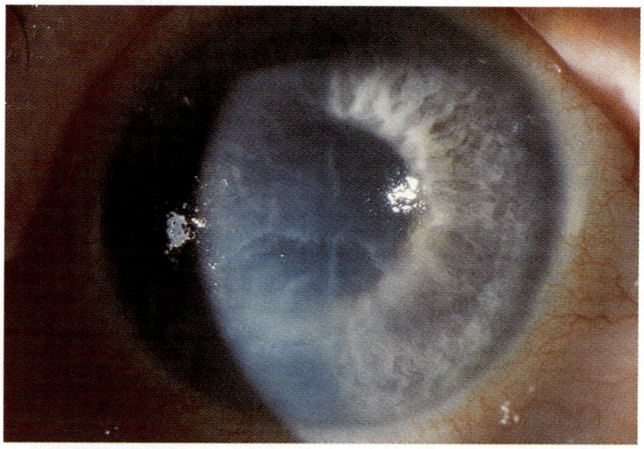
Plate 4-69

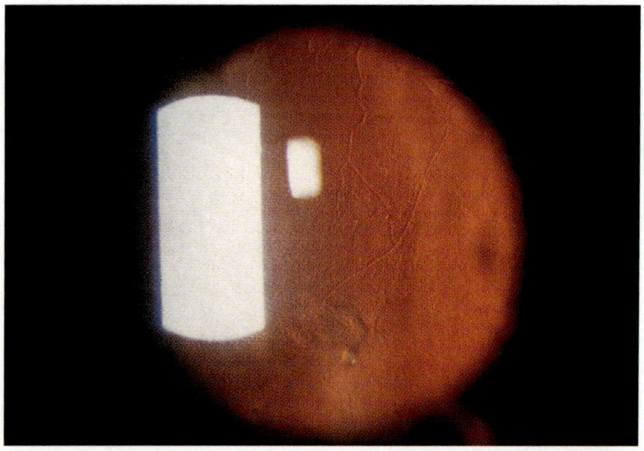
Plate 4-82

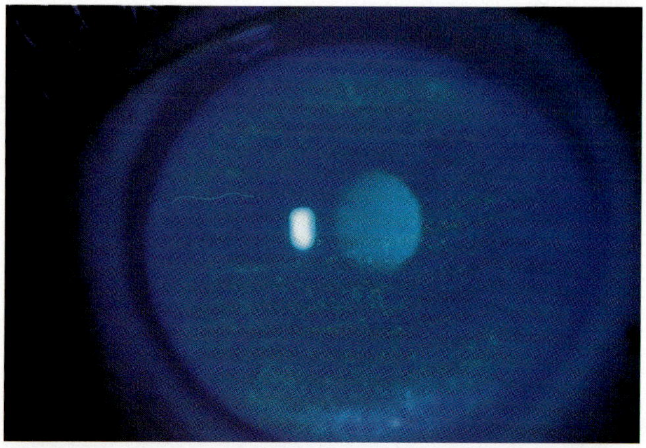
Plate 4-93

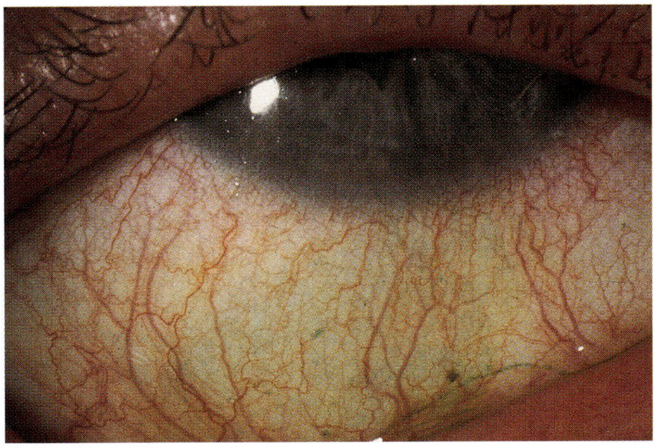

Plate 4-95

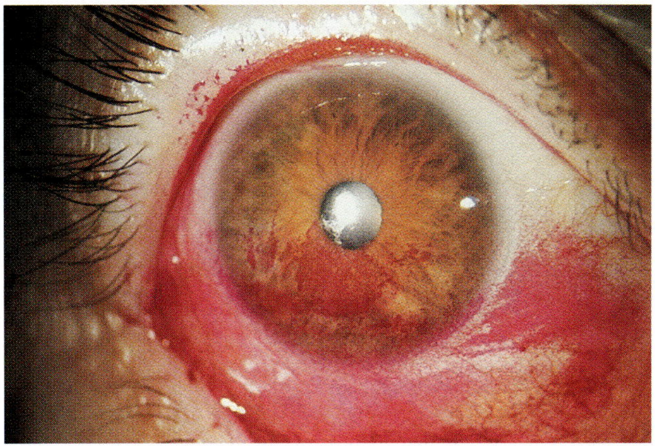

Plate 4-96

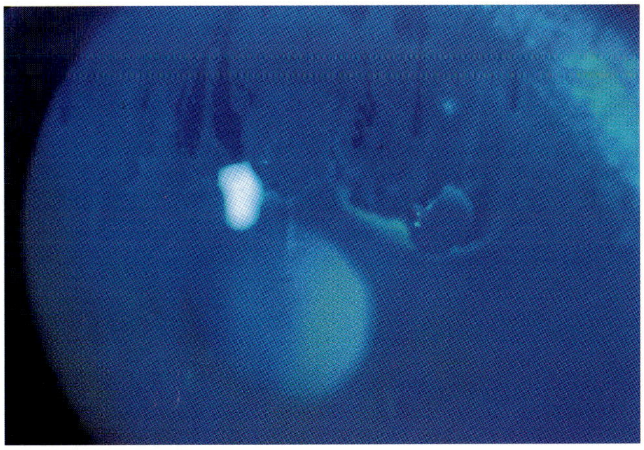

Plate 4-97

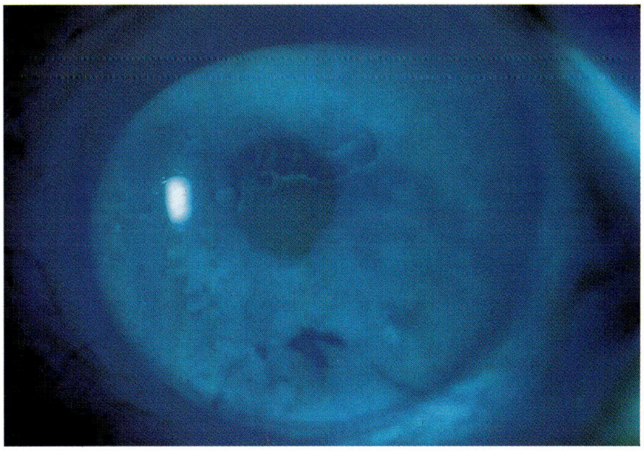

Plate 4-104

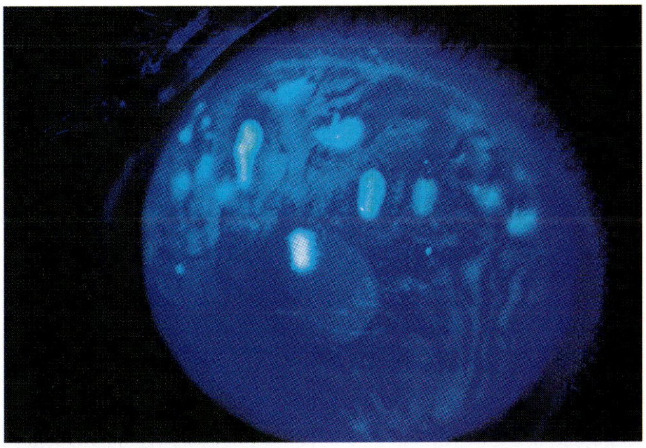

Plate 4-113

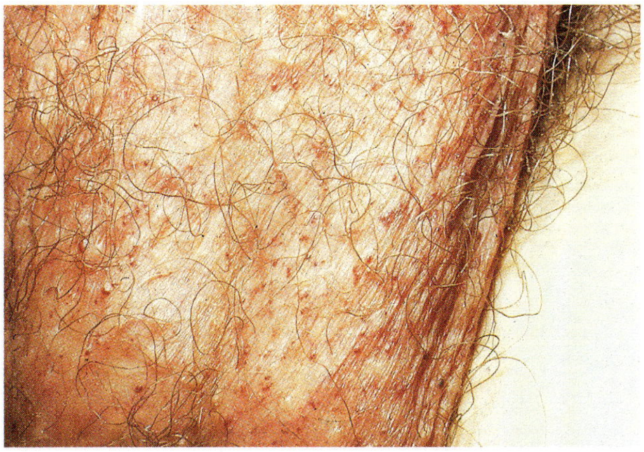

Plate 5-4

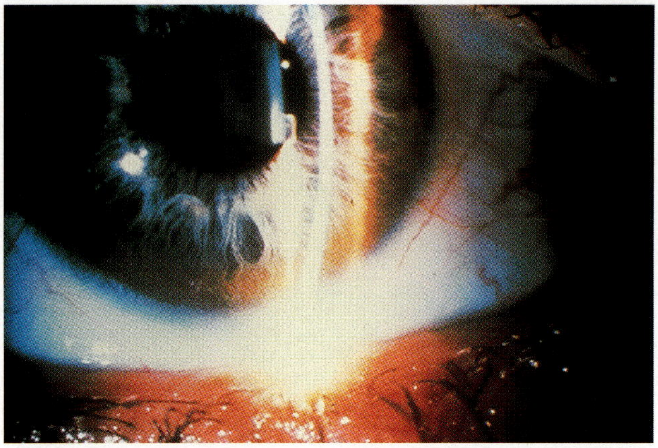

Plate 5-9

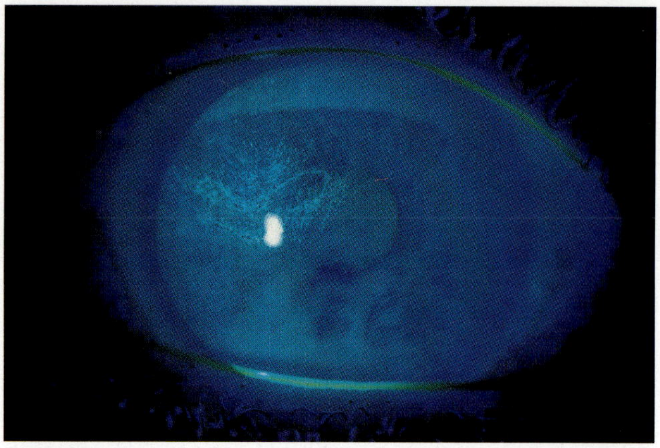

Plate 5-14

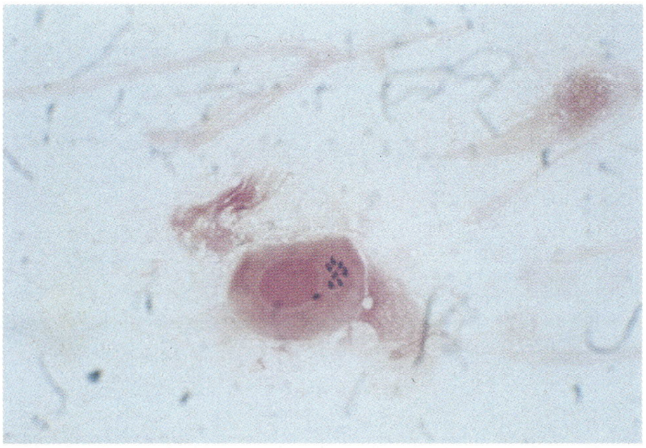

Plate 5-23

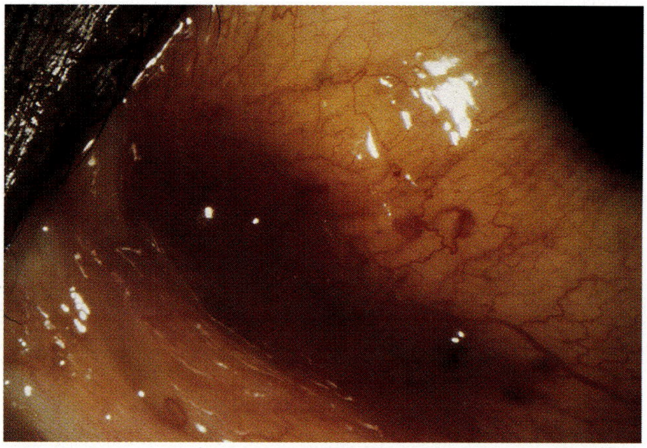

Plate 5-24

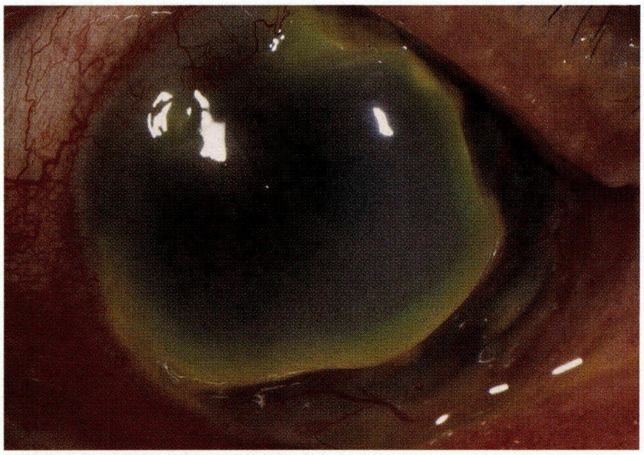

Plate 5-40

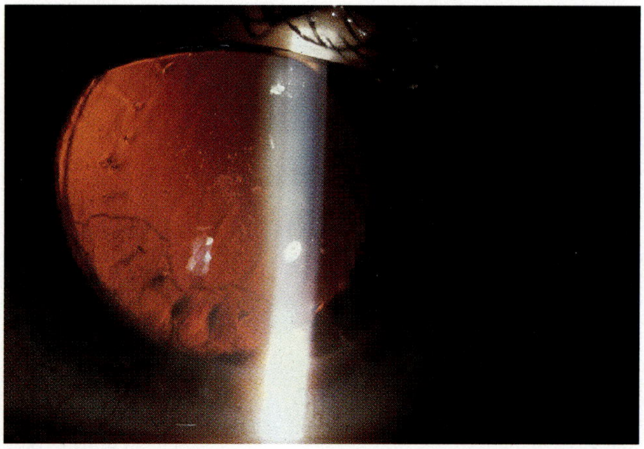

Plate 5-52

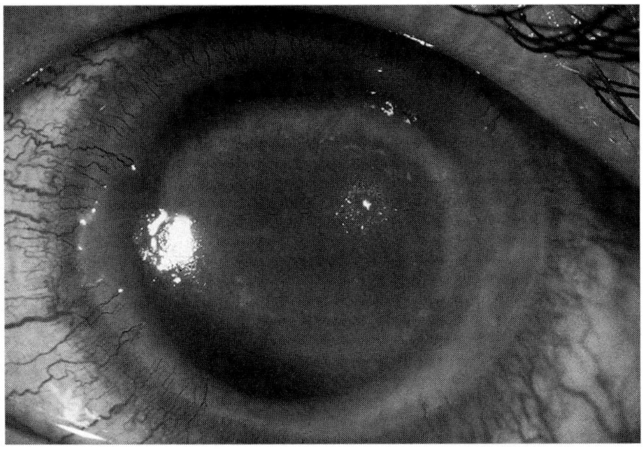

Fig. 4-28 *Acanthamoeba* keratitis. A dense ring infiltrate is present in this eye with *Acanthamoeba* keratitis. Typically, at least 3 to 6 weeks of infection are required for a ring infiltrate to develop.

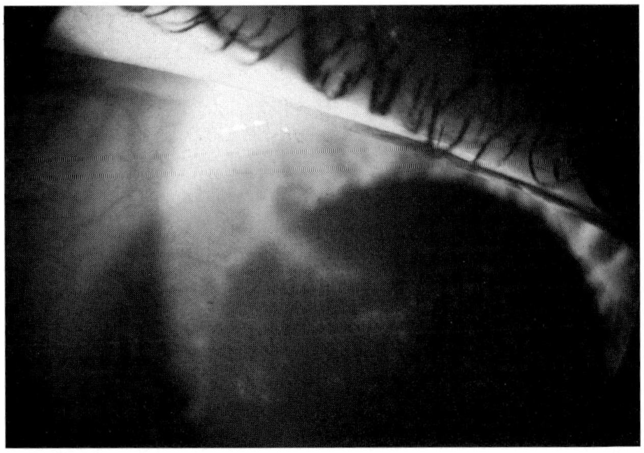

Fig. 4-29 *Acanthamoeba* keratitis. Radial infiltrates surrounding corneal nerves can be seen in *Acanthamoeba* keratitis.

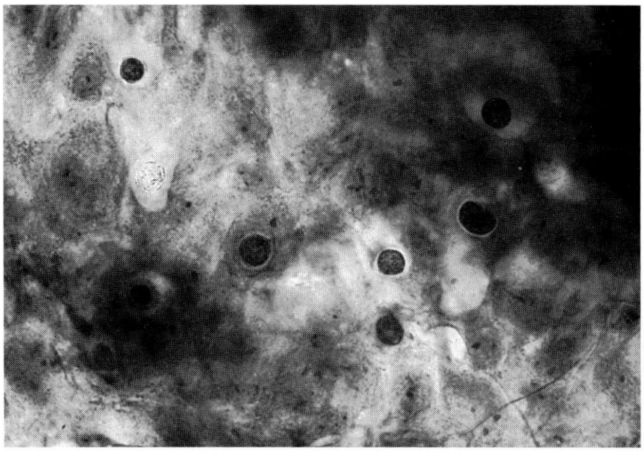

Fig. 4-30 *Acanthamoeba* keratitis. Multiple *Acanthamoeba* cysts are readily apparent on this epithelial scraping with Giemsa stain. (Courtesy of Ralph C. Eagle, Jr., M.D.)

Box 4-8 Agents Used to Treat *Acanthamoeba* Infections

DIAMIDINES

Propamidine
Dibromopropamidine

ANTISEPTICS

Polyhexamethylene biguanide
Chlorhexidine

AMINOGLYCOSIDES

Neomycin

IMIDAZOLES

Clotrimazole
Ketoconazole
Miconazole
Fluconazole
Itraconazole

The treatment and prognosis of *Acanthamoeba* keratitis are greatly aided by early diagnosis. The organism is very resistant to most available agents, and infection may be difficult to eradicate because of a medication-induced transformation to the cyst form, which is even more resistant to therapy. As medications are gradually withdrawn, these cysts may transform themselves back to active trophozoites, producing a recurrence. As a result medical therapy is prolonged, usually lasting months. Several classes of agents have been found to be effective against *Acanthamoeba* organisms (Box 4-8). Most of these agents are not commercially available as topical medications and must be compounded by a pharmacist. Therapy usually involves a combination of two or more agents from different classes, such as propamidine and polyhexamethylene biguanide. An optimal combination has not been established. Systemic therapy with itraconazole or fluconazole may be helpful. Because concomitant bacterial or fungal infection may develop, they should be ruled out by culture and treated if they are present. The medications are typically used at least every hour around the clock for several days to start and are slowly tapered according to the clinical response. Because most of the topical medications are toxic to the epithelium and are used for months, drug toxicity can occur but may be difficult to differentiate from ongoing infection. It may be necessary to decrease the drop frequency and to observe the patient closely to determine whether drug toxicity has occurred.

The usefulness of topical corticosteroids in the management of *Acanthamoeba* keratitis is unclear. Suppression of the host inflammatory reaction by corticosteroids may enhance survival of the organism, worsening the infection. However, corticosteroids may reduce tissue damage caused by the inflammatory response and have been reported to reduce or prevent encystment of the organism, enhancing the efficacy of medical therapy. In general, corticosteroids are not added until clinical improvement is established with the anti-*Acanthamoeba* regimen.

Pain control is a necessary adjunct to antiamoebic therapy because of the severe pain often produced by this protracted infection. Nonsteroidal antiinflammatory agents such as sulindac have been effective in many patients and should be considered as first-line therapeutic agents. The use of narcotic agents, though occasionally necessary, should be kept to a minimum.

Surgical management includes epithelial debridement, cryotherapy, and penetrating keratoplasty. Epithelial debridement combined with medical therapy may be helpful in the early, superficial stages of infection to reduce parasitic load and to enhance medication penetration. Cryotherapy is also effective in eliminating trophozoites, but it is less effective against cysts and may result in corneal opacification, thinning, and necrosis. Therefore it is usually combined with penetrating keratoplasty. Corneal transplantation for visual rehabilitation is ideally postponed until more than 6 months after the infection has been eradicated. It may be required, however, for progressive infection that cannot be controlled by maximal medical therapy. Recurrent infection, typically in the remaining cornea and at the graft-host junction because of peripheral spread along the corneal nerves, may continue to be a serious problem after corneal transplantation. *Acanthamoeba* infection may also recur in the body of the graft.

Atypical Mycobacteria Keratitis

Atypical mycobacteria are the species of mycobacteria other than *Mycobacterium tuberculosis* and *Mycobacterium leprae*. These organisms are ubiquitous and may be found in soil, water (including municipal tap water), and dust. They are a rare cause of ocular infection. *Mycobacterium fortuitum* and *Mycobacterium chelonei* are the most frequently reported organisms of this group associated with infectious keratitis.

Atypical mycobacteria tend to be pathogenic when host defenses are compromised. It is therefore not surprising that most cases of atypical mycobacterial keratitis are associated with trauma, surgery (including refractive surgery), and contact lens use. Clinically, it presents with a slowly progressive, indolent keratitis. Often the antecedent trauma is days or weeks (rarely months or years) prior to presentation. Examination reveals a slowly progressive, minimally suppurative infiltrate. The base of early infiltrates may exhibit radiating lines into the stroma to give it the appearance of a cracked windshield. An immune ring, satellite lesions, or an endothelial plaque may also occasionally be present (Fig. 4-31).

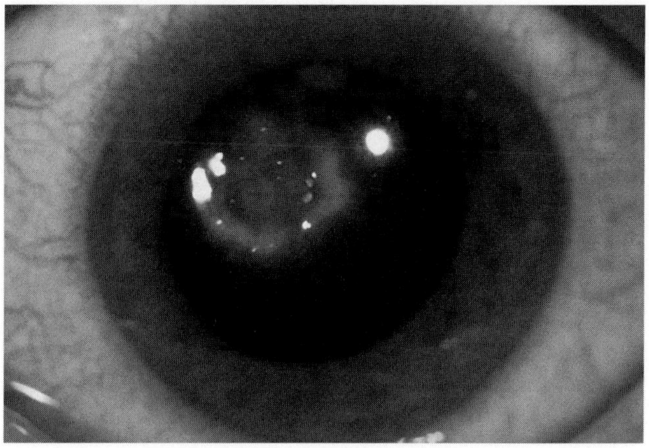

Fig. 4-31 Atypical mycobacteria keratitis. A large stromal infiltrate, denser at the edge, has a central epithelial defect. Note the projections into the stroma at the periphery of the infiltrate.

The differential diagnosis of this infection includes those organisms that also produce indolent ulcers—fungi, anaerobes (e.g., *Propionibacterium acnes*), *Nocardia*, and herpes simplex virus. The diagnosis of atypical mycobacterial keratitis is made by the demonstration of acid-fast organisms on a smear of corneal scrapings stained with Ziehl-Neelsen acid-fast stain (Fig. 4-32). Löwenstein-Jensen culture medium is recommended, though these organisms occasionally grow on blood or chocolate agar. Cultures may become positive within 7 days, but growth is sometimes delayed for several weeks.

The mainstay of therapy for atypical mycobacterial ulcers is 10 to 20 mg/ml topical amikacin. This preparation is not available commercially and must be compounded by a pharmacist. Initial topical amikacin therapy may be supplemented with a subconjunctival injection of 20 mg amikacin if clinically indicated. Other antibiotics that may be effective against certain species of atypical mycobacteria include the fluoroquinolones (especially against *M. fortuitum*), erythromycin, clarithromycin, doxycycline, imipenem, and kanamycin. The initial response to treatment is often slow, and therapy is prolonged. Surgical therapy includes debridement, which may be helpful if patients respond poorly, or therapeutic penetrating keratoplasty if medical treatment fails or if perforation occurs.

Viral Keratitis

Herpes simplex keratitis Herpes simplex keratitis is one of the most common infectious causes of corneal blindness in the United States. Humans are the only natural hosts for the herpes simplex virus (HSV), and

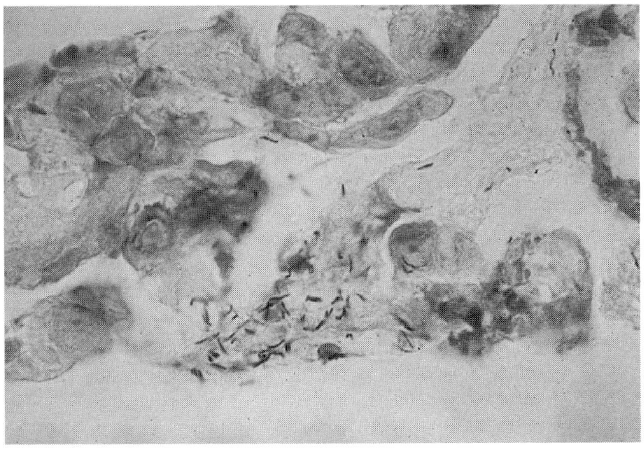

Fig. 4-32 Atypical mycobacteria keratitis. A Ziehl-Neelsen acid-fast stain demonstrates atypical mycobacteria in this deep corneal scraping. (Courtesy of Ralph C. Eagle, Jr., M.D.) (See color plate.)

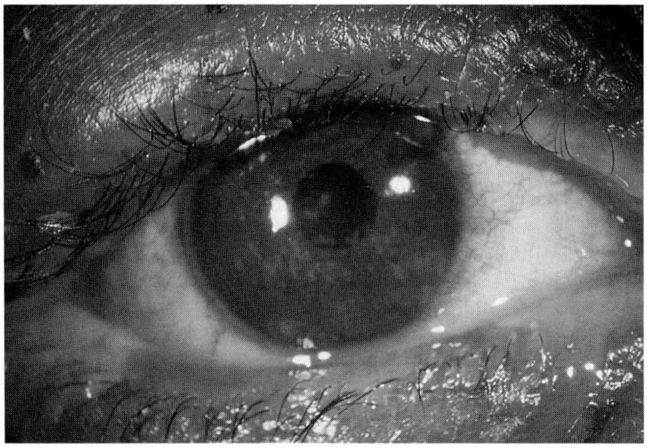

Fig. 4-34 Primary herpes simplex infection. The right eye of the patient seen in Fig. 4-33 demonstrates eyelid margin ulceration and a microdendritic epithelial keratitis.

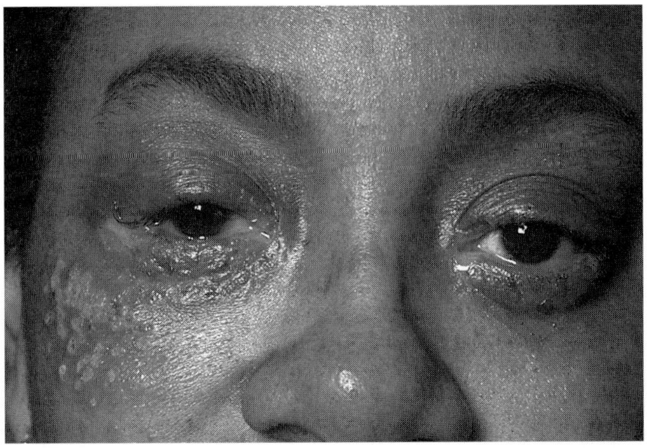

Fig. 4-33 Primary herpes simplex infection. Fever and flulike symptoms developed in this patient because of primary herpes simplex infection. Vesicular eruptions of the skin and eyelid margins are seen in the right eye more than in the left eye.

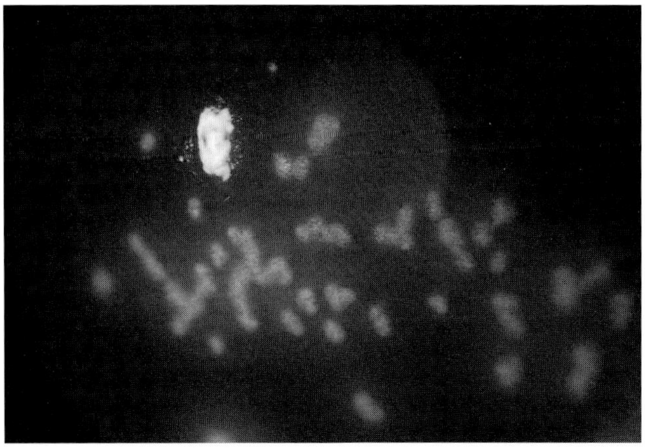

Fig. 4-35 Primary herpes simplex infection. The microdendrites seen in Fig. 4-34 are highlighted with fluorescein dye. In primary herpes simplex keratitis, the dendrites are often smaller and more numerous than they are in recurrent epithelial disease. (See color plate.)

approximately 90% of the population carries antibodies to it. HSV type 1 typically produces oral or labial infection, whereas HSV type 2 is usually associated with genital infection. Ocular herpes simplex infection is caused primarily by HSV type 1, though HSV type 2 is occasionally isolated.

Primary HSV infection usually occurs in childhood and is typically subclinical. Features often include fever, flulike symptoms, and a vesicular eruption on the eyelids (Fig. 4-33), sometimes associated with follicular conjunctivitis, preauricular adenopathy, or dendritic keratitis (Figs. 4-34 and 4-35). Primary HSV infection can be unilateral or bilateral. The initial infection is usually self-limited and is followed by a latent period during which the virus remains dormant in the trigeminal ganglion.

Most clinical herpes simplex ocular infections are recurrences. Many factors are associated with the reactivation of the virus, including physical and emotional stress, ocular trauma (including surgery), fever, menstruation, exposure to ultraviolet light, and concurrent infectious disease. Once reactivated, the virus travels from the ganglion through the nerve fibers to the target tissue. The site of the primary infection may not necessarily be the site of a recurrence. Primary infection in the oral region may present with recurrent ocular disease because both regions are enervated by neurons that originate in the trigeminal ganglion.

Recurrent herpes simplex infection may affect the eyelids, conjunctiva, cornea, or uveal tract (Box 4-9). Eyelid involvement is characterized by typical grouped vesicles that become ulcerated and crusted before healing without scarring (Figs. 4-36, 4-37, and 4-38).

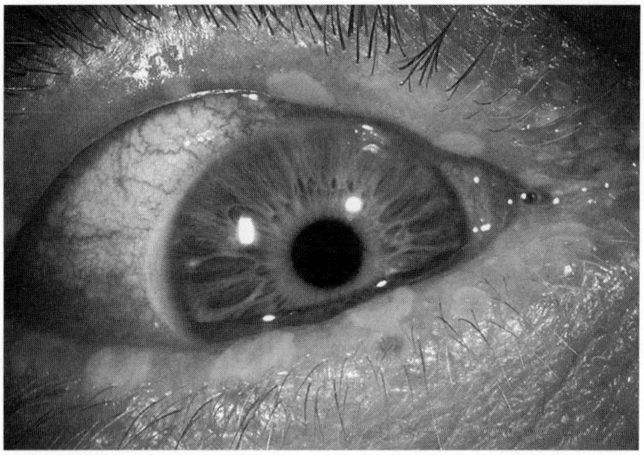

Fig. 4-36 Herpes simplex dermatitis. Multiple vesicular eruptions of the eyelid margin are present in this patient with a history of herpes simplex keratitis.

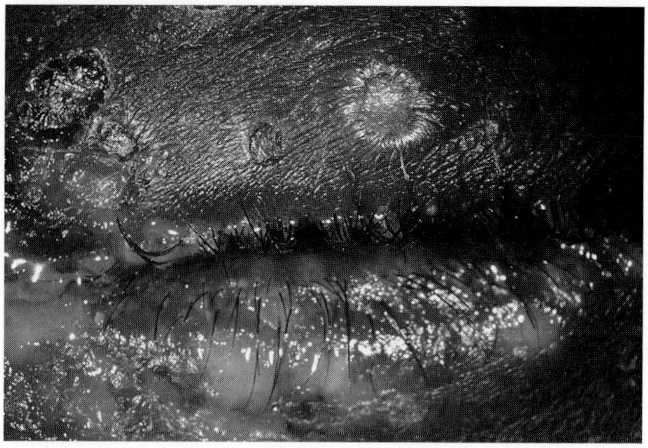

Fig. 4-37 Herpes simplex dermatitis. Multiple herpetic lesions are seen on the skin and eyelid margin in this patient with recurrent herpes simplex infection.

Box 4-9 Anterior Segment Manifestations of Recurrent Herpes Simplex

EYELIDS

Vesicular blepharitis (resolves without scarring)

CONJUNCTIVA

Follicular conjunctivitis
Dendritic conjunctival ulcer

CORNEA

Intraepithelial vesicles
Macropunctate keratitis
Dendritic epithelial keratitis
Marginal ulcer
Neurotrophic keratopathy
Necrotizing stromal keratitis
Disciform keratitis (endotheliitis)
Nonnecrotizing stromal keratitis
Limbal vasculitis
Linear endotheliitis
Diffuse endotheliitis

UVEA

Iritis
Iridocyclitis
Trabeculitis

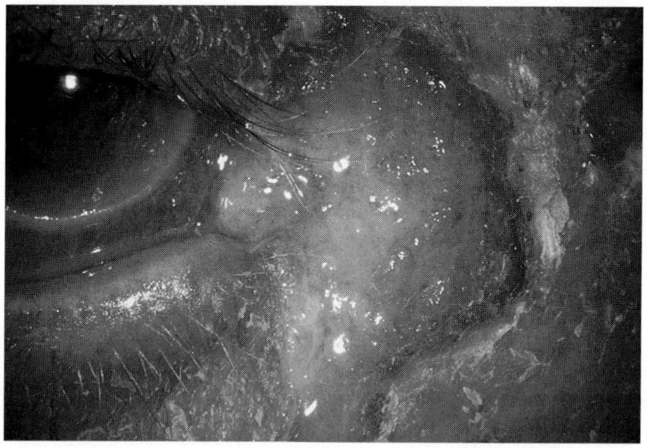

Fig. 4-38 Herpes simplex dermatitis and keratitis. A large area of ulcerated skin involving the medial canthal and lateral nose region is caused by herpes simplex infection. Limbal keratitis can also be seen.

Conjunctival infection may present with or without eyelid or corneal involvement as a recurrent follicular conjunctivitis or by a dendritic ulcer on the bulbar or palpebral conjunctiva that stains with fluorescein (Fig. 4-39). The most common location for recurrent ocular HSV disease is the cornea, where it may produce epithelial, stromal, or endothelial disease, either alone or in combination. Curiously, more than 90% of the time, recurrent ocular HSV is a unilateral phenomenon.

Classically, HSV infection of the corneal epithelium produces a linear or a serpiginous branching dendritic ulcer (Fig. 4-40). These lesions have swollen epithelial borders that contain live virus and stain with rose bengal (Fig. 4-41), but they are depressed at the base, which is ulcerated and stains with fluorescein. The end of each dendritic branch may enlarge and appear rounded, forming a "terminal end bulb" (Figs. 4-42 and 4-43). The depressed and ulcerated appearance of HSV dendrites and the presence of terminal bulbs help to differentiate herpes simplex dendrites from the elevated, plaquelike "pseudodendrites" of herpes zoster. In contrast, however, herpes simplex conjunctival dendrites lack the terminal end bulbs. Occasionally, in the very early stages of epithelial infection, intraepithelial vesicles that contain live virus and do not stain are observed. These micro-

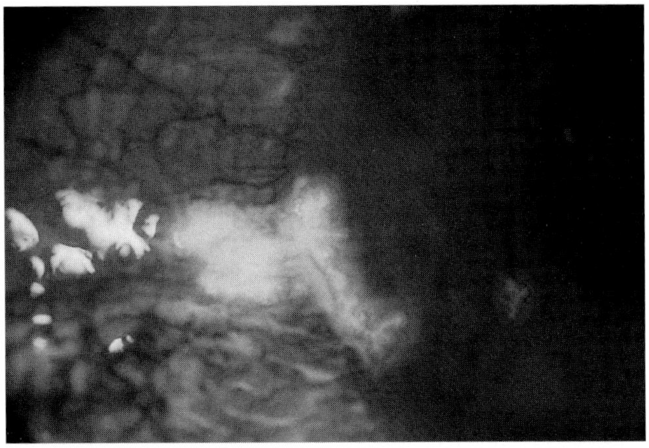

Fig. 4-39 Herpes simplex conjunctival dendrite. A limbal epithelial dendrite involving the cornea and the conjunctiva can easily be seen using fluorescein dye. The branching pattern and terminal end bulbs are not as apparent on the conjunctiva as they are on the cornea. (See color plate.)

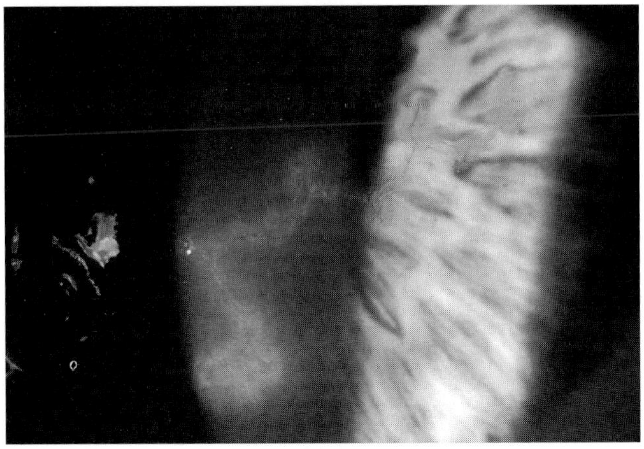

Fig. 4-40 Herpes simplex corneal dendrite. A classic branching corneal dendrite is present. The heaped-up edges, depressed base, and terminal end bulbs are seen.

cysts may coalesce to form typical dendritic ulcers. Dendritic ulcers may progress to form larger amoeboid or maplike geographic ulcers (Fig. 4-44). An underlying stromal reaction is usually minimal or absent, though occasionally a moderate stromal inflammatory reaction may be seen, with subsequent dendritiform scarring known as *ghost dendrites* (Fig. 4-45). Ghost dendrites may be a helpful diagnostic clue if a patient has recurrent keratitis or keratouveitis of obscure origin.

An uncommon manifestation of HSV epithelial keratitis is the formation of a marginal ulcer, which may appear as a peripheral infiltrate (Fig. 4-46) with an overlying epithelial defect (which may be dendritic) and dilated limbal vasculature. It is caused by active viral epithelial infection, which then induces a significant underlying stromal inflammatory reaction resulting from the proximity of the limbal vasculature. Peripheral corneal

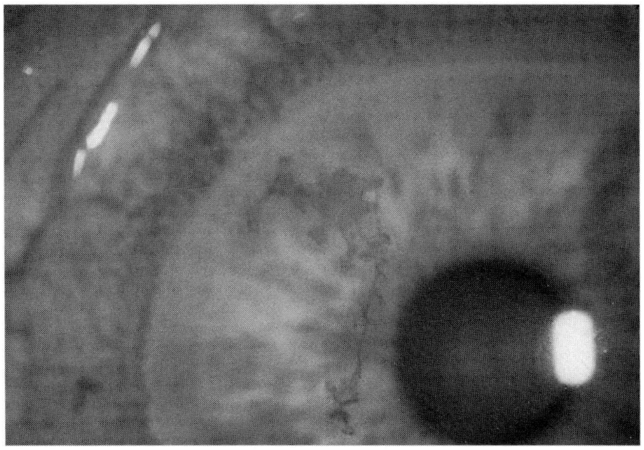

Fig. 4-41 Herpes simplex corneal dendrite. Rose bengal staining of a corneal dendrite. (See color plate.)

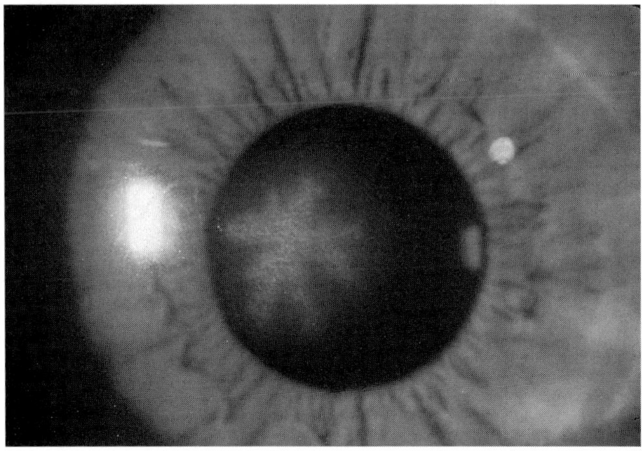

Fig. 4-42 Herpes simplex corneal dendrite. This dendrite demonstrates stellate corneal inflammation.

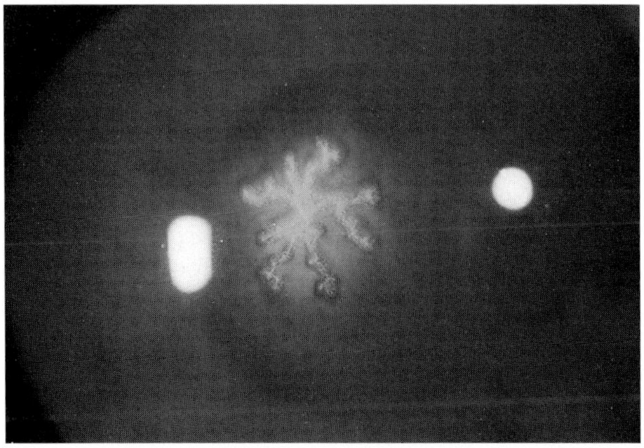

Fig. 4-43 Herpes simplex corneal dendrite. Fluorescein staining of the dendrite seen in Fig. 4-42. The branching pattern, heaped-up edges, depressed base, and terminal end bulbs are seen. (See color plate.)

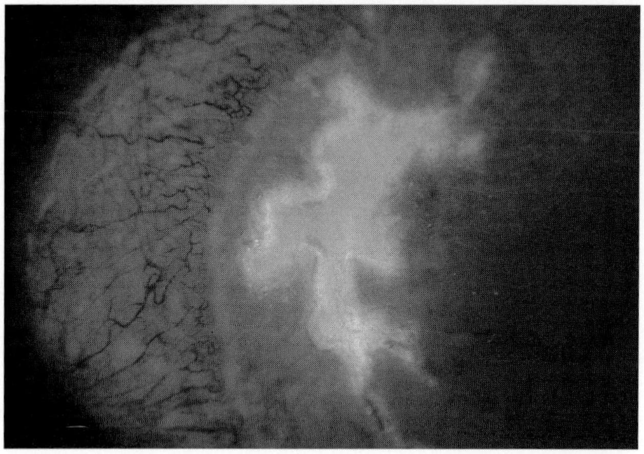

Fig. 4-44 Herpes simplex geographic ulcer. This dendrite has expanded and formed a maplike geographic ulcer, seen with fluorescein dye. (See color plate.)

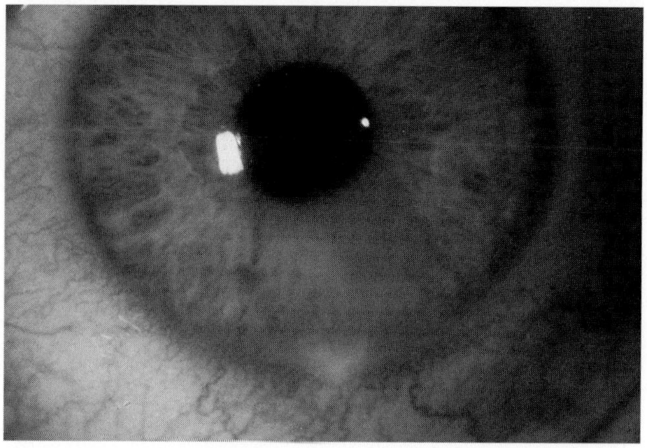

Fig. 4-46 Herpes simplex marginal infiltrate. Limbal corneal infiltrate with adjacent conjunctival injection are seen, as can moderate surrounding corneal edema.

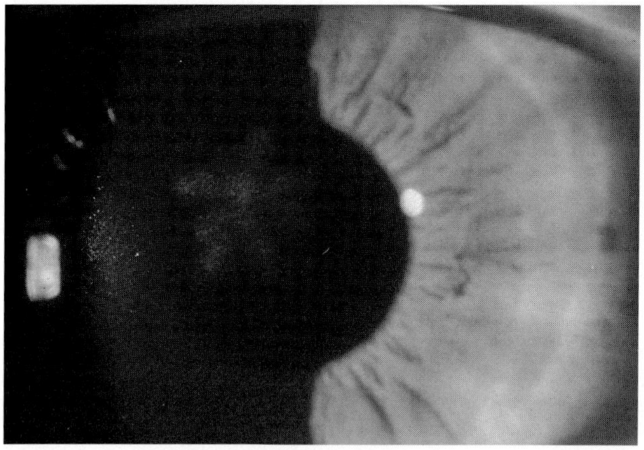

Fig. 4-45 Herpes simplex "ghost dendrite." After resolution of the acute epithelial dendrite seen in Figs. 4-42 and 4-43, a mild degree of stromal haze in the shape of the previous dendrite is still seen.

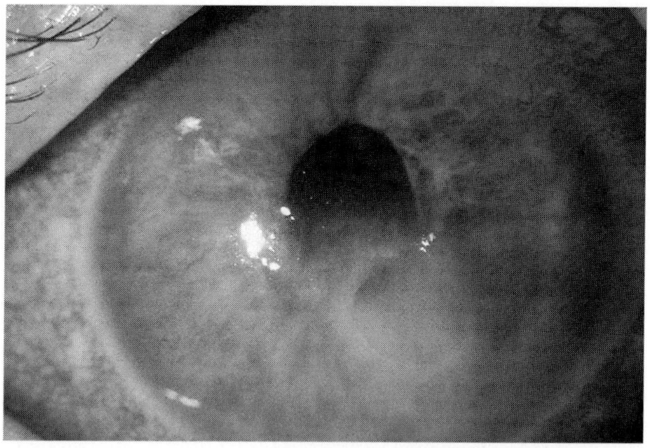

Fig. 4-47 Herpes simplex neurotrophic keratitis. A neurotrophic corneal ulcer demonstrating a large epithelial defect with rolled edges and moderate haze in the base of the ulcer is seen. Note the surrounding corneal edema and mild corneal thinning.

neovascularization may also be present. Although these lesions may resemble peripheral staphylococcal hypersensitivity keratitis, infiltrates of the latter condition usually do not cause epithelial defects until late in their course.

Recurrent HSV infection may produce corneal hypoesthesia, which may contribute to the formation of sterile, nonhealing ulcers known as neurotrophic keratopathy. These lesions either evolve from a previously treated dendritic lesion or arise de novo. They may initially present as a small epithelial erosion and progress to become a large, oval epithelial defect with swollen, rolled edges, typically central or paracentral in location. Diffuse stromal haze and thinning may be present at the base of prolonged ulcerations (Fig. 4-47). It is thought that a combination of reduced corneal sensation, decreased tear production, toxicity from antiviral medication, and inflammation contributes to the formation of these lesions. If left untreated they lead to significant scarring, neovascularization, secondary infection, thinning, or perforation.

Stromal HSV disease may present either in a necrotizing or nonnecrotizing form (see Box 4-9). Necrotizing stromal keratitis is characterized by a white, necrotic stromal infiltrate with an overlying epithelial defect that may progressively thin and perforate (Fig. 4-48). This rare manifestation of HSV keratitis is probably caused by a severe stromal inflammatory reaction to viral antigens, perhaps associated with viral infection of the stroma. Microbial superinfection must be ruled out in these patients.

Nonnecrotizing stromal keratitis is thought to be an immune rather than an infectious process and presents as interstitial keratitis or disciform keratitis. Immune

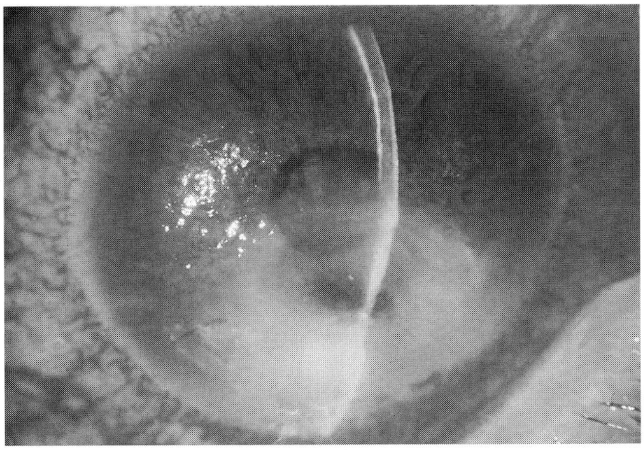

Fig. 4-48 Herpes simplex necrotizing stromal keratitis. A large area of necrotizing stromal keratitis is seen. Observe the significant thinning with a central perforation and a flat anterior chamber.

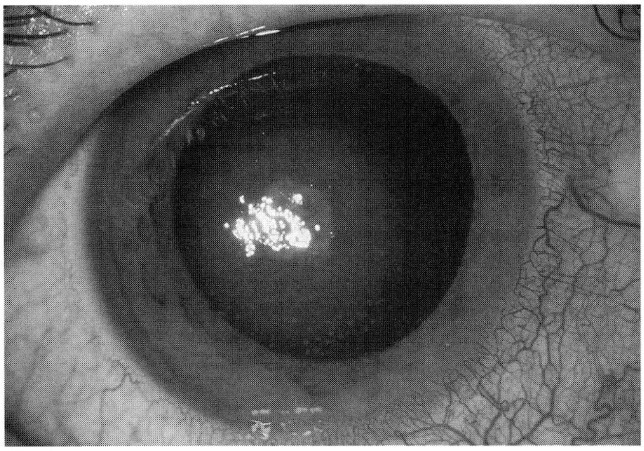

Fig. 4-49 Herpes simplex disciform keratitis (endotheliitis). A large circular area of stromal edema with underlying keratic precipitates is classic for disciform keratitis (endotheliitis).

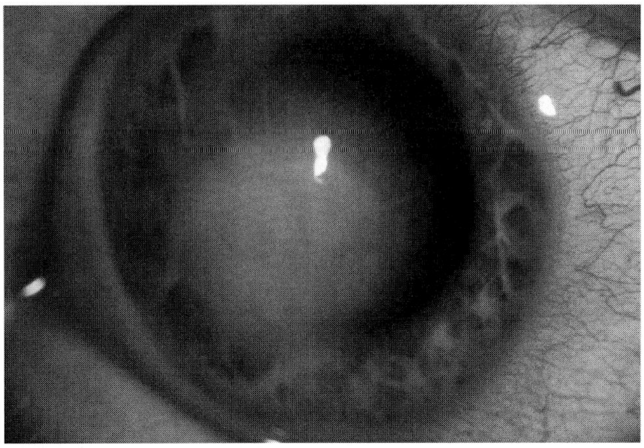

Fig. 4-50 Herpes simplex disciform keratitis (endotheliitis). Significant stromal edema with Descemet's folds are evident in this eye with disciform keratitis (endotheliitis).

stromal keratitis (interstitial keratitis) may present with stromal haze or blotchy white infiltrates, neovascularization, an intact epithelium, and occasionally an immune ring. Stromal edema may accompany the infiltrate, and keratic precipitates may be present. It may occur without a known history of a dendritic ulcer, or it may occur weeks or months after an epithelial infection. It is thought to result from an antigen-antibody-mediated inflammatory reaction to viral antigens in the stroma. Chronic or recurrent inflammation may lead to visual loss because of increased neovascularization, lipid deposition, scarring, and thinning.

The term *disciform keratitis* has been used to describe any disc-shaped swelling of the cornea after herpes simplex epithelial keratitis. It is the most common form of stromal HSV disease. However, several different viruses may produce a disciform keratitis, including herpes varicella/zoster, vaccinia, and mumps. Clinically, it presents with a circular area of stromal edema, keratic precipitates localized to the area of edema, and a mild anterior chamber reaction (Fig. 4-49). If the stroma is sufficiently edematous, Descemet's folds and epithelial edema may also be present (Figs. 4-50 and 4-51). Intraocular pressure is sometimes elevated. Disciform keratitis also represents an immune response to viral antigens, the location of which has historically been thought to be the stroma. However, because of the relative absence of stromal inflammation in this entity and the presence of an inflammatory response that appears to be directed against the endothelium, it has recently been suggested that the primary target of the inflammatory reaction is the endothelium, not the stroma. It has therefore been suggested that this entity be reclassified as a form of endotheliitis rather than a form of stromal keratitis and that the term *disciform endotheliitis* replace *disciform keratitis*.

HSV endotheliitis may also present in either a linear or diffuse form. Linear endotheliitis presents with a line of keratic precipitates that may progress across the cornea, with overlying stromal edema, much like endothelial corneal transplant rejection. This condition may be difficult to manage, and it requires topical corticosteroids and antivirals. Diffuse endotheliitis presents with keratic precipitates across virtually the entire corneal endothelium, associated with overlying stromal edema and a significant anterior chamber reaction (Fig. 4-52).

Limbal vasculitis or limbitis is another immune manifestation of HSV disease that may produce one or more quadrants of intense limbal hyperemia and swelling (Fig. 4-53). It may be associated with an inflammatory Wessely ring, and it is generally responsive to topical corticosteroids.

Herpes simplex iridocyclitis can present with or without simultaneous keratitis. A known history of HSV ker-

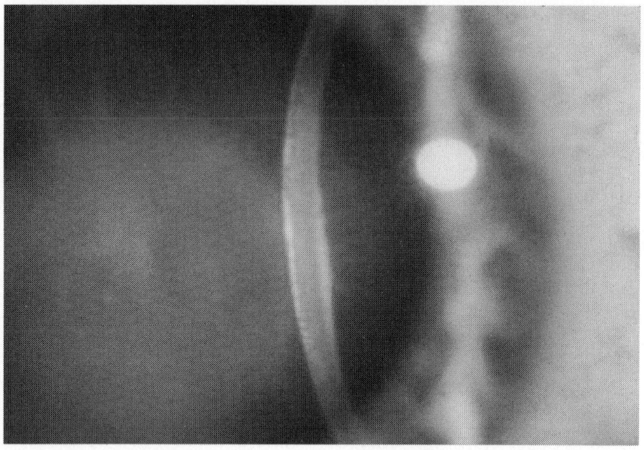

Fig. 4-51 Herpes simplex disciform keratitis (endotheliitis). A slit-beam view of the eye in Fig. 4-50 reveals significant corneal edema.

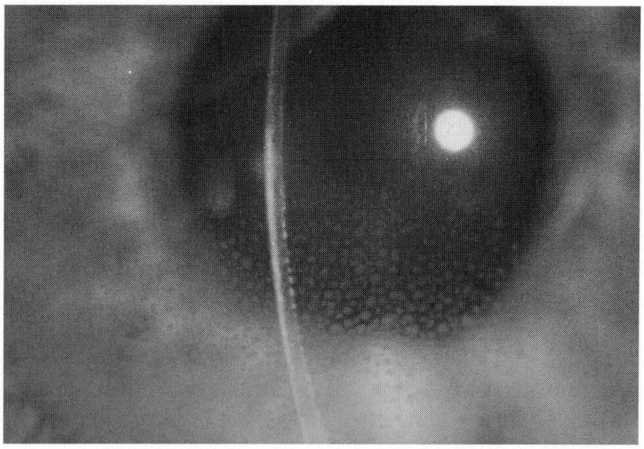

Fig. 4-52 Herpes simplex diffuse endotheliitis. Myriad keratic precipitates are readily apparent in this eye with a history of herpes simplex keratitis. A significant anterior chamber reaction occurred. Often the intraocular pressure is elevated.

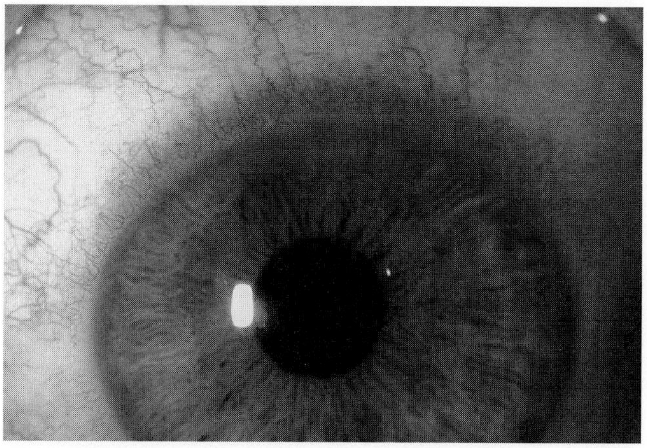

Fig. 4-53 Herpes simplex limbitis. Significant superior limbal inflammation is present in this eye with known herpes simplex keratitis.

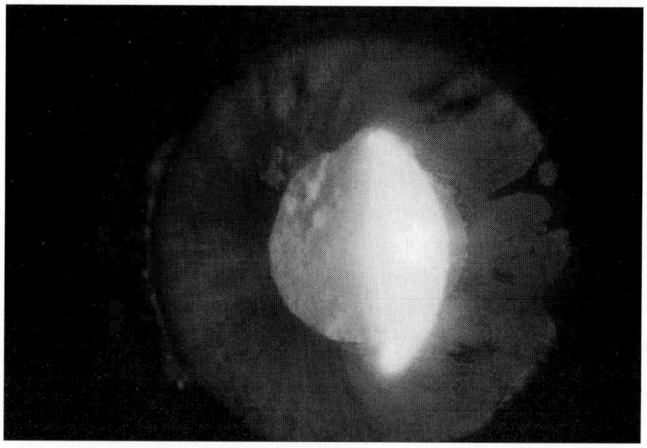

Fig. 4-54 Herpes simplex iris atrophy. Retroillumination off the retina reveals severe diffuse iris atrophy in this eye after multiple episodes of herpes simplex keratouveitis. (See color plate.)

atitis may be absent in some patients. It is typically unilateral, with ciliary flush, a moderate to severe anterior chamber reaction, and keratic precipitates. Sectorial or diffuse iris atrophy is a common finding, probably because of ischemic necrosis from a vasculitic process (Fig. 4-54). Concomitant trabeculitis produces secondary glaucoma. Because iridocyclitis is generally associated with lower than normal intraocular pressure, if it develops in a patient with elevated intraocular pressure, the cause may be herpes simplex or herpes zoster.

The diagnosis of herpes simplex keratitis is almost always made clinically, through a complete history and examination. Elements of the history typically include episodes of oral sores (fever blisters) and facial sores, previous unexplained episodes of a unilateral red eye, corticosteroid use, or previously documented HSV ocular disease. If the diagnosis is still in doubt after the examination, scrapings of eyelid, corneal, or conjunctival lesions may undergo Giemsa or Papanicolaou staining to look for multinucleated giant cells and eosinophilic intranuclear inclusion bodies. These findings, however, support both herpes simplex and herpes zoster infection. Scrapings should be taken from the base of a skin lesion or from the edge of a corneal or conjunctival lesion. Viral cultures may be taken and are positive in approximately 70% of patients with HSV keratitis if they have not undergone previous antiviral therapy. Viral cultures should be taken before the instillation of rose bengal stain, which is toxic to HSV and may reduce the yield. Polymerase chain reaction techniques and electron microscopy are also sensitive and specific in the detection of HSV DNA or virions, but these techniques are expensive, technically involved, and not widely available.

Two categories of antiviral agents are effective against the herpes simplex virus: purine and pyrimidine nucleosides (Box 4-10). Idoxuridine (IDU) is a pyrimidine

Box 4-10 Antiviral Agents Effective Against Herpes Simplex Virus

PYRIMIDINES

Idoxuridine (IDU)
Trifluorothymidine

PURINES

Vidarabine
Acyclovir
Famciclovir
Valacyclovir

nucleoside, and it was the first agent used to treat HSV. Although it is effective against HSV, its poor solubility and corneal surface toxicity have limited its use. The most notable noncorneal toxic reactions to idoxuridine include follicular conjunctivitis, punctal edema, and punctal stenosis. Vidarabine, which is better tolerated, is a purine nucleoside available only in ointment form for topical use. It is considered less potent than other available agents, however, and is a second-line agent for cases resistant to other antiviral medications or a first-line agent when an ointment is preferred (e.g., in a child). Trifluorothymidine is a fluorinated pyrimidine nucleoside analogue that has become the drug of choice for HSV epithelial keratitis. It has been shown to be more effective than idoxuridine or vidarabine against HSV dendritic ulcers. Like idoxuridine, it may be associated with significant surface toxicity, follicular conjunctivitis, punctal occlusion, and contact dermatitis. Acyclovir is a purine nucleoside activated by viral phosphorylation, and it is specific for virus-infected cells. It has good ocular penetration with systemic therapy, producing therapeutic dosages in tears and aqueous. It is well tolerated and is as effective as other antiviral agents, but it is less toxic. It is therefore a useful therapeutic alternative for infectious epithelial keratitis that is complicated by surface toxicity, that is not responsive to trifluorothymidine, or when topical therapy is difficult. It is unavailable as a topical preparation in the United States, but it is available as a topical preparation in Europe and elsewhere.

The treatment of ocular herpes simplex infection must be tailored to the particular presentation of the disease. As a general rule, infectious forms are treated with antiviral medication, and immune or inflammatory manifestations require corticosteroids, usually with antiviral prophylaxis. When in doubt, avoid the use of topical corticosteroids.

Herpes simplex blepharitis generally resolves on its own without scarring. If lesions do develop on or near the eyelid margin, a prophylactic topical antiviral agent (such as trifluorothymidine or vidarabine) should be used 5 times a day to guard against corneal infection. A 7- to 10-day course of oral acyclovir (400 mg 5 times a day) may be considered for primary HSV infection. Systemic acyclovir may shorten the duration of severe infection, but this has not been proven. Some physicians use topical antibiotic ointment to prevent superinfection of the skin lesions, whereas others use acyclovir ointment to treat skin lesions away from the eye.

HSV conjunctivitis is an active viral infection of the conjunctival epithelium, and it should be treated with a topical antiviral medication 5 times a day until the lesions resolve, typically in 7 to 10 days.

The mainstay of treatment for HSV epithelial keratitis is trifluorothymidine 5 to 9 times a day or vidarabine ointment 5 times a day. Acyclovir ointment is also effective but is not available for ocular use in the United States. The usual duration of treatment is 10 to 14 days, though the medications are usually tapered after 5 to 7 days, depending on the clinical response. Gentle epithelial debridement of the ulcer with a sterile spatula or a cotton-tipped applicator may be considered, especially for centrally located lesions, to decrease the viral load and potentially to reduce the chances of stromal scarring and ghost dendrite formation. Debridement must be accompanied by antiviral therapy. Corticosteroids should not be used in the treatment of infectious epithelial keratitis because they tend to potentiate the infection. Occasionally, if a severe underlying inflammatory reaction results, a weak topical corticosteroid may be considered after several days of antiviral therapy have been initiated and the infection is responding.

A major problem with prolonged antiviral use is the development of toxicity. Epithelial toxicity may result in delayed healing of the epithelial defect or in a persistent epithelial defect, filamentary keratopathy, and diffuse punctate keratopathy. Toxic conjunctivitis and corneal stromal ulceration, scarring, and neovascularization may also occur. If epithelial closure is delayed after prolonged treatment of a dendritic ulcer, antiviral toxicity should be considered. The antiviral agent should be stopped, preservative-free lubrication should be started, and the patient should be closely observed.

Because the pathogenesis of stromal keratitis and iritis is thought to be related to viral antigens remaining from previous episodes of viral proliferation, such as dendritic keratitis, it was hypothesized that the addition of oral acyclovir to trifluorothymidine for the treatment of epithelial keratitis might help prevent stromal keratitis or iritis. However, results of the Herpetic Eye Disease Study recently showed that for patients with infectious epithelial keratitis being treated with trifluorothymidine, the addition of acyclovir provided no additional benefit in the prevention of stromal keratitis or iritis (Box 4-11).

The therapy for neurotrophic keratopathy should be oriented toward the promotion of epithelial healing by the elimination of toxic agents that may interfere with

Box 4-11 Major Conclusions of the Herpetic Eye Disease Study (HEDS)

Topical corticosteroids were significantly better than placebo in reducing the persistence and progression of herpes simplex stromal keratitis when also treated with prophylactic trifluorothymidine.

Oral acyclovir provided no additional statistical or clinical benefits to patients with herpes simplex stromal keratitis who were already using corticosteroids and trifluorothymidine.

Oral acyclovir may be beneficial in the treatment of herpes simplex virus iridocyclitis.

For patients with herpes simplex epithelial keratitis treated with trifluorothymidine, the addition of oral acyclovir provided no additional benefit in the prevention of stromal keratitis or iritis.

Oral acyclovir decreases the frequency of recurrent herpes simplex virus keratitis, especially in patients with a history of stromal disease.

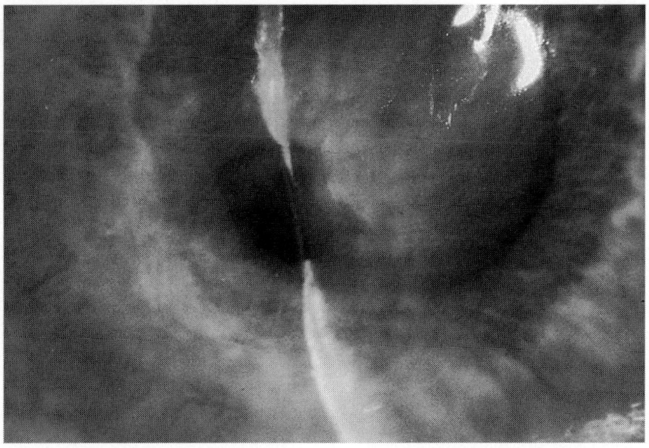

Fig. 4-55 Herpes simplex necrotizing keratitis. This corneal perforation resulted from herpes simplex necrotizing keratitis. It was too large to treat with cyanoacrylate tissue glue and instead was managed with penetrating keratoplasty.

epithelial closure and by increasing lubrication. Because neurotrophic keratopathy is not an infectious manifestation of HSV keratitis, antiviral medication should be discontinued. Corticosteroids should be avoided, if possible, because they may promote collagenase activity and stromal melting. Sometimes, however, they are helpful if a patient has a significant stromal inflammatory reaction at the base of the ulcer impeding reepithelialization. Treatment of this condition is difficult, and options include frequent antibiotic or lubricating ointments, artificial tears without preservatives, patching, bandage contact lenses, temporary or permanent tarsorrhaphy, and a conjunctival flap. Cyanoacrylate tissue glue is often effective for small impending or frank perforations.

Immune stromal keratitis, disciform keratitis (endotheliitis), and iritis all respond well to topical corticosteroids. The minimum effective corticosteroid dosage should be used, along with concurrent prophylactic antiviral therapy. If a full-strength topical corticosteroid (e.g., 1% prednisolone acetate) is used more than once a day, topical antiviral therapy should be prescribed at a dosage similar to that for topical corticosteroids to prevent recurrent viral infection. The efficacy of topical corticosteroids in the management of stromal keratitis was evaluated by the Herpetic Eye Disease Study. The results of this study demonstrated that topical corticosteroids were significantly better than placebo in reducing the duration and progression of stromal keratitis but that they did not have to be started immediately. Another arm of this study showed that oral acyclovir provided no additional statistical or clinical benefits to patients with stromal keratitis who were already using corticosteroids and trifluorothymidine. Oral acyclovir was found to be effective at decreasing the recurrences of HSV keratitis, with the greatest benefit going to patients with a history of stromal disease.

Surgical intervention in HSV disease is usually reserved for patients who no longer have active infectious or inflammatory disease but who have been left with significant stromal scarring and reduced visual acuity. Penetrating keratoplasty is usually required for these patients because of the depth of the scarring. If the stromal scarring is limited to the anterior stroma and corneal thinning is minimal, a superficial procedure such as excimer laser phototherapeutic keratectomy may be considered. Any surgical intervention carries a significant risk for the reactivation of infection, and it is recommended that systemic antiviral therapy (e.g., 400 mg acyclovir PO bid) be used for at least 1 year after penetrating keratoplasty.

Surgical intervention for active HSV disease is rarely necessary. If a patient has a persistent epithelial defect or neurotrophic keratopathy, temporary or permanent tarsorrhaphy may be helpful. Occasionally, a conjunctival flap may be required. Small perforations may be sealed with the application of cyanoacrylate tissue glue. Larger perforations may require a lamellar patch graft or penetrating keratoplasty (Figs. 4-55 and 4-56).

Herpes zoster keratitis The varicella zoster virus is a herpes virus that causes the clinical syndrome of chicken pox after primary infection (usually in childhood). This infection produces a self-limited vesicular rash. During primary infection the virus migrates through nerve fibers in a retrograde fashion to the sensory nerve ganglia, where it enters a latent phase, similar to the herpes simplex virus. Months, years, or decades

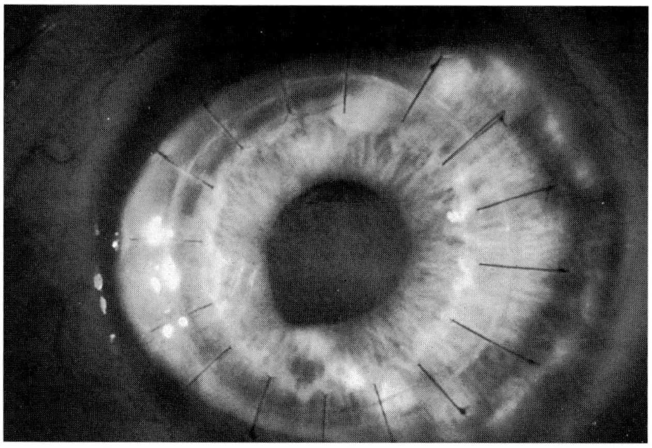

Fig. 4-56 Herpes simplex penetrating keratoplasty. Three months after emergency corneal transplantation for the perforated ulcer seen in Fig. 4-55, the graft is clear with moderate whorl punctate staining.

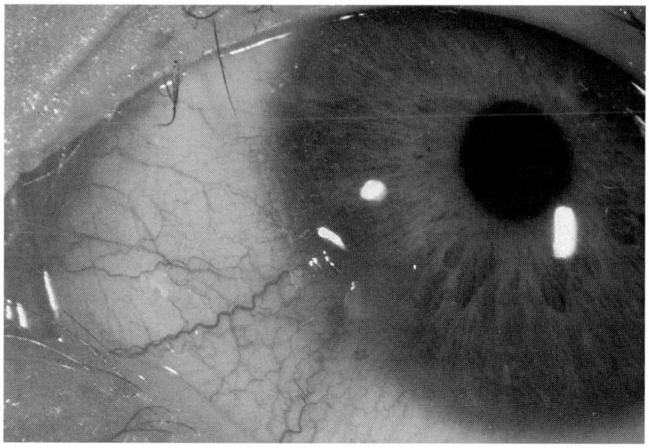

Fig. 4-57 Varicella (chicken pox) vesicle. A limbal chicken pock can be seen in this 2-year-old child with chicken pox.

later the virus in the ganglion may reactivate, producing a vesicular eruption in the dermatome supplied by the ganglion. This dermatomal reactivation is known as an episode of shingles. Although any dermatome may be affected by a reactivation, typically the involved dermatome is on the trunk. However, in approximately 15% to 20% of patients, the trigeminal nerve distribution is affected, producing the clinical syndrome of herpes zoster ophthalmicus.

Primary varicella infection occasionally involves the eye. Vesicles may form on the eyelids, where they can cause scarring. Vesicles may also be seen on the conjunctiva or limbus (Fig. 4-57). Rarely a superficial punctate or dendritiform keratopathy may be present (Fig. 4-58). Occasionally, weeks or months later, an immune disciform keratitis (endotheliitis) similar to that seen after a herpes simplex virus (HSV) infection may occur.

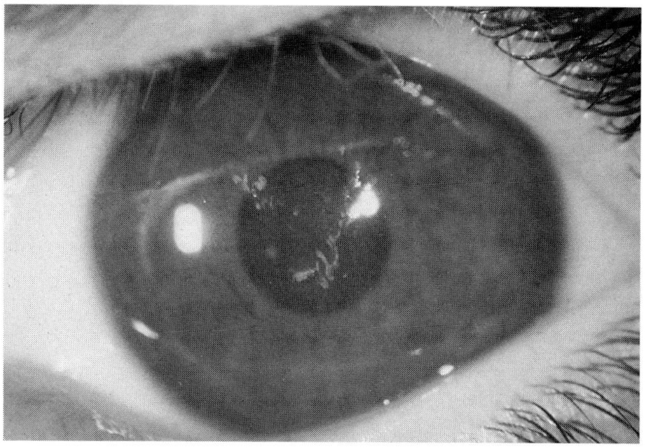

Fig. 4-58 Varicella (chicken pox) dendrite. An epithelial dendrite is present in this patient with chicken pox.

Box 4-12 Anterior Segment Manifestations of Herpes Zoster Ophthalmicus

EYELIDS AND PERIORBITAL SKIN

Dermatomal vesicular eruption (leads to scarring)
Postherpetic neuralgia

CONJUNCTIVA

Hyperemia
Follicular conjunctivitis

CORNEA

Punctate epithelial keratitis
Microdendritic epithelial keratitis
Delayed-onset pseudodendritic mucous plaques
Neurotrophic keratopathy
Anterior stromal infiltrates
Immune stromal keratitis
Disciform keratitis (endotheliitis)

SCLERA

Episcleritis
Scleritis

UVEA

Iridocyclitis
Trabeculitis

Herpes zoster ophthalmicus can affect virtually every anatomic component of the eye, from the eyelid to the optic nerve (Box 4-12). Of the three divisions of the trigeminal nerve, the ophthalmic division is most frequently affected, and of this division, the frontal nerve branch is the most often involved. This nerve supplies the upper eyelid, superior conjunctiva, forehead, and

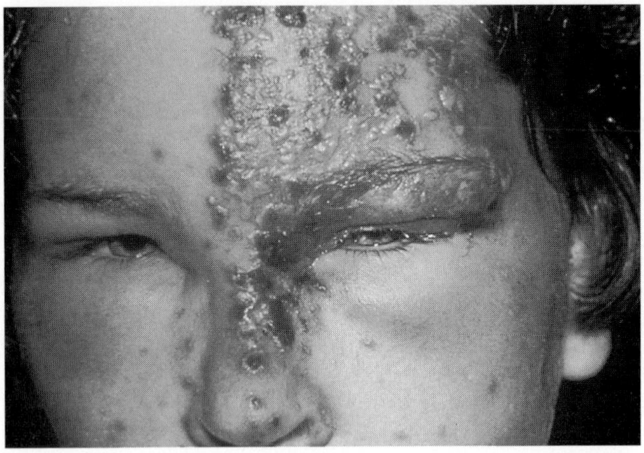

Fig. 4-59 Herpes zoster dermatitis. A vesicular rash involving the ophthalmic division of the trigeminal nerve (V_1) is seen. Herpes zoster dermatitis is unilateral and obeys the midline. Hutchinson's sign, the presence of vesicles on one side of the tip of the nose, indicates involvement of the nasociliary branch and may forecast ocular involvement.

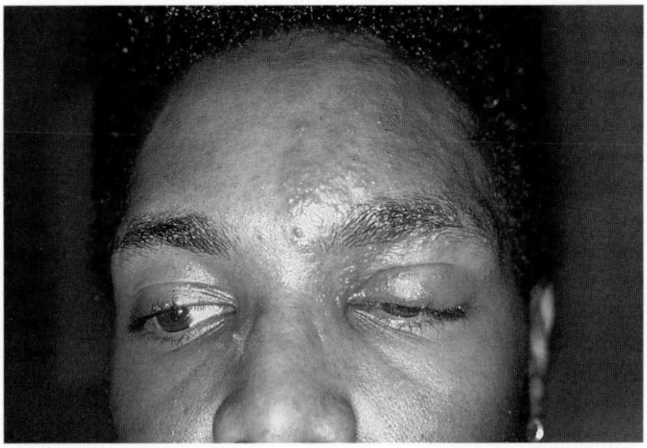

Fig. 4-60 Herpes zoster dermatitis. A rash involving the frontal branch of V_1 is seen in this patient with human immunodeficiency virus. The rash reached the scalp region. (Courtesy of Guy F. Webster, M.D., Ph.D.)

scalp (be sure to look for lesions beyond the hairline). The nasociliary branch enervates the rest of the conjunctiva, sclera, uveal tract, anterior and posterior ethmoid sinuses, and the skin on the tip of the nose. Hutchinson's sign is the presence of vesicles on the side of the tip of the nose that may herald future ocular involvement.

Eyelid involvement is characterized by a typical vesicular eruption in the dermatomal pattern of the involved branch (Figs. 4-59 and 4-60). The presence of this vesicular rash, which does not cross the midline, makes the diagnosis easy. Often it is preceded by a burning, tingling, or warm sensation in that distribution in the days before the skin eruption. There may also be a prodrome consisting of fever, chills, headache, and malaise. Vesicles rupture, crust over, and resolve in 2 to 3 weeks. However, these lesions can leave behind significant scarring, which may result in pitting, trichiasis, entropion, ectropion, or cicatrization and lead to corneal exposure.

Conjunctival involvement is usually in the form of hyperemia associated with a watery discharge, though occasionally vesicles may develop. It usually occurs early in the disease and is associated with the skin eruption.

Herpes zoster is manifested in various ways in the cornea. In the early stages of infection, there may be SPK or, more commonly, microdendritic keratitis (Fig. 4-61). These small dendrites consist of swollen epithelial cells in a stellate pattern that resemble herpes simplex dendrites. These early herpes zoster virus (HZV) dendrites tend to be more peripheral and smaller but more numerous than classic HSV dendrites. The lesions usually clear in a few days without any therapy. Occasionally, a mild anterior stromal haze may remain after the lesions resolve. Herpes zoster virus has been cultured from these lesions. Delayed-onset mucous plaque pseudodendrites

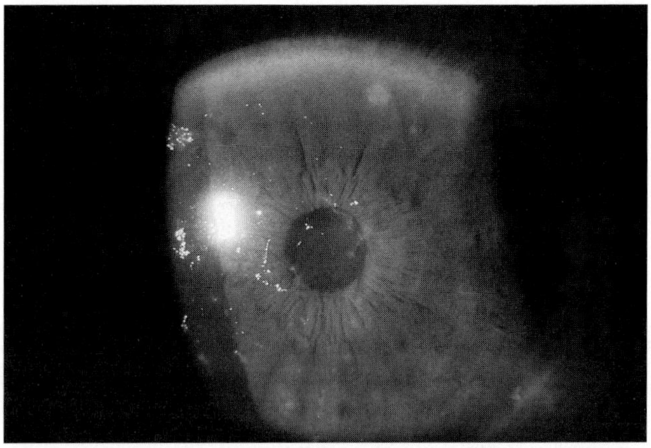

Fig. 4-61 Herpes zoster microdendritic keratitis. Multiple small dendrites are seen early in the course of herpes zoster, even before the skin rash develops.

may develop weeks or months after the initial ocular infection. They are elevated, coarse, gray-white dendritiform lesions, larger and coarser than classic HSV dendrites (Figs. 4-62 and 4-63). They lack the round terminal end bulbs and stain moderately with fluorescein (Figs. 4-64 and 4-65). They may be described as "painted" or "stuck" to the surface of the cornea. They tend to be migratory around the cornea, and they may sometimes be wiped from the surface, leaving a relatively intact epithelium. Viral cultures of these lesions usually are negative. Although they are self-limited, it may take months for them to disappear. Treatment is with aggressive lubrication and occasionally topical corticosteroids. Rarely, especially in immunocompromised hosts, topical or systemic antiviral agents may be helpful.

Anterior stromal infiltrates are another common manifestation of herpes zoster keratitis in which single or multiple granular anterior stromal infiltrates are found. They

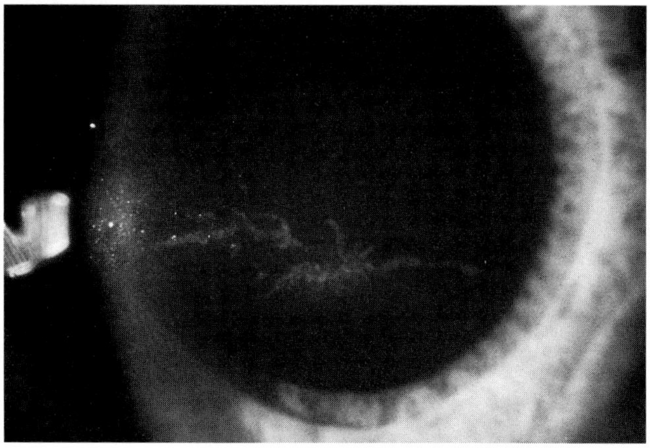

Fig. 4-62 Herpes zoster pseudodendrites. Coarse, gray-white, elevated mucous plaque lesions of the epithelium are occasionally found weeks or months after a herpes zoster ocular infection. It typically occurs in a dendritiform pattern.

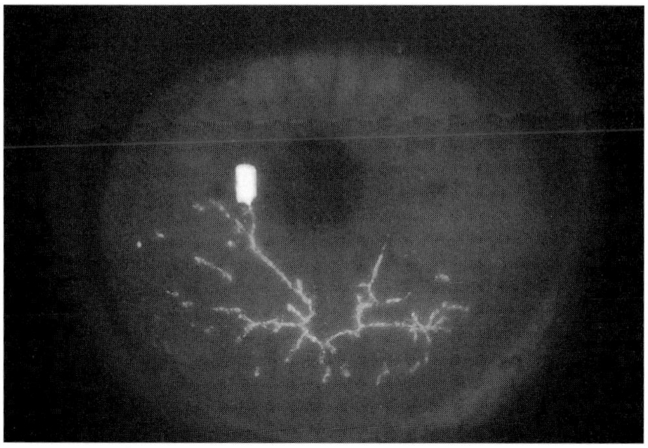

Fig. 4-63 Herpes zoster pseudodendrites. Fluorescein dye highlights these lesions. They can be differentiated from herpes simplex true dendrites because pseudodendrites do not have ulcerated centers, and they lack terminal end bulbs. (See color plate.)

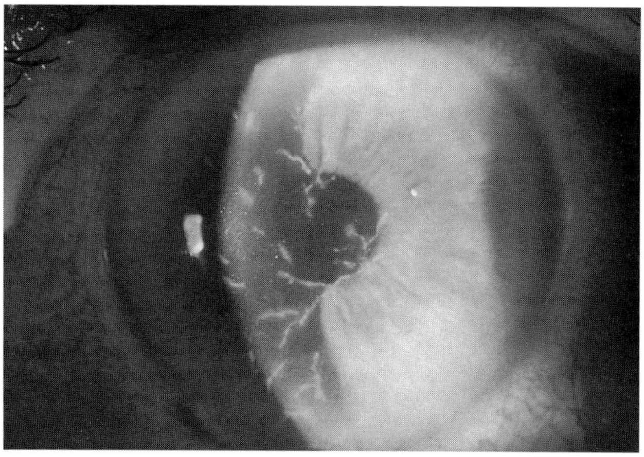

Fig. 4-64 Herpes zoster pseudodendrites. The pseudodendrites appear "stuck" onto the surface of the cornea.

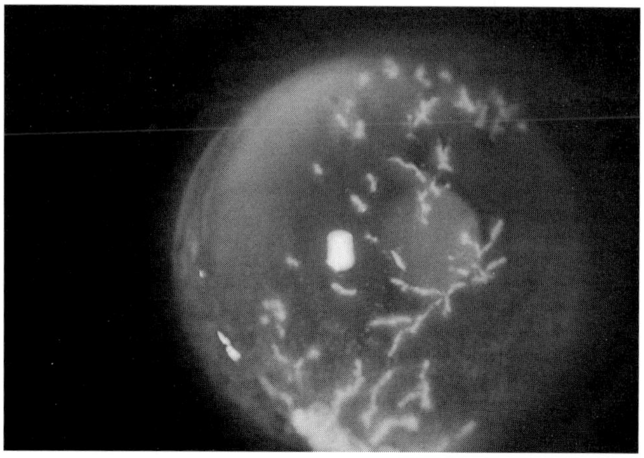

Fig. 4-65 Herpes zoster pseudodendrites. Fluorescein dye staining of the cornea seen in Fig. 4-64. (See color plate.)

represent an inflammatory reaction to the viral antigens from the preceding infection and may leave a round scar. This condition is referred to as nummular keratitis. The infiltrates generally respond to low-dose topical corticosteroids, which must be tapered very slowly.

Stromal keratitis may develop weeks or months after the initial ocular infection, and it may clinically resemble HSV disciform keratitis (endotheliitis). A localized round or disc-shaped area of corneal edema, mild stromal inflammation, and localized keratic precipitates with an intact epithelium are seen (Fig. 4-66). An immune ring may also develop. It, too, is thought to be caused by an inflammatory reaction to viral antigens in the stroma or endothelium. Repeated episodes may result in visually significant stromal scarring, thinning, calcific degeneration, vascularization, and lipid deposition (Fig. 4-67). Necrotizing keratitis sometimes develops (Fig. 4-68).

Neurotrophic keratopathy is a potentially dangerous development in patients with herpes zoster infections. It is clinically similar to, but often more severe than, that seen in herpes simplex keratitis. Corneal anesthesia, likely a result of destructive ganglionitis, may be profound. It may develop immediately or it may evolve over the initial few weeks after infection. Sensation returns for some patients in the next few months, but most have a permanent decrease in corneal sensation. Neurotrophic keratopathy eventually may develop in as many as 25% of patients. Clinically, it begins as a hazy or irregular epithelium or as a coarse, punctate epitheliopathy. This condition may then progress to form a round or oval depressed epithelial defect and ulceration, with heaped-up, rolled edges (Figs. 4-69 and 4-70). The lesions can produce severe scarring and vascularization, and they may progressively melt or perforate. Superinfection with

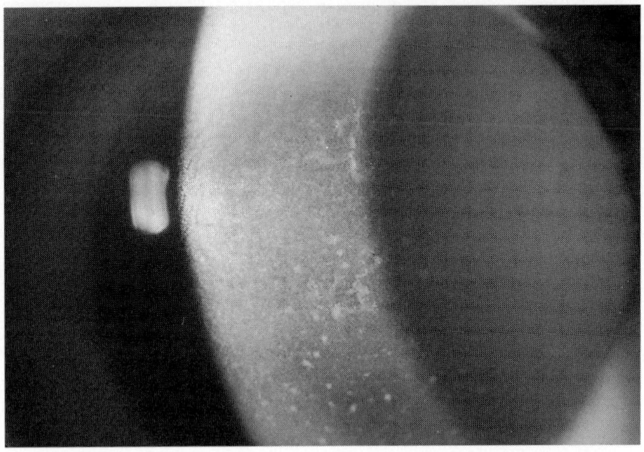

Fig. 4-66 Herpes zoster stromal keratitis (endotheliitis) and uveitis. Diffuse corneal stromal haze and multiple keratic precipitates are seen. Small, faint "pseudodendrites" are also present.

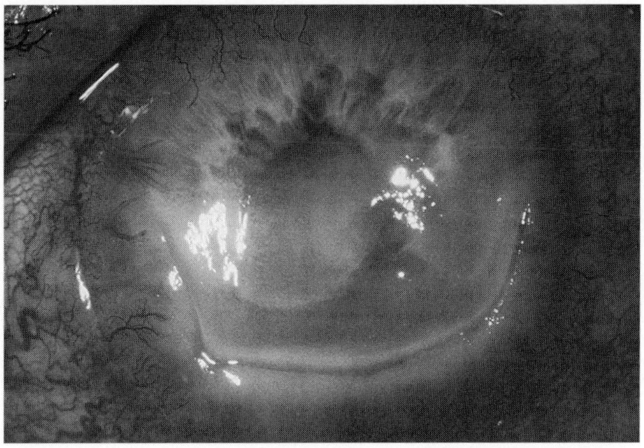

Fig. 4-68 Herpes zoster necrotizing keratitis. Peripheral ulcerative keratitis is seen inferiorly. Additionally, diffuse central stromal edema and significant peripheral corneal neovascularization have developed.

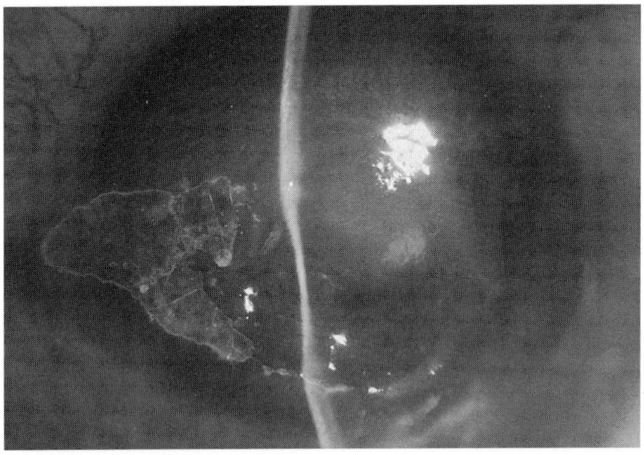

Fig. 4-67 Herpes zoster scarring. Significant corneal scarring, thinning, and calcific degeneration are present in this eye with chronic inflammation from herpes zoster keratitis.

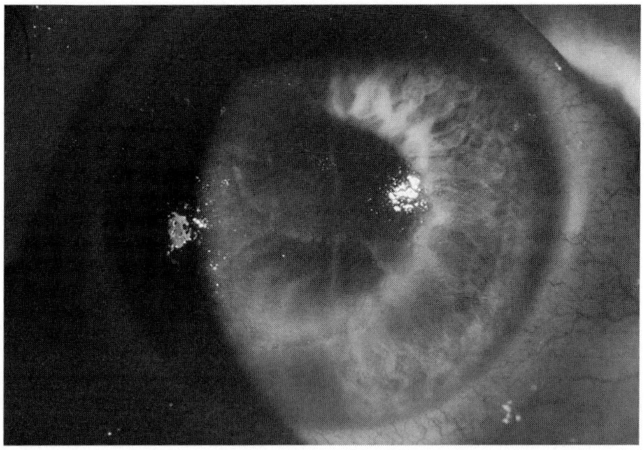

Fig. 4-69 Herpes zoster neurotrophic keratitis. A chronic oval epithelial defect is present inferiorly with moderate underlying stromal edema and haze. (See color plate.)

bacteria, fungus, or atypical mycobacteria may develop. The pathogenesis of this condition is thought to be a combination of factors, including reduced sensation (hence reduced neurotransmitters, which may play a key role in epithelial maintenance and healing), reduced tear formation, and reduced blinking. Postinfectious structural changes to the eyelid that aggravate this condition include trichiasis, cicatricial changes resulting in corneal exposure, entropion, and ectropion.

Iridocyclitis is a frequent finding in herpes zoster infection, either in isolation or in association with other abnormalities. Clinically, it may present as either a granulomatous or nongranulomatous anterior uveitis with keratic precipitates and posterior synechia formation. Occasionally, a hypopyon or a hyphema may be seen. A focal vasculitic phenomenon may cause ischemic necrosis of the iris, resulting in late sectorial iris atrophy. The iritis is frequently associated with glaucoma because of trabeculitis, synechial-angle closure, trabecular clogging with inflammatory debris, or a combination of these factors.

Episcleritis, scleritis, necrotizing retinitis (especially in immunocompromised patients), cranial nerve palsies, extraocular muscle palsies, optic neuropathy, and fatal cranial arteritis are other possible manifestations of herpes zoster infection. Rarely, chronic, recurrent iridocyclitis with iridoplegia may be caused by HZV even if the patient has no history of a dermatomal skin rash.

The mainstay of treatment of herpes zoster ophthalmicus is systemic therapy with an antiviral agent such as acyclovir or, more recently, famciclovir or valacyclovir. Studies have shown that acyclovir treatment (800 mg PO 5 times a day for 7 to 10 days) reduced acute pain, duration of skin lesions, new lesion formation, and duration

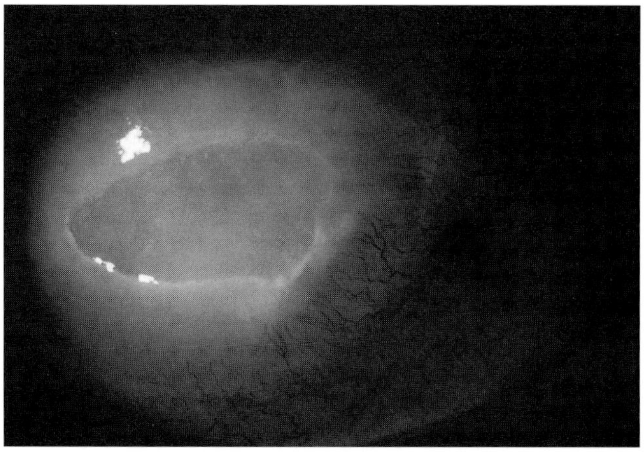

Fig. 4-70 Herpes zoster neurotrophic keratitis. The rolled, heaped-up epithelial edges are apparent in this neurotrophic ulcer after instillation of fluorescein dye using a cobalt blue light.

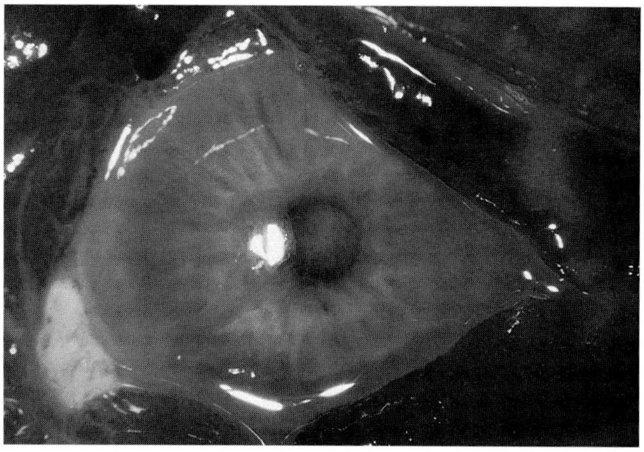

Fig. 4-71 Adenoviral keratoconjunctivitis. Severe hemorrhagic follicular keratoconjunctivitis is seen. A moderate amount of superficial corneal haze and stromal edema is present.

of viral shedding. It also sped resolution of the lesions, particularly if treatment was instituted within 72 hours of onset. Acyclovir treatment has been shown to reduce the incidence of pseudodendritic keratitis, stromal keratitis, and uveitis. Patients who are immunosuppressed may require intravenous therapy. Famciclovir (500 mg tid) and valacyclovir (1 g tid) have potential advantages over acyclovir, including increased antiviral potency and a lower pill-per-day requirement. The role of systemic corticosteroid administration for the prevention of postherpetic neuralgia remains controversial.

The inflammatory complications of zoster infections such as anterior stromal infiltrates, stromal keratitis, episcleritis, iridocyclitis, and trabeculitis generally respond to topical corticosteroid therapy. However, topical corticosteroid therapy may be prolonged, and recurrences are common. The minimum dosage of corticosteroid required to achieve the desired clinical effect should be used. Chronic low-dose topical corticosteroids (as low as 1 drop/week) may be necessary to prevent inflammatory recurrences.

Corneal pseudodendrites or late-onset mucous plaques are generally transient, do not respond to antivirals (except occasionally in immunocompromised hosts), and should be treated with lubrication. Gentle debridement and topical corticosteroids may also be considered.

The treatment of neurotrophic keratopathy from herpes zoster is similar to that of HSV-related neurotrophic ulcers and involves frequent lubrication with preservative-free tears or ointments, patching, bandage contact lenses, temporary or permanent lateral tarsorrhaphy, or a conjunctival flap. Progressive melting and impending perforation may require cyanoacrylate tissue adhesive and a bandage soft contact lens. Frank perforations may require tissue adhesive if they are small or a patch graft or penetrating keratoplasty if they are large.

One of the most difficult long-term problems associated with herpes zoster infections is the development of postherpetic neuralgia. It is often defined as the persistence of pain beyond 1 month after the resolution of the dermatitis. The severity of the pain is debilitating in some patients. It generally subsides within 1 year of the initial infection, but it may persist longer for some patients. Various agents have been used to help reduce the pain, including antidepressants, cimetidine, and capsaicin or doxepin creams. Stellate ganglion nerve blocks may be helpful, but some patients do not find relief from any of the therapeutic modalities.

Other viral keratitis

Adenovirus Adenoviruses are a group of DNA viruses with 47 serotypes. They are a common cause of ocular infection, with peak outbreaks occurring in the midwinter (associated with upper respiratory infection) and midsummer (associated with swimming pool use). The virus is primarily spread by contact or by fomites. Serotypes 3, 4, and 7 (pharyngoconjunctival fever [PCF]) and 8, 11, 19, and 37 (epidemic keratoconjunctivitis [EKC]) account for most ocular disease. Ocular infection usually presents in the form of a follicular conjunctivitis, which is discussed in detail in Chapter 1 (Fig. 4-71).

Corneal involvement from adenoviral infection is often associated with epidemic keratoconjunctivitis, but it may also occur with other adenoviral infectious syndromes such as pharyngoconjunctival fever. Corneal infection usually follows a typical pattern, beginning with fine, diffuse punctate keratitis that may be evident several days after the onset of follicular conjunctivitis (Fig. 4-72). This punctate epithelial keratitis represents viral infection and replication within the corneal epithelium.

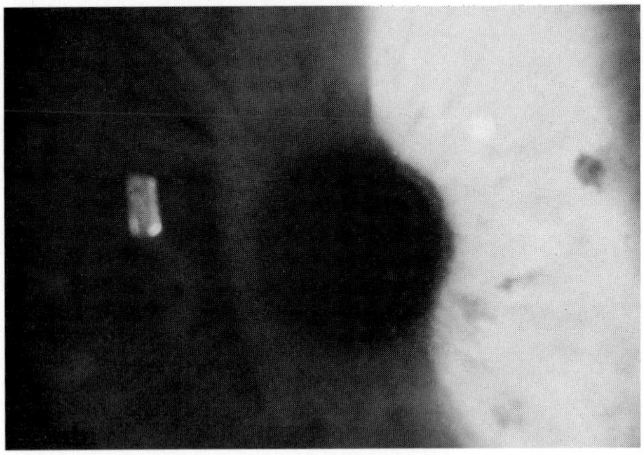

Fig. 4-72 Adenoviral keratoconjunctivitis. Fine, diffuse punctate epithelial keratitis can be seen in this eye with adenoviral conjunctivitis.

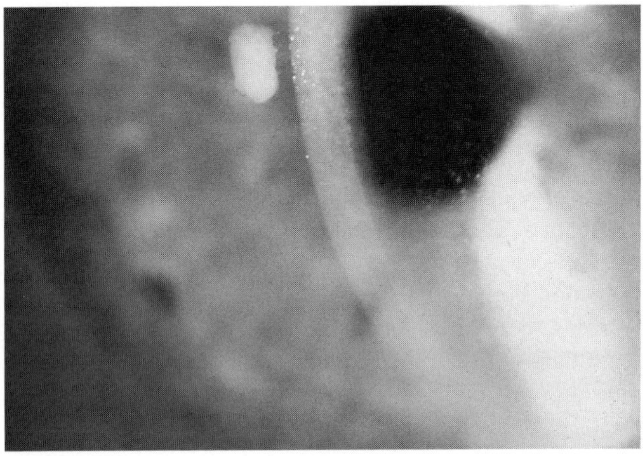

Fig. 4-73 Adenoviral keratoconjunctivitis. With retroillumination off the iris, large, coarse, elevated epithelial lesions are seen.

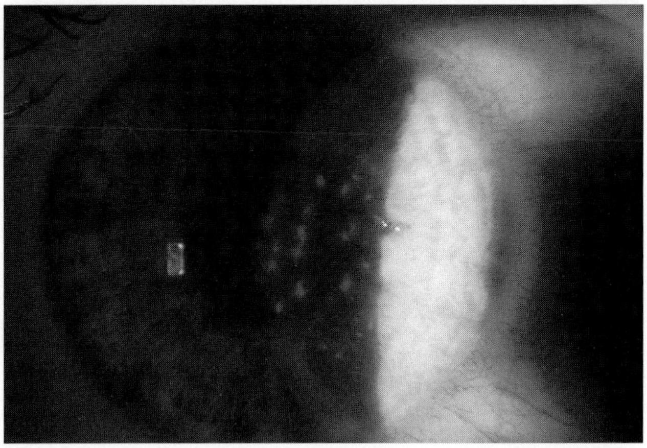

Fig. 4-74 Adenoviral subepithelial infiltrates. Multiple subepithelial infiltrates are present several weeks after adenoviral conjunctivitis. These active subepithelial infiltrates stain minimally with fluorescein.

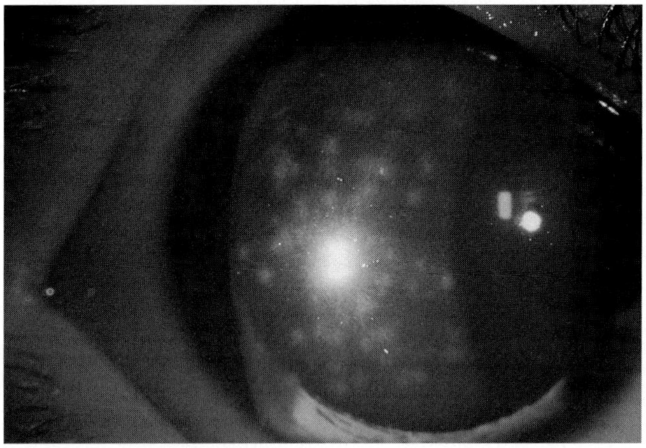

Fig. 4-75 Adenoviral subepithelial infiltrates. Numerous subepithelial infiltrates are seen. The corneal surface is smooth and without fluorescein staining.

During the first week, the lesions may coalesce into larger, coarse, elevated epithelial lesions (Fig. 4-73) that stain with fluorescein. They are usually centrally located and symptomatic, producing photophobia, foreign body sensation, and tearing or pain, and they usually persist into the second week. Rarely, large epithelial defects result. In severe cases, pseudomembranous conjunctivitis can also occur. Typically, by the end of the second week of infection, the host immune system has cleared the remaining replicating virus. As the focal, elevated epithelial lesions begin to resolve, discrete circular subepithelial gray-white opacities may begin to appear. These lesions are typically small (0.5 to 1.0 mm), multiple, centrally located, and do not stain or stain minimally with fluorescein dye (Fig. 4-74). There may be a few to as many as 50 to 75 of these subepithelial infiltrates scattered across the cornea (Fig. 4-75). Although they may be asymptomatic, these lesions can reduce vision if located in the visual axis, and can produce photophobia and glare symptoms. These lesions are thought to result from an immune-mediated response to adenoviral antigens that remain in the region of Bowman's membrane after epithelial infection. In general, the lesions slowly resolve over weeks to months, but some persist for years.

The treatment of acute adenoviral conjunctivitis and early keratitis is largely supportive. Because no commercially available antiadenoviral agent exists, initial therapy usually consists of cool compresses, lubrication with preservative-free artificial tears, and occasionally mild topical vasoconstrictors. Topical nonsteroidal antiinflammatory agents may be helpful for pain. In general, topical corticosteroids should be avoided because the disease is self-limited and because corticosteroids may suppress the host immune response, thus promoting viral replication and enhancing viral shedding. Additionally, the use of corticosteroids exposes the patient to potential corticosteroid-related complications or to potential exacerbation of the infection should the initial diagnosis be incorrect (e.g., HSV). However, topical corticosteroids may be necessary if patients have severe discomfort, pseudomembrane formation, iritis, or corneal erosions. An ointment should be used because drops are quickly washed out from profuse tearing.

The role of topical corticosteroids in the treatment of subepithelial infiltrates is controversial. Usually, the infiltrates resolve without treatment in weeks to months (rarely years). Although topical corticosteroids are effective at eliminating these opacities, they may recur as corticosteroids are tapered, leading to a pattern of treatment, remission, recurrence, and retreatment. This cycle may significantly prolong the course of the disease. Therefore the initiation of topical corticosteroid therapy as the initial treatment of subepithelial infiltrates should be deferred unless the infiltrates are severe, appear in the visual axis, or cause other symptoms. In those cases, the lowest clinically effective dose of topical corticosteroid (e.g., 0.1% fluorometholone) should be used, and therapy should be tapered slowly. If a patient has a recurrence after corticosteroid withdrawal, consideration should be given to withholding the reinstitution of topical corticosteroid therapy if the infiltrates are not in the visual axis or producing significant symptoms.

A topical antiviral drug, cidofovir, is being tested for efficacy against adenoviral keratoconjunctivitis in humans; it showed significant efficacy in experimental animals. Phase 2 studies have been completed, but it will probably be several years before the medication is approved by the Food and Drug Administration even if phase 3 studies show clinical efficacy.

Epstein-Barr virus The Epstein-Barr virus (EBV) is a herpesvirus known to cause infectious mononucleosis. Exposure to the virus is widespread, and some studies have shown EBV-specific antibodies in more than 90% of the study population. EBV infection in younger children may present with few clinical signs, although exposure later in life may manifest as the fever, sore throat, malaise, lymphadenopathy, hepatosplenomegaly, arthralgia, and myalgia of infectious mononucleosis.

Ocular manifestations of EBV infection are not commonly reported, but they may involve all segments of the eye. The conjunctiva is affected most often with follicular conjunctivitis. The follicular response may be intense, and it may be associated with ipsilateral preauricular and cervical lymphadenopathy, known as Parinaud's oculoglandular syndrome.

Corneal epithelial involvement in the form of dendritiform epithelial keratitis has been reported. These lesions tend to be self-limited and do not require treatment. Corneal stromal involvement takes the form of subepithelial infiltrates similar to those seen in adenoviral keratoconjunctivitis or of deeper multifocal stromal keratitis producing well-demarcated pleomorphic round or ring-shaped opacities. Peripheral keratitis with vascularization has also been reported. All these inflammatory lesions respond well to topical corticosteroids, though stromal scarring may remain after the resolution of keratitis.

EBV may also produce scleritis, dacryoadenitis, uveitis, multifocal choroiditis, optic neuropathy, and optic nerve swelling, and it has been implicated as a possible causative factor in Sjögren's syndrome and iridocorneal endothelial syndrome.

The diagnosis of EBV infection is made using serologic tests for EBV viral capsid antigen, EBV nuclear antigen, and EBV early antigen. IgM antibodies to viral capsid antigen or a fourfold rise in IgG antibodies to EBV nuclear antigen is diagnostic of recent EBV infection.

Vaccinia virus The vaccinia virus is a poxvirus used in the worldwide inoculation against smallpox. Since the eradication of smallpox and the discontinuation of the inoculation program, vaccinia infection is rarely encountered.

Ocular involvement from vaccinia was largely caused by autoinoculation after administration of the vaccine. It produces pustules on the eyelids and conjunctiva and eyelid erythema and swelling that make it resemble periorbital cellulitis. Corneal involvement, if it occurs at all, may be manifested as superficial punctate keratitis, dendritiform epithelial keratitis, stromal keratitis, or disciform keratitis (endotheliitis).

Although vaccinia is self-limited, therapy may shorten its course and reduce the severity of infection. Treatment modalities include intramuscular injections of vaccinia immunoglobulin, vidarabine, idoxuridine, or trifluorothymidine. Corticosteroids may be helpful for the resolution of stromal keratitis, but only after the resolution of epithelial infection and while maintaining concurrent antiviral prophylaxis.

Measles (rubeola) and mumps Measles (rubeola) is a highly contagious viral disease that, though uncommon in the United States, is a continued cause of morbidity and mortality in developing countries. Infection typically occurs in childhood, and it may present with fever, cough, flulike symptoms, Koplik's spots (gray-white pinpoint dots on an erythematous base) on the oral mucosa, and conjunctivitis. A maculopapular rash may then develop.

The ocular manifestations of measles infection include conjunctivitis and epithelial keratitis. The conjunctivitis typically presents with conjunctival injection, chemosis, and a watery discharge, without a marked papillary or follicular reaction. Occasionally, conjunctival epithelial lesions may be found. Lesions similar in appearance to oral Koplik's spots have also been reported on the conjunctiva. Corneal involvement usually takes the form of superficial punctate keratitis. All these findings are generally self-limited and require only supportive therapy.

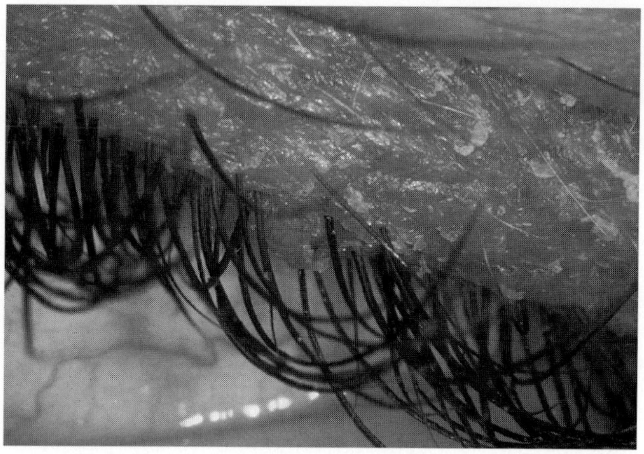

Fig. 4-76 Molluscum contagiosum. An umbilicated molluscum lesion of the upper eyelid margin is seen.

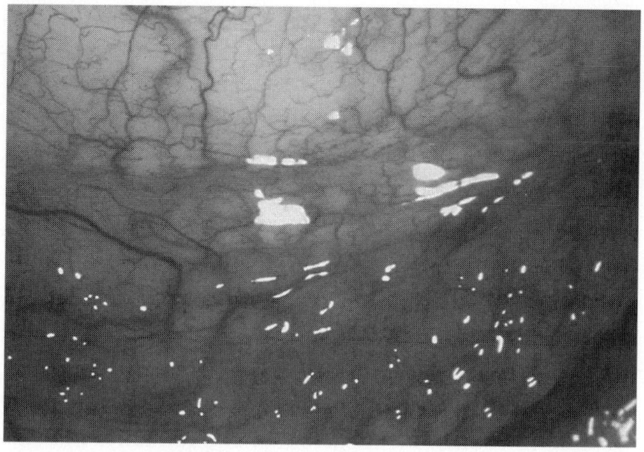

Fig. 4-77 Molluscum contagiosum. This severe follicular conjunctivitis was caused by a toxic reaction to the viral particles shed from the eyelid margin lesion seen in Fig. 4-76.

In developing countries, the measles virus has been associated with corneal blindness in children. However, it is likely that most corneal blindness attributed to measles is caused by a combination of severe malnutrition and vitamin A deficiency, traditional folk therapies, and secondary bacterial or herpes simplex infection along with measles keratitis.

Mumps is another contagious viral disease, primarily affecting children, characterized by bilateral swelling of the parotid glands. A patient may have a prodrome of fever, malaise, headache, and anorexia. After the parotitis, orchitis may develop in males, though this finding is more common in infections developing after puberty.

The most common ocular manifestation of mumps infection is dacryoadenitis. It produces painful swelling of the lacrimal glands that may cause mild proptosis simultaneously with the parotitis. Conjunctival injection or follicular conjunctivitis may be present. Corneal involvement usually presents as a painless, unilateral, full-thickness infiltration of the stroma with an intact epithelium, and associated iritis may develop. These findings usually appear the week after the onset of the parotitis, and they typically resolve spontaneously within 3 weeks without vascularization or significant reduction in visual acuity. Topical corticosteroids may hasten their resolution. Scleritis, anterior uveitis, neuroretinitis, and optic neuropathy have also been associated with mumps infection.

Molluscum contagiosum The molluscum contagiosum virus is a poxvirus that produces round, umbilicated lesions on the skin (Fig. 4-76). These lesions are generally painless, but they may produce chronic follicular conjunctivitis (Fig. 4-77) because of a toxic reaction to viral shedding into the tear film when present on the eyelids. This condition is discussed in detail in Chapter 1. Toxic reactions have also been reported to affect the cornea, producing punctate epithelial keratopathy, pseudodendritic epitheliopathy, pannus formation resembling trachoma, or subepithelial infiltrates.

Molluscum lesions usually resolve spontaneously over months to years in immunocompetent patients, but new lesions may develop. In immunocompromised patients the lesions may be larger, more numerous, and have a protracted course, but the conjunctivitis is less severe. Lesions are removed surgically by simple excision or incision and curettage. Cryotherapy, electrocautery, and chemical cauterization are also effective in eliminating these lesions in most patients.

Interstitial Keratitis

Syphilitic interstitial keratitis *Interstitial keratitis* is a term used to describe any nonulcerative inflammatory infiltration of the corneal stroma without significant involvement of the epithelium or endothelium. It may result in corneal vascularization, scarring, and thinning. After resolution of the keratitis, these vessels often regress, leaving empty vascular channels known as *ghost vessels.* Although interstitial keratitis has many causes, congenital and acquired syphilis remain the most common, especially in developing countries.

Syphilis is caused by infection with the spirochete *Treponema pallidum.* Congenital infection may occur by transplacental transmission of the spirochete; acquired infection is usually transmitted sexually but rarely by direct contact with an infected mucocutaneous lesion. Ocular involvement, including interstitial keratitis, may be a manifestation of congenital or acquired syphilis and may occur early and late in the course of the disease.

Interstitial keratitis of congenital syphilis usually develops in the first or second decade. Clinically, it

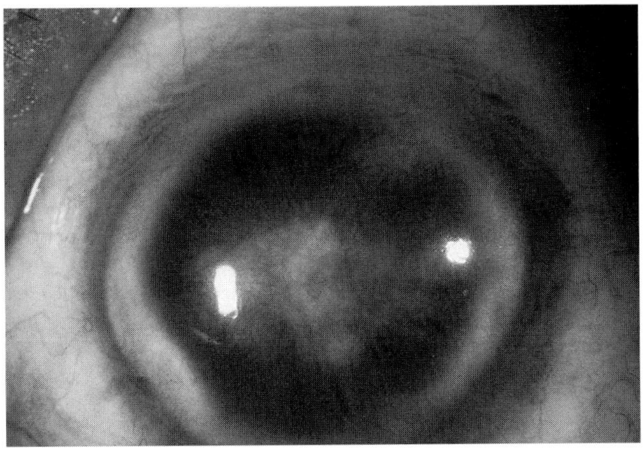

Fig. 4-78 Syphilitic interstitial keratitis. Patchy stromal scarring is typical of interstitial keratitis.

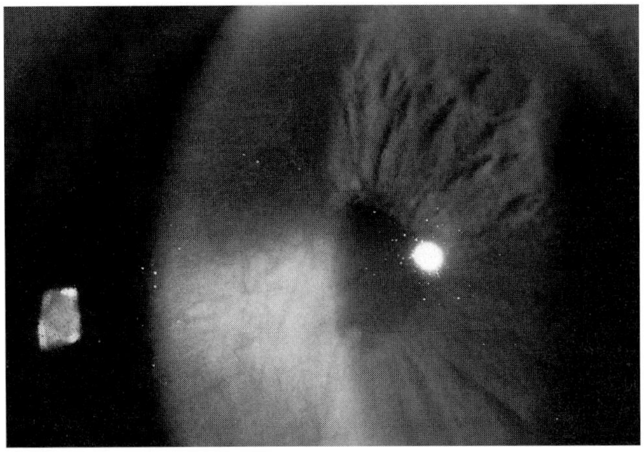

Fig. 4-79 Syphilitic interstitial keratitis. A dense corneal scar from congenital syphilis is seen. Ghost vessels are visible superiorly as white lines and in the scar as lucent lines.

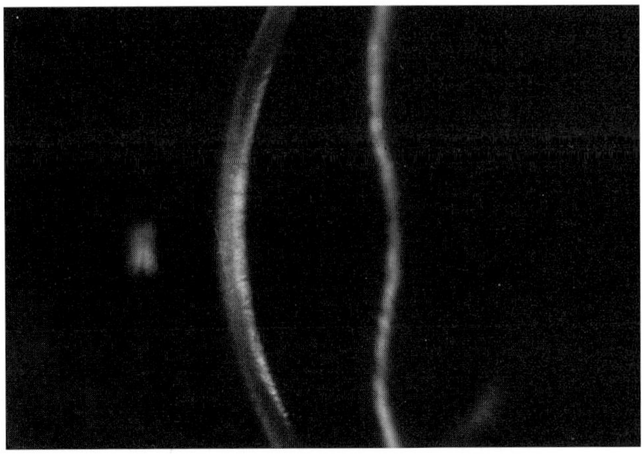

Fig. 4-80 Syphilitic interstitial keratitis. A slit-beam view of the cornea seen in Fig. 4-79 reveals the scarring to be in the posterior cornea.

presents with a diffuse inflammatory infiltration in the deep stroma, giving the cornea a "ground-glass" appearance, or patchy stromal infiltrates, which may enlarge, become confluent, and advance centrally with deep corneal neovascularization. Stromal infiltration over deep stromal neovascularization produces a dull red color known as a *salmon patch*. Corneal edema is usually present. Patients have pain, photosensitivity, and reduced visual acuity. More than 80% of the cases of interstitial keratitis caused by congenital syphilis are bilateral; however, weeks or months may separate episodes in each eye. If left untreated, the stromal inflammation and neovascularization may progress to involve the entire cornea and may persist for weeks or months prior to regressing spontaneously. Regression usually begins peripherally and advances centrally. Sequelae of interstitial keratitis include deep stromal scarring (Figs. 4-78, 4-79, and 4-80), thinning, ghost vessels (Figs. 4-81 and 4-82), Descemet's folds or scrolls, and stromal lipid deposition.

Treatment with topical corticosteroids significantly speeds resolution of the keratitis, reduces neovascularization, and improves the visual outcome. If there has been no history of previous treatment, systemic penicillin therapy is required to prevent systemic complications, although it may not alter the course of the ocular disease.

Corneal involvement is uncommon in patients with acquired syphilis. During primary syphilis infection, a conjunctival chancre occasionally is found, and peripheral corneal extension may incite a stromal inflammatory response. Peripheral corneal infiltrates have also been reported in some patients with secondary syphilis. However, the most common manifestation of acquired syphilis infection is unilateral interstitial keratitis, which usually develops during the latent phase of syphilis infection, without any other overt signs of active disease. The average time from initial infection to the onset of interstitial keratitis is 10 years. The antigenic stimulus for the development of keratitis is unknown. Clinical manifestations of acute interstitial keratitis in acquired syphilis are similar to those of congenital syphilis, though the inflammation typically resolves more quickly and is associated with less neovascularization. Interstitial keratitis caused by acquired syphilis is usually unilateral, but in as many as 40% of patients it is bilateral. As in congenital syphilis, the keratitis is very responsive to topical corticosteroid therapy and should be accompanied by systemic antitreponemal therapy if the patient has no history of adequate previous treatment. In contrast to congenital syphilis, the stromal keratitis may be somewhat responsive to systemic antitreponemal therapy.

Postinflammatory corneal sequelae include stromal scarring, especially posterior, with middle and deep stromal ghost vessels. Significant corneal thinning is often present. A small clear zone may surround the

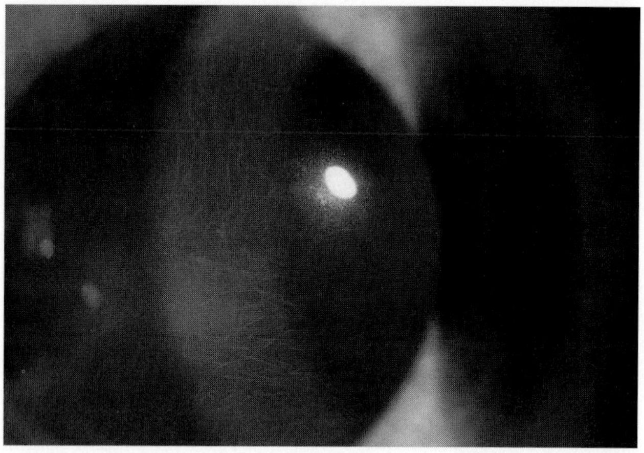

Fig. 4-81 Syphilitic interstitial keratitis. Multiple ghost vessels traverse the entire cornea.

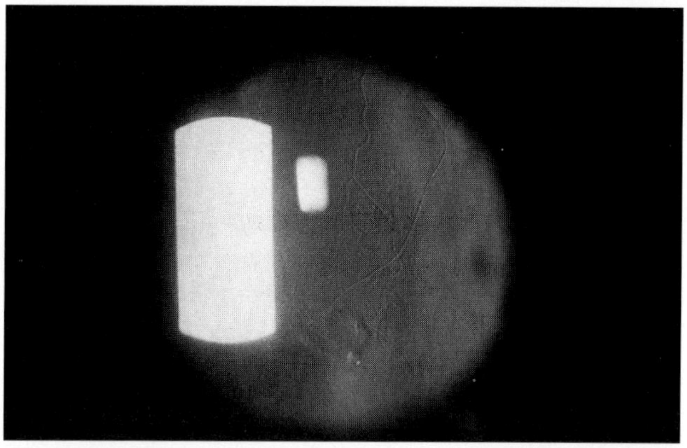

Fig. 4-82 Syphilitic interstitial keratitis. Retroillumination off the retina highlights the ghost vessels. (See color plate.)

ghost vessels, and lipid keratopathy may develop. Postinflammatory endothelial damage may stimulate the formation of Descemet's ridges or scrolls and predispose the cornea to future edema. In badly scarred or edematous corneas, penetrating keratoplasty may be required for visual rehabilitation.

The diagnosis of syphilis is based on patient history, clinical presentation, and serologic test results. Corneal findings consistent with active interstitial keratitis or the sequela of past interstitial keratitis should prompt an investigation. Elements of the patient's history that may suggest syphilis include a prolonged episode of sensitivity to light during childhood and previous venereal disease in the patient or in the patient's mother during pregnancy. Physical examination may reveal other stigmata of syphilitic infection, both ocular and nonocular, among them nasal deformity, abnormal dentition, and deafness. Finally, these tests should be performed as part of the workup: Venereal Disease Research Laboratory (VDRL) or rapid plasma reagin (RPR) (both revert to normal after treatment) *and* fluorescein treponemal antibody (FTA) or microhemagglutination-*Treponema pallidum* (MHA-TP) (once positive, remains positive for both). Patients with positive results on the FTA or MHA-TP test should be considered for treatment with systemic penicillin, generally while under the simultaneous care of an internist or an infectious disease specialist. Patients with positive results on the FTA or MHA-TP test and negative results of the VDRL or RPR test who have a history of appropriate past treatment do not usually require retreatment.

Nonsyphilitic interstitial keratitis Although interstitial keratitis is classically associated with syphilitic infection, it may be caused by other infectious and inflammatory conditions (Box 4-13). Herpes simplex and herpes zoster are two major causes of nonsyphilitic interstitial keratitis and are discussed earlier in this chapter. Several of the other more important conditions associated with interstitial keratitis are discussed in this section.

Box 4-13 Infectious and Inflammatory Conditions Associated with Interstitial Keratitis

BACTERIAL

Syphilis
Lyme disease
Brucellosis

MYCOBACTERIAL

Tuberculosis
Leprosy
Atypical mycobacteria

VIRAL

Herpes simplex
Herpes zoster
Epstein-Barr
Measles (rubeola)
Mumps

CHLAMYDIAL

Lymphogranuloma venereum

PARASITIC

Onchocerciasis
Cysticercosis
Leishmaniasis
Trypanosomiasis

SYSTEMIC CONDITIONS

Cogan's syndrome
Sarcoidosis
Lymphoma
Kaposi's sarcoma

Cogan's syndrome Cogan's syndrome is defined as the association of nonsyphilitic interstitial keratitis with vestibuloauditory disturbances similar to Ménière's disease (vertigo, tinnitus, nausea, vomiting, and ultimately hearing loss). Cogan's syndrome has also been associated with systemic vasculitic processes such as polyarteritis nodosa, Wegener's granulomatosis, and rheumatoid arthritis. As many as 10% of patients with Cogan's syndrome may have serious vasculitic complications such as aortitis and aortic insufficiency, coronary arteritis, or systemic necrotizing vasculitis.

The cause of Cogan's syndrome remains unknown. No associated infectious disease has been identified. The pathogenesis is probably caused by an autoimmune response to a common antigen in the cornea and the inner ear.

Clinically, these patients present with the typical findings of interstitial keratitis: patchy stromal infiltration that may incite neovascularization. Corneal infiltrates may at first appear superficial and may resemble those seen in adenoviral infections. Later the infiltrates involve the more posterior portion of the cornea. At the time of presentation, patients typically complain of the sudden onset of pain, photophobia, and tearing. Vestibuloauditory symptoms may be present at the time of initial presentation, or may develop within the next 6 months.

The differential diagnosis of Cogan's syndrome includes other potential causes of interstitial keratitis and hearing loss, particularly congenital syphilis. Cogan's syndrome may be differentiated from congenital syphilis in that syphilitic interstitial keratitis is usually associated with a slow, gradual onset, serologic test results positive for syphilis, and systemic stigmata of syphilitic infection. Tuberculosis, herpes zoster, measles, mumps, and systemic inflammatory conditions associated with vasculitis should also be considered in the differential diagnosis of Cogan's syndrome.

The treatment of Cogan's syndrome includes topical corticosteroids for the corneal disease and, if the patient has auditory dysfunction, systemic corticosteroids. Untreated Cogan's syndrome may result in permanent sensorineural hearing loss. Systemic corticosteroids or other immunosuppressive agents may be required, under the guidance of an internist or a rheumatologist, if systemic vasculitis develops.

Mycobacterial infection Mycobacterial infection, including that caused by *M. tuberculosis* or *M. leprae,* rarely produces interstitial keratitis. Tuberculosis may produce interstitial keratitis that is typically unilateral and sectorial within the cornea. Stromal infiltration is followed by neovascularization that lasts weeks. It is responsive to topical corticosteroid therapy, but antituberculous agents are required to treat the systemic disease.

M. leprae infection may produce SPK, corneal nerve infiltration, focal avascular keratitis, or interstitial keratitis. Focal avascular keratitis indicates the development of lepromas within the cornea that contain *M. leprae* organisms. Lepromas are usually asymptomatic and present as peripheral, focal, white subepithelial opacities. Interstitial keratitis may develop and may lead to significant scarring; it is thought to represent a response to active infection within the cornea, in contrast to other forms of interstitial keratitis. *M. leprae* organisms may also infiltrate corneal nerves, producing a characteristic beaded or "string of pearls" appearance that is pathognomonic of leprosy and may be associated with corneal hypesthesia. The treatment regimen includes systemic antilepromatous agents and topical corticosteroids and cycloplegics as necessary for interstitial keratitis and iritis. Because of the decreased corneal sensation that accompanies this infection, the corneal epithelium must be monitored carefully for the development of neurotrophic keratopathy.

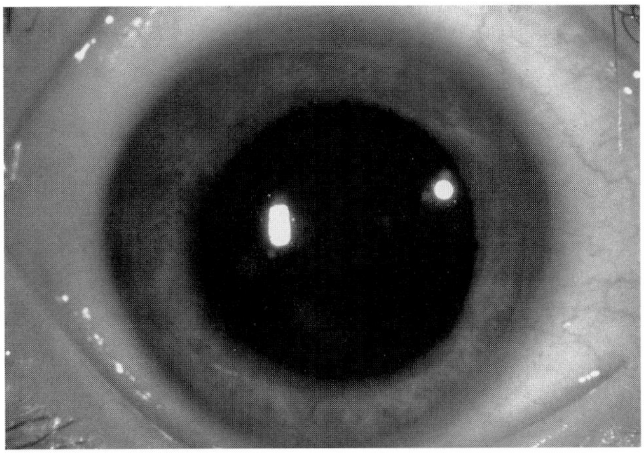

Fig. 4-83 Lyme keratitis. Several nummular corneal infiltrates are seen inferiorly in this patient with Lyme disease. Treatment for Lyme disease improved the patient's systemic symptoms, but the keratitis continued.

Lyme disease Lyme disease is produced by a spirochete, *Borrelia burgdorferi*, carried by *Ixodes* ticks. Infection produces a systemic disease characterized by three stages. Stage 1 presents with an erythematous, progressively enlarging "bull's-eye" skin rash known as erythema chronicum migrans. Stage 2 is characterized by disseminated infection and may result in cardiac and neurologic complications. Stage 3 includes rheumatologic or central nervous system manifestations. Treatment with systemic antibiotics is required. Ocular involvement is usually absent in stage 1 disease. Episcleritis, interstitial keratitis, uveitis, vasculitis, exudative retinal detachment, and optic disc edema (resulting from Lyme meningoencephalitis) have all been reported in association with late (stage 2 or 3) infection. Interstitial keratitis is usually bilateral and is characterized by multiple "nummular" stromal infiltrates with indistinct borders at all levels of the stroma (Figs. 4-83, 4-84, and 4-85). It does

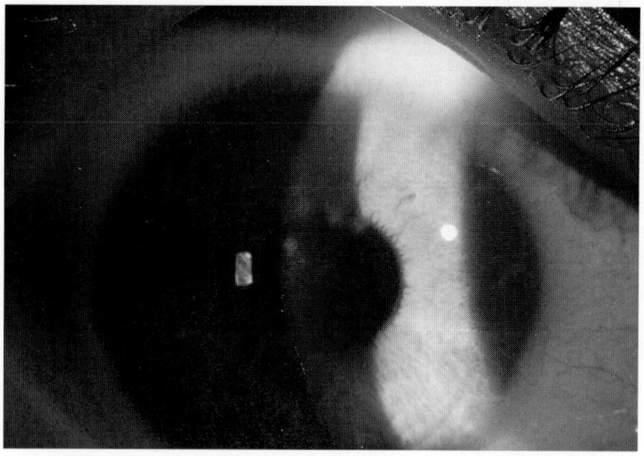

Fig. 4-84 Lyme keratitis. The same eye seen in Fig. 4-83 seven years later demonstrates nummular corneal infiltrates in a superior location.

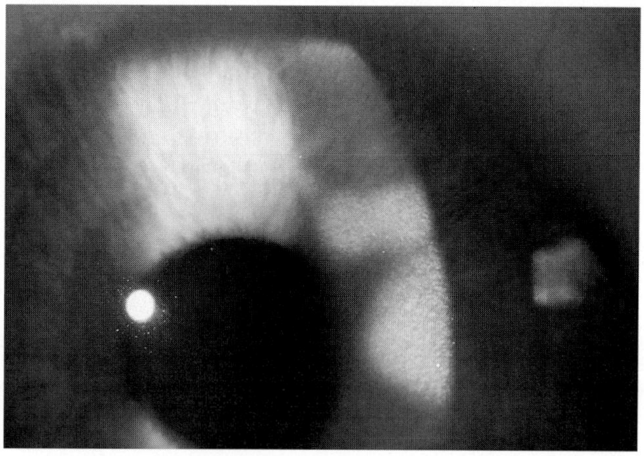

Fig. 4-85 Lyme keratitis. The fellow eye of the patient seen in Figs. 4-83 and 4-84 reveals several large, circular subepithelial infiltrates.

not respond to the administration of systemic antibiotics alone, and it requires the addition of topical corticosteroids to prevent progression of the inflammation to scarring and vascularization.

Onchocerciasis Onchocerciasis, also known as river blindness, has been one of the major causes of infectious corneal blindness worldwide, but it is expected to be eradicated in the next 20 years. The causative organism is a filarial parasite known as *Onchocerca volvulus*. The disease is transmitted by the bite of the *Simulium* species of blackfly, whose breeding grounds are in flowing rivers. Once a patient is infected, microfilariae migrate throughout the body and may enter the eye along scleral vessels and nerves, hematogenously or by direct invasion from the conjunctiva. Microfilariae may be seen in the cornea, anterior chamber, vitreous, and retina. Early corneal infection is characterized by live microfilariae in the cornea or by dead parasites surrounded by a small, punctate, inflammatory stromal infiltrate. More advanced corneal disease is characterized by peripheral stromal haze advancing centrally from the nasal and temporal limbus in the interpalpebral zone until the entire cornea becomes opaque and vascularized. The infiltration is usually superficial, and the leading edge is usually infiltrated by microfilariae. This pattern has been referred to as sclerosing keratitis. The primary therapy for onchocerciasis is with the antiparasitic agent ivermectin. This agent is effective against microfilariae but not against adult worms, and therefore it must be administered repeatedly until all adult worms have died. Community action is also required to reduce the parasitic reservoir and thus the rate of reinfection.

SURFACE DISEASES

Contact Lens–Related Disorders

Contact lenses are worn by millions of persons and are a safe and effective means to correct refractive error. However, complications related to contact lens wear are not infrequent and may result in significant ocular morbidity. Contact lens-related microbial keratitis is the most destructive complication of contact lens use and is discussed earlier in this chapter. Corneal hypoxia related to tight lens syndrome, toxic reactions to contact lens solutions, giant papillary conjunctivitis, corneal warpage, corneal neovascularization, and pseudo-superior limbic keratoconjunctivitis (pseudo-SLK) syndrome are additional complications of contact lens wear.

Tight lens syndrome Corneal oxygenation during contact lens wear is dependent primarily on the replenishment of the tear film through and around the lens with each blink. Soft contact lenses of high water content allow greater oxygen transmissibility (Dk/L) through the lens than contact lenses of low water content. A tight lens, whether soft or hard, results in decreased or no lens movement during a blink, significantly reducing oxygen penetration into the anterior cornea. This syndrome often develops shortly after the patient has been fit for contact lenses, though it may occur later, particularly if there has been an unnoticed change in the lens-cornea relationship. Patients generally present with pain, photophobia, decreased vision, or foreign body sensation that typically starts several hours after lens insertion. For users of extended wear contact lenses, symptoms may present after overnight wear. Examination with the lens in place reveals little to no lens movement. An impression of the lens on the cornea (for rigid lenses) or on the conjunctiva (for soft lenses) often remains after the lens is removed (Fig. 4-86). Perilimbal injection, SPK, anterior stromal infiltrates, stromal edema (Fig. 4-87), anterior chamber reaction, or even a hypopyon may develop.

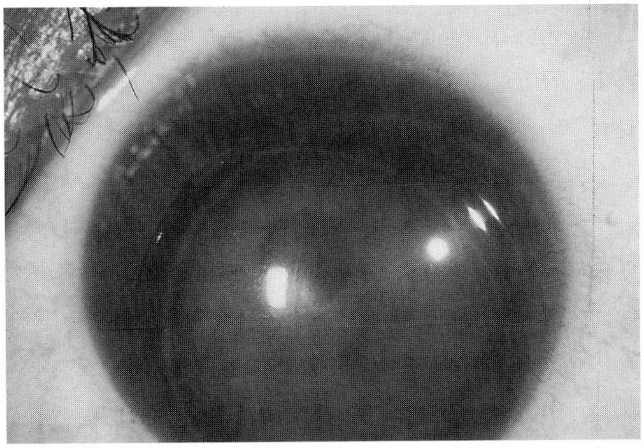

Fig. 4-86 Tight lens syndrome. The imprint of a tight "stuck-on," rigid, gas-permeable contact lens is still seen on this cornea 10 minutes after removal of the lens. Moderate underlying corneal edema is present.

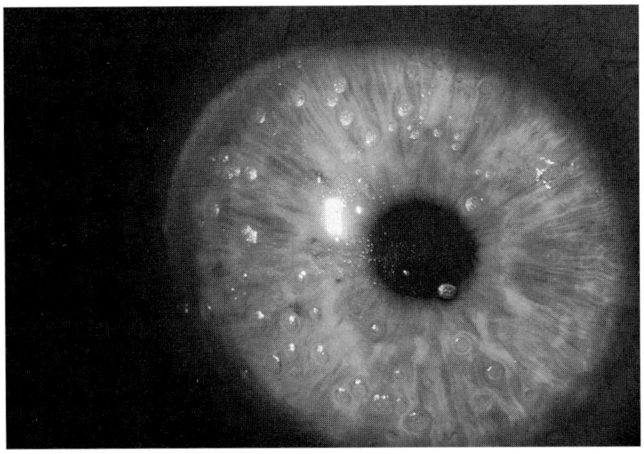

Fig. 4-88 Contact lens deposits. Numerous proteinaceous deposits are seen on this soft contact lens.

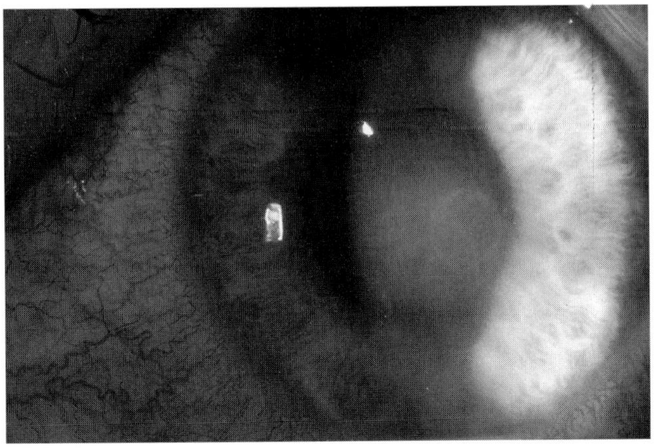

Fig. 4-87 Tight lens syndrome. Tight lenses or lens overwear can cause stromal edema, as seen in this eye. A small, circular, immune ring is present.

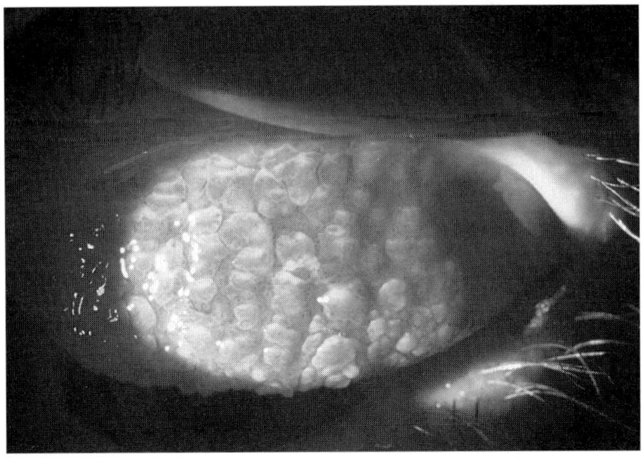

Fig. 4-89 Giant papillary conjunctivitis. Multiple giant papillae are present under the upper eyelid of this rigid, gas-permeable contact lens wearer.

Treatment consists of the discontinuation of contact lens wear, the administration of cycloplegics if a patient has an anterior chamber reaction, and observation. Consider topical antibiotic therapy if a punctate keratopathy is present. After the syndrome has resolved, the patient must be fitted with a looser lens before contact lens use can be resumed.

Giant papillary conjunctivitis Giant papillary conjunctivitis (GPC) is a common complication of contact lens wear that affects as many as 5% of contact lens users. This clinical syndrome is also seen in association with ocular prostheses and exposed sutures.

The cause of this syndrome has been linked to the protein deposits that form on the surface of contact lenses. Soft contact lenses accumulate more of these deposits than hard lenses, and soft lenses of high water content accumulate more deposits than soft lenses of low water content (Fig. 4-88). Type 1 hypersensitivity resulting in mast cell degranulation, delayed-type hypersensitivity, and chronic mechanical trauma have all been implicated in the pathogenesis of this condition.

Clinically, these patients present with a history of itching, foreign body sensation (especially with the lens in place), mucoid discharge, decreased wearing time, or complete intolerance of the contact lenses. Patients may be asymptomatic when the contact lens is out. Examination usually reveals giant papillae (Fig. 4-89), larger than 1 mm on the superior palpebral conjunctiva, but sometimes smaller papillae measuring 0.3 to 1.0 mm are present (this form may represent an earlier stage of GPC). Occasionally ptosis is also present. The lens may be high riding or coated with protein deposits, or both.

In addition to pharmacologic treatment, the main focus of therapy for GPC is aimed at reducing the accumulation of lens deposits and decreasing the exposure time of the conjunctiva to these substances. Reduction in the accumulation of lens deposits may be accomplished by better lens care practices, including the use of a daily surfactant lens cleaner, cold chemical disinfection, and weekly or semiweekly enzymatic cleaning. If this regimen is unsuccessful, switching to a disposable contact lens system may be a helpful alternative for soft contact lens wearers. Daily disposable contact lenses would allow for the least accumulation of lens deposits. Switching to rigid lenses may be an alternative for some patients. Reduced wearing time, especially changing from extended wear to daily wear, is indicated. Effective pharmacologic agents include 4% cromolyn, lodoxamide, and olopatidine, which are mast cell stabilizers. The use of topical corticosteroids, though effective, should be minimized because of the risk for infection, cataracts, and glaucoma from a chronic condition that does not threaten sight. For mild to moderate GPC, a combination of frequent lens replacement, better lens cleaning, reduced wearing time, and a mast cell stabilizer 2 to 4 times a day may be sufficient. However, more severe cases may require the temporary cessation of lens wear in addition to the above regimen. Patients should be observed every few weeks, and resolution of the symptoms and eventual flattening of the papillae, often with mild residual subepithelial fibrosis, should be monitored.

Corneal neovascularization Superficial corneal neovascularization is another common complication of contact lens wear. It is more prevalent among users of soft contact lenses, especially extended wear lenses. Additionally, hybrid lenses (rigid center, soft skirt) and aphakic soft lenses—which are thicker, less oxygen permeable, and do not move as well—increase the risk for neovascularization. It is usually an asymptomatic development noted incidentally on routine examination, unless it has become so extensive as to involve the visual axis. Clinically, it may present superiorly as a superficial vascular ingrowth from the limbus, which advances centripetally (Fig. 4-90). However, the neovascular process may not be limited to the superior limbus and may extend completely around the peripheral cornea. Corneal hypoxia from extended lens wear, tight lenses, and low oxygen permeability is thought to be the stimulus for the vascular ingrowth (Fig. 4-91).

As much as 2 mm of superficial corneal neovascularization may be tolerated. Once discovered, however, progression should be carefully monitored, and measures should be taken to reduce the hypoxic stimulus for progression. Consideration should be given to reducing lens-wearing time by changing from extended wear to daily wear or by reducing daily wear time. Tight lenses should be refit and made looser or lenses with greater oxygen permeability should be used. Rigid lenses may be substituted for aphakic or high-minus soft contact lenses. If neovascularization has extended beyond 2 mm from the limbus despite the above measures, consideration should be given to the discontinuation of contact lens

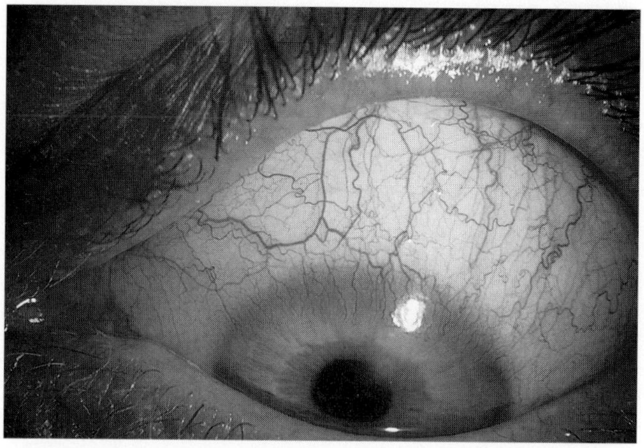

Fig. 4-90 Corneal neovascularization. 2 to 3 mm of superior corneal neovascularization is seen in this soft contact lens wearer.

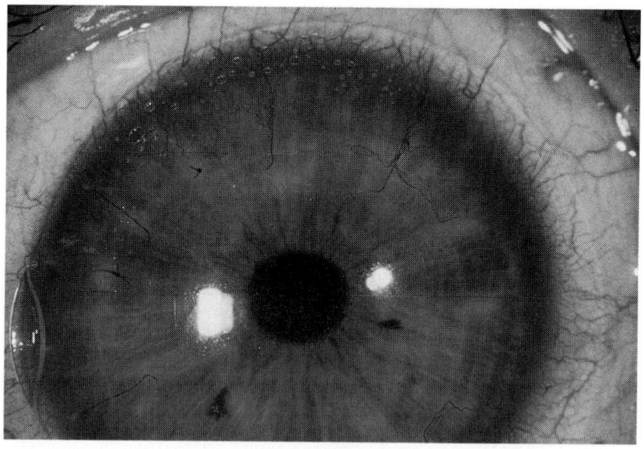

Fig. 4-91 Corneal neovascularization. Significant corneal neovascularization is present in this eye of a wearer of hybrid contact lenses (rigid center, soft skirt) after corneal transplantation. Note the tracking of the vessels into the corneal transplant wound.

use altogether. Topical corticosteroids (after discontinuation of lens wear) may be used to treat extensive neovascularization, especially in patients who have undergone or are considering corneal transplantation (in whom the neovascular ingrowth increases the risk for graft rejection) or when the vascularization is associated with stromal infiltrates. After successful treatment, determined by regression of the active blood vessels, the lens fit or wearing time should be adjusted to prevent recurrence.

Toxicity to solutions Toxicity and hypersensitivity reactions to contact lens solutions are frequent complications of contact lens use. Saline solutions and multipurpose solutions with preservatives, especially those containing thimerosal (no longer widely used), chlorhexidine, polyhexamethylene biguanide, or polyquaternium, are associated with toxicity. Occasionally, inadequate rinsing of daily cleaners or enzymes, accidental substitution of disinfecting solution for saline, or failure to neutralize hydrogen peroxide may result in the unintended introduction of toxic chemicals to the surface of the eye.

Toxicity and allergic reactions may affect the eyelids, conjunctiva, or cornea. These conditions may present acutely after solutions are changed, but usually they develop after several months. Patients present with mild pain, photophobia, burning, and a red eye. Corneal findings include SPK or multiple sterile, peripheral, anterior stromal infiltrates similar to those found in staphylococcal hypersensitivity keratitis. Skin findings are less common, but contact dermatitis can develop on the eyelids and the eyelid margins. Conjunctival reactions include hyperemia, chemosis, and a mixed papillary and follicular response. Occasionally, a patient has solution-induced superior limbal hypertrophy and pannus formation with associated SPK resembling SLK.

Treatment involves the cessation of lens wear until the condition resolves. Lubrication with preservative-free artificial tears may provide additional symptomatic relief. When the condition clears, the use of new lenses, peroxide-based disinfection systems, and preservative-free saline prevents recurrences.

Corneal warpage Corneal warpage is a complication of contact lens use in which prolonged contact lens wear produces an alteration in corneal curvature. This change in shape induces irregular astigmatism, which may, in turn, reduce visual acuity. This complication is more commonly seen among long-term wearers of polymethylmethacrylate lenses, though it may develop in those who wear rigid gas-permeable and soft contact lenses. Patients report satisfactory vision with lenses in place but reduced visual acuity with glasses (spectacle blur). Eventually the condition may cause decreased vision both with glasses and with contacts. Contact lens discomfort or intolerance may also occur because of the altered lens-cornea relationship.

The diagnosis of corneal warpage may be suspected by the presence of irregular keratometry mires or irregular astigmatism on computed corneal topography, where none had existed before. However, no corneal thinning or other signs of keratoconus are found on slit-lamp examination. Treatment consists of the cessation of contact lens wear until corneal regularity returns. Normalization of corneal curvature may take several weeks, or even months, and should be followed by refitting of the contact lenses.

Pseudo–superior limbic keratoconjunctivitis Occasionally contact lens wear produces keratopathy that is similar to or misdiagnosed as SLK. Clinically pseudo-SLK presents primarily with hyperemia and fluorescein staining of the superior bulbar conjunctiva (Fig. 4-92). There may be superficial infiltrates in the superior cornea, and superior corneal pannus may develop. These infiltrates are thought to result from a toxicity or hypersensitivity reaction to preservatives in the contact lens solutions, especially thimerosal. Conjunctival scrapings may demonstrate eosinophils, which are not found in true SLK and suggest an allergic mechanism. Corneal filaments and a superior tarsal papillary reaction, notable features of SLK, are usually absent in this syndrome. Contact lens wear improves SLK symptoms, whereas discontinuing contact lens wear improves pseudo-SLK symptoms.

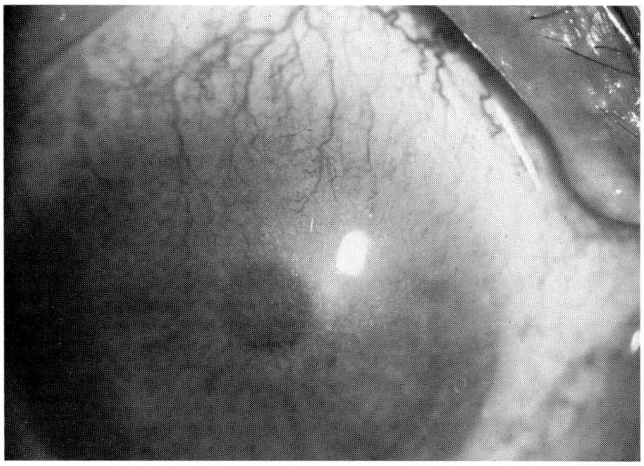

Fig. 4-92 Pseudo–superior limbic keratoconjunctivitis. Significant superior conjunctival injection and corneal neovascularization and haze mimic true superior limbic keratoconjunctivitis.

Treatment of pseudo-SLK consists of discontinuing contact lens wear and using preservative-free artificial tears to increase lubrication. Topical corticosteroids may be used to treat subepithelial infiltrates, though they should be used with caution in any contact lens–related problem and only if infection seems unlikely. Once the condition is resolved, the lens should be replaced and a hydrogen peroxide–based disinfection system should be used.

Bandage Soft Contact Lenses

In addition to the correction of refractive errors, contact lenses have been used for a variety of therapeutic applications. Therapeutic indications for the use of bandage soft contact lenses include enhancement of drug delivery, reduction of discomfort in ocular surface disorders, facilitation of wound healing, and corneal surface protection. Although the use of therapeutic lenses is associated with the risk for contact lens–related complications, particularly in patients who already have underlying ocular disease, the risks can be minimized by careful patient selection, lens fitting, and monitoring.

Bandage contact lenses may be indicated for various ocular surface diseases including recurrent corneal erosions, bullous keratopathy, filamentary keratopathy, SLK, and Thygeson's superficial punctate keratopathy (SPK) and for persistent epithelial defects such as in exposure and neurotrophic keratopathy. Bandage lenses may also be useful for corneal protection in patients with trichiasis or entropion until surgical correction can be performed. After ocular surgery patients may benefit from bandage lens placement to help seal a small wound leak or to provide relief from exposed sutures that cannot be removed. They are also often used after certain types of refractive surgery, notably excimer laser photorefractive keratectomy. Bandage contact lenses are required after the application of cyanoacrylate tissue adhesive to provide comfort and to prevent premature dislodging of the adhesive.

Because many conditions requiring bandage lens placement also require extended treatment, it is important to avoid a tight-fitting lens and to observe the patient closely. The lens should have adequate, though not excessive, movement and should feel comfortable.

Bandage soft contact lenses carry the same potential complications as conventional soft lenses, but patients who require the bandage lenses are even more susceptible to infection. The most devastating complication is microbial keratitis. Particularly severe infections, occasionally caused by unusual organisms including fungi and mycobacteria, may develop in compromised eyes. Patients with bandage lenses should be observed closely, and prophylactic antibiotics can be considered. Sterile infiltrates or hypopyons have been associated with bandage lens use and are usually a result of tight-fitting lenses and hypoxia. Infectious causes must be ruled out. Less serious complications include corneal edema (usually from hypoxia), neovascularization, and GPC.

In general, bandage soft lenses are a useful adjunct or an alternative therapy for numerous ocular surface or postsurgical conditions. They are more effective for short-term rather than chronic use. Disposable soft contact lenses work well for this purpose. Because there may be significant morbidity attached to their use, careful patient selection, judicious application, and close follow-up are required.

Superficial Punctate Keratopathy

Various clinical entities may present with a superficial punctate keratopathy (SPK), which appears as pinpoint, depressed corneal epithelial defects that stain with fluorescein (Fig. 4-93). It typically presents with foreign body sensation, pain, photophobia, tearing, or redness. They are nonspecific findings indicative of ocular surface irritation caused by trauma, toxicity, tear film abnormality or insufficiency, exposure, or infection (Box 4-14). Superficial punctate keratopathy is separate from the coarse, elevated punctate keratitis seen in Thygeson's SPK to be discussed later in this chapter.

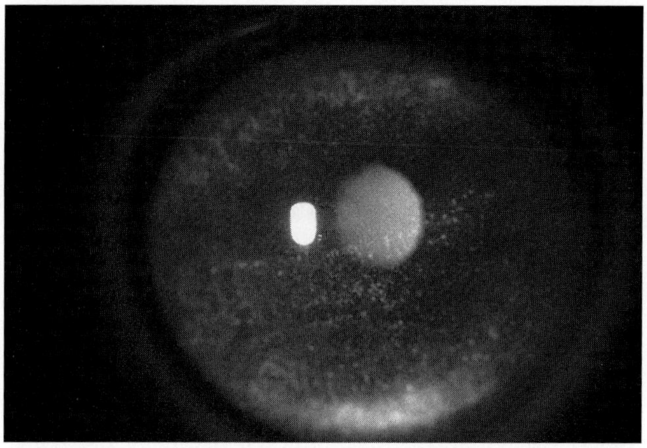

Fig. 4-93 Superficial punctate keratopathy. Multiple pinpoint epithelial defects are seen with fluorescein dye and the cobalt blue light. (See color plate.)

Box 4-14 Conditions Associated with a Superficial Punctate Keratopathy

TRAUMA

Eye rubbing
Trichiasis/misdirected lashes
Foreign body
Contact lenses
Mucus fishing syndrome

TOXICITY

Topical medications or preservatives
Vapors or smoke
Chemical injury
Ultraviolet light

TEAR FILM

Meibomian gland dysfunction
Dry eye syndrome (aqueous deficiency)
Mucin deficiency

EXPOSURE

Bell's palsy
Entropion or ectropion
Proptosis
Nocturnal lagophthalmos
Eyelid trauma or surgery

INFECTION

Bacterial conjunctivitis
Viral keratoconjunctivitis

Any condition that results in a disturbance of the components of the tear film may produce SPK. For example, meibomian gland dysfunction in blepharitis, dry eye caused by aqueous layer deficiency (as in Sjögren's syndrome), or mucin layer deficiency (as in ocular cicatricial pemphigoid or Stevens-Johnson syndrome) may result in corneal epithelial damage and SPK. Examination of the eyelid margins, tear lake, tear break-up time, and conjunctiva is helpful to determine the cause of the SPK. Schirmer's testing for tear insufficiency may also be revealing. SPK limited to the interpalpebral zone suggests the possibility of exposure keratopathy or dry eyes, and careful attention should be paid to the presence of eyelid retraction (as in thyroid ophthalmopathy), and eyelid excursion with each blink. It may aid in the diagnosis to know whether the patient sleeps with the eyes partially open (nocturnal lagophthalmos).

Surface toxicity caused by exogenous agents may also present with SPK, often in a central whorl pattern. These agents include any ophthalmic preparations with preservatives, including contact lens solutions, antibiotic drops, over-the-counter antihistamine/decongestant drops, and even artificial tears. Surface toxicity may also result from exposure to toxic vapors, smoke, or frank chemical injury to the eye. Ultraviolet light exposure, as seen occasionally in welders or in users of sun lamps, may produce diffuse and painful SPK.

Trauma is a frequent cause of SPK, and it may result from many factors, including eye rubbing, contact lens wear, mucus fishing syndrome, floppy eyelid syndrome, trichiasis, or a foreign body. It is important to flip the eyelids to examine their tone and the appearance of the tarsal conjunctiva and to look for foreign bodies. If a patient wears contact lenses, the condition (deposits, tears, trapped debris) and the fit of the lens should be evaluated.

Infection may also be a cause. Bacterial or viral conjunctivitis may be associated with SPK, and the presence of pseudomembranes may particularly predispose a patient to this complication. Rarely, an early bacterial keratitis, especially due to *Pseudomonas* in association with contact lens use, may present in this fashion.

The management of SPK begins by attempting to determine and treat the underlying cause. Often, however, the treatment is nonspecific and supportive. Lubrication with preservative-free artificial tears may be used and combined with a lubricating ointment at night if necessary. More severe cases may be treated with the addition of antibiotic drops or ointment.

Contact lens wearers with significant SPK should be prescribed antibiotic drops that provide adequate *Pseudomonas* treatment. Drops should be applied 4 to 8 times a day, contact lens wear should be discontinued, and the patient should be observed frequently until the ocular surface demonstrates significant improvement. These patients should not be patched. An antibiotic ointment at bedtime and a short-acting cycloplegic may also be considered, depending on the severity of the symptoms.

Dry Eye Syndrome and Sjögren's Syndrome

Dry eye syndrome, or keratoconjunctivitis sicca, may result from clinical entities that cause decreased tear production, increased tear evaporation, or both.

The tear film is composed of three interrelated layers, each of which is produced by a different portion of the eye. Although these layers have no distinct boundaries, it is helpful to consider them separately. The innermost layer, which is closest to the corneal epithelium, is the mucin layer. It is formed by the goblet cells of the conjunctiva, and it adheres to the glycoproteins on the surface of the corneal epithelium. Its hydrophilic properties create a wettable surface on the corneal epithelium. The middle layer of the tear film is the aqueous layer, formed by the main and accessory lacrimal glands. It is responsible for 90% of the thickness of the tear film, and it contains all the water-soluble components of tears including lactoferrin, lysozyme, inorganic salts, and glucose. It is this layer that is primarily deficient in Sjögren's syndrome. The outermost layer of the tear film is the lipid layer, which is formed by the meibomian glands in the eyelids and is secreted at the eyelid margins. The lipid layer serves to reduce surface tension of the tear film to facilitate tear spreading and to retard evaporation. The tear film is renewed by blinking, which delivers new aqueous and lipid components to the corneal surface and pumps out the tear lake through the lacrimal drainage system. The normal blink rate is approximately 6 to 10 times per minute; the tear film must remain intact across the ocular surface between blinks.

The causes of dry eye syndrome may be broadly classified as aqueous tear deficiency states and evaporative disorders (Box 4-15). An associated mucin layer, or lipid-layer deficiency, may also be present in certain conditions, contributing to the pathophysiology of the dry eye. The classic cause of aqueous tear deficiency is Sjögren's syndrome, though other conditions may reduce aqueous tear production.

Sjögren's syndrome is a disorder that is characterized by the association of keratoconjunctivitis sicca and xerostomia (dry mouth). Primary Sjögren's syndrome refers to dry eyes and dry mouth without any associated autoimmune disease, whereas secondary Sjögren's syndrome refers to dry eyes and dry mouth associated with a systemic autoimmune disease such as rheumatoid arthritis (Fig. 4-94). Sjögren's syndrome affects women more frequently than men. Because dry eyes and dry mouth are nonspecific symptoms that may be associated with numerous conditions, a more specific set of diagnostic criteria for Sjögren's syndrome has been proposed (Box 4-16).

The pathophysiology of this condition involves lymphocytic infiltration of the lacrimal glands and the parotid glands. This infiltration eventually destroys and replaces the acini and ducts of the glands, reducing the production and flow of tears and saliva.

Clinically, these patients usually present complaining of ocular or oral dryness, or both. Other symptoms consist of intermittent or constant burning or a dry, gritty, foreign body sensation. These symptoms are

Box 4-15 Conditions Associated with Dry Eye Syndrome

- Mucin deficiency states (often associated with aqueous tear deficiency)
  - Stevens-Johnson syndrome
  - Ocular cicatricial pemphigoid
  - Vitamin A deficiency
- Aqueous tear deficiency states
  - Sjögren's syndrome
    - Primary Sjögren's syndrome
    - Secondary Sjögren's syndrome
      - Collagen vascular diseases
      - Hashimoto's thyroiditis
      - Raynaud's phenomenon
  - Postradiation treatment
  - Lacrimal gland disease
  - Neurotrophic keratopathy
  - Pharmacologic
    - Antihistamines
    - Antidepressants
    - Beta-blockers
    - Alpha-blockers
  - Systemic diseases
    - Sarcoidosis
    - Human immunodeficiency virus
    - Graft-versus-host disease
    - Trachoma
    - Amyloidosis
    - Lymphoma
    - Hepatitis B and C
- Increased evaporative loss
  - Meibomian gland dysfunction/ocular rosacea
  - Blink disorders
    - Bell's palsy
    - Nocturnal lagophthalmos
  - Abnormalities of eyelid/globe interaction
    - Ectropion
    - Entropion
    - Proptosis
    - Blepharoplasty or ptosis surgery

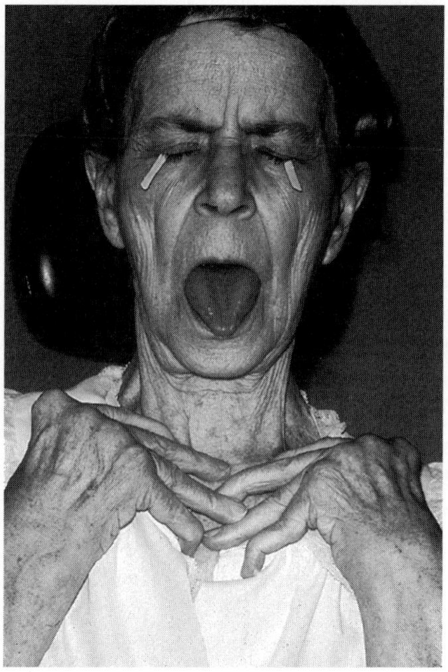

Fig. 4-94 Sjögren's syndrome. This patient with severe Sjögren's syndrome is undergoing a Schirmer's test. Note the dry mouth and rheumatoid arthritic changes in the hands.

Box 4-16 Diagnostic Criteria for Sjögren's Syndrome*

1. Keratoconjunctivitis sicca as evidenced by low results of Schirmer's test, fluorescein or rose bengal corneal staining, and decreased tear break-up time.
2. Reduced salivary gland flow rate.
3. Lymphocytic infiltration of salivary glands obtained from a lip biopsy.
4. Systemic autoimmune process demonstrated by specific serum autoantibodies (ANA, RF, or SS-A/SS-B).

*Three of the four criteria are necessary to make a diagnosis of probable Sjögren's syndrome, whereas all four make the diagnosis of definite Sjögren's syndrome.

usually at their peak when the patient attempts to read or concentrate on a task (thus reducing blink rate), and they worsen throughout the day. Vision reduction depends on the severity of the condition. Particularly dry exterior environments, such as airplane cabins, tend to exacerbate the symptoms. Patients may also have excessive production of stringy mucus, which may dry overnight and produce crusting in the morning. Clinical examination typically reveals SPK that stains with fluorescein, lissamine green (Fig. 4-95), or rose bengal (Fig. 4-96). The staining pattern may extend onto the conjunctiva in the nasal and temporal interpalpebral zones. Filamentary keratopathy may also be present, and thick, stringy mucus is often found in the fornices. The intermarginal tear lake may be notably reduced or absent. Not infrequently, however, patients complain of bouts of overflow tearing. If this happens, it is likely that the SPK was so severe that it caused intense reflex tearing. Occasionally, keratoconjunctivitis sicca is so profound that it causes a frank epithelial defect and superficial sterile ulceration of the cornea, often in a paracentral location, that progressively melts and perforates. Because of chronic epithelial damage, these eyes are susceptible to secondary infection, particularly with unusual organisms such as fungi or atypical mycobacteria.

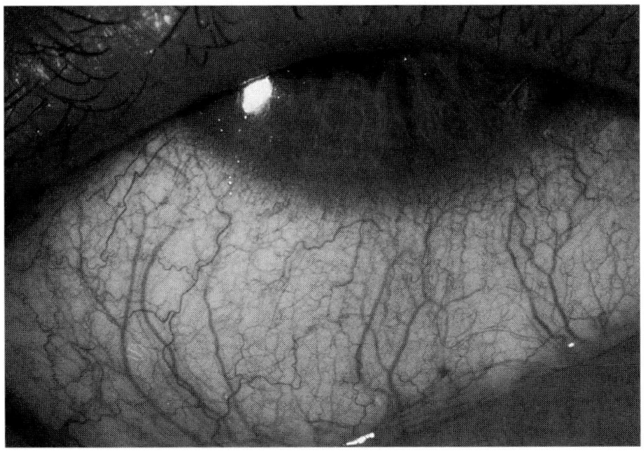

Fig. 4-95 Dry eye syndrome with lissamine green stain. Lissamine green staining of the inferior conjunctiva in a patient with dry eye syndrome. (See color plate.)

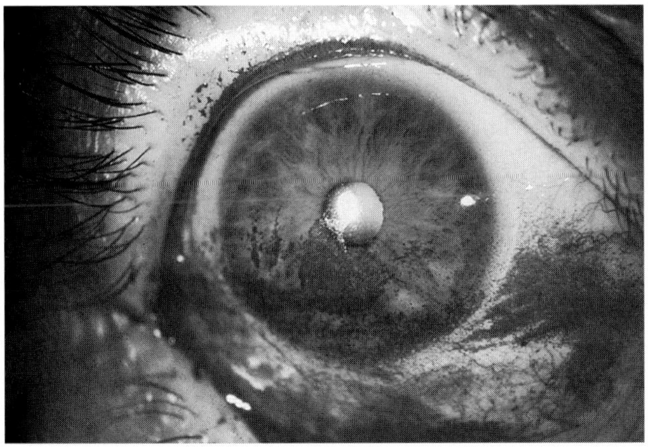

Fig. 4-96 Dry eye syndrome with rose bengal stain. Rose bengal dye uptake in the inferior half of the cornea and the inferior conjunctiva indicates significant epithelial damage from dry eye syndrome. (See color plate.)

Oral symptoms include dryness, difficulty swallowing, altered taste, and dental problems. Systemic disease involving the skin, gastrointestinal tract, genitourinary tract (especially in women), or respiratory tract may also develop. Vasculitic phenomena affecting the skin and central nervous system and an increased risk for lymphoproliferative disorders including lymphoma have also been reported in association with Sjögren's syndrome.

The diagnosis of dry eye syndrome is made after clinical evaluation and diagnostic testing. Clinical examination may reveal a reduced or absent tear meniscus and a rapid tear break-up time (Fig. 4-97). The normal tear meniscus measures approximately 0.5 to 1.0 mm in height above the eyelid margin, and the normal tear break-up time is approximately 10 seconds or longer. Tear break-up time is measured by instilling fluorescein into the lower fornix and observing the fluorescein-stained

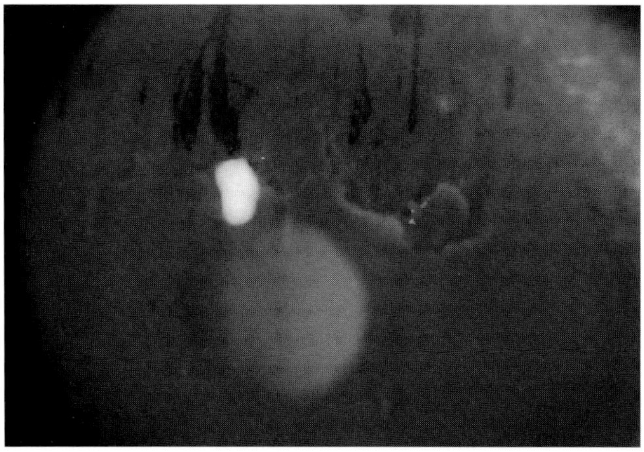

Fig. 4-97 Dry eye syndrome with rapid tear break-up time. After fluorescein dye is placed in the eye, the patient is told not to blink. The cornea is evaluated with the cobalt blue light for the development of breaks in the tear film, as seen superiorly in this patient with dry eyes. Some anterior basement membrane changes have occurred in this patient. (See color plate.)

tear film under the cobalt blue light while the patient refrains from blinking. The time from the last blink to the appearance of the first defect in the fluorescein-stained tear film is the break-up time. These findings are nonspecific signs of dry eye, and they may be caused by decreased aqueous production, lipid or mucin layer disturbances, or epithelial disease such as anterior basement membrane dystrophy.

Schirmer's testing provides an objective, rapid, and simple assessment of dry eyes that is specific for decreased aqueous production. It is performed by placing a strip of filter paper in the inferior fornix of each eye to absorb the tears produced (Fig. 4-98). These strips are left in place for 5 minutes, after which the wet length of each strip is recorded in millimeters. To avoid falsely elevated results, it is important to gently dry any collected tears or retained fluid from the inferior fornix before placing the strips. This test may be performed with or without topical anesthesia. Testing without anesthesia (Schirmer 1 test) produces mild irritation and thus measures basal and reflex tearing, whereas testing with anesthesia (basic secretion test) relieves this component and tests predominantly basal tear production. Conducting the Schirmer 1 test while stimulating the nasal mucosa (Schirmer 2 test) may provide a more specific assessment of reflex tearing. Although no consensus exists on what constitutes a positive test result, it is generally agreed that lengths of wetness smaller than 5 mm are strongly suggestive of decreased tear production. Values greater than 15 mm for Schirmer's tests without anesthesia and greater than 10 mm for tests with anesthesia are considered normal and must be correlated with other evidence of aqueous deficiency to support a diagnosis of Sjögren's syndrome. Values between 5 and 10 mm are

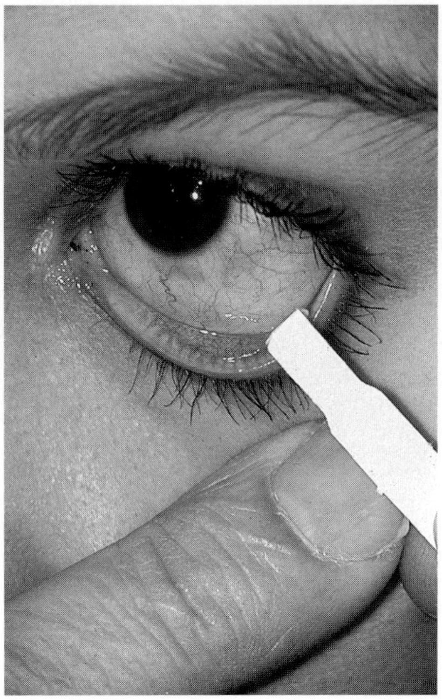

Fig. 4-98 Schirmer's test. After topical anesthesia is given and the eye is balloted dry, Schirmer's filter paper is placed in the inferior fornix for 5 minutes. The amount of wetting is then measured.

suggestive of mild aqueous deficiency, but they must be correlated with other clinical data.

There are other laboratory tests for aqueous tear deficiency, including tear film osmolarity and lysozyme or lactoferrin concentration. Tear film osmolarity has been shown to increase in patients with aqueous tear deficiency, and this test may be a sensitive and specific diagnostic tool. However, the high cost and limited availability of this analysis have minimized the usefulness of this technology. Tear film lactoferrin and lysozyme concentrations are reduced in patients with aqueous deficiency, but their correlation with clinical symptoms is unclear, and questions remain regarding specificity and interpretation of results. Impression cytology is another technique used to examine the secondary changes to the conjunctival surface caused by chronic dry eye and thus to confirm the clinical diagnosis, but it is only a research tool.

If dry eye state is suspected, it is important to distinguish between conditions caused by decreased tear production and those caused by increased tear evaporation, though they frequently overlap. In addition to performing the clinical workup described, it is necessary to look for signs of meibomian gland disease and eyelid or blink abnormalities, all of which may contribute to increased evaporative loss. Observe the eyelid excursion with each blink under the slit lamp to ensure that the cornea is covered each time. Ask about previous eyelid surgery

Box 4-17 Systemic Autoimmune Workup for Decreased Aqueous Tear Production

Rheumatoid factor
Sjögren's syndrome A and B (SS-A, SS-B)
Antinuclear antibody
Angiotensin-converting enzyme

(cosmetic or otherwise) that may contribute to blink abnormalities and increased evaporation, and ask whether the patient's eyes are partially open while sleeping. These frequently overlooked conditions are common causes of increased evaporative loss. Once a diagnosis of decreased tear production has been suggested, the differential diagnosis may be separated into Sjögren's syndrome (primary or secondary) or non-Sjögren's causes (see Box 4-15). A systemic workup for autoimmune diseases can be helpful in narrowing the differential diagnosis (Box 4-17).

The mainstay of treatment for dry eye is artificial tear replacement and tear conservation. Each of many artificial tear preparations on the market has a different formulation and viscosity, and some contain buffers and electrolytes. These agents are available in formulations with and without preservatives. Patients may use these preparations frequently during the day to provide symptomatic relief, but for constant use (more than 4 times a day), a preservative-free product is recommended to reduce surface toxicity. Tear ointment preparations are also available and are highly useful, especially for overnight relief. Daytime ointments are available, but patients tend to avoid them because of the temporarily blurred vision and stickiness they cause. A slow-release artificial tear insert (hydroxypropyl cellulose) is also available as a small rod that is placed daily in the inferior fornix. Because this rod slowly dissolves in 6 to 12 hours, it provides continuous lubrication. Although these inserts may be helpful for patients with mild to moderate aqueous tear deficiency, they are poorly tolerated by some because of the resultant foreign body sensation or blurred vision. In addition, patients with a severe aqueous deficiency may not have sufficient moisture to dissolve the rods adequately.

Although no artificial tear preparation has been shown to have therapeutic effect on the ocular surface changes that may result from long-standing keratoconjunctivitis sicca, a recently developed electrolyte-based tear preparation (TheraTears; Advanced Vision Research, Woburn, Mass.) increases goblet cell density and corneal glycogen levels in rabbits. This increase has not been associated with a significant reduction in symptoms different from that of other tear preparations, and the clinical significance of these findings is undetermined.

In addition to tear replacement, tear conservation plays an important role in the management of dry eye. The primary method for increasing tear retention is punctal occlusion. Punctal occlusion may be performed by several methods, including temporary or permanent plugs, thermocautery, laser cautery, or suture closure. These procedures allow increased retention of the tear film on the ocular surface. Temporary punctal occlusion is performed for diagnostic purposes through the use of collagen punctal plugs. These dissolvable rods are placed in the punctum, where they expand and occlude the canaliculus before dissolving over several days. Their major disadvantage is that the degree and duration of punctal occlusion are variable and cannot always be ascertained. Reversible permanent punctal occlusion is best accomplished with the use of silicone punctal plugs. Several styles are available. They are placed in the punctal opening or deep within the canaliculus. Although they may be left in place indefinitely, surface plugs are easily removed and canalicular plugs can be flushed out should the procedure have to be reversed. Punctal closure may be achieved by thermocautery of the punctum and canaliculus with a handheld cautery device. This method produces permanent scarring and closure of the system, and, though it may occasionally reopen, it should be regarded as an irreversible procedure. It is important to establish reliably the need for permanent punctal closure before performing this procedure. Collagen (dissolvable) or silicone (removable) plugs are used before permanent occlusion to help ensure that symptomatic overflow tearing does not develop. Permanent punctal closure can also be performed using the argon laser, but this procedure tends to result in reopening more often than thermocautery. Although the argon laser method offers the potential advantage of titrating the amount of tissue shrinkage and punctal closure, it offers no clinically significant advantages over thermocautery for complete punctal occlusion, and it is significantly more expensive. Closure of the punctum with an interrupted nylon suture is another effective means of long-term punctal closure, which can be reversed by suture removal, if necessary. Conservation is possible through the addition of side shields to the patient's glasses and through the use of moisture chambers; both methods reduce tear evaporation.

Besides aqueous deficiency, other ocular and nonocular causes of increased evaporative loss, whether the primary cause or a contributing factor of the dry eye syndrome, should be addressed. Blepharitis and meibomian gland disease should be treated with warm compresses, eyelid scrubs, antibiotic ointment at night, and occasionally systemic tetracycline medications. Similarly, eyelid malpositions or other causes of exposure should be addressed. Exogenous factors such as sitting near ventilation ducts, pointing car vents toward the face, and using medications that may decrease aqueous tear production should be eliminated, if possible (Box 4-18).

Several agents that increase tear production (known as secretagogues), including oral and topical pilocarpine, have been used in patients with dry eyes, but the clinical results have been mixed. Recently, topical cyclosporine solution has been associated with increased tear production, and it is under evaluation for its efficacy in the treatment of keratoconjunctivitis sicca.

Recurrent Corneal Erosion

Recurrent corneal erosion, or recurrent erosion syndrome, is characterized by recurrent episodes of pain, photophobia, and tearing caused by spontaneous microscopic or macroscopic corneal epithelial defects. Onset is usually sudden, particularly when the patient opens the eyes during the night or in the morning, and the pain can be profound. Often a patient has a history (sometimes remote) of a traumatic corneal abrasion to the affected eye, perhaps from a fingernail, a tree branch, or a paper cut.

Recurrent corneal erosion may result from several underlying conditions, such as anterior basement membrane or superficial stromal corneal dystrophies, previous corneal trauma, or chronic corneal edema in which there is abnormal adhesion of the epithelium to basement membrane and Bowman's membrane (Box 4-19).

One of the most frequent causes of recurrent corneal erosion is anterior basement membrane dystrophy (map-dot-fingerprint dystrophy) (Fig. 4-99). This condition results in the production of an abnormal basement membrane that adheres poorly to Bowman's membrane and to which the overlying epithelium is loosely adherent. As a result these areas are at a higher risk for spontaneous sloughing, thus producing corneal erosion. Nonetheless, only 10% of people with anterior basement membrane dystrophy have recurrent corneal erosions, though approximately 50% of those with recurrent erosion syndrome may have underlying anterior basement membrane dystrophy.

Corneal trauma that produces a corneal abrasion can also cause recurrent erosion syndrome months or years after the original episode. It is thought that in some patients the normal attachment complexes, which generally redevelop over several weeks after epithelial healing, fail to form properly and create a predisposition to recurrent erosions in that location. Epithelial basement membrane damage at the time of the injury may also play a role.

Clinically, these patients present with a sudden onset of pain. There may be a history of repeated episodes in the same eye, although the severity varies. Patients may

Box 4-18 Major Medications Associated with Decreased Aqueous Tear Production

ANTIHISTAMINES
Diphenhydramine hydrochloride
Chlorpheniramine
Pheniramine

DECONGESTANTS
Phenylephrine
Ephedrine
Pseudoephedrine

ANTIDEPRESSANTS
Amitriptyline
Nortriptyline
Phenelzine
Imipramine
Doxepin
Desipramine
Tranylcypromine
Sertraline

BETA-BLOCKERS
Propranolol
Atenolol
Metoprolol
Labetalol
Timolol

ALPHA-BLOCKERS
Clonidine
Prazosin

NEUROLEPTICS
Chlorpromazine
Thioridazine
Prochlorperazine
Fluphenazine

ANXIOLYTICS
Diazepam
Chlordiazepoxide

ANTIARRHYTHMICS
Disopyramide
Mexiletine
Quinidine

ANTICHOLINERGICS
Atropine
Homatropine
Scopolamine

HISTAMINE 2–BLOCKERS
Cimetidine

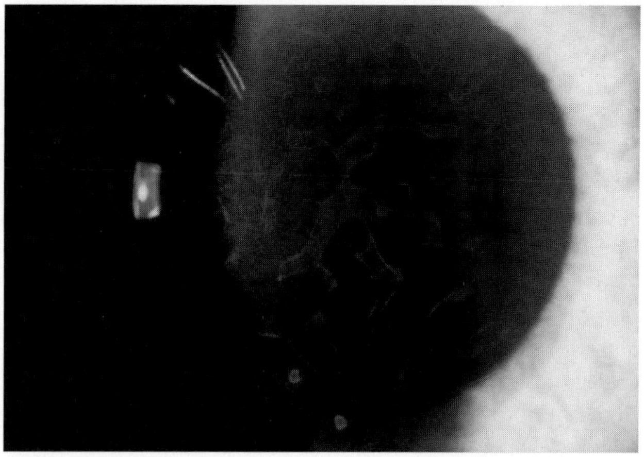

Fig. 4-99 Anterior basement membrane dystrophy. Diffuse map changes of anterior basement membrane dystrophy are seen. Two Cogan's microcysts are evident inferiorly.

Box 4-19 Major Conditions Associated with Recurrent Corneal Erosions

TRAUMA
Corneal abrasion
Previous corneal surgery

CORNEAL DYSTROPHIES
Anterior basement membrane
Meesmann's
Corneal dystrophies of Bowman's membrane
Granular
Lattice

CHRONIC CORNEAL EDEMA
Pseudophakic or aphakic bullous keratopathy
Fuchs' dystrophy

SYSTEMIC DISEASE
Diabetes mellitus

report chronic, usually mild, discomfort or a foreign body sensation in the eye between erosion episodes. Examination typically reveals a mildly to severely irregular epithelium or a small or large epithelial defect, often with a surrounding flap of loose epithelium (Fig. 4-100). The epithelial irregularity is often best seen by "negative staining" revealed after fluorescein instillation or by retroillumination off the retina (Figs. 4-101 and 4-102). Epithelial inspection may demonstrate other characteristics of anterior basement membrane dystrophy such as microcysts, "maps," or "fingerprint" lines. Examination of the fellow cornea for evidence of anterior basement

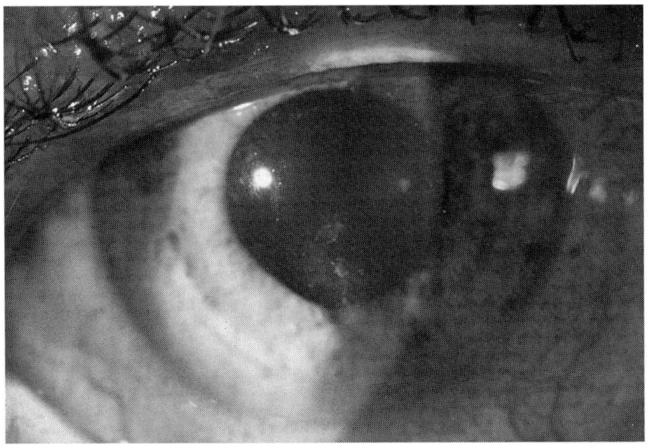

Fig. 4-100 Recurrent erosion syndrome. An area of loose irregular epithelium can be seen in this patient who noted pain on awakening that morning.

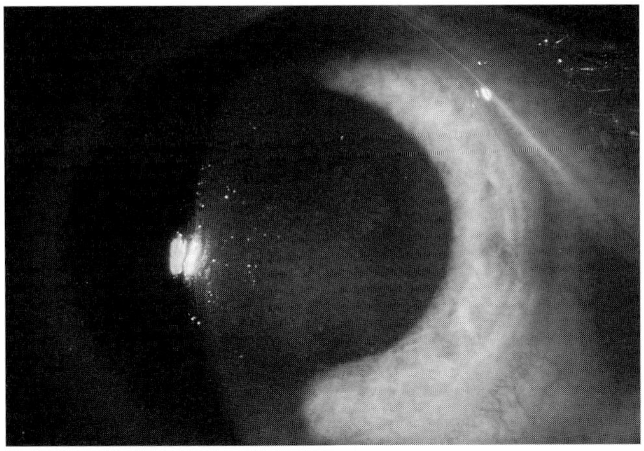

Fig. 4-101 Recurrent erosion syndrome. A large central area of irregular gray-white epithelium is present. It is so loose that it moves with each blink.

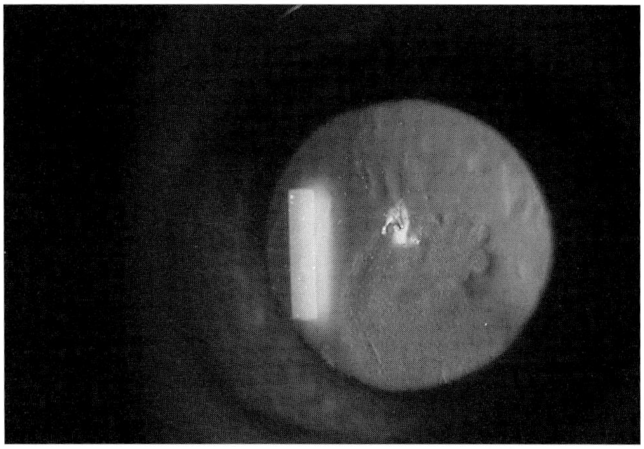

Fig. 4-102 Recurrent erosion syndrome. Using retroillumination off the retina, the irregular epithelium can be seen extremely well. Occasionally, in eyes with healed erosions, direct illumination is unrevealing, but irregular epithelium may be seen on retroillumination.

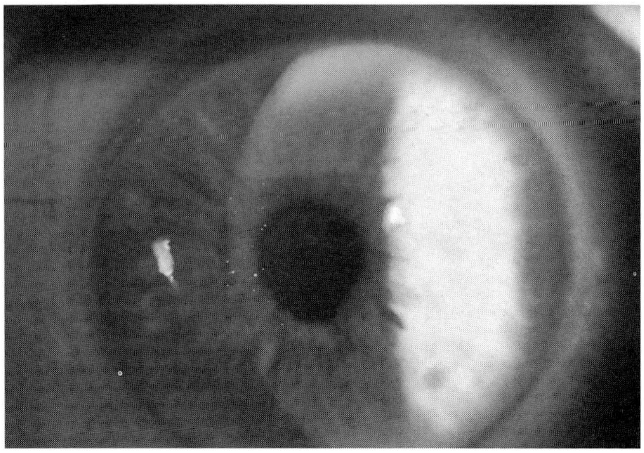

Fig. 4-103 Anterior basement membrane dystrophy. Mild map changes of anterior basement membrane dystrophy are seen centrally.

membrane changes may be helpful (Figs. 4-103 and 4-104). Occasionally, erosions are small enough that they have already healed by the time the patient arrives in the office. Signs of an epithelial healing pattern, localized brawny edema (anterior stromal granularity), or evidence of anterior basement membrane dystrophy is diagnostically helpful in these patients.

The management of recurrent corneal erosions initially involves the acute treatment of the epithelial defect with antibiotic ointment, with or without pressure patching and a cycloplegic. Pressure patching significantly decreases the pain in some patients, whereas others find the frequent use of an ointment more comfortable. Patching may have to be repeated daily for large erosions. If loose corneal epithelium impedes healing, it should be gently debrided. Once the acute epithelial defect is healed, a variety of medical and surgical approaches may be used to prevent subsequent episodes.

Medical therapy is instituted initially, and it consists of daily lubrication with an artificial tear preparation and an artificial tear ointment at night. This treatment increases surface lubrication, especially at night and while opening the eyes in the morning, thereby reducing mechanical epithelial trauma from the eyelids. Lubrication therapy should be continued for at least 3 to 6 months after an erosion. Hypertonic saline (5% sodium chloride) drops and ointment may be substituted for standard tear and ointment preparations, or it may be used secondarily if the patient has another episode of erosion while using standard tears and ointment. Hypertonic solutions may

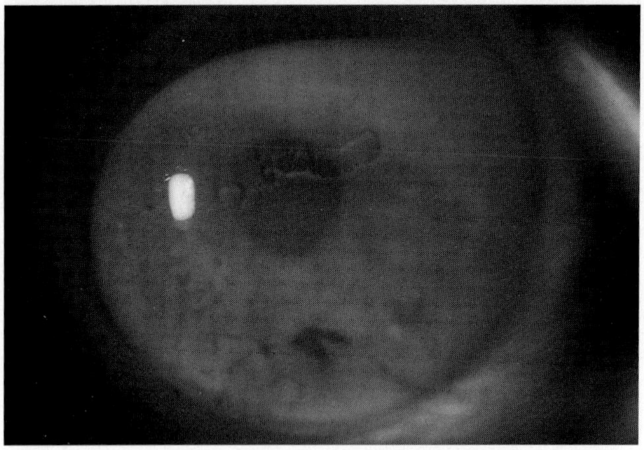

Fig. 4-104 Anterior basement membrane dystrophy. Using fluorescein dye and the cobalt blue light, "negative staining" over the irregular epithelium in the eye with ABM dystrophy in Fig. 4-103 is apparent. (See color plate.)

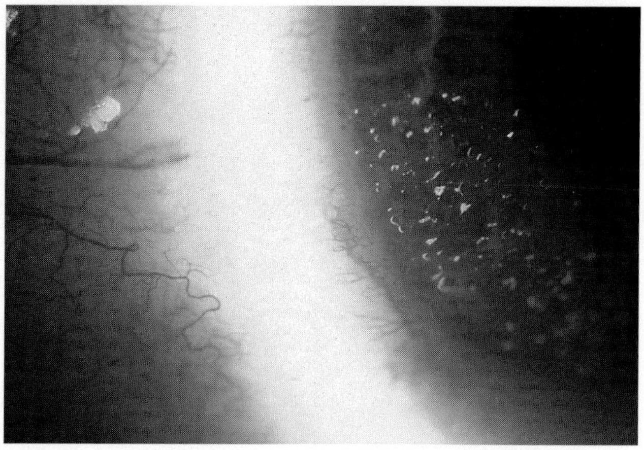

Fig. 4-106 Anterior stromal micropuncture. Examination with sclerotic scatter highlights the numerous puncture marks.

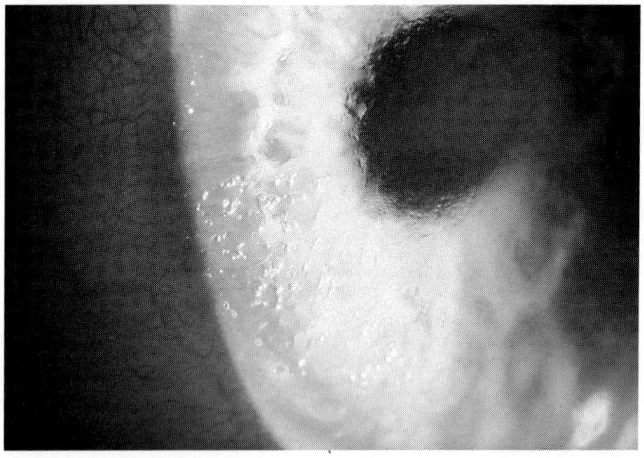

Fig. 4-105 Anterior stromal micropuncture. Multiple punctures have been made with a 25-gauge needle to approximately 10% to 15% of the stroma in an area of loose epithelium. This eye had recurrent erosion syndrome, a result of trauma from a child's fingernail.

relieve epithelial edema, which is thought to develop at night when tear evaporation is reduced, thus decreasing the likelihood of erosion formation and adding to the benefits of lubrication described above. Bandage soft contact lenses have been used to aid in healing the acute defect and in preventing subsequent recurrent erosions. However, these lenses are associated with an increased risk for microbial keratitis and tight-lens reactions, and they may not provide any increased long-term success over medical treatment.

Surgery is often necessary when erosions recur despite aggressive medical therapy. Surgical options include epithelial debridement, diamond burr polishing of Bowman's membrane, anterior stromal micropuncture, Nd:YAG laser photoadhesion, and excimer laser phototherapeutic keratectomy.

Epithelial debridement removes loose epithelial flaps that may interfere with healing It is performed with a sterile cotton swab or a blunt or sharp instrument at the slit lamp. Often the apparently normal surrounding epithelium is loose and comes off easily, yielding a much larger epithelial defect than expected. The epithelium should be debrided until a healthy edge of adherent epithelium is encountered. The success of this procedure in preventing future erosions may be enhanced by debriding the epithelium and basement membrane with a blade (taking great care not to incise the cornea) to remove any adherent basement membrane complexes. Perhaps a safer and more effective method is to use a large (e.g., 5-mm diameter) diamond burr and gently polish Bowman's membrane after epithelial debridement. This treatment efficiently cleans Bowman's membrane and provides a fresh substrate onto which epithelium can regrow and establish attachment complexes.

Anterior stromal micropuncture is another useful technique to reduce recurrent erosions. Especially effective for localized erosions caused by trauma outside the visual axis, it involves the creation of multiple punctures in the anterior stroma of the affected area of the cornea using a 25-gauge needle (Figs. 4-105 and 4-106). This procedure may be accomplished rapidly at the slit lamp with topical anesthesia and a standard 25-gauge needle or a commercially manufactured stromal puncture needle with a prebent tip. The advantages of the prebent tip are that it provides a standard, reproducible depth with each puncture and that it prevents perforation. Anterior stromal micropuncture may be performed during an episode of acute erosion, through an epithelial defect or an intact epithelium, or even between episodes of erosion (Fig. 4-107). It produces fine anterior stromal scars

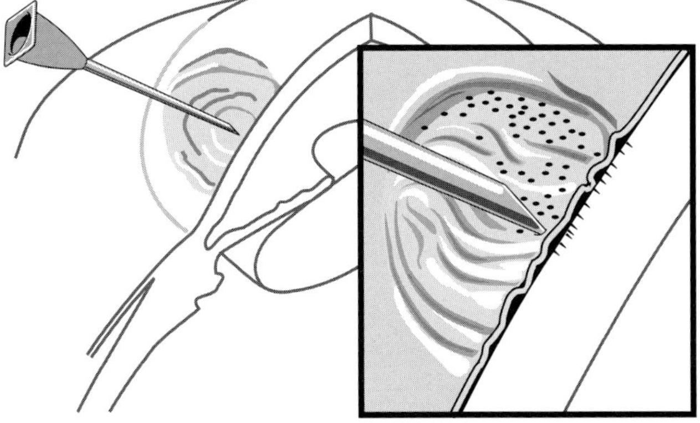

Fig. 4-107 Anterior stromal micropuncture procedure. A 25-gauge needle with a straight or bent tip is applied through the epithelium (or an epithelial defect) into the superficial (10% to 15%) stroma. Treatment should be continued approximately 1 mm into the normal epithelium. Ideally, treatments are made outside the visual axis.

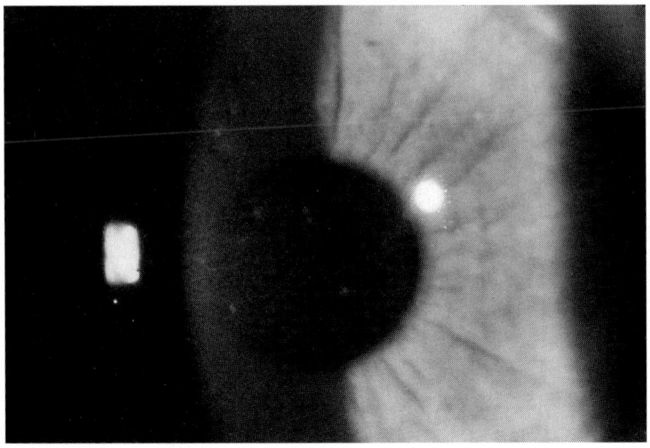

Fig. 4-108 Thygeson's SPK. Multiple small, elevated, gray-white epithelial dots can be seen centrally.

resulting in strong adhesion between the epithelium and the underlying stroma, and it is highly effective. The scars formed from this treatment often, but not always, fade after several months. Therefore this procedure should be avoided or used with great caution in the visual axis. Infection and perforation after this procedure are rare, but they do occur. Preoperative antibiotic drops may be considered, and postoperative antibiotics should be given until the surface has healed.

Nd:YAG laser photoadhesion is another technique, similar to stromal puncture, that uses the Nd:YAG laser rather than a needle to perform the so-called punctures. It essentially produces the same effect, leaves a minimal amount of scarring, and may be performed through an intact epithelium. However, because it is a more involved and expensive option, it is seldom used in the treatment of recurrent erosions.

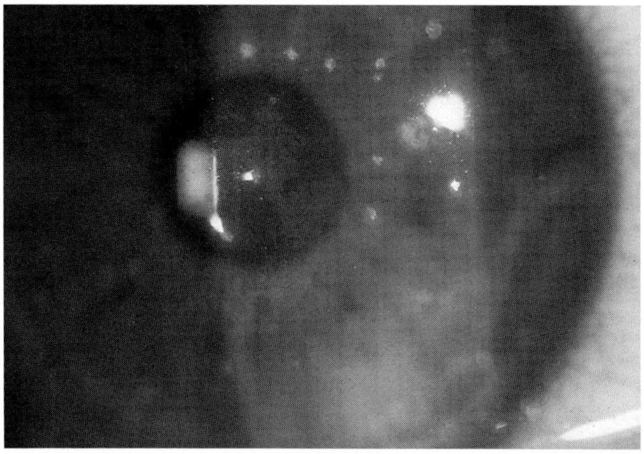

Fig. 4-109 Thygeson's SPK. Fluorescein dye highlights the lesions because they may stain mildly. The stellate nature of the dots is apparent.

Excimer laser PTK is also an effective means of treating recurrent corneal erosions. This technique involves debridement of all loose epithelium followed by a superficial (5 μm) excimer laser ablation of Bowman's membrane. It allows the precise removal of all adherent abnormal basement membrane, and it permits new epithelium to establish healthy adherence complexes on a fresh substrate. The minimal depth of the ablation usually results in an insignificant refractive shift, though the procedure may be combined with photorefractive keratectomy if the patient has underlying myopia. The success rate of PTK is excellent, but it may not be significantly better than less expensive techniques previously mentioned. A modification of this technique, however, where abnormal anterior stroma is ablated, may be superior for recurrent erosions caused by anterior stromal dystrophies. All of these procedures work well (90% to 95% success rates) for the treated areas, but recurrent erosions outside the treatment zone can continue to be problematic.

Thygeson's Superficial Punctate Keratopathy

Thygeson's SPK is a chronic, recurrent form of epithelial keratitis consisting of multiple, small, discrete, elevated, granular, gray-white epithelial lesions in an otherwise quiet eye (Figs. 4-108 and 4-109). Retroillumination off the retina may help highlight the lesions (Figs. 4-110 and 4-111). Typical symptoms are mild photophobia, foreign body sensation, burning, or tearing. There may be few or many lesions present, and the location of the lesions can vary from week to week. The patient's usual age of onset is between the first and fourth decades of life, and most cases are bilateral.

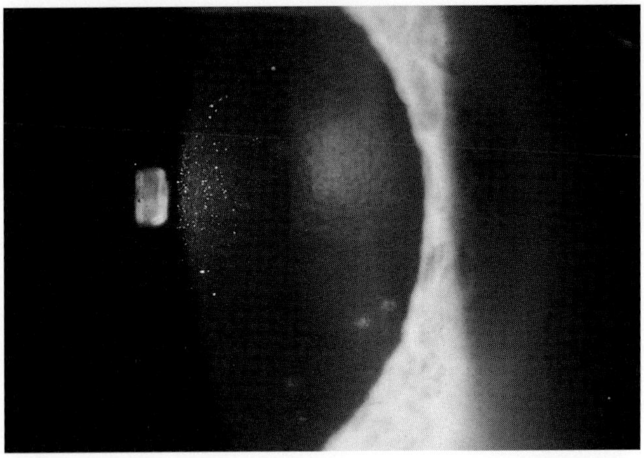

Fig. 4-110 Thygeson's SPK. Several discrete lesions are evident inferiorly.

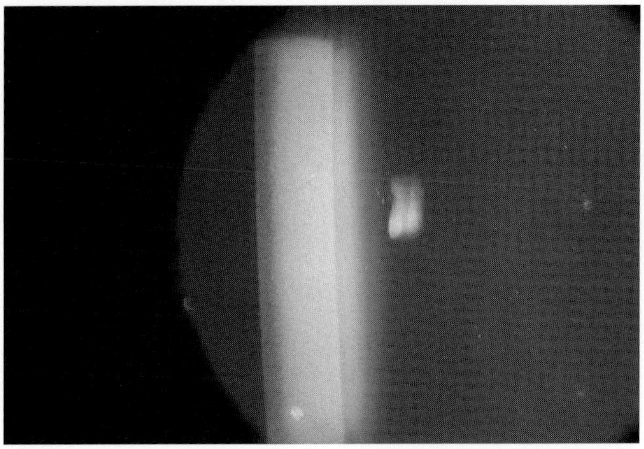

Fig. 4-111 Thygeson's SPK. Retroillumination off the retina can be used to identify lesions.

The cause is unclear. The morphologic resemblance of these lesions to those seen in other viral infections (such as adenovirus, measles, mumps, and rubella) has suggested a viral etiology, but no such association has been confirmed.

Untreated, the condition tends to be chronic and relapsing, with each episode lasting several weeks to months. Total duration of the disease may be many years. Treatment with weak topical corticosteroids during acute exacerbations generally hastens the resolution, though it may prolong the overall course of the disease. Therefore mild cases are treated with supportive therapy only, such as artificial tears and ointment. For more severe or symptomatic cases, the lowest effective dose of topical corticosteroid to achieve a therapeutic effect should be used and then slowly tapered. A bandage contact lens may be considered if corticosteroid therapy fails or when lenses are needed for refractive correction.

Filamentary Keratopathy

Filamentary keratopathy consists of multiple short, mucoid strands adherent to the corneal surface (Fig. 4-112). These strands consist of degenerated epithelial cells and mucus attached to the cornea at one end. They may be seen in a variety of pathological ocular conditions (Box 4-20). The pathophysiology of filament formation is not certain, but it is thought to result from a combination of relatively increased goblet cell mucus production, caused by diminished aqueous tears, and ocular surface epithelial damage, seen often in dry eye conditions.

Patients with a filamentary keratopathy present with a foreign body sensation or burning, or with significant pain aggravated by blinking that is occasionally associated with reflex tearing and blepharospasm. The filaments stain with fluorescein (Fig. 4-113). Strands may be seen to move or twist with each blink, thus producing the pain frequently associated with this syndrome. There

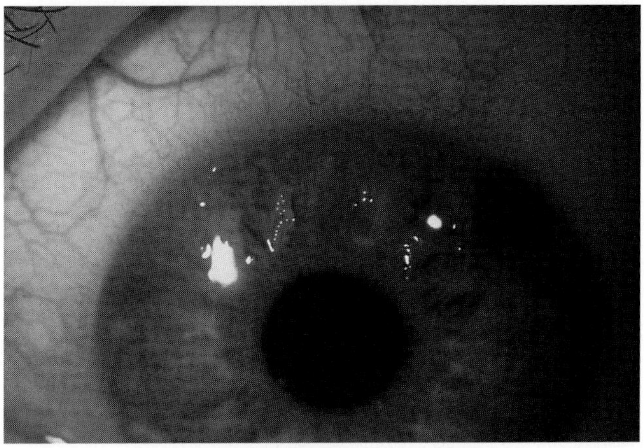

Fig. 4-112 Filamentary keratopathy. Multiple short mucoid strands are seen attached to the corneal surface superiorly.

may be other signs of dry eye, including SPK, small tear lake, or decreased tear break-up time. Superior limbic keratoconjunctivitis, another common cause of filamentary keratopathy, includes superior filaments, conjunctival injection, and tarsal papillary reaction. Filaments may be associated with previous epithelial trauma or recent ocular surgery such as penetrating keratoplasty. Filaments also develop in patients with ptosis or neurotrophic keratopathy and after pressure patching. Corneal sensation should be tested in patients thought to have filamentary keratopathy from a neurotrophic disorder.

Unless the underlying cause of filamentary keratopathy is easily treated, the management of corneal filaments is difficult because of multiple recurrences. Mechanical removal of the filaments may be accomplished under topical anesthesia with either fine forceps or a cotton-tipped applicator. Filaments must be removed at their base to allow proper epithelial healing. Although removal may be helpful for a moderate number of filaments, it is not practical for large numbers

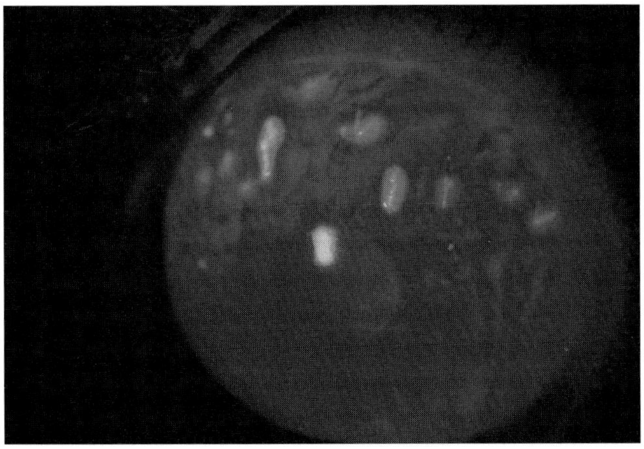

Fig. 4-113 Filamentary keratopathy. The filaments stain brightly with fluorescein dye and cobalt blue light. (See color plate.)

Box 4-20 Major Conditions Associated with Filamentary Keratopathy

KERATOCONJUNCTIVITIS SICCA

SUPERIOR LIMBIC KERATOCONJUNCTIVITIS

POSTSURGICAL STATES
Cataract extraction
Penetrating keratoplasty

NEUROTROPHIC KERATOPATHY

PTOSIS

POSTPATCHING

TRAUMA
Corneal abrasion
Recurrent erosion
Contact lens

of filaments throughout the cornea. Frequent lubrication with preservative-free artificial tears during the day and tear ointment at bedtime is usually necessary to promote epithelial healing and to improve the symptoms of underlying dry eye usually associated with the development of filaments. The use of 5% sodium chloride solutions and ointments is helpful. Refractory filaments may be amenable to treatment with mucolytic agents such as 10% *N*-acetylcysteine. Bandage contact lenses may be considered (except in patients with severe dry eyes), though extreme caution must be taken because of the risk for infection. Frequent lubrication and follow-up are necessary if bandage lenses are used.

Box 4-21 Major Conditions Contributing to Exposure Keratopathy

PROPTOSIS
Thyroid ophthalmopathy
Orbital mass

NOCTURNAL LAGOPHTHALMOS

NEUROGENIC
Central or peripheral facial nerve palsy

EYELID MALPOSITION
Ectropion
Entropion
Cicatricial scarring
- Herpes zoster
- Trauma
- Chemical or thermal injury

POSTSURGERY
Blepharoplasty
Ptosis repair

Exposure Keratopathy

Exposure keratopathy refers to the drying of the ocular surface because of inadequate eyelid closure or inadequate eyelid/globe interaction. It may result from a variety of conditions (Box 4-21).

One of the classic causes of exposure keratopathy is Bell's (seventh nerve) palsy, which may reduce or prevent eyelid closure on the affected side. As a result the tear film is inadequately spread across the surface of the cornea, and the surface is insufficiently protected from drying. If a patient has a preserved Bell's reflex that allows the eye to roll upward under the upper eyelid during attempted blinking, some surface lubrication is provided even if the eyelid does not close completely, thus reducing exposure-related problems.

Decreased eyelid excursion during normal blinking, whether natural or the result of previous eyelid surgery (e.g., ptosis repair, cosmetic blepharoplasty) or of disease (e.g., Parkinson's) is another common cause of corneal exposure. Similarly, nocturnal lagophthalmos may allow exposure keratopathy to develop during sleep, resulting in symptoms on awakening and throughout the day. Proptosis may prevent normal eyelid closure across the entire ocular surface during normal blinking because of the anterior displacement of the globe, thus producing exposure. Proptosis is frequently seen in patients with thyroid ophthalmopathy, and it may be aggravated by eyelid retraction associated with this condition. Eyelid malpositions such as entropion, ectropion, or cicatricial changes (as seen after trauma, burns, or herpes zoster infection) may also disrupt the normal eyelid/globe interaction or excursion and result in corneal exposure.

Clinical examination of these patients reveals SPK, usually in a horizontal band in the lower third of the cornea. If SPK is localized to the inferior cornea, it should suggest the possibility of exposure as a cause. Patients may have symptoms of burning, tearing, photophobia, or foreign body sensation that are usually worse in the morning. The history should include questions regarding previous eyelid surgery and nocturnal lagophthalmos. Examination should include a search for evidence of eyelid disease or malposition and an evaluation of the patient's normal eyelid excursion during a blink. It is also important to look for evidence of secondary infection or ulceration of the cornea from chronic exposure (Fig. 4-114). If proptosis is suspected, exophthalmometry measurements should be performed.

Treatment consists of supportive therapy with lubrication using preservative-free artificial tears and ointments until the underlying structural disorder (if present) is corrected. Often Bell's palsy resolves or sufficiently improves after several months to allow adequate corneal coverage. Occasionally, lateral tarsorrhaphy or gold weights in the upper eyelid are necessary for residual eyelid closure deficits. Eyelid taping or patching at night may help. Abnormalities in the eyelid structure should be repaired, and exophthalmos (as in thyroid ophthalmopathy) may require eyelid lowering or orbital decompression. Persistent exposure complicated by sterile corneal ulceration and refractory to all other treatment modalities is rare but may require a conjunctival flap.

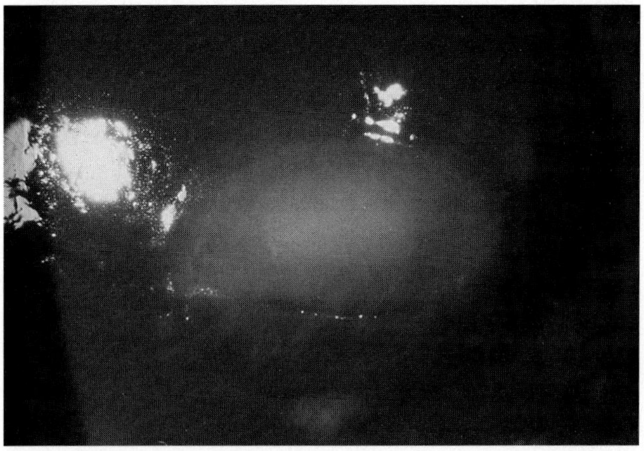

Fig. 4-114 Exposure keratopathy. Chronic exposure caused by a brain tumor caused a persistent epithelial defect as seen by the rolled-up epithelial edges. Underlying corneal infiltration and ulceration and surrounding corneal edema are also present.

Neurotrophic Keratopathy

Neurotrophic keratopathy results from the loss of corneal sensation, leading to epithelial breakdown and impaired epithelial healing. Corneal epithelial maintenance, integrity, and mitosis are positively influenced by the presence of neurotransmitters, such as acetylcholine and substance P, within the epithelium. Therefore the depletion of these substances in denervated or partially denervated corneas is thought to play a major role in the pathophysiology of this condition. Additionally, decreased reflex tearing leads to a dry eye condition.

The most common causes of reduced corneal sensation and neurotrophic keratopathy are ocular herpes simplex and zoster infections. These infections are discussed in detail earlier in this chapter. Reduced corneal sensation from trigeminal nerve damage is another important cause of neurotrophic keratopathy. This nerve damage may result from tumor, aneurysm, previous surgery, or congenital disorders (Box 4-22). Occasionally, these disorders are associated with seventh cranial nerve palsy

Box 4-22 Major Conditions Associated with Reduced Corneal Sensation

INFECTIOUS

Herpes simplex
Herpes zoster
Leprosy

NEUROLOGIC

Stroke
Trigeminal nerve dysfunction
- Postsurgical (e.g., for trigeminal neuralgia)
- Postirradiation
- Compression from tumor or aneurysm

TOPICAL MEDICATIONS AND DEVICES

Beta-blockers
Anesthetics
Nonsteroidal antiinflammatory medications
Contact lenses

CONGENITAL

Familial dysautonomia (Riley-Day syndrome)
Möbius syndrome

POSTSURGICAL

Penetrating keratoplasty
Cataract extraction
Refractive surgery

caused by the proximity of these structures and resulting in exposure keratopathy, thus significantly worsening the corneal prognosis. Topical medications including beta-blockers and nonsteroidal antiinflammatory agents have been associated with reduced corneal sensation. Anesthetic abuse is another well-recognized cause of severe neurotrophic keratopathy. Fumes reaching the eye from the chronic use of crack cocaine have also been reported to cause neurotrophic keratopathy.

Clinically, these patients present initially with surface abnormalities that range from decreased tear production (caused by the absence of neural stimulation from the cornea), loss of corneal luster, SPK, and epithelial breakdown to frank ulceration, thinning, and perforation. The classic neurotrophic defect is a round or oval, central or paracentral epithelial defect with gray or white heaped-up, rolled epithelial edges. The base of the ulcer may be clear or it may develop a diffuse haze. The underlying stroma is usually edematous. Secondary infection is common and, if suspected, should be ruled out with scrapings for culture.

To confirm the diagnosis, corneal sensation should be tested either with a Cochet-Bonnet esthesiometer or a sterile cotton wisp before the application of topical anesthesia. The results in the unaffected eye should be used for comparison. Examination should include a careful evaluation of eyelid function, excursion, and tear production (Schirmer's test) because corneal exposure and dry eye syndrome significantly worsen the visual prognosis. Any structural abnormalities should be corrected, if possible. After a thorough history and examination, if no evidence has surfaced either of active or previous herpes simplex or herpes zoster infection or of other causes of reduced sensation, consider computed tomography or magnetic resonance imaging to rule out a lesion of the central nervous system that may produce trigeminal nerve dysfunction.

The treatment of neurotrophic keratopathy is often difficult. Initial therapy for mild cases consists of the frequent application of preservative-free artificial tears and ointments. Small epithelial defects may respond to frequent antibiotic ointments or pressure patching. Large, persistent neurotrophic defects often respond well to tarsorrhaphy. Additional treatment includes punctal occlusion, bandage soft contact lens, or conjunctival flap. Amniotic membrane grafts may aid reepithelialization. Small perforations may be amenable to repair with cyanoacrylate tissue adhesive and a bandage lens, but large perforations may require lamellar or penetrating keratoplasty combined with lateral tarsorrhaphy.

Ultraviolet and Radiation Keratopathy

Radiation keratopathy refers to corneal damage caused by the effects of various forms of radiant energy. Corneal damage may result from ultraviolet, infrared, or ionizing radiation.

Ultraviolet light occupies the 200- to 400-nm range of the electromagnetic spectrum. The cornea absorbs wavelengths between 200 nm and 300 nm, whereas the lens absorbs wavelengths from 300 nm to 400 nm. Corneal damage is frequent in welders who work without masks and in those who sit under sunlamps without adequate ocular protection. Symptoms generally do not develop until several hours after exposure. Patients then report sharp pain or burning, red eyes, photophobia, and tearing. Examination may reveal heavy or confluent SPK throughout the interpalpebral zone. The treatment regimen includes cycloplegia and frequent antibiotic ointment or pressure patching for severe cases. Milder cases may only require antibiotic ointments or drops without cycloplegia or patching. Oral pain medication is sometimes required for severe cases. Although the corneal surface usually recovers quickly, chronic ultraviolet exposure may ultimately lead to the development of pterygia or spheroidal degeneration.

Infrared radiation may contribute to corneal injury, though this is rare. Glass blowers and operators of blast furnaces are occasionally exposed to rapid intense blasts of heat to the face and eyes, which may produce damage. This type of infrared exposure has been associated with true exfoliation of the lens capsule, where it can be seen to peel back in partial-thickness scrolls. Infrared radiation may also produce thermal damage to the corneal epithelium and sometimes to the stroma. These injuries are treated in a similar fashion to those caused by ultraviolet radiation.

Other forms of ionizing radiation, such as those used to treat ocular and periocular neoplasms, can produce corneal damage, but the corneal damage is usually associated with or caused by conjunctival damage. Radiation may produce significant cicatricial alterations in the conjunctiva, resulting in profound mucin deficiency, which may be combined with an aqueous tear deficiency if the lacrimal gland ducts become obliterated. The resultant surface disease may produce severe corneal opacification and vascularization.

Dellen

A delle is a peripheral thinning or dimpling of the cornea adjacent to an elevated lesion, typically at the limbus (Fig. 4-115). Dellen are usually asymptomatic and result from inadequate wetting of the corneal surface because of the closely located elevated lesion. Often the limbal elevation results from postoperative conjunctival hemorrhage or chemosis or from a high bleb after glaucoma filtration surgery. Pingueculae, pterygia, subconjunctival hematomas, and limbal conjunctival masses may also produce this condition. The impaired eyelid/

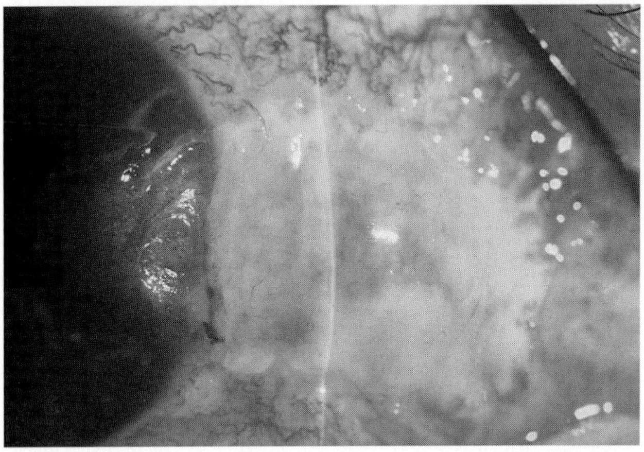

Fig. 4-115 Delle. A small area of peripheral corneal drying and thinning is seen adjacent to a swollen conjunctival graft 1 week after a pterygium excision and conjunctival autograft was performed.

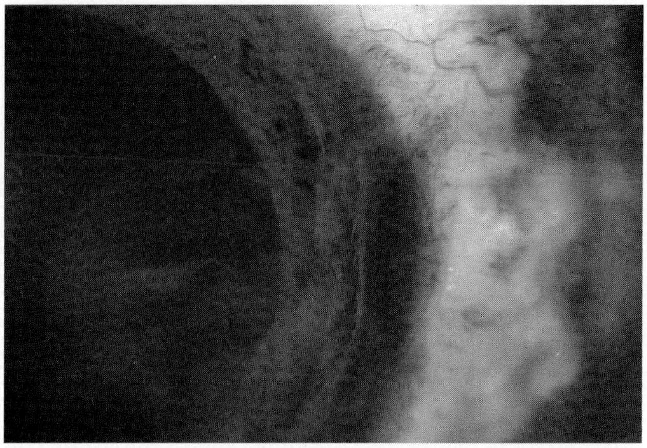

Fig. 4-116 Delle. A moderately large area of peripheral corneal desiccation results from conjunctival elevation 4 days after pars plana vitrectomy surgery.

globe interaction in the area of the cornea immediately adjacent to the elevated lesion leads to poor tear film spread into this area and to localized corneal drying and thinning (Figs. 4-116 and 4-117). Fluorescein may pool over the depression, but the area stains minimally. All layers of the cornea are intact in this area, but they are thinned because of desiccation. Treatment consists of lubrication with antibiotics or artificial tear ointment and pressure patching, if necessary. Lubrication must be continued until the limbal elevation subsides or is removed.

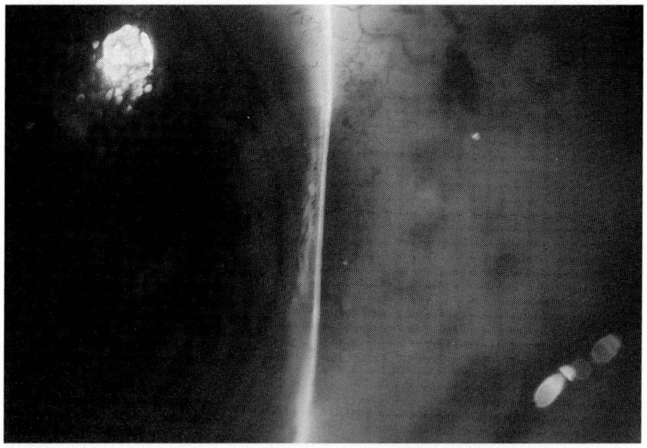

Fig. 4-117 Delle. A slit-beam view of the delle seen in Fig. 4-116. Approximately 50% corneal thinning is present.

Aphakic and Pseudophakic Bullous Keratopathy

Aphakic bullous keratopathy (ABK) and pseudophakic bullous keratopathy (PBK) are postsurgical conditions characterized by corneal edema after cataract surgery. In the United States they are a leading indication for penetrating keratoplasty.

Bullous keratopathy may result from direct surgical trauma to the endothelium, resulting in either persistent corneal edema after surgery or delayed-onset edema as the remaining endothelial cells gradually fail. Delayed-onset edema may result from persistent injury or irritation of the corneal endothelium from vitreous touch or from a poorly designed or positioned intraocular lens. Chronic uveitis may contribute to the development of corneal edema. Preexisting endothelial disease, such as endothelial dystrophy, predisposes the patient to corneal decompensation after surgery.

Intraoperative factors that may add to the development of bullous keratopathy include direct endothelial damage from surgical instrumentation, lens fragments, or intraocular lenses. Endothelium may be directly damaged by ultrasonic energy from phacoemulsification. Phacoemulsification in the posterior chamber or within the capsular bag significantly reduces ultrasound-induced endothelial damage. Vitreous loss during cataract surgery may enhance endothelial loss by increased surgical time and manipulation and by vitreous/endothelial touch.

Stripping of Descemet's membrane is an uncommon, though serious, complication of intraocular surgery. If it is left untreated and it does not improve spontaneously, it may result in bullous keratopathy. It may occur because of the repeated insertion of instruments through the surgical wound that may catch, and eventually strip, the posterior cornea. The flap may be a barely perceptible layer flapping freely into the anterior chamber from the superior wound, or it may be a large flap encompassing most of the posterior cornea (Fig. 4-118). These flaps may be repaired with the instillation of an air bubble or

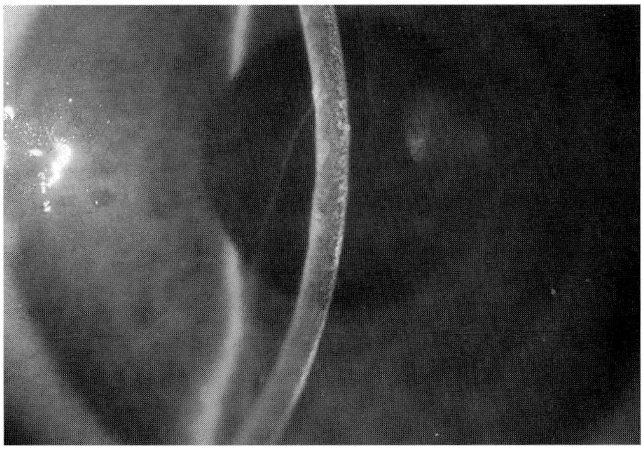

Fig. 4-118 Descemet's detachment. A large planar detachment of Descemet's membrane and a moderate amount of corneal edema have developed.

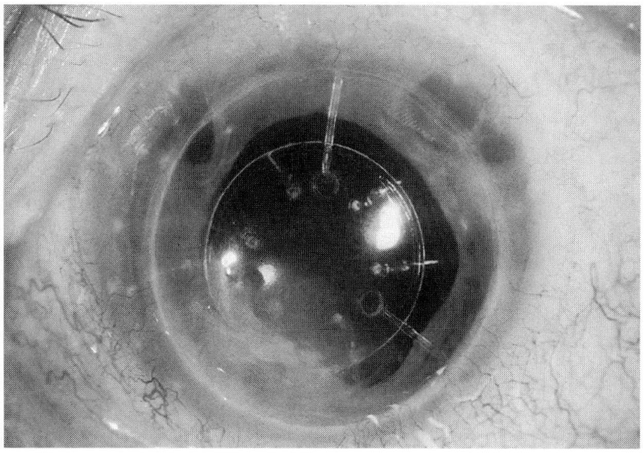

Fig. 4-120 Anterior chamber intraocular lens and pseudophakic bullous keratopathy. This Fyodorov "Sputnik" iris-clip anterior chamber intraocular lens had three sticks with rounded ends placed anteriorly to the iris and three closed loops placed posteriorly to the iris. This corneal graft is developing corneal edema inferiorly.

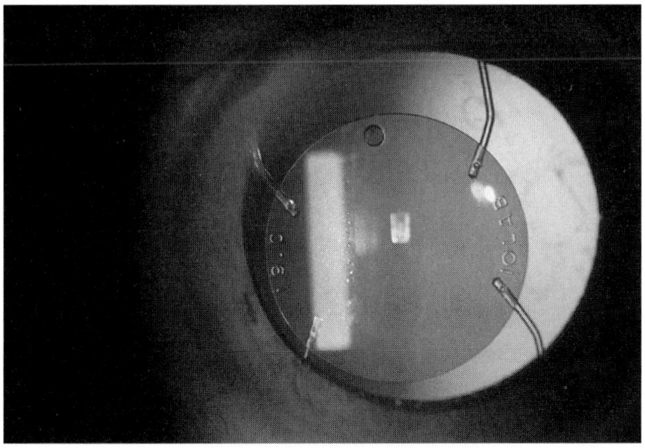

Fig. 4-119 Anterior chamber intraocular lens. This closed-loop anterior chamber intraocular lens (Iolab, Azar 91Z) was associated with the development of corneal decompensation.

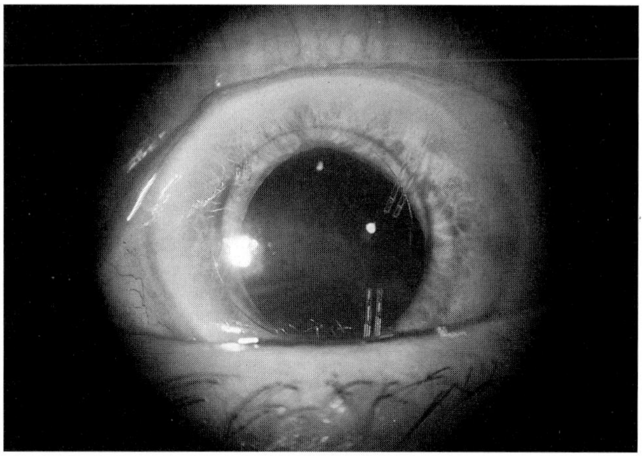

Fig. 4-121 Anterior chamber intraocular lens and pseudophakic bullous keratopathy. A Stableflex, closed-loop, anterior chamber intraocular lens is seen with moderate corneal edema. This lens has four L-shaped, closed hoop haptics that are particularly difficult to explant.

with nonexpansile concentrations of gas (e.g., 18% SF_6 or 14% C_3F_8) into the anterior chamber, which remains after surgery until it reabsorbs. Occasionally, direct suturing of the membrane to the corneal stroma may be required. Small Descemet's flaps and even large flaps not scrolled onto themselves often resolve spontaneously, though it may take weeks to months.

Delayed postoperative causes of bullous keratopathy are usually related to the combined effects of surgical endothelial cell loss, age-related endothelial cell loss, and the presence of an intraocular lens. Complicated surgery may hasten endothelial loss and the onset of edema. Vitreous in the anterior chamber with endothelial touch, caused by either an intracapsular procedure or a complicated extracapsular procedure, may accelerate endothelial cell loss and precipitate the onset of edema. Chronic inflammation can produce the same effect. However, one of the major causes of delayed-onset corneal edema is related to chronic endothelial trauma produced by older-style anterior chamber intraocular lenses (Figs. 4-119 and 4-120). These lens types were usually of a rigid or closed-loop design that produced chronic low-grade inflammation, peripheral endothelial trauma, and eventual corneal decompensation (Figs. 4-121 and

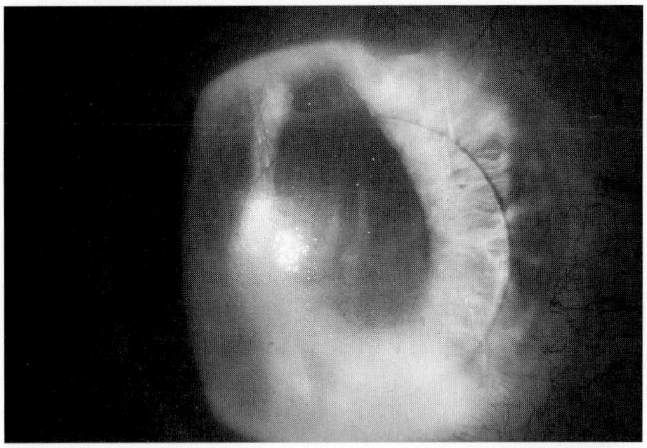

Fig. 4-122 Anterior chamber intraocular lens and pseudophakic bullous keratopathy. This Leiske, anterior chamber, intraocular lens has two closed-loop haptics. Corneal edema with Descemet's folds has developed centrally.

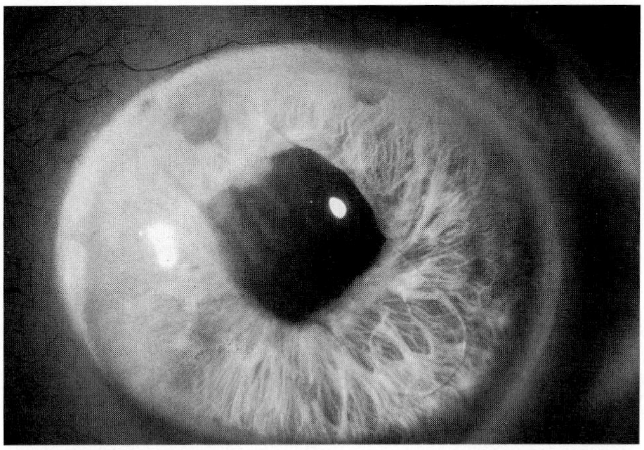

Fig. 4-123 Anterior chamber intraocular lens and pseudophakic bullous keratopathy. This Copeland iris-plane lens has a windmill shape with two solid haptics posterior to the iris and two haptics anterior to the iris. Corneal edema with Descemet's folds are present superiorly.

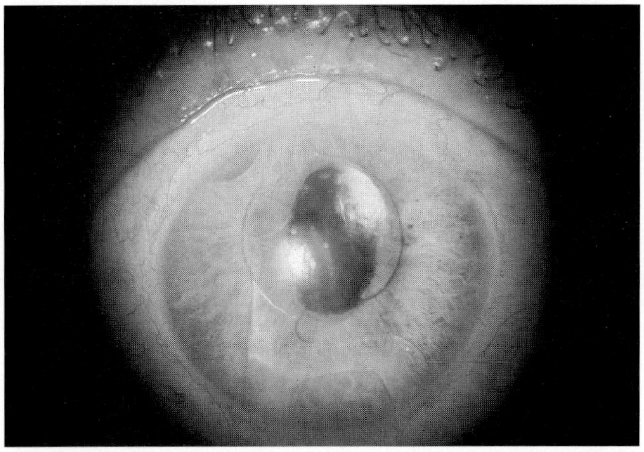

Fig. 4-124 Anterior chamber intraocular lens and pseudophakic bullous keratopathy. Corneal decompensation in this eye was related to this rigid Kelman, anterior chamber, intraocular lens.

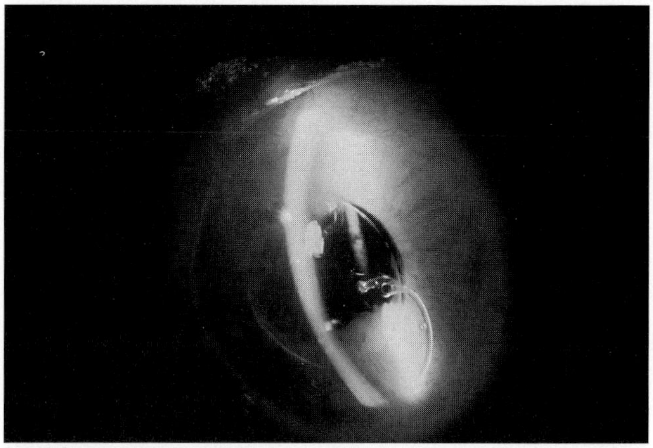

Fig. 4-125 Anterior chamber intraocular lens and pseudophakic bullous keratopathy. A Binkhorst iris-clip lens and corneal edema are present.

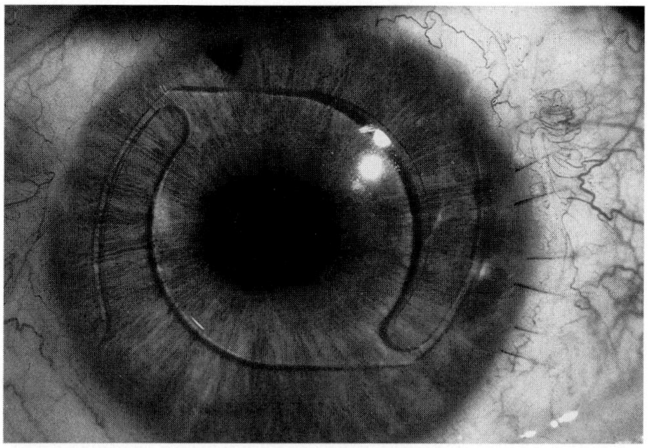

Fig. 4-126 Open-loop, anterior chamber, intraocular lens. This Kelman-style, multiflex, open-loop, anterior chamber, intraocular lens was placed as a secondary implant to correct aphakia. This type of lens is not associated with a significantly greater risk for corneal edema than posterior chamber intraocular lenses.

4-122). Other older-style anterior chamber and iris-supported lenses are also associated with bullous keratopathy (Figs. 4-123, 4-124, and 4-125). Modern, flexible, open-loop designs do not appear to be associated with a significantly increased rate of bullous keratopathy (Fig. 4-126).

Clinically, patients with bullous keratopathy present with decreasing vision in the affected eye. Examination reveals stromal edema sometimes associated with Descemet's folds. Mild cases may present with localized, peripheral edema with a clear central cornea (known as Brown-McLean syndrome) (Fig. 4-127). Stromal edema may be associated with epithelial edema and the formation of epithelial bullae, which may rupture and produce pain (Figs. 4-128 and 4-129). These ruptured bullae are risk factors for infection. These corneas can develop an-

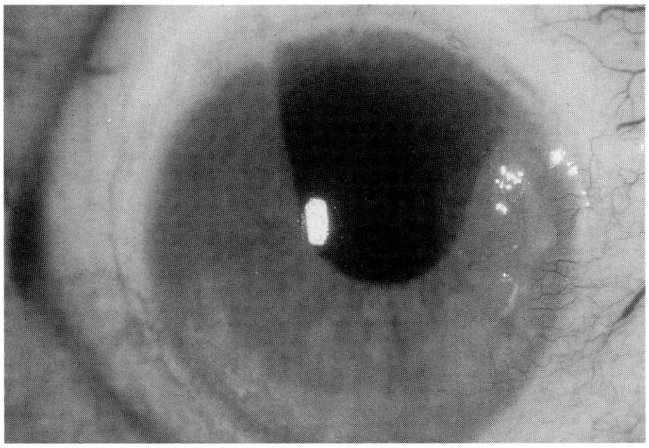

Fig. 4-127 Brown-McLean syndrome. Peripheral corneal edema, initially sparing the central cornea and vision, is present in this aphakic eye. Brown-McLean syndrome occurs more often in aphakic eyes but has been seen in pseudophakic eyes, too.

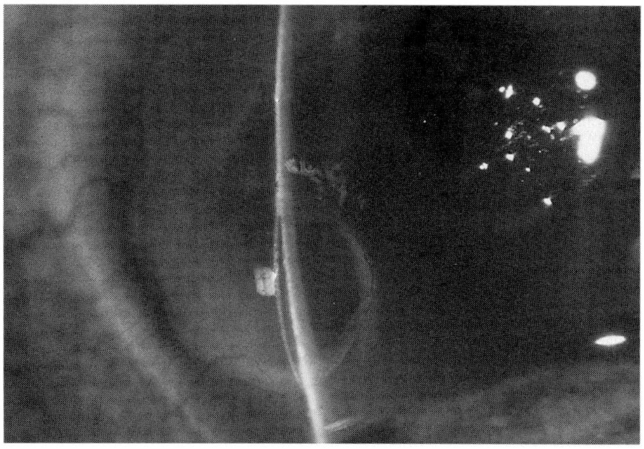

Fig. 4-129 Aphakic bullous keratopathy. This eye with aphakic bullous keratopathy has significant stromal and epithelial corneal edema. Note the large epithelial bulla in the slit beam.

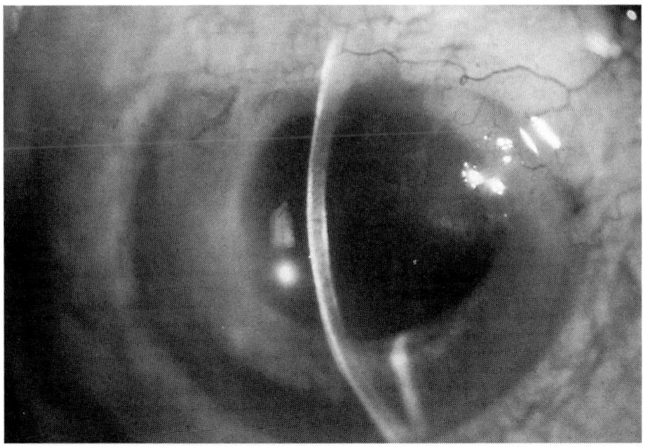

Fig. 4-128 Pseudophakic bullous keratopathy. Corneal edema can be seen in this eye with a posterior chamber intraocular lens. The patient underwent previous extracapsular cataract extraction and posterior chamber lens placement with glaucoma surgery. The cornea was clear for several years after surgery but then decompensated.

terior basement membrane dystrophy changes, degenerative pannus, deep vascularization, and opacification.

Treatment of bullous keratopathy depends on its severity. Initially, if the edema is mild, decreased vision and symptoms related to bullae formation and rupture may be minimized by the use of 5% sodium chloride drops and ointment. Lowering elevated intraocular pressure may improve corneal edema. As the edema worsens, penetrating keratoplasty is the treatment of choice for pain relief and visual rehabilitation. This surgery should be combined with vitrectomy or intraocular lens exchange or removal, if indicated.

Patients who experience significant pain from ruptured bullae may benefit from anterior stromal micropuncture or PTK, which are effective in reducing bullae formation but do not generally improve vision. These techniques are identical to that described for recurrent erosion syndrome. Anterior stromal micropuncture can be applied directly through the bullae. These procedures can provide pain relief for those who want to defer surgery, or these may serve as an adjunct to provide relief for those awaiting surgery. Bandage soft contact lenses may also be used to reduce the pain from ruptured bullae, though they carry a significantly increased risk for infectious keratitis, particularly in compromised corneas, and their use should be minimized. A conjunctival flap may be considered to establish a stable ocular surface and for pain relief in eyes that have poor visual potential or are otherwise not candidates for penetrating keratoplasty.

Patients who are not in significant discomfort and who have good vision in the other eye may want to defer surgery. However, they must be made aware that chronically sick corneas, such as those with bullous keratopathy, are at a higher risk for microbial keratitis. Ulcerative keratopathy in these corneas may result in severe infections that heal slowly and produce complications such as corneal neovascularization, which may reduce the prognosis for future corneal transplantation.

CONCLUSION

Many infectious and inflammatory conditions cause corneal disease. These diseases can also be exacerbated by other corneal surface disorders. Understanding the various diseases and interrelationships between the cornea, conjunctiva, eyelids, and various systemic abnormalities can aid in the diagnosis and treatment of this complex group of conditions.

MAJOR POINTS

The corneal epithelium is the most important mechanical defense against the development of ulcerative keratitis.

Trauma and contact lens wear are the most common risk factors for microbial keratitis.

Contact lens-related epithelial defects should be considered high risks for the development of ulcerative keratitis and should not be patched. They should be treated with frequent antibiotic therapy that includes adequate coverage for *Pseudomonas.*

Cultures should be performed on ulcers that are large (>1 to 2 mm), central, associated with a hypopyon, or atypical in history or appearance. Cultures should be inoculated directly onto the appropriate growth media.

Hyperacute conjunctivitis caused by *Neisseria gonorrhoeae* requires urgent systemic treatment with ceftriaxone.

Corneal ulcers should be treated aggressively with antibiotic therapy every 30 to 60 minutes and should be monitored closely for clinical response.

Trauma, especially with vegetable matter, and chronic ocular disease are major risk factors for fungal keratitis.

Fungus grows on Sabouraud's agar (without cycloheximide), blood agar, or chocolate agar at room temperature.

Fungal cultures should be held for 3 weeks to allow for late growth.

Natamycin is the drug of choice for filamentous fungi, whereas topical amphotericin B is the drug of choice for yeasts.

Acanthamoeba organisms are found in tap water, swimming pools, hot tubs, ponds and lakes, sea water, and soil.

The major risk factors for *Acanthamoeba* keratitis include infrequent and ineffective contact lens disinfection. Patients should not wear contact lenses while swimming. Contact lenses should be disinfected before reinsertion.

Early *Acanthamoeba* keratitis may produce a dendritiform epithelial defect resembling herpes simplex keratitis.

Pain out of proportion to the clinical findings is associated with *Acanthamoeba* keratitis. A ring infiltrate and radial keratoneuritis are also highly suggestive of an advanced *Acanthamoeba* infection.

Acanthamoeba organisms may be demonstrated by Gram stain, Giemsa stain, or calcofluor white stain.

Most herpes simplex ocular infections are recurrent disease.

Herpes simplex virus epithelial dendrites are serpiginous, branching lesions with elevated edges and ulcerated centers. They may have terminal end bulbs, and they represent active viral infection.

Nonnecrotizing herpes simplex virus stromal keratitis in the forms of disciform keratitis or endotheliitis (more common) and immune stromal keratitis (less common) are immune-mediated reactions and do not generally represent active viral infection.

Corticosteroids should not be used in the treatment of herpes simplex virus epithelial keratitis because they potentiate the infection.

Herpes zoster mucous plaque pseudodendrites are elevated, stellate lesions that lack terminal end bulbs.

Congenital or acquired syphilis, herpes simplex, and herpes zoster are major causes of interstitial keratitis.

Cogan's syndrome is the association of nonsyphilitic interstitial keratitis with vestibular abnormalities and, ultimately, with hearing loss. As many as 10% of patients may have associated systemic vasculitis.

Noninfectious, typically peripheral, corneal infiltrates may be produced by tight contact lens syndrome or by solution toxicity/hypersensitivity.

Although bandage soft contact lenses are useful in certain clinical situations, they are associated with an increased risk for contact lens–related complications, including microbial keratitis, and they necessitate careful patient selection and lens fitting and close follow-up.

Dry eye syndrome may be produced by conditions that reduce aqueous tear production, increase tear evaporation, or both.

Recurrent corneal erosions may occur in 10% of patients with anterior basement membrane dystrophy, though approximately 50% of patients with recurrent corneal erosions have underlying anterior basement membrane dystrophy.

Pseudophakic bullous keratopathy is a leading indication for penetrating keratoplasty in the United States.

Historically, older-style rigid and closed-loop anterior chamber and iris-fixated intraocular lenses were associated with delayed-onset bullous keratopathy.

Modern, flexible, open-loop anterior chamber intraocular lenses do not appear to be associated with an increased incidence of delayed-onset bullous keratopathy.

SUGGESTED READINGS

Books

Burd EM, Ogawa GSH, Hyndiuk RA: Bacterial keratitis and conjunctivitis. In Smolin G and Thoft RA, editors: *The cornea: scientific foundations and clinical practice*, New York, 1994, Little, Brown.

Holland EJ, Mozayeni RM, Schwartz GS: Herpes simplex keratitis. In Krachmer JH, Mannis MJ, and Holland EJ, editors: *Cornea*, St Louis, 1997, Mosby.

Liesegang TJ: Herpes zoster keratitis. In Krachmer JH, Mannis MJ, and Holland EJ, editors: *Cornea*, St Louis, 1997, Mosby.

Pflugfelder SC, Whitcher JP, Daniels TE: Sjögren syndrome. In Pepose JS, Holland GN, and Wilhelmus KR, editors: *Ocular infection and immunity*, St Louis, 1996, Mosby.

Journals

Alfonso E, Mandelbaum S, Fox MJ, Forster RK: Ulcerative keratitis associated with contact lens wear, *Am J Ophthalmol* 101:429-433, 1986.

Allansmith MR, Korb DR, Greiner JV, et al: Giant papillary conjunctivitis in contact lens wearers, *Am J Ophthalmol* 83: 697-708, 1977.

Barron BA, Gee L, Hauck HH, et al on behalf of the Herpetic Eye Disease Study Group: Herpetic Eye Disease Study: a controlled trial of oral acyclovir for herpes simplex stromal keratitis, *Ophthalmology* 101:1871-1882, 1994.

Bower KS, Kowalski MS, Gordon YJ: Fluoroquinolones in the treatment of bacterial keratitis, *Am J Ophthalmol* 121:712-715, 1996.

Brady SE, Cohen EJ: Acanthamoeba keratitis, *Ophthalmol Clin North Am* 3: 537-544, 1990.

Clemmons CS, Cohen EJ, Arentsen JJ, et al: *Pseudomonas* ulcers following patching of corneal abrasions associated with contact lens wear, *CLAO J* 13:161-164, 1987.

Cobo LM: Corneal complications of herpes zoster ophthalmicus, *Cornea* 7:50-56, 1988.

Cogan DG: Syndrome of nonsyphilitic interstitial keratitis and vestibuloauditory symptoms, *Arch Ophthalmol* 42:42-49, 1949.

Dawson CR, Hanna L, Wood TR, Despain R: Adenovirus type 8 keratoconjunctivitis in the United States, *Am J Ophthalmol* 69:473-480, 1970.

Fox RI, Robinson CA, Curd JG, et al: Sjögren's syndrome: proposed criteria for classification, *Arthritis Rheum* 29:577-585, 1986.

Friedlander MH: Ocular manifestations of Sjögren's syndrome: keratoconjunctivitis sicca, *Rheum Dis Clin North Am* 18: 591-608, 1992.

The Herpetic Eye Disease Study Group: Acyclovir for the prevention of herpes simplex virus eye disease, *N Engl J Med* 339:300-306, 1998.

The Herpetic Eye Disease Study Group: Herpetic Eye Disease Study: a controlled trial of oral acyclovir for the prevention of stromal keratitis or iritis in patients with herpes simplex virus epithelial keratitis, *Arch Ophthalmol* 115:703-712, 1997.

Illingworth CD, Cook SD: Acanthamoeba keratitis, *Surv Ophthalmol* 42:493-508, 1998.

Laibson PR: Ocular adenoviral infections, *Int Ophthalmol Clin* 24:49-64, 1984.

Laibson PR, Oconer JT, Chiri S, Ortolan G: Corneal infiltrates in epidemic keratoconjunctivitis: response to double blind corticosteroid therapy, *Arch Ophthalmol* 84:36-40, 1970.

Lemp MA: General measures in the management of the dry eye, *Int Ophthalmol Clin* 27:36-43, 1987.

Levey SB, Cohen EJ: Methods of disinfecting contact lenses to avoid corneal disorders, *Surv Ophthalmol* 41:245-251, 1996.

Liesegang TJ: Corneal complications from herpes zoster ophthalmicus, *Ophthalmology* 92:316-324, 1985.

Musch DC, Sugar A, Meyer RF: Demographic and predisposing factors in corneal ulceration, *Arch Ophthalmol* 101:1545-1548, 1983.

Piebenga LW, Laibson PR: Dendritic lesions in herpes zoster ophthalmicus, *Arch Ophthalmol* 90:268-270, 1973.

Poggio EC, Glenn RJ, Schein OD, et al: The incidence of ulcerative keratitis among users of daily-wear and extended-wear soft contact lenses, *N Engl J Med* 321:779-783, 1980.

Schein OD, Buehler PO, Stamler JF, et al: The impact of overnight wear on the risk of contact lens–associated ulcerative keratitis, *Arch Ophthalmol* 112:186-190, 1994.

Schein OD, Glynn RJ, Poggio EC, et al on behalf of the Microbial Keratitis Study Group: The relative risk of ulcerative keratitis among users of daily-wear and extended-wear soft contact lenses, *N Engl J Med* 321:773-778, 1989.

Sendele DD, Kenyon KR, Mobila EF, et al: Superior limbic keratoconjunctivitis in contact lens wearers, *Ophthalmology* 90:616-622, 1983.

Wilhelmus KR, Gee L, Hauck HH, et al on behalf of the Herpetic Eye Disease Study Group: Herpetic Eye Disease Study: a controlled trial of topical corticosteroids for herpes simplex stromal keratitis, *Ophthalmology* 101:1883-1896, 1994.

CHAPTER 5

Systemic and Immunologic Conditions Affecting the Cornea

Many systemic diseases produce abnormalities in the anterior segment of the eye. In general these conditions can be divided into diseases that produce deposits and those that produce inflammatory reactions. Deposits are usually accumulations of a substance from an inherited metabolic error or a neoplastic process. The overabundant substance is deposited in the cornea or the conjunctiva and less commonly in the deeper ocular structures. Immune-mediated complications of systemic disease may produce inflammation or ulceration in the conjunctiva, sclera, or cornea. Occasionally these inflammatory complications are associated with life-threatening systemic vasculitis, and they may even be the first manifestations of systemic disease. In certain circumstances this finding may provide the ophthalmologist with the unique opportunity to both diagnose systemic disease and even save a life.

CORNEAL MANIFESTATIONS OF SYSTEMIC DISEASE

Metabolic Diseases

Mucopolysaccharidoses Mucopolysaccharidoses (MPS) constitute a group of lysosomal storage diseases resulting from a deficiency in one or more of the enzymes required for the metabolism of mucopolysaccharides (primarily keratan sulfate, dermatan sulfate, and heparan sulfate). Consequently these substances and their abnormal metabolic products accumulate primarily within connective tissues throughout the body. Because the corneal stroma is comprised of approximately 4% mucopolysaccharides (chondroitin sulfate and keratan sulfate), it is frequently involved in these disorders, clinically presenting as progressive corneal clouding (Figs. 5-1 and 5-2 and Table 5-1). Accumulations of heparan sulfate may produce retinal, optic nerve, or central nervous system abnormalities. Each of the mucopolysaccharidoses is associated with a distinct pattern of systemic findings and morphologic features. All of these conditions are autosomal recessive with the exception of Hunter syndrome, which is X-linked recessive. Histopathologically, mucopolysaccharide accumulation within keratocytes may be demonstrated in specimens stained with colloidal iron or Alcian blue.

Hurler syndrome (MPS IH) produces a progressive clinical syndrome consisting of dwarfism, deafness, mental retardation, joint contractures, hepatosplenomegaly, and a typical facies. Ophthalmic findings include diffuse corneal clouding throughout the stroma with scattered punctate opacities, as well as a pigmentary retinopathy, optic disc swelling, or optic atrophy. No effective therapy has been found for this condition, and it usually results in death within the first decade.

Scheie syndrome (MPS IS) results from a partial deficiency of the same enzyme responsible for Hurler syndrome, and it produces a less severe clinical syndrome. Patients usually have normal intelligence, normal life span, and normal stature. Although the typical facies of Hurler syndrome may be absent, patients have coarse facial features, hepatosplenomegaly, stiff joints, and aortic insufficiency. Corneal clouding may be present in patients with Scheie syndrome, starting peripherally and progressing centrally, as may a pigmentary retinopathy and optic atrophy.

Hunter syndrome (MPS II) is an X-linked recessive syndrome characterized by deafness, short stature, hepatosplenomegaly, pigmentary retinopathy, optic nerve swelling, optic nerve atrophy, and typical facial features, though clinically significant corneal clouding is absent.

Of the remaining mucopolysaccharidoses, corneal clouding may be a feature of Morquio syndrome (MPS IV), Maroteaux-Lamy syndrome (MPS VI), and Sly syndrome (MPS VII), but it is generally absent in Sanfilippo syndrome (MPS III). Corneal transplantation may be considered for some patients if retinopathy and optic atrophy are not advanced. Recurrence of corneal clouding in the graft, however, may limit the long-term prognosis (Fig. 5-3).

Macular corneal dystrophy also results from the accumulation of keratan sulfate within corneal keratocytes, but, because no systemic associations have been reported with this condition (unlike the systemic muco-

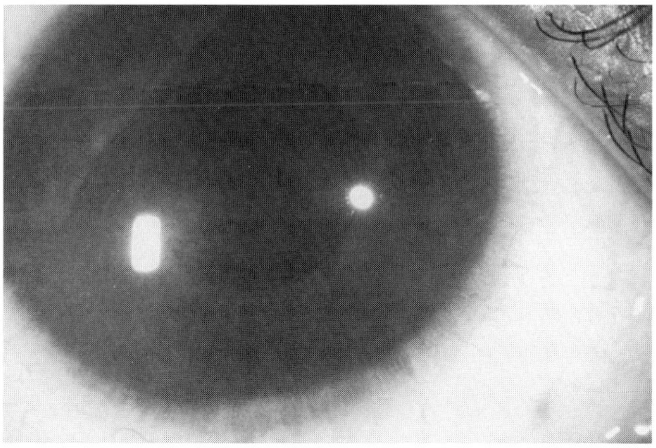

Fig. 5-1 Maroteaux-Lamy syndrome. Significant diffuse corneal clouding is seen in this eye of a child with Maroteaux-Lamy syndrome.

Table 5-1 Corneal clouding in the systemic mucopolysaccharidoses

Disorder	Corneal clouding	Inheritance
Hurler syndrome (MPS IH)	+	Autosomal recessive
Scheie syndrome (MPS IS)	+	Autosomal recessive
Hunter syndrome (MPS II)	–	X-linked recessive
Sanfilippo syndrome (MPS III)	–	Autosomal recessive
Morquio syndrome (MPS IV)	+	Autosomal recessive
Maroteaux-Lamy syndrome (MPS VI)	+	Autosomal recessive
Sly syndrome (MPS VII)	+	Autosomal recessive

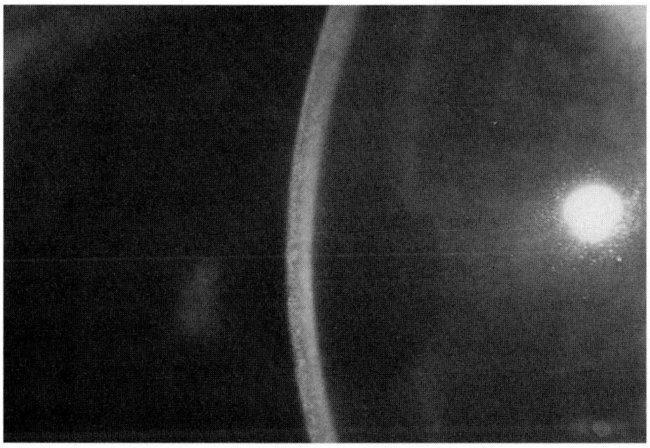

Fig. 5-2 Maroteaux-Lamy syndrome. Slit-beam view of the eye seen in Fig. 5-1 reveals full-thickness corneal involvement.

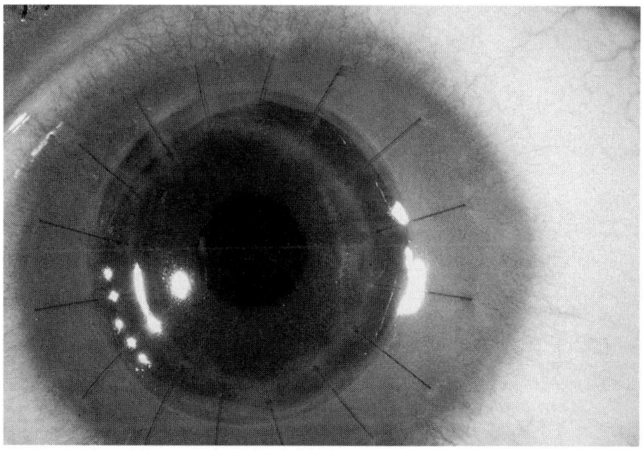

Fig. 5-3 Maroteaux-Lamy syndrome. A clear graft is present 3 months after corneal transplantation in the eye seen in Figs. 5-1 and 5-2.

polysaccharidoses), it appears to be a localized phenomenon. The exact enzyme deficiency responsible for macular dystrophy is unknown. This condition is discussed in further detail in Chapter 3.

Lipidoses The lipidoses are systemic disorders of lipid metabolism, primarily gangliosides (gangliosidoses) and sphingomyelin (sphingolipidoses). The resultant lipid accumulation within tissues produces a variety of systemic, primarily neurologic, syndromes. Ocular involvement is usually limited to the posterior segment and includes a macular cherry red spot and optic atrophy. Corneal involvement may be seen in Fabry's disease, generalized gangliosidosis, and multiple sulfatase deficiency. All of these syndromes are autosomal recessive except Fabry's disease, which is X-linked recessive.

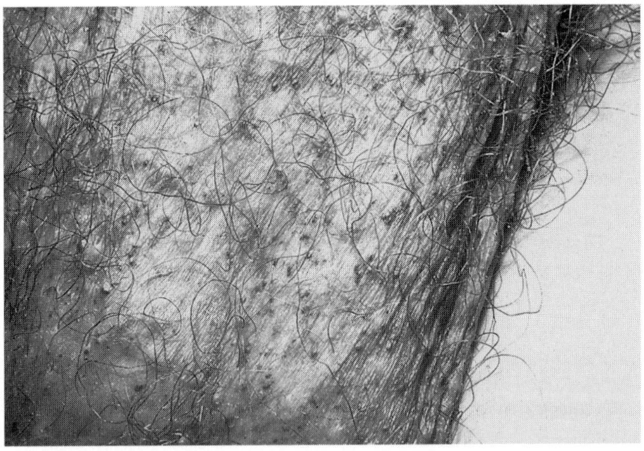

Fig. 5-4 Fabry's disease. Multiple small, cutaneous angiokeratomas are seen on the skin of a patient with Fabry's disease. (See color plate.)

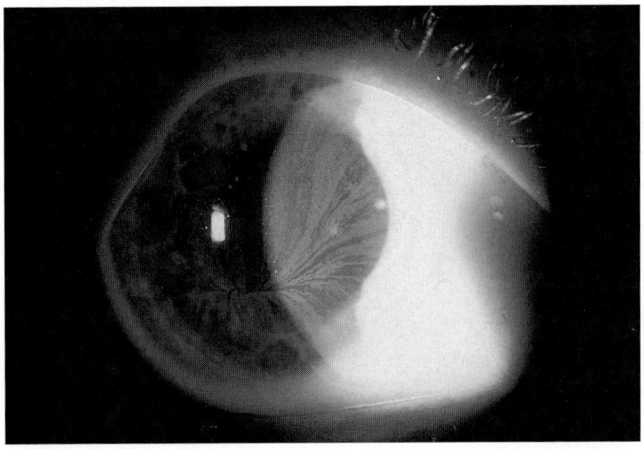

Fig. 5-5 Fabry's disease cornea verticillata. A fine tan-brown branching pattern is seen in the epithelium of this patient with Fabry's disease. It appears to originate from a point or a line in the inferior cornea and to spread superiorly and inferiorly from that location.

Although the cardiovascular and renal systems are primarily involved, Fabry's disease is a multisystem condition. Clinically, these patients present with cutaneous angiokeratomas (rough, hard-surfaced vascular papules) (Fig. 5-4), renal failure, painful peripheral neuropathy, cardiovascular disease, and neurologic abnormalities.

Ocular findings in patients with Fabry's disease are common and distinctive. Corneal involvement is typical and presents in the form of a verticillate keratopathy (also called *cornea verticillata*). Clinically, fine, brown, branching, linear epithelial opacities that seem to emanate from a common point, usually in the inferior paracentral cornea, are found (Fig. 5-5). These findings are usually apparent in the first decade of life in affected males, although they are also found in carrier females. These opacities do not generally affect visual acuity. Deposits are similar to those found in patients receiving chronic medications such as amiodarone, chloroquine, or indomethacin (Box 5-1). Other ocular findings include periorbital edema, tortuous conjunctival vessels with small aneurysms (Fig. 5-6), spokelike posterior cataracts,

Box 5-1 Differential Diagnosis of Cornea Verticillata

Fabry's disease
Amiodarone
Chloroquine
Hydroxychloroquine
Indomethacin
Phenothiazines
Atovaquone

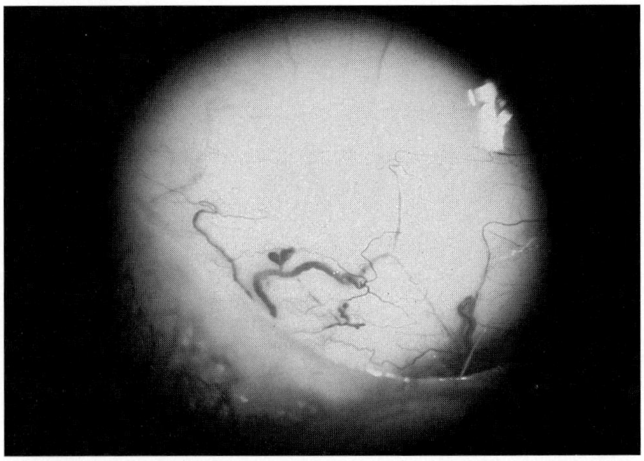

Fig. 5-6 Fabry's disease. Tortuous conjunctival vessels with small aneurysms are present in this patient with Fabry's disease.

optic nerve swelling, retinal vascular tortuosity, and optic atrophy.

Mucolipidoses Mucolipidoses are metabolic disorders in which both mucopolysaccharides and lipids accumulate, resulting in clinical features of both the mucopolysaccharidoses and the lipidoses (Box 5-2).

Mucopolysaccharides may accumulate in the cornea, whereas sphingolipids accumulate in the retina and the central nervous system. Corneal clouding, macular cherry-red spot, or optic atrophy may be features of several of these disorders.

Hyperlipoproteinemias Five categories of hyperlipoproteinemia may produce systemic disease, most notably premature coronary artery and peripheral vascular disease. Although nonspecific, the early onset of corneal arcus or xanthelasma may be associated with these conditions, and the presence of either should prompt further evaluation. Hyperlipoproteinemias are categorized by the primary lipoprotein elevated in the serum (Table 5-2).

Hypolipoproteinemias In addition to the hyperlipoproteinemias, several conditions resulting in hypolipoproteinemia may also produce corneal deposits or a cloudy cornea. Tangier disease is a rare autosomal recessive condition that causes enlarged tonsils, splenomegaly, hepatomegaly, peripheral neuropathy, and corneal clouding. Corneal findings include diffuse stromal clouding that increases with age, though small punctate opacities develop in the deeper stroma. Corneal arcus is absent.

Box 5-2 Mucolipidoses

- Mucolipidosis I type 1
- Mucolipidosis I type 2
- Mucolipidosis II
- Mucolipidosis III (pseudo-Hurler syndrome)
- Mucolipidosis IV (Berman's syndrome)
- Goldberg's syndrome
- Mannosidosis
- Fucosidosis

Lecithin-cholesterol acyltransferase (LCAT) deficiency is another rare condition affecting plasma lipoproteins that produces anemia and proteinuria. Ocular findings include diffuse stromal clouding with a peripheral annular opacity resembling corneal arcus.

Cystinosis Cystinosis is a rare autosomal recessive disease in which cystine accumulates in the bone marrow, lymph nodes, liver, and spleen because of a defective lysosomal transport system. Deposits are also found in the renal tubular cells, producing gradual renal failure. The disease appears in three different forms: infantile (nephropathic), adolescent (intermediate), and adult (benign). Ocular manifestations may be seen in all forms of this condition, and include diffuse cystine crystalline deposits throughout the cornea and conjunctiva. The corneal crystals are glistening and polychromatic, and are deposited in the stroma; the deposits are more dense peripherally than centrally (Figs. 5-7 and 5-8). The deposits may appear as early as 6 months of age, and can produce significant photophobia. Corneal sensation is typically decreased, and visual acuity is usually minimally affected. Intracellular crystals have also been found in the iris, lens, ciliary body, choroid, and retinal pigment epithelium. Ophthalmoscopic evaluation may reveal peripheral retinal degeneration and macular crystals.

Infantile (nephropathic) cystinosis presents in the first decade of life with Fanconi syndrome (renal tubular disease producing generalized aminoaciduria, renal glycosuria, and phosphaturia combining to produce hypophosphatemia), dwarfism, rickets, and renal failure requiring kidney transplantation. Ocular findings are most severe in the infantile form of the disease. Significant corneal opacity can develop in patients with this form of the disease as they live longer because of kidney transplantation.

Adolescent (intermediate) cystinosis is characterized by onset in the second decade of life and mild renal involvement. Ocular manifestations are somewhat milder than in the infantile form, and retinopathy is usually not found.

Adult (benign) cystinosis involves little or no renal disease, and ocular findings may therefore represent the

Table 5-2 Serum abnormalities and ocular findings in the hyperlipoproteinemias

Type	Serum elevation	Corneal arcus	Xanthelasma	Lipemia retinalis
1	Chylomicrons	–	+	+
2	Beta-lipoproteins and cholesterol	+	+	–
3	Triglycerides, cholesterol, beta-lipoproteins	+	+	+
4	Very low density lipoproteins, triglycerides	+	+	+
5	Chylomicrons, very low density lipoproteins	–	+	+

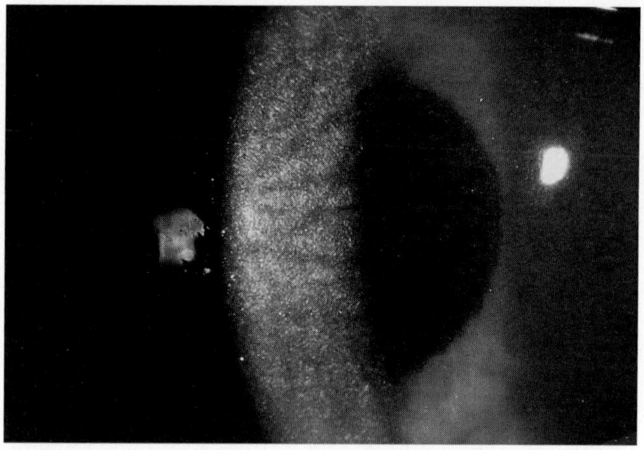

Fig. 5-7 Cystinosis. Myriad corneal crystals are present throughout the cornea of this patient with infantile cystinosis. He had previously undergone renal transplantation.

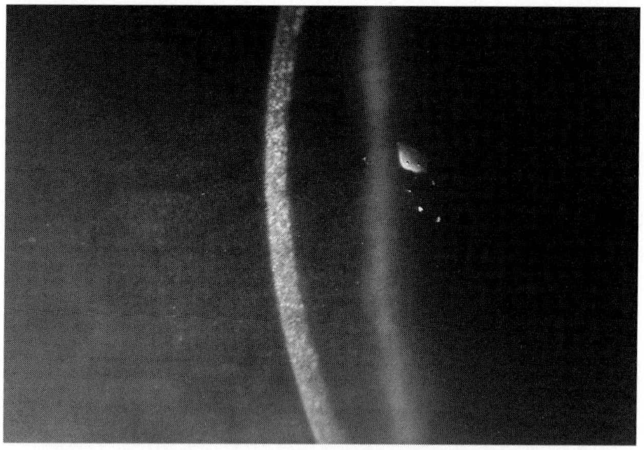

Fig. 5-8 Cystinosis. A slit-beam view of the eye seen in Fig. 5-7 demonstrates the crystals in all layers of the cornea.

only clinical manifestations of this form of the condition. Life expectancy is normal.

Cystinosis must be differentiated from other conditions associated with a "crystalline-like" corneal deposition, such as lattice dystrophy, multiple myeloma, and other monoclonal gammopathies (Box 5-3). The diagnosis of cystinosis may be confirmed by conjunctival biopsy, if necessary.

Because visual acuity is usually not significantly affected in the adult or adolescent forms of this condition, no treatment is necessary. Cysteamine eye drops have been used in the infantile form to clear the corneal crystals. Rarely, corneal transplantation may be required in adults with infantile cystinosis.

Diabetes mellitus In general, few corneal changes are caused by diabetes mellitus. However, decreased corneal sensation, punctate staining, and neurotrophic corneal ulcerations occur more frequently in persons with diabetes than in those without. Poor epithelial healing and persistent epithelial defects are not uncommon in patients with diabetes, especially after epithelial removal during vitrectomy. Regarding the cornea, patients with diabetes fare as well as those without it after cataract surgery and corneal transplantation.

Box 5-3 Differential Diagnosis of Corneal Crystals

Cystinosis
Schnyder's crystalline dystrophy
Multiple myeloma
Infectious crystalline keratopathy
Gout
Monoclonal gammopathies
Waldenström's macroglobulinemia
Cryoglobulinemia
Bietti's crystalline dystrophy
Lattice dystrophy
Avellino dystrophy

Wilson's Disease

Wilson's disease (hepatolenticular degeneration) is a rare autosomal recessive disorder resulting in a deficiency of ceruloplasmin (a serum copper-binding protein). As a result, copper is deposited throughout the body, especially in the liver, basal ganglia, kidneys, and eyes.

Clinically, patients with Wilson's disease present with ataxia, hepatosplenomegaly, cirrhosis, and progressive neurologic degeneration. Ocular abnormalities result from copper deposits in the basement membranes and include the classic Kayser-Fleischer ring (brown-gold to green copper deposits in peripheral Descemet's membrane) (Fig. 5-9) and a "sunflower" cataract. Early Kayser-Fleischer rings may only be visible gonioscopically. Other rare causes of copper deposits in the cornea include a retained copper intraocular foreign body, primary biliary cirrhosis, chronic active hepatitis, intrahepatic cholestasis of childhood, and multiple myeloma or lung tumors involving copper transport proteins.

The diagnosis of Wilson's disease may be suspected clinically by the constellation of hepatic and neurologic findings, and can be confirmed by demonstrating a depression or absence of serum ceruloplasmin, increased urinary copper excretion, or the presence of a Kayser-Fleischer ring. If left untreated, this condition can be fatal. Treatment with copper chelating agents such as penicillamine can significantly improve the prognosis and lead to the elimination of the Kayser-Fleischer ring.

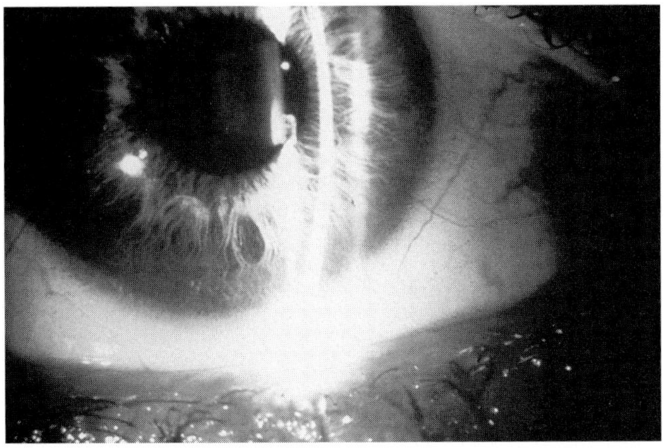

Fig. 5-9 Wilson's disease and Kayser-Fleischer ring. A tan-brown ring is seen in the corneal periphery of this patient with Wilson's disease. The slit beam highlights its deep location. (See color plate.)

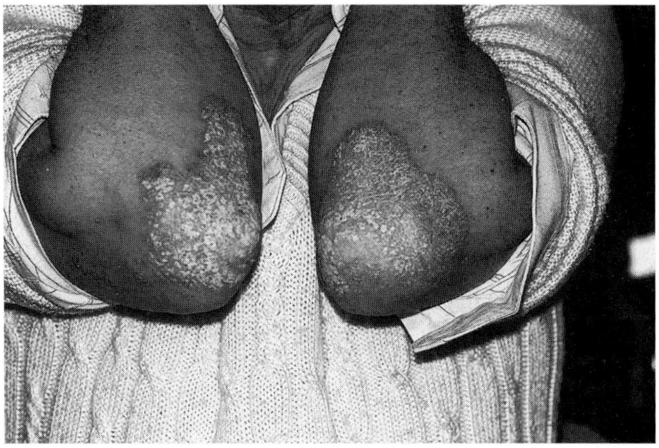

Fig. 5-11 Psoriasis. Scaly erythematous plaques are seen on the elbows of this patient with psoriasis. (Courtesy of Ira J. Udell, M.D.)

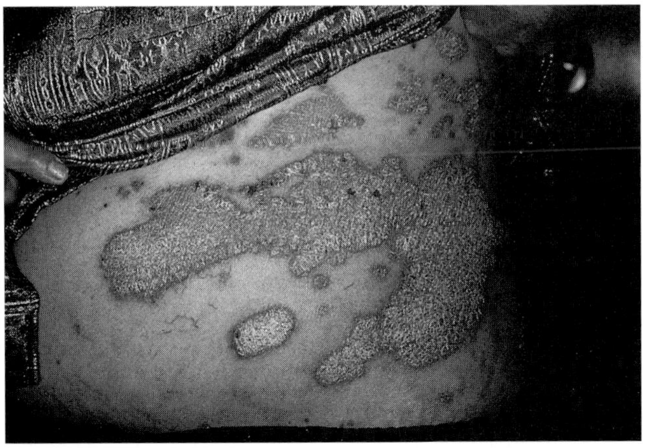

Fig. 5-10 Psoriasis. Multiple well-demarcated, silvery, scaly plaques are present on the trunk of this patient with psoriasis. (Courtesy of Guy F. Webster, M.D., Ph.D.)

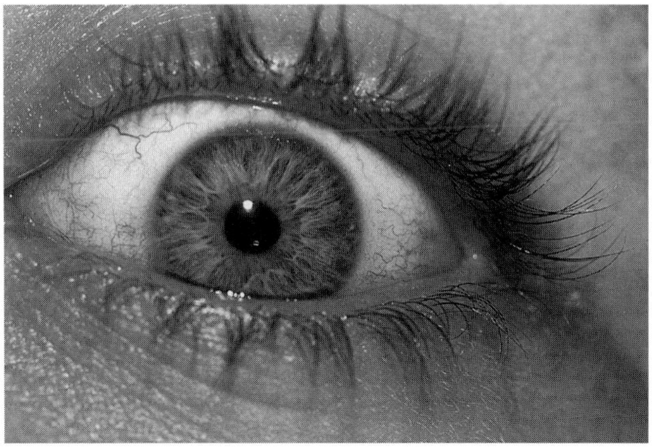

Fig. 5-12 Psoriasis. Scaly psoriatic plaques are present in the lateral canthal region and on the lower eyelid.

Dermatologic Diseases

Psoriasis Psoriasis vulgaris is a common, relapsing skin disease characterized by erythematous and scaly plaques on the skin and occasionally associated with nail and joint involvement. It may affect as much as 3% of the population.

Psoriasis appears in several different forms, all of which share classic skin lesions consisting of well-demarcated, erythematous plaques with silvery scales on the surface (Fig. 5-10). The elbows, knees, and sacrum are most commonly affected, though any area of the body can be involved (Fig. 5-11). Facial lesions are uncommon, but ophthalmic manifestations may be found in as many as 10% of patients.

Ocular manifestations of psoriasis can involve the eyelids, conjunctiva, cornea, and uveal tract. Eyelid findings include psoriatic eyelid plaques and blepharitis (Fig. 5-12). Conjunctival manifestations include injection, primary psoriatic lesions that appear as yellowish conjunctival plaques, or limbal conjunctival nodules (Fig. 5-13). Keratoconjunctivitis sicca has developed in more than 15% of patients with psoriasis. Reported corneal findings are hypertrophic, dysplastic-appearing epithelial lesions, peripheral corneal infiltrates, and superficial vascularization (Fig. 5-14). Iritis is a well-described association with psoriasis, which is more common in patients with psoriatic arthritis.

Treatment modalities for the skin lesions include topical corticosteroids, and tars, as well as systemic therapy

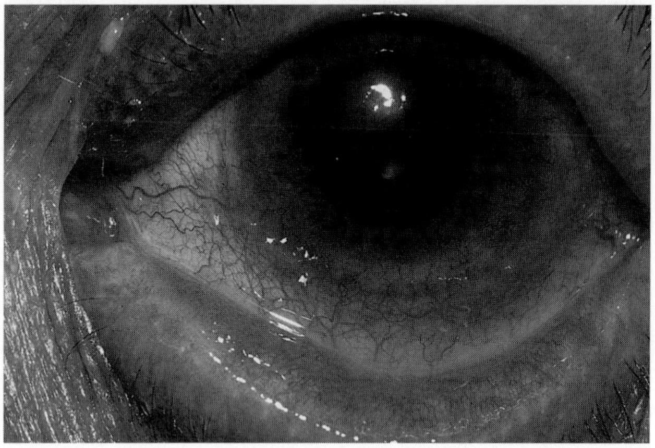

Fig. 5-13 Psoriasis. Moderate conjunctival injection with limbal nodules is seen in this patient with psoriasis.

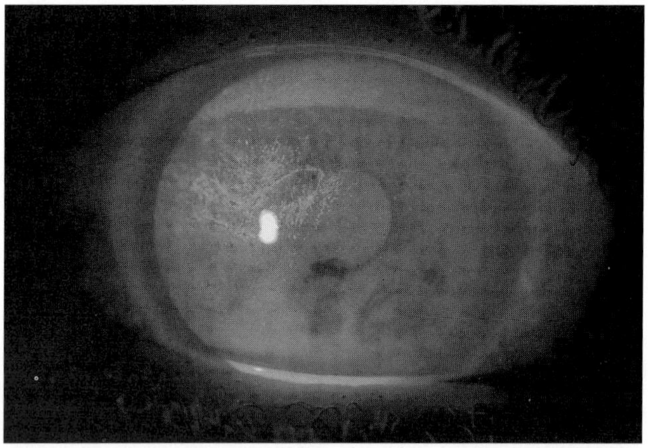

Fig. 5-14 Psoriasis. Epithelial irregularity and superficial staining are highlighted with fluorescein dye and cobalt blue filter in this patient with psoriasis. (See color plate.)

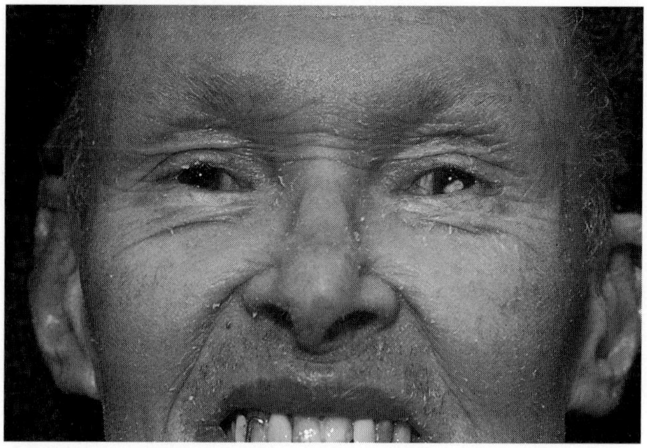

Fig. 5-15 Ichthyosis. Fine powdery scales appear on the entire body of this patient with ichthyosis vulgaris. A corneal ulcer in the left eye left a dense scar.

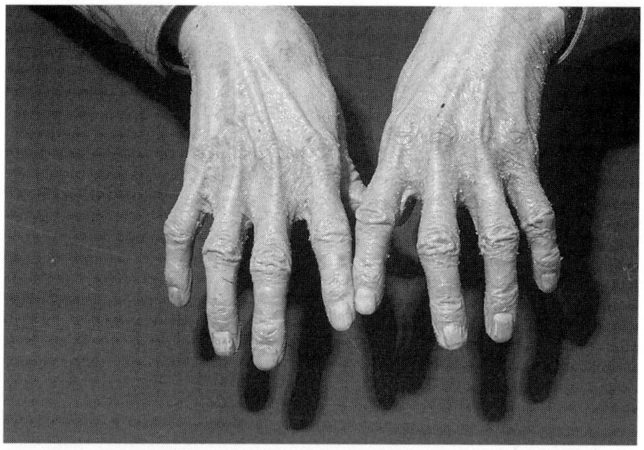

Fig. 5-16 Ichthyosis. Fine powdery scales seen on the hands of the patient in Fig. 5-15.

with oral retinoids, immunosuppressives, and psoralen/ultraviolet light therapy known as PUVA therapy. Care must be taken to protect the eyes during PUVA therapy to guard against cataract formation. Most of the inflammatory ocular conditions respond to topical corticosteroids, and the sicca symptoms respond to artificial tears and lubricating ointments.

Ichthyosis Ichthyosis is a term used to refer to a group of inherited dermatologic disorders that produce scaling of the skin. The four major clinical entities in this category are ichthyosis vulgaris (autosomal dominant), X-linked recessive ichthyosis, lamellar ichthyosis (autosomal recessive), and epidermolytic hyperkeratosis (autosomal dominant).

Ichthyosis vulgaris, the most common form of these disorders, typically produces fine, powdery scales on the trunk and extensor surfaces that initially appear in the first decade (Figs. 5-15 and 5-16). An association with atopy has been noted. Ocular involvement is usually limited to scales on the eyelids and eyelashes (Fig. 5-17).

X-linked recessive ichthyosis produces darker, more prominent scales than ichthyosis vulgaris that cover most of the body (Fig. 5-18). Scales are usually apparent at birth or shortly thereafter. Ocular findings include multiple tiny, punctate, gray-white opacities in the posterior part of the corneal stroma that are also found in female carriers (Fig. 5-19).

Lamellar ichthyosis produces severe, coarse, polygonal scales throughout the body. It is usually apparent at birth. Eyelid involvement can produce secondary ectropion and lagophthalmos because of the tautness of the involved eyelid skin. Secondary conjunctival changes caused by exposure may include hyperemia, thickening, and keratinization. The resultant chronic corneal exposure can produce exposure keratopathy, scarring, ulceration, and neovascularization.

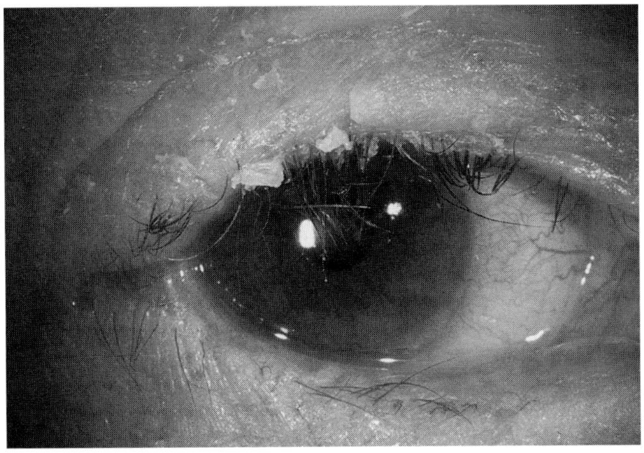

Fig. 5-17 Ichthyosis. The right eye of the patient seen in Figs. 5-15 and 5-16 develops extensive crusting and flaking of the eyelid skin.

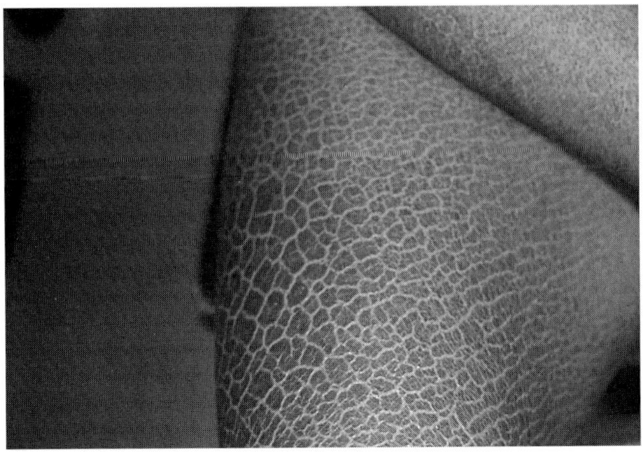

Fig. 5-18 Ichthyosis. Dark polygonal scales are present on the leg of this patient with X-linked recessive ichthyosis.

Epidermolytic hyperkeratosis produces a blistered, erythematous appearance to the skin at birth, which then becomes covered with coarse scales. Ocular involvement is usually limited to scales on the eyelids and eyelashes.

Incontinentia pigmenti Incontinentia pigmenti is an X-linked dominant disorder that affects multiple systems throughout the body. It is seen primarily in females because of the high incidence of lethality in affected male embryos. Clinically it may present with dermatologic, dental, ophthalmologic, and occasionally neurologic abnormalities.

Infants with this disorder have vesiculobullous lesions on the skin during the first weeks of life. This manifestation evolves into a verrucous stage that is followed by the formation of hyperpigmented, irregular lesions on the torso and extremities.

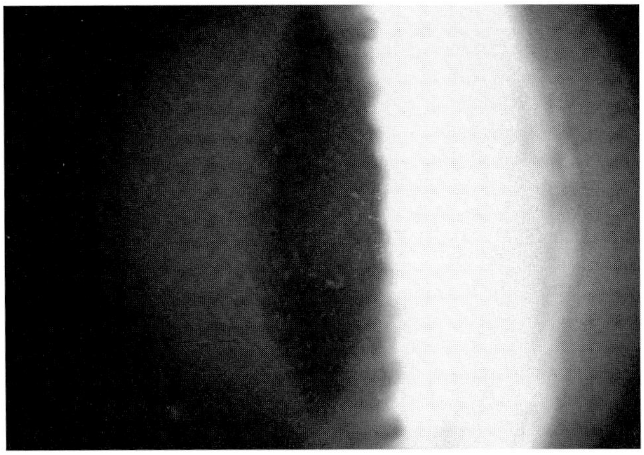

Fig. 5-19 Ichthyosis. Tiny gray-white opacities in the posterior cornea are seen in this patient with X-linked recessive ichthyosis.

Ocular manifestations of incontinentia pigmenti include focal conjunctival hyperpigmentation, rare corneal opacities, microphthalmos, cataracts, strabismus, and peripheral retinal vascular abnormalities with ischemia and neovascularization.

Multiple Myeloma

Multiple myeloma is a malignant neoplasm of plasma cells resulting in their monoclonal proliferation and the secretion of excessive immunoglobulin. Excessive monoclonal immunoglobulin secretion is responsible for the typical protein spike demonstrated on serum protein electrophoresis (SPEP) studies in these patients.

Ophthalmic manifestations are usually secondary to immunoglobulin deposits or hyperviscosity and may involve the conjunctiva, cornea, uveal tract, retina, optic nerve, and orbit. Conjunctival findings include a sludging of red blood cells in the conjunctival vasculature because of hyperviscosity and crystalline deposits. Corneal involvement can include a fine, scintillating, crystalline deposition of immunoglobulins. The crystals are deposited throughout the stroma; the deposits are usually heaviest peripherally and are occasionally the first manifestation of the disease (Fig. 5-20). They may gain access to the cornea through the limbal vasculature or the tear film. Noncrystalline epithelial deposits of immunoglobulins presenting as gray-white or translucent opacities have also been described. Hypercalcemia associated with multiple myeloma may produce band keratopathy. Copper deposits in Descemet's membrane and crystalline deposits in the lens have also been reported. Uveal involvement can take the form of pars plana cysts filled with myeloma proteins (these cysts turn white after fixation in formalin) or choroidal masses.

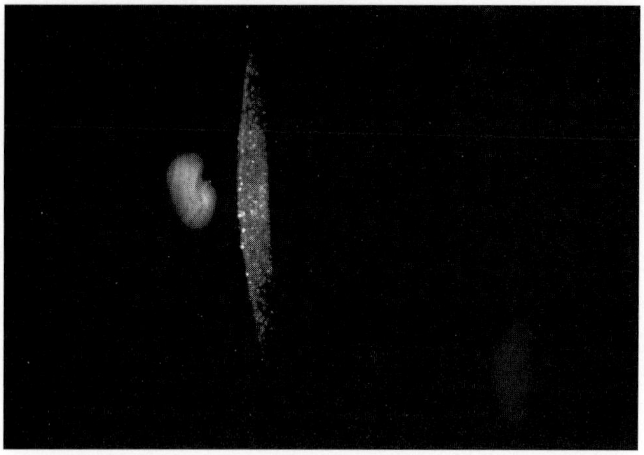

Fig. 5-20 Multiple myeloma. Slit-beam examination demonstrates the crystalline deposition of immunoglobulins throughout the cornea of this patient with multiple myeloma.

Box 5-4 Major Ocular Findings in Graves' Disease

No symptoms
Eyelid
- Eyelid retraction
- Lagophthalmos (especially nocturnal)

Conjunctiva
- Injection
- Chemosis

Cornea
- Superficial punctate keratopathy
- Exposure keratopathy
- Corneal ulceration

Orbit
- Proptosis
- Motility limitation
- Strabismus
- Compressive optic neuropathy

THYROID OPHTHALMOPATHY

Thyroid ophthalmopathy refers to a constellation of ocular signs and symptoms frequently encountered in patients with Graves' disease. Graves' disease is a specific form of hyperthyroidism caused by autoantibodies that stimulate thyroid function (thyroid-stimulating immunoglobulin). Although eye abnormalities may be found in hyperthyroidism not caused by Graves' disease, Graves' disease accounts for most cases of thyroid ophthalmopathy.

Clinically, Graves' disease is a combination of hyperthyroidism, diffuse goiter, and ophthalmopathy. Classic symptoms of hyperthyroidism, such as weight loss, palpitations, nervousness, and diarrhea, may accompany these findings, and the diagnosis can usually be confirmed by thyroid function tests. However, it is important to note that although most patients will present with abnormal thyroid function test results consistent with hyperthyroidism, occasionally patients may be euthyroid at presentation. Furthermore, patients who undergo treatment for Graves' disease and are rendered euthyroid or even hypothyroid are still at risk for the development of thyroid ophthalmopathy.

Ocular manifestations of Graves' disease are largely caused by the enlargement of the extraocular muscles that accompanies this condition (Box 5-4). The pathogenesis of this enlargement is unclear, but it seems to be related to the effects of autoantibodies directed against the antigens in extraocular muscles. The stages of thyroid ophthalmopathy have several different classifications. One of the best-known classification systems was developed by Werner, and it uses the acronym *"NOSPECS"* to represent six stages of the disorder. It is important to note, however, that not all findings develop in all patients and that the stages need not present in succession. Initially patients may present with **no** signs or symptoms of thyroid ophthalmopathy or only **s**igns of eyelid retraction or eyelid lag in downgaze, with or without any symptoms. Other eye findings include **p**roptosis, **e**xtraocular muscle involvement producing motility limitation or diplopia, **c**orneal exposure, and **s**ight loss resulting from compressive optic neuropathy.

Corneal and anterior segment findings are largely related to eyelid retraction, proptosis, or both. Eyelid retraction in primary gaze can produce the classic thyroid "stare" and may contribute to an inadequate eyelid excursion with each blink. This eyelid retraction can produce poor tear film spread over the cornea, usually greatest inferiorly. Examination reveals increased scleral show above and below the limbus, often accompanied by punctate fluorescein or rose bengal staining of the inferior cornea. Nocturnal lagophthalmos frequently accompanies this finding, producing chronic exposure keratopathy. Concomitant proptosis caused by extraocular muscle enlargement can significantly aggravate this process. Patients may have a dry, gritty, or foreign body sensation, burning, photophobia, redness, and tearing that are worse in the morning. If left untreated, chronic exposure can result in corneal opacification or ulceration and vision loss.

Initial treatment of the anterior segment findings includes frequent lubrication with preservative-free artificial tears during the day and lubricating ointment at night. If no significant improvement results or the keratopathy worsens, lateral tarsorrhaphy or upper eyelid-lowering procedures may be considered. Orbital decompression, systemic corticosteroids (acutely), or radiation therapy can be considered for patients with chronic exposure keratopathy associated with proptosis, or patients with diplopia or optic nerve compression. Systemic therapy for the underlying thyroid disease should be coordinated with the patient's internist or endocrinologist.

HUMAN IMMUNODEFICIENCY VIRUS

Acquired immunodeficiency syndrome (AIDS) is caused by human immunodeficiency virus (HIV) type 1 and has been recognized as a clinical entity since 1981. Initial infection may produce a nonspecific viral syndrome that is followed by a symptom-free period, which may last 10 years or longer. During this period CD4+ T-cell counts fall until constitutional symptoms and eventually opportunistic infections arise.

HIV has been demonstrated in the tear film, cornea, and conjunctiva, and therefore concerns are valid about possible disease transmission during office examination and during corneal transplantation. Tonometer tips are adequately disinfected by wiping them with 70% isopropyl alcohol and then air drying them, and trial contact lenses are adequately disinfected by chemical systems. No cases have been reported of HIV transmission through the office practice of ophthalmology. Potential corneal donors are screened thoroughly for the risk factors for HIV, and the blood of the donor is tested for HIV antibodies before transplantation. Although it is theoretically possible for a donor who has not yet undergone seroconversion to pass undetected through the screening process, no cases have been documented of HIV transmission through corneal transplantation.

Ocular manifestations of HIV infection are largely related to the many opportunistic infections and neoplasms that may arise as immune function deteriorates (Box 5-5). However, HIV retinopathy (cotton wool spots, blot hemorrhages, white-centered hemorrhages, or perivasculitis in a patient with HIV) and keratoconjunctivitis sicca are probably caused by HIV itself. Cytomegalovirus infection is the most prevalent intraocular opportunistic infection associated with AIDS, and it generally appears with posterior segment findings. Opportunistic infections and neoplasms may affect every ocular structure, from the eyelids to the optic nerve.

The most common anterior segment complication of HIV infection is caused by the herpes zoster virus (HZV). Herpes zoster ophthalmicus may develop in as many as 4% of patients with AIDS, and it has been suggested that it is an indicator of possible underlying HIV infection if it appears in young, otherwise healthy patients. It has also been shown to be predictive of an increased risk for clinical AIDS in patients with HIV. The spectrum of eye findings related to herpes zoster infection in patients with HIV is similar to that in immunocompetent patients and is discussed in detail in Chapter 4. However, the external disease and the ocular manifestations of herpes zoster infection may be atypical or prolonged in patients with AIDS who are significantly immunocompromised. Severe complications such as disseminated HZV infection, acute retinal necrosis or progressive outer retinal necrosis, and cerebral arteritis are more common in HIV-positive patients.

Box 5-5 Major Anterior Segment Complications of Human Immunodeficiency Virus (HIV) Infection

PRIMARY

Keratoconjunctivitis sicca

SECONDARY

Herpes zoster virus
Herpes simplex virus
Bacterial and fungal keratitis
Microsporidia
Molluscum contagiosum
Kaposi's sarcoma

Systemic antiviral therapy with acyclovir, famciclovir, or valacyclovir is used to treat acute herpes zoster infections in patients with HIV infection. Severe or disseminated HZV infections may require intravenous antiviral administration, and prolonged therapy is often necessary. Systemic corticosteroids should be avoided (if possible) in these patients because of their already immunocompromised states and the possibility for the potentiation of other ocular or systemic opportunistic infections. Pseudodendritic, stromal, or neurotrophic keratitis and iritis are treated as they are in immunocompetent patients (see Chapter 4).

Ocular herpes simplex virus (HSV) infections develop in patients with HIV with approximately the same frequency as in patients without HIV. As with herpes zoster, atypical presentations or prolonged infections may be found in these patients, and therefore prolonged therapy is often required. Interestingly, immune-mediated HSV stromal keratitis is less frequent in these patients, perhaps because of the T-cell depletion and dysfunction that accompany HIV infection. Treatment is similar to that for immunocompetent patients (see Chapter 4).

Microsporidiosis is another opportunistic infection that develops in patients with AIDS, and it may cause chronic diarrhea in as many as 30% of patients in the advanced stages of AIDS. The ophthalmic manifestations of microsporidiosis appear in two forms: stromal keratitis (usually found in patients without HIV) or chronic keratoconjunctivitis associated with diffuse, coarse, punc-

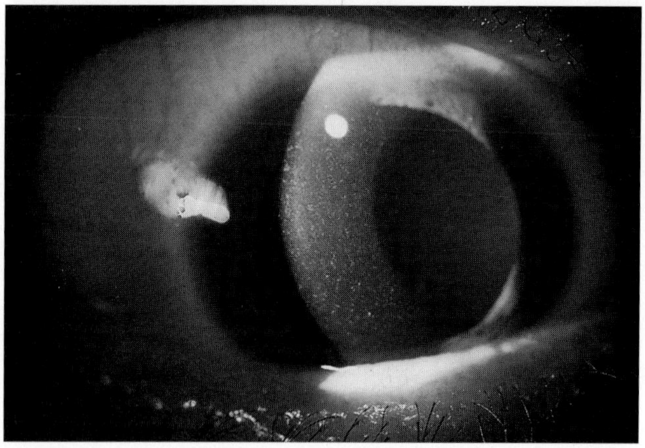

Fig. 5-21 Microsporidiosis. Diffuse punctate epithelial keratitis is seen in this patient with microsporidiosis.

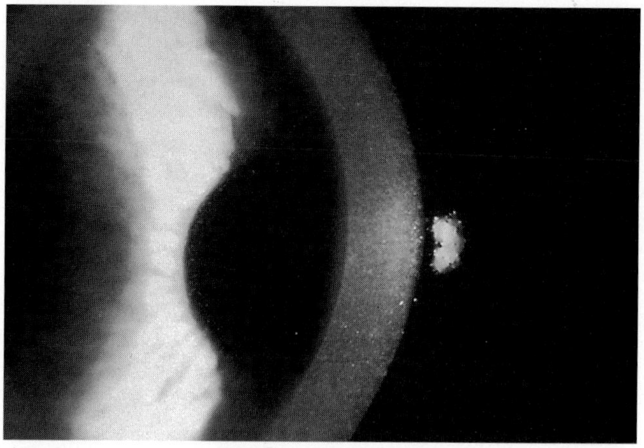

Fig. 5-22 Microsporidiosis. The diffuse epithelial lesions are highlighted using retroillumination off the iris, seen best at the edge of the pupil. (Courtesy of Gaurav Shah, M.D.)

tate corneal epitheliopathy (usually seen in patients with HIV). The chronic conjunctivitis and epithelial keratitis seen in patients with AIDS appears as bilateral, diffuse, coarse, elevated punctate epithelial keratopathy that stains with fluorescein (Figs. 5-21 and 5-22). An associated conjunctival injection and occasionally a mild conjunctival papillary reaction develop. Vision may be diminished, and patients have pain, photophobia, and tearing. The diagnosis may be confirmed by the demonstration of intracellular organisms on Gram or Giemsa staining of a scraping of the conjunctiva or cornea (Fig. 5-23). Several different agents have been used to treat this infection with variable or poor results, among them topical metronidazole, thiabendazole, propamidine, oral itraconazole, and albendazole. Fumagillin (Fumadil B), used to treat microsporidian disease in honeybees, has been found recently to be a moderately effective treatment when used topically in concentrations ranging from 3 to 10 mg/ml. The disease may recur, however, when treatment discontinues. The best treatment is improvement in the patient's immune status.

Bacterial and fungal infections of the cornea can also occur in AIDS patients, and are often secondary to ocular surface disease from herpes simplex or zoster keratitis, HIV-associated keratoconjunctivitis sicca, or radiation therapy for localized neoplasms such as Kaposi's sarcoma. These infections may be severe and fulminant, and they often require prolonged intensive therapy.

Molluscum contagiosum is also seen in patients with AIDS. It is caused by a poxvirus that produces round, umbilicated lesions on the skin of the eyelids or face. These lesions are usually painless, but if they develop on the eyelids, they can produce chronic follicular conjunctivitis caused by a toxic reaction to viral shedding into the tear film. This condition is discussed in detail in Chapter 1. In immunocompetent patients, infection usually results in 10 or fewer lesions on the face. In patients with AIDS, numerous lesions, many of them larger than normal, may appear on the face and eyelids, and the conjunctival follicular reaction may be absent. Molluscum lesions usually resolve spontaneously in several months in immunocompetent patients (though new lesions may develop), but their duration may be prolonged or they may recur in patients with AIDS. The greater number of lesions makes eradication by excision difficult.

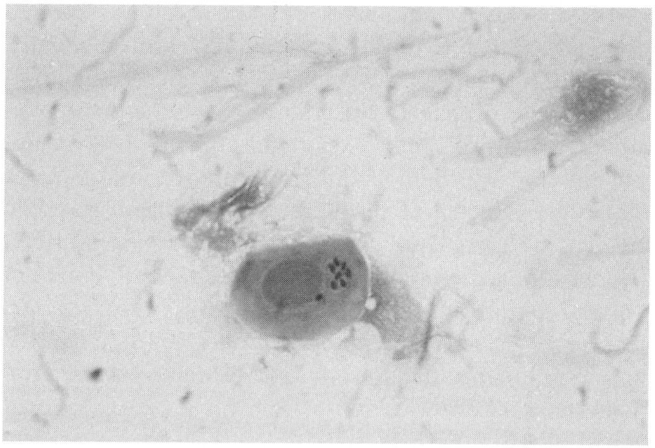

Fig. 5-23 Microsporidiosis. Gram stain of an epithelial scraping reveals multiple gram-positive organisms within the epithelial cells, consistent with microsporidiosis. (See color plate.)

Kaposi's sarcoma is the most common AIDS-related neoplasm of the eye and has been reported in as many as 2% of patients with AIDS. It usually develops on the eyelids or conjunctiva as a slow-growing red or violaceous lesion (Figs. 5-24 and 5-25), and it is often confused with subconjunctival hemorrhage. Although the treatment of systemic Kaposi's sarcoma lesions is chemotherapy, eyelid or conjunctival lesions do not necessarily require any therapy if they do not obstruct vision. Lesions that obscure vision may be treated with local excision, cryotherapy, radiation therapy, or systemic chemotherapy.

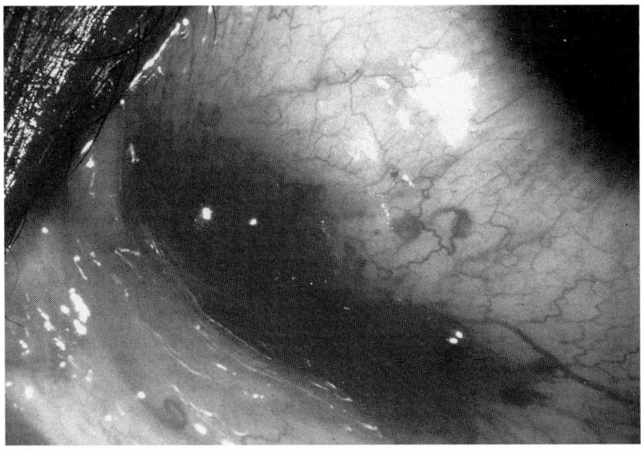

Fig. 5-24 Kaposi's sarcoma. A deep red conjunctival mass is present in the inferior fornix of this patient with HIV. Kaposi's sarcoma may be misdiagnosed as subconjunctival hemorrhage. (See color plate.)

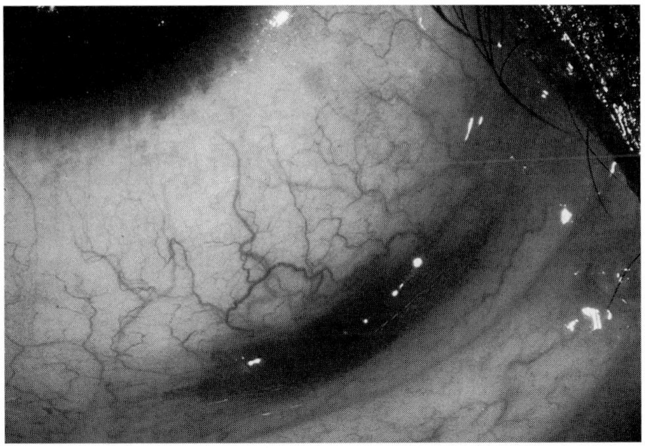

Fig. 5-25 Kaposi's sarcoma. The fellow eye of the patient seen in Fig. 5-24 has a smaller Kaposi's sarcoma lesion in the inferior fornix.

The most common posterior segment opportunistic infection in patients with AIDS is cytomegalovirus (CMV). One of the herpesviruses, CMV classically produces hemorrhagic, necrotizing retinitis in immunocompromised patients. It may develop in at least 20% of patients with AIDS, but it is a late event in the course of HIV infection, usually occurring after CD4+ T-cell counts fall below 50 cells/μl. Anterior segment findings are few, but the virus has been isolated from the conjunctiva. Diffuse, fine, stellate, corneal endothelial deposits consisting of fibrin and macrophages may be seen in patients with CMV retinitis and, more recently, in patients with HIV but without CMV retinitis. This finding may be medication related.

Ocular toxoplasmosis, herpes zoster retinitis in the form of either acute retinal necrosis or progressive outer retinal necrosis, fungal chorioretinitis, syphilitic retinitis, tuberculous chorioretinitis, and *Pneumocystis* choroiditis are other posterior segment opportunistic infections associated with HIV infection and are discussed elsewhere in this series.

CORNEAL DISEASE IN COLLAGEN VASCULAR DISORDERS

Rheumatoid Arthritis

Rheumatoid arthritis is a common, chronic, systemic, autoimmune disease that produces symmetric, erosive, and deforming polyarthritis. It affects approximately 1% of the population and is more common in women than in men. Any joint may be affected, but the metacarpophalangeal and interphalangeal joints are most commonly involved. In advanced cases, ligamentous changes associated with arthritis can result in joint subluxation and angulation, producing the characteristic "swan neck" deformity of the digits. Larger joints such as the wrists, shoulders, or knees may also be affected. In addition to these findings, numerous extraarticular inflammatory manifestations involve multiple organ systems and affect as many as 25% of patients with rheumatoid arthritis. Although rheumatoid arthritis is thought to be an autoimmune condition, the exact inciting stimulus for the immunologic response remains unknown. Genetic susceptibility and exogenous stimuli such as infectious agents have been implicated.

Ocular manifestations of rheumatoid arthritis most frequently affect the anterior segment; they include keratoconjunctivitis sicca, episcleritis, scleritis, sclerosing keratitis, stromal keratitis, paracentral keratolysis, peripheral ulcerative keratitis, and limbal furrowing (Box 5-6). Posterior segment findings are less frequent and include posterior scleritis, choroidal effusion, and retinal vasculitis.

The most common ocular manifestation of rheumatoid arthritis is keratoconjunctivitis sicca, which may affect as many as 25% of patients with rheumatoid arthritis. When keratoconjunctivitis sicca appears with xerostomia and an autoimmune disease such as rheumatoid arthritis, it is referred to as secondary Sjögren's syndrome. Autoimmune involvement of the lacrimal glands produces an aqueous tear deficiency resulting in dry eye syndrome. Clinically, patients may present with a foreign body sensation, burning, mucous discharge, pain, and photophobia. Examination may reveal a thick accumulation of mucus, superficial punctate keratopathy, or filamentous keratopathy (Fig. 5-26). Sjögren's syndrome (Fig. 5-27) and aqueous tear deficiency are discussed in detail in Chapter 4.

Episcleritis either alone or associated with an underlying scleritis is also seen in patients with rheumatoid arthritis. It can present in simple or nodular forms, and

Box 5-6 Major Anterior Segment Manifestations of Rheumatoid Arthritis

CORNEA
- Keratoconjunctivitis sicca
- Sclerosing keratitis
- Stromal keratitis
- Peripheral ulcerative keratitis (marginal keratolysis)
- Paracentral keratolysis
- Limbal guttering

EPISCLERA
- Episcleritis
  - Simple
  - Nodular

SCLERA
- Scleritis
  - Diffuse
  - Nodular
  - Necrotizing with inflammation
  - Necrotizing without inflammation (scleromalacia perforans)
  - Posterior

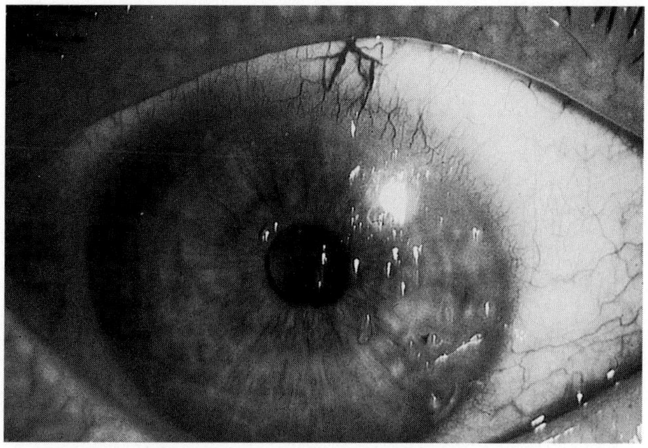

Fig. 5-26 Rheumatoid arthritis. Multiple corneal filaments are present in this patient with severe dry eye syndrome and rheumatoid arthritis.

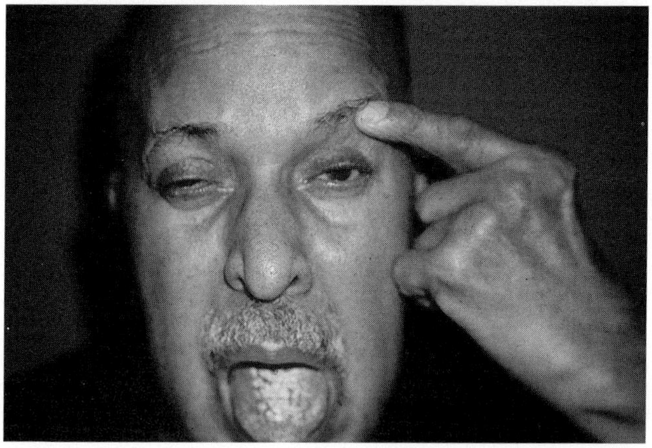

Fig. 5-27 Sjögren's syndrome. This patient with Sjögren's syndrome has severe dry eyes, dry mouth, and rheumatoid arthritis, as seen in his hands.

clinically it appears as injection of the radial episcleral vasculature. It is usually accompanied by mild pain and tenderness, though it may be painless. Affected areas blanch after the application of topical phenylephrine, thus helping to distinguish episcleritis from scleritis. Episcleritis and scleritis are discussed in greater detail in Chapter 6.

Scleritis is the next most common ocular manifestation of rheumatoid arthritis after keratoconjunctivitis sicca, and its presence may have serious implications regarding the systemic course of the disease. Scleritis can present in an anterior form or a posterior form and it is reported in approximately 6% of patients with rheumatoid arthritis. Anterior scleritis can present in either a diffuse (most common form), nodular, or necrotizing form. Although other systemic autoimmune or infectious conditions can also produce scleritis, rheumatoid arthritis is the most common underlying cause. Clinically, patients present with a deep, boring pain that may radiate through the orbit or to the temple and jaw. Examination reveals diffuse scleral injection and swelling (diffuse form) or localized tender nodules of scleral inflammation (nodular form) (Fig. 5-28). The involved areas have a violaceous hue (seen best by gross inspection in natural light) and are associated with overlying conjunctival and episcleral injection. It is often difficult to distinguish between episcleritis and scleritis. Patients with scleritis tend to have more severe pain, and the involved areas do not blanch well with topical phenylephrine.

Necrotizing anterior scleritis is the least common form of anterior scleritis, and it may occur with or without inflammation. Necrotizing anterior scleritis *with* inflammation typically presents with intense scleritis and severe pain. Involved areas exhibit signs of scleral necrosis, usually with an overlying conjunctival epithelial defect. Choroidal pigment may become apparent as the sclera thins. The presence of necrotizing anterior scleritis with inflammation is an ominous sign. As many as 40% to 60% of these patients can lose vision, and clinically it is an indicator for life-threatening systemic complications. Without adequate systemic immunosuppression, 30% to 50% or more of these patients may die within 5 to 10 years of the onset of scleritis because of complications related to severe systemic vasculitis.

Necrotizing anterior scleritis *without* inflammation is termed *scleromalacia perforans*. It is found in patients who have had long-standing, severe rheumatoid arthritis.

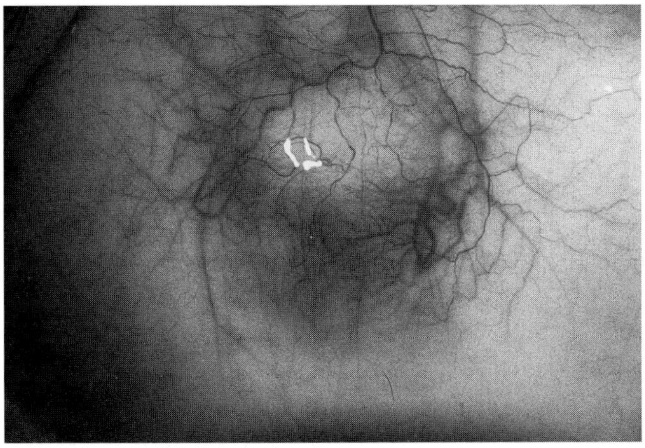

Fig. 5-28 Rheumatoid arthritis. Nodular scleritis is present superiorly. Several areas of gray sclera indicate previous episodes of scleritis.

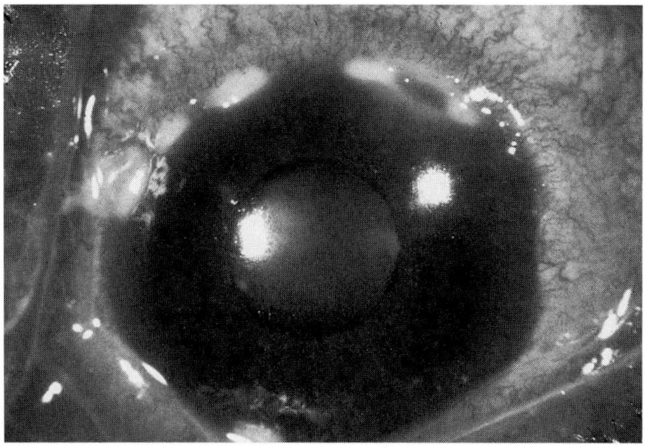

Fig. 5-29 Rheumatoid arthritis. Multiple dense, peripheral corneal infiltrates are seen in this patient with rheumatoid arthritis. The lesion at the 1 o'clock position is ulcerated and shows significant corneal thinning.

Clinically, it presents as painless necrotic scleral lesions in a relatively quiet eye. These active lesions generally produce no notable ocular inflammation or discomfort, and they result in areas of extensive scleral thinning, often with visible or protruding underlying choroid. Perforation rarely occurs. Patients may seek treatment for a newly noted discoloration on the eye or because of blurred vision secondary to induced astigmatism.

Corneal manifestations of rheumatoid arthritis are also seen, either with scleritis or as isolated findings. These changes may be categorized as nonulcerative and ulcerative. Nonulcerative corneal manifestations include sclerosing keratitis and acute stromal keratitis, whereas ulcerative manifestations include peripheral ulcerative keratitis (marginal keratolysis), paracentral keratolysis, and limbal guttering (terminology may vary between texts). Sclerosing keratitis is a frequent corneal finding associated with scleritis that clinically presents as peripheral corneal thickening and opacification adjacent to an area of active scleritis. It may progress centrally into the cornea and become vascularized. Long-term sequelae of untreated sclerosing keratitis include corneal scarring and lipid deposition. Stromal keratitis is another corneal manifestation of rheumatoid arthritis which presents with peripheral stromal infiltrates and edema with an intact epithelium, usually associated with scleritis. Untreated, these infiltrates may coalesce and produce epithelial breakdown and stromal melting, resembling peripheral ulcerative keratitis, vascularization, and scarring.

Peripheral ulcerative keratitis is characterized by corneal ulceration that can occur in isolation or in association with necrotizing scleritis. Clinically, the ulcer appears as an area of peripheral infiltration and thinning with an epithelial defect (Fig. 5-29), which may extend circumferentially and progress centrally. Associated limbal and conjunctival injection often develops. If left untreated, these lesions can progressively thin to descemetocele formation or perforation (Figs. 5-30 and 5-31). Limbal guttering is a similar condition and produces peripheral corneal thinning, usually with an intact epithelium and variable degrees of thinning.

Paracentral keratolysis is characterized by acute, severe paracentral corneal ulceration (often without a significant infiltrate) and melting that usually occurs with associated necrotizing scleritis, keratoconjunctivitis sicca, or both. The lesions typically involve previously clear cornea and may rapidly progress to descemetocele formation and perforation.

It is important to note that all of the above findings are not unique to rheumatoid arthritis, and may be found in other collagen vascular diseases. Their presence should alert the clinician to the possibility of underlying systemic autoimmune disease. If an underlying disease is not known, a systemic workup should be initiated.

Treatment of the ocular manifestations of rheumatoid arthritis varies according to the specific condition. Keratoconjunctivitis sicca may be treated initially with preservative-free artificial tears and tear ointments. Punctal occlusion, moisture shields, moisture chambers, and lateral tarsorrhaphy are helpful adjuncts. Adequate and aggressive treatment of dry eye is essential, especially if associated inflammatory complications such as necrotizing scleritis or corneal ulceration develop. When treatment is required, episcleritis may respond to topical or systemic nonsteroidal antiinflammatory drugs (NSAIDs), or to topical or systemic corticosteroids.

The treatment of scleritis, in contrast, is not straightforward. In general, topical therapy is ineffective for scleritis, and systemic therapy is necessary. Oral NSAIDs such as ibuprofen, naproxen, or indomethacin may be effective in mild or moderate cases, though more severe

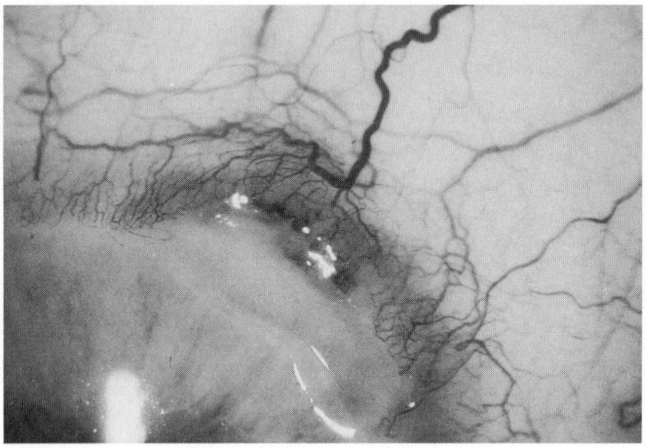

Fig. 5-30 Rheumatoid arthritis. Peripheral ulcerative keratitis adjacent to an area of conjunctival and scleral inflammation is present superiorly. Moderate corneal ulceration and thinning have occurred.

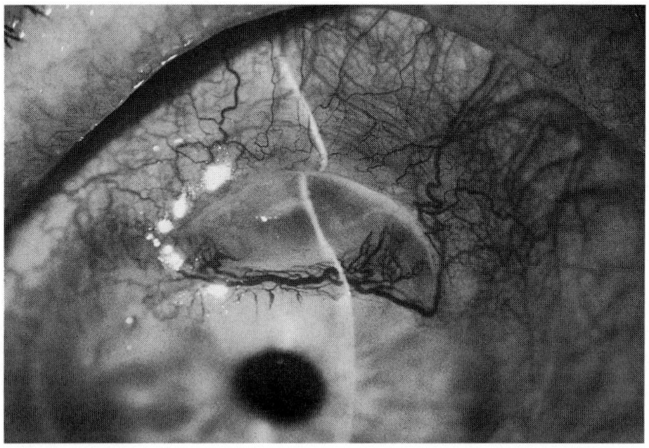

Fig. 5-31 Rheumatoid arthritis. This eye with chronic corneal inflammation has an area of deep ulceration. Adjacent scleral and conjunctival inflammation develops with an overhanging ledge.

cases often require systemic corticosteroids or other immunosuppressive agents. Therapy must usually be continued for weeks, or even months, with gradual tapering of the antiinflammatory medications. Periocular corticosteroids are generally contraindicated and may increase the risk for scleral melting or perforation. Necrotizing scleritis should be considered both an ocular and a medical emergency. It represents an ocular manifestation of systemic vasculitis, and it requires prompt rheumatologic evaluation and the institution of systemic immunosuppression to reduce ocular and systemic morbidity. Systemic corticosteroids provide rapid immunosuppression, but the side effects of long-term maintenance doses are problematic for many patients. Systemic methotrexate, azathioprine, cyclophosphamide, and cyclosporine are potent immunosuppressive agents and can be effective in the treatment of necrotizing scleritis as well as severe nonnecrotizing scleritis unresponsive to

Box 5-7 Agents with Anticollagenase Activity

Tetracyclines
N-Acetylcysteine (e.g., Mucomyst)
Medroxyprogesterone

other therapy. The goal of therapy is to limit tissue destruction by reducing inflammation and to promote epithelial healing. Therefore aggressive treatment of the dry eye component of this ocular disease is also essential. Severe tissue loss may compromise the integrity of the globe, and tectonic surgical procedures such as scleral, pericardial, or fascia lata patch grafts may be required for some patients. It is also important to be aware that secondary bacterial, fungal, or atypical mycobacterial infections may complicate these lesions and that suspicious areas should be cultured and aggressively treated before the administration of high-dose immunosuppression, if possible.

Sclerosing keratitis and stromal keratitis are usually associated with scleritis and respond to topical corticosteroid administration. The treatment of the associated scleritis as outlined above is also required, and it aids in the resolution of the corneal disease.

Peripheral ulcerative keratitis and paracentral keratolysis are thought to be related, in part, to the increased activity of collagenase. Initial therapy should be aimed at the promotion of epithelial healing with aggressive lubrication by means of preservative-free tears and tear ointments. In general, corneal melting stops when the epithelial defect is healed. Punctal occlusion or lateral tarsorrhaphy may be helpful or necessary adjuncts. Topical corticosteroids should be used cautiously in these conditions because of their tendency to enhance collagenase activity, thereby hastening tissue loss and perforation. The minimal effective dose should be employed, and the patient should have frequent follow-up examinations. Patients already receiving topical corticosteroids should undergo gradual tapering. Periocular corticosteroid therapy is contraindicated because of the inability to withdraw the drug should progressive melting occur. Topical cyclosporine theoretically offers the advantages of local immunosuppression without the enhancement of collagenase activity. Topical and systemic agents with anticollagenase activity may be helpful in some patients (Box 5-7). Systemic immunosuppression, either with prednisone or with other agents outlined above, may also be required. Surgical options for peripheral ulcerative keratitis include conjunctival resection or recession adjacent to the involved cornea to keep the conjunctival collagenases away from the cornea. Lamellar patch grafting may be required if perforation seems likely. Cyanoacrylate glue

Box 5-8 Major Autoimmune Conditions Affecting the Anterior Segment

Rheumatoid arthritis
Sjögren's syndrome
Systemic lupus erythematosus
Wegener's granulomatosis
Polyarteritis nodosa
Relapsing polychondritis
Scleroderma
Sarcoidosis
Inflammatory bowel disease
Cogan's syndrome

with a bandage soft contact lens is useful for small perforations in either peripheral or central ulcers, but larger perforations may require penetrating keratoplasty.

Other Collagen Vascular Diseases

Other collagen vascular diseases may present with inflammatory complications in the eye (Box 5-8).

Systemic lupus erythematosus Systemic lupus erythematosus (SLE) is a collagen vascular disease that may affect multiple organ systems. Clinical manifestations include arthralgia, skin rashes (Fig. 5-32), glomerulonephritis, and central nervous system manifestations. The diagnosis can be made based on the presence of antinuclear antibodies, anti-double-stranded DNA antibodies, and other autoantibodies.

Ocular manifestations of SLE may involve both the anterior and posterior segments (Box 5-9). The cutaneous manifestations of SLE include chronic blepharitis and a typical lupus rash on the eyelids. Conjunctival injection and symblepharon have been infrequently reported, and SLE may also produce a secondary Sjögren's syndrome in as many as 25% of patients. Corneal involvement is uncommon but may include stromal keratitis and neovascularization. Episcleritis and scleritis are associated with SLE. Scleritis may be an indication of the severity of the systemic disease, and it may occasionally be the initial manifestation of the condition. Cataracts can develop secondary to chronic systemic corticosteroid use. Posterior segment findings are usually related to vasculitis and include cotton wool spots, retinal hemorrhages, and retinal vasculitis.

Wegener's granulomatosis Wegener's granulomatosis (WG) is an autoimmune disease producing a systemic vasculitis. Classically it affects the upper and lower respiratory tracts as well as the kidneys, though other organ systems may be involved. Systemic manifestations include sinusitis, pulmonary infiltrates, hemoptysis, and glomerulonephritis. A common ophthalmic manifestation of WG is rapidly progressive orbital inflammation. Anterior segment ocular findings usually result from complications of focal vasculitis, and include localized or diffuse conjunctival and episcleral injection, peripheral subepithelial and anterior stromal infiltrates, as well as scleritis and peripheral ulcerative keratitis (Box 5-10). Wegener's granulomatosis should be considered in all patients with necrotizing sclerokeratitis (Figs. 5-33 and 5-34). As in other collagen vascular diseases, scleritis and peripheral ulcerative keratitis often signify more serious systemic vasculitis. Necrotizing scleritis can produce profound tissue loss, and peripheral ulcerative keratitis may progress circumferentially and centrally, resembling a Mooren's ulcer. Secondary Sjögren's syndrome that produces keratoconjunctivitis sicca is also a frequent finding.

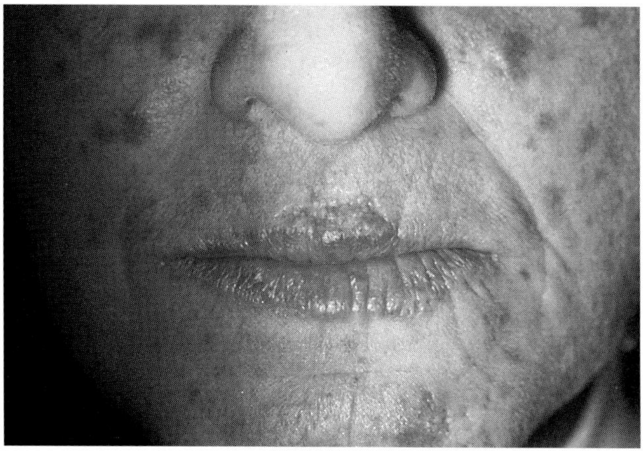

Fig. 5-32 Lupus erythematosus. A blotchy facial rash is evident in this patient with discoid lupus erythematosus. (Courtesy of Guy F. Webster, M.D., Ph.D.)

Box 5-9 Major Anterior Segment Manifestations of Systemic Lupus Erythematosus

EYELID
Cutaneous (discoid) lupus plaques
Blepharitis

EPISCLERA
Episcleritis

SCLERA
Scleritis (nodular form most common)

CORNEA
Keratoconjunctivitis sicca
Stromal keratitis
Peripheral ulcerative keratitis

UVEAL TRACT
Uveitis

Box 5-10 Major Anterior Segment Manifestations of Wegener's Granulomatosis

EPISCLERA

Episcleritis

SCLERA

Scleritis

CORNEA

Peripheral ulcerative keratitis
Focal peripheral stromal keratitis

UVEAL TRACT

Anterior and posterior uveitis

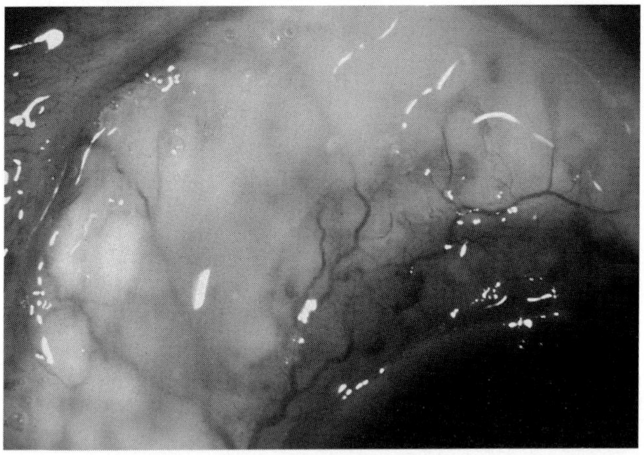

Fig. 5-33 Wegener's granulomatosis. Acute necrotizing sclerokeratitis is present superiorly with no known systemic illness. Emergency systemic evaluation demonstrates otitis media, pulmonary infiltrates, and glomerulonephritis, and the workup reveals antineutrophil cytoplasmic antibodies.

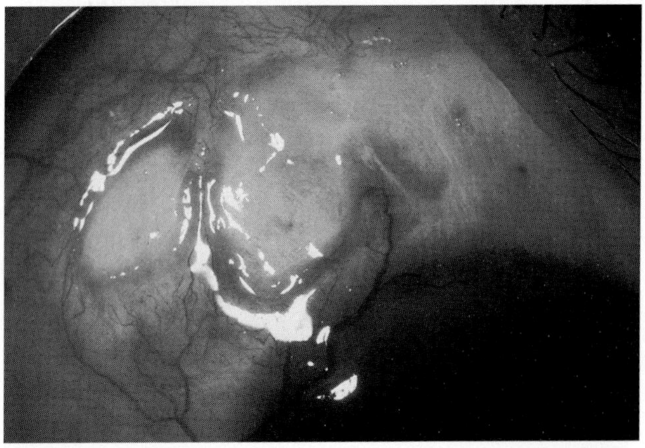

Fig. 5-34 Wegener's granulomatosis. After 5 weeks of treatment with systemic cyclophosphamide and prednisone, the patient seen in Fig. 5-33 shows ocular and systemic improvement. The necrotizing scleritis is no longer active, and the sclera is almost completely reepithelialized.

The diagnosis of WG may be confirmed by the presence of antineutrophil cytoplasmic antibodies (ANCA). ANCA appears in two forms, each with a different staining pattern and disease specificity. The cytoplasmic staining pattern (C-ANCA) is more specific for WG, and the perinuclear staining pattern (P-ANCA) is less specific and may be seen in polyarteritis nodosa, inflammatory bowel disease, rheumatoid arthritis, and other inflammatory conditions. As in other autoimmune conditions, the ocular manifestations of WG are managed primarily by treating the systemic disease with corticosteroids and other immunosuppressive agents, most commonly cyclophosphamide. Keratoconjunctivitis sicca should be aggressively treated with preservative-free tears, lubricating ointments, punctal occlusion, and lateral tarsorrhaphy (if necessary). Conjunctivitis and episcleritis may respond to topical corticosteroids, but their use should be minimized in patients with ulcerative keratitis because of possible corneal melting. In addition to systemic therapy, surgical options for peripheral ulcerative keratitis and necrotizing scleritis include conjunctival recession or resection, or tectonic lamellar or full-thickness keratoplasty and scleral patch grafting.

Autoimmune diseases such as polyarteritis nodosa, scleroderma, relapsing polychondritis, and dermatomyositis may also produce anterior segment findings similar to those in the above conditions, including keratoconjunctivitis sicca, episcleritis, scleritis, peripheral ulcerative keratitis, and uveitis. This wide variety of conditions demonstrates the importance of a complete review of systems and systemic autoimmune workup in patients who present with these findings. Not infrequently, an initial workup is unrevealing. If the clinical suspicion for an autoimmune disease remains high, a workup should be repeated 6 to 12 months later. This second workup is often diagnostic.

GRAFT-VERSUS-HOST DISEASE

Graft-versus-host disease (GVHD) is a systemic illness that may develop after bone marrow transplantation from a donor. It is most likely the result of systemic sensitization of the donor cells, which recognize the recipient as foreign. It has many of the characteristics of autoimmune conditions.

The most frequent ocular finding is severe dry eyes. Conjunctival scarring can also result. The primary mode of treatment is immunosuppression with systemic corticosteroids and with other immunosuppressive agents. Local ocular treatment is directed at keeping the eye moist and includes preservative-free tear drops and ointments. Prevention and treatment of ocular infection are also important.

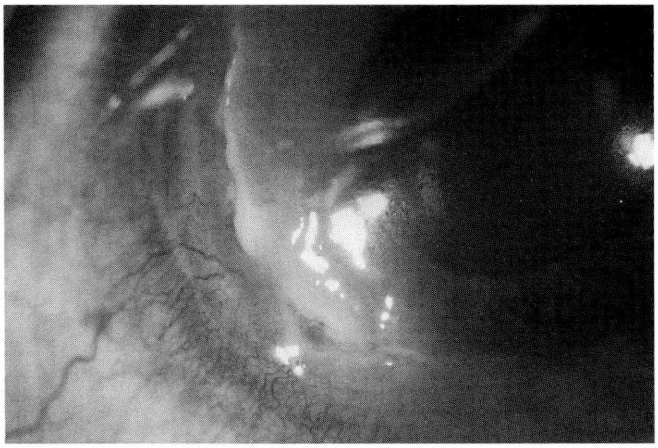

Fig. 5-35 Mooren's ulceration. Peripheral ulcerative keratitis of no known cause is considered a Mooren's ulcer. This eye has the classic linear ulceration with an overhanging infiltrate at the central edge. Peripheral to the active lesion is corneal scarring and neovascularization, evidence of previous inflammation.

MOOREN'S ULCERATION

Mooren's ulcer refers to chronic, painful, progressive, peripheral ulcerative keratitis in the absence of an underlying cause such as systemic collagen vascular disease, infection, or trauma. Clinically it presents as a peripheral corneal infiltration that evolves into an ulceration with an epithelial defect (Fig. 5-35). The ulcer progresses centrally and circumferentially, typically with an overhanging central ledge that is gray and infiltrated (Figs. 5-36 and 5-37). The ulcer is usually painful and may progress entirely around the corneal periphery. The surrounding conjunctiva, episclera, and sclera are usually hyperemic. As the chronic ulceration progresses centrally, peripheral areas may heal with vascularization and scarring. Spontaneous perforation is rare but has been reported, though these eyes are more susceptible to perforation with minor trauma because of profound tissue loss.

Two distinct types of Mooren's ulcer have been described (Table 5-3). The first type occurs in older patients and is usually unilateral, less painful, and responds reasonably well to therapy. The second type occurs more frequently in younger patients and is usually bilateral, more painful, and relentlessly progressive despite medical and surgical therapy (Figs. 5-38, 5-39, 5-40, and 5-41).

By definition the cause of Mooren's ulceration is unknown, though presumably the pathogenesis is immunologically based. The differential diagnosis includes those autoimmune conditions that can produce sterile ulcerative keratitis (Box 5-11), and a complete workup for collagen vascular disease should be performed on these patients (Box 5-12). Hepatitis C infection is recently associated with Mooren's ulceration, and serologic testing for this infection should be included in the workup. Infectious scleritis must be ruled out, and suspected cases should be cultured and treated appropriately. This condition is easily distinguished from Terrien's marginal degeneration in which the peripheral thinning is often bilateral, noninflamed, and slowly progressive with an intact epithelium and without an overhanging edge (Table 5-4).

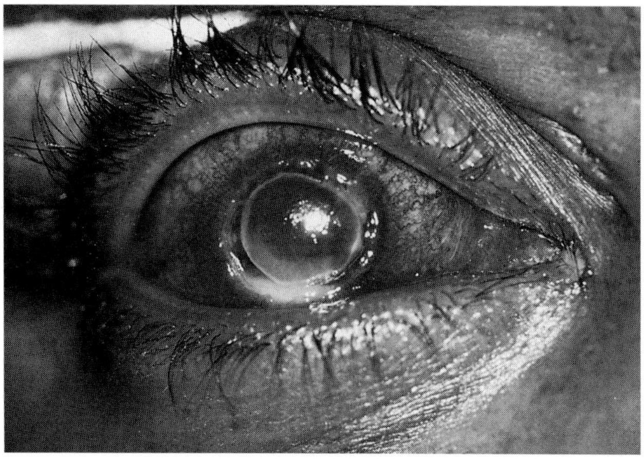

Fig. 5-36 Mooren's ulceration. A 360° peripheral corneal ulcer is seen. The limbal cornea is severely thinned, and a large hypopyon is present.

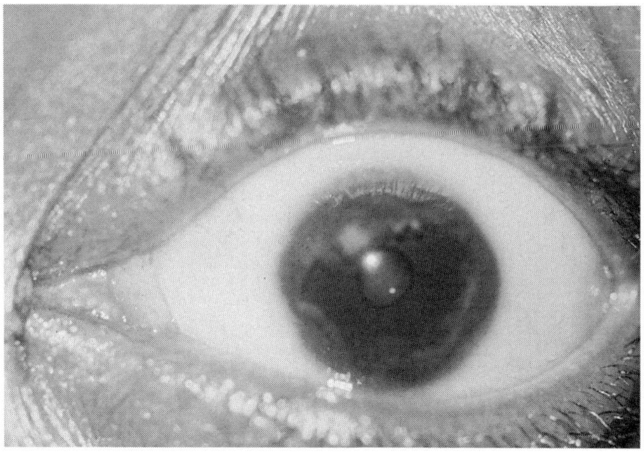

Fig. 5-37 Mooren's ulceration. The fellow eye of the patient seen in Fig. 5-36 demonstrates a healed Mooren's ulcer.

Several medical and surgical treatment options are used for Mooren's ulcers. Once microbial superinfection has been ruled out, topical corticosteroids may be used initially; these tend to work well for ulcers of the type 1 variety. As with any peripheral ulcerative keratitis, however, topical corticosteroid therapy must be closely monitored because of the possibility of the enhancement of collagenase activity and the resultant potentiation of stromal melting. Topical cyclosporine has also been used with some success. Bilateral or type 2 disease may be refractory to topical therapy, and systemic immunosuppressive agents such as prednisone, cyclophosphamide,

Table 5-3 Comparison of Mooren's ulceration types 1 and 2

Feature	Type 1	Type 2
Laterality	Usually unilateral	Usually bilateral
Age	Older patients	Younger patients
Race	More commonly white	More commonly black
Progression	Slowly progressive	May be rapidly progressive
Pain	Minimal	Moderate to severe
Response to treatment	Responds well to therapy	Poor response to therapy

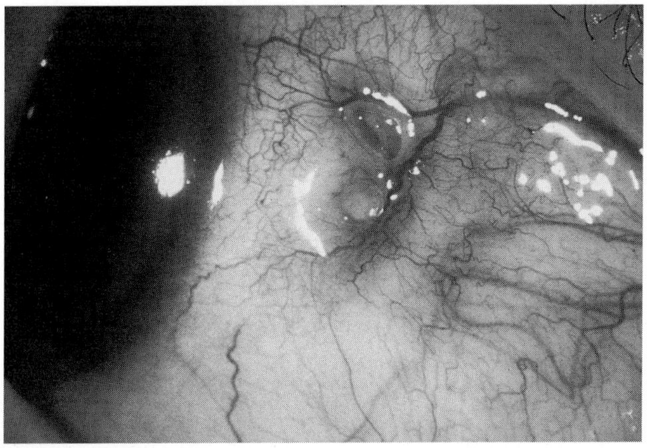

Fig. 5-38 Mooren's ulceration. This eye has two localized areas of necrotizing scleritis of unknown cause.

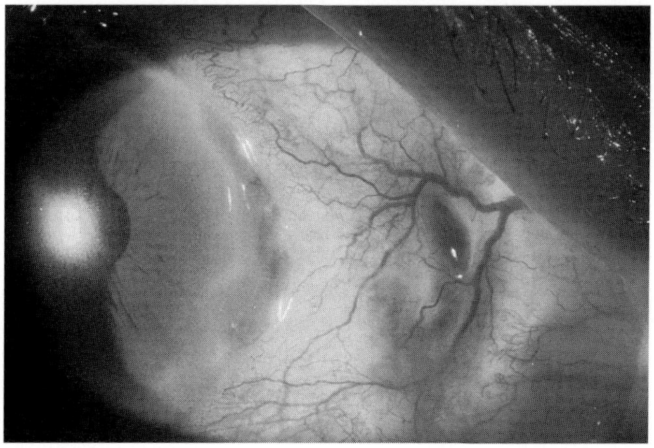

Fig. 5-39 Mooren's ulceration. The active scleritis seen in the eye in Fig. 5-38 resolves, but peripheral ulcerative keratitis develops.

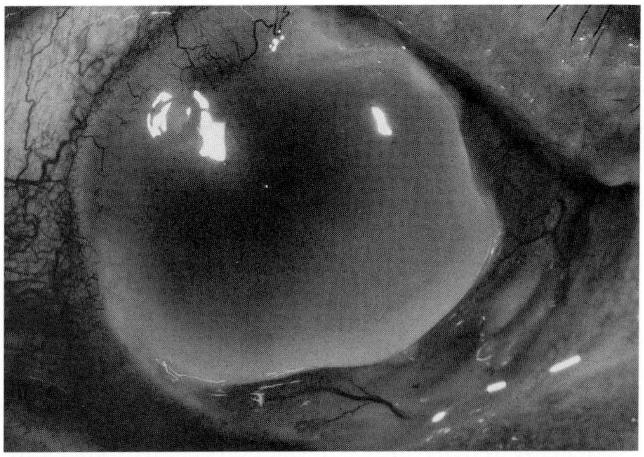

Fig. 5-40 Mooren's ulceration. The peripheral ulcerative keratitis seen in Fig. 5-39 has progressed despite aggressive topical and systemic treatment. (See color plate.)

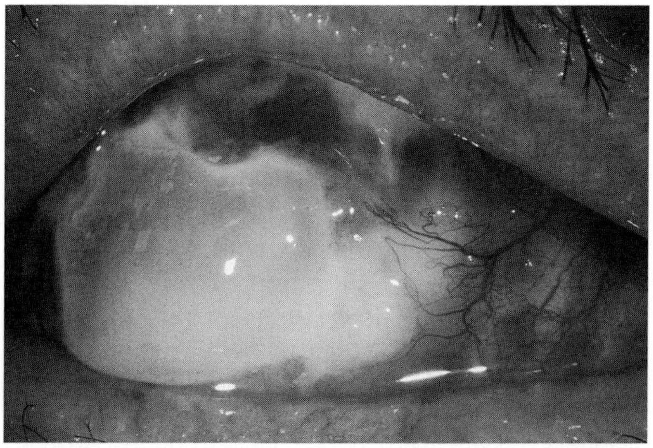

Fig. 5-41 Mooren's ulceration. The peripheral ulcerative keratitis seen in Figs. 5-39 and 5-40 continues to worsen and eventually develops a large hypopyon.

Table 5-4 Comparison of major features of Mooren's ulceration and Terrien's marginal degeneration

Feature	Mooren's ulceration	Terrien's marginal degeneration
Thinning	Peripheral corneal ulceration	Peripheral corneal thinning
Laterality	Unilateral or bilateral	Usually bilateral
Inflamed eye	Present	Absent
Pain	Present	Absent
Progression	May progress quickly	Progresses slowly
Epithelial defect	Present	Absent
Ulceration	Present	Absent
Edge	Overhanging edge	Lipid infiltration of leading edge, not overhanging
Neovascularization	Minimal peripheral vascularization	Peripheral vascularization

Box 5-11 Conditions That May Produce Sterile Ulcerative Keratitis

Rheumatoid arthritis
Sjögren's syndrome
Systemic lupus erythematosus
Wegener's granulomatosis
Polyarteritis nodosa
Relapsing polychondritis
Scleroderma
Inflammatory bowel disease
Giant cell arteritis
Psoriasis
Rosacea
Hepatitis C
Idiopathic (Mooren's ulceration)

Box 5-12 Autoimmune Workup for Sterile Ulcerative Keratitis

Rheumatoid factor (RF)
Antinuclear antibody (ANA)
Angiotensin-converting enzyme (ACE)
Antineutrophil cytoplasmic antibody (C & P ANCA)
Sjögren's syndrome (SS-A & SS-B)
Erythrocyte sedimentation rate (ESR)
Complete blood count (CBC)
Hepatitis C antibody

methotrexate, azathioprine, or cyclosporine may be required. Conjunctival resection or recession, which theoretically moves the source of conjunctival anticorneal stromal antibodies and collagenases away from the cornea, has also been performed with limited success. Occasionally corneal cyanoacrylate glue, patch grafting, or full-thickness corneal transplantation may be required for severe thinning or perforation. If the patient has a positive hepatitis C serology result, systemic treatment with interferon alfa-2b has been reported to be effective in treating the associated peripheral ulcerative keratitis.

PHLYCTENULOSIS

Phlyctenulosis refers to a localized, immune-related lesion in the conjunctiva or cornea. It is usually a limited, noninfectious process that is commonly found in children or young adults. Clinically, the lesions appear as round, elevated focal infiltrates, most commonly at the limbus, though conjunctival and corneal lesions may be found. Conjunctival and limbal lesions appear as small, elevated, hyperemic, pink or gray nodules, which tend to have an ulcerated center that stains with fluorescein (Fig. 5-42). Corneal phlyctenules may initially appear at the limbus or may appear primarily in the cornea as focal, elevated, anterior stromal infiltrates. These lesions are connected to the limbus by blood vessels without an intervening clear space (Fig. 5-43). The central portion of the lesion may be ulcerated and stain with fluorescein. These lesions may slowly heal in 1 to 2 weeks leaving a stromal scar, or they may progress centrally, drawing blood vessels into the cornea behind them. They may take on a wedge shape with the base toward the limbus and may cause variable degrees of corneal thinning. During acute attacks, patients usually present with pain, photophobia, and tearing.

The pathogenesis of phlyctenules is thought to be caused by a type IV hypersensitivity (cell-mediated immunity) response to microbial antigens (Box 5-13). Classically, this reaction was associated with tuberculosis infection, and this remains a common cause of the condition worldwide. However, currently *Staphylococcus* organisms associated with staphylococcal blepharitis are thought to be the most common associated organism in the United States. Other implicated agents include

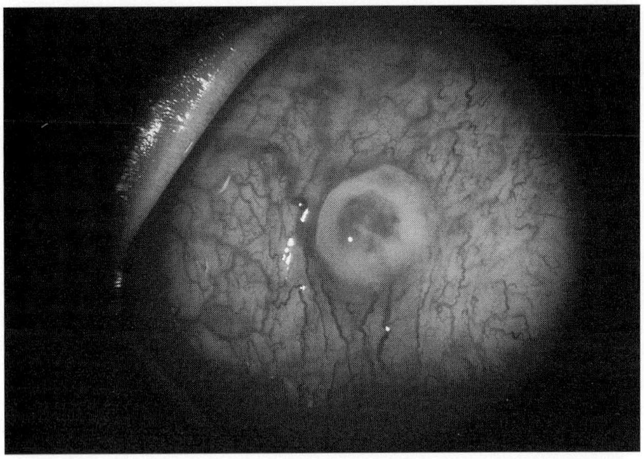

Fig. 5-42 Phlyctenulosis. An elevated conjunctival phlyctenule with an ulcerated center caused by staphylococcal blepharitis is seen.

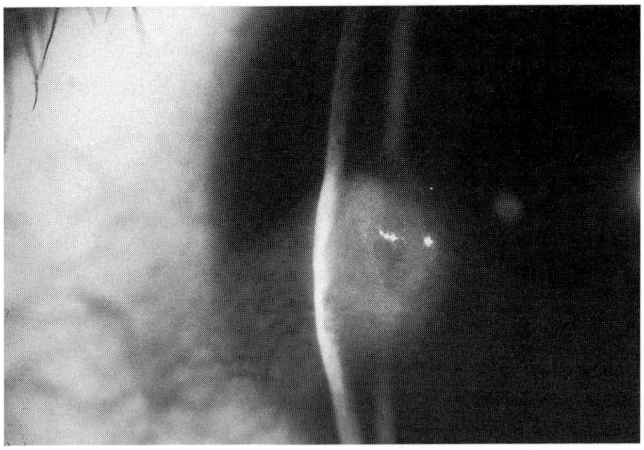

Fig. 5-43 Phlyctenulosis. An elevated corneal phlyctenule with a leash of blood vessels is present. This patient, from a developing country, tests positive for tuberculosis.

Chlamydia, Coccidioides, Candida, HSV, and nematodes. Rosacea dermatitis and blepharitis may produce similar findings. Patients with phlyctenules should therefore be tested for tuberculosis, and chlamydial infection should be suspected in recurrent cases, particularly in younger patients.

The treatment of phlyctenulosis is directed both at eliminating the underlying cause, as well as at the inflammatory lesion itself. Staphylococcal blepharitis should be aggressively treated with eyelid hygiene and antibiotic ointment. Oral tetracycline, doxycycline, minocycline, or erythromycin may also be helpful in patients with associated meibomian gland dysfunction or chlamydial infection. Systemic tuberculosis, if present, should be treated with the appropriate antituberculous regimen. The phlyctenular lesions are responsive to topical corticosteroids, but topical antibiotics should be used simultaneously if an epithelial defect appears over the lesion (Fig. 5-44).

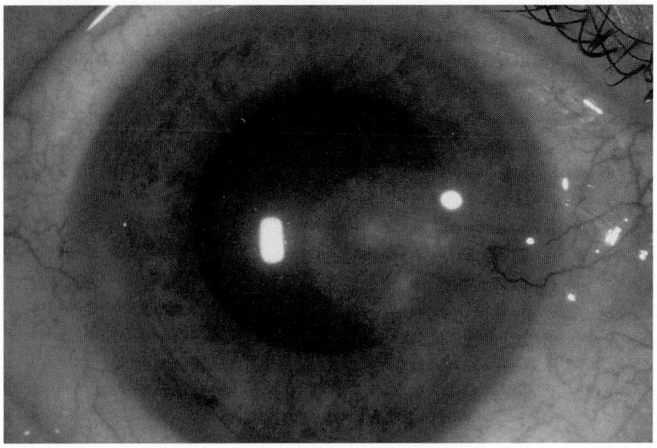

Fig. 5-44 Phlyctenulosis. A healed phlyctenule with residual corneal scarring and neovascularization is seen at the 3 o'clock position.

Box 5-13 Microbial Agents Associated with Phlyctenulosis

Staphylococcus
Mycobacterium tuberculosis
Chlamydia
Coccidioides
Candida
Herpes simplex virus
Nematode infections

STAPHYLOCOCCAL HYPERSENSITIVITY KERATITIS

One of the most common peripheral corneal disorders is staphylococcal hypersensitivity keratitis, also known as catarrhal marginal keratitis. It usually presents associated with a staphylococcal blepharitis, and it is thought to be an immune response in the cornea to staphylococcal antigens. Patients usually present with mild pain, photophobia, and tearing. Clinical findings include peripheral, localized, corneal stromal infiltrates, usually less than 1 × 1 mm, with intervening clear zones between the infiltrates and the limbus (Fig. 5-45). The infiltrates may be single or multiple, and are more commonly located where the eyelid margins cross the limbus (10, 2, 4, and 8 o'clock positions). Multiple small infiltrates may coalesce into larger ones. Initially these lesions lack an overlying epithelial defect, but with prolonged inflammation, the epithelium may break down (Fig. 5-46). When an epithelial defect occurs, the underlying stroma may thin and become secondarily infected. Prolonged inflammation may promote vascularization of these lesions.

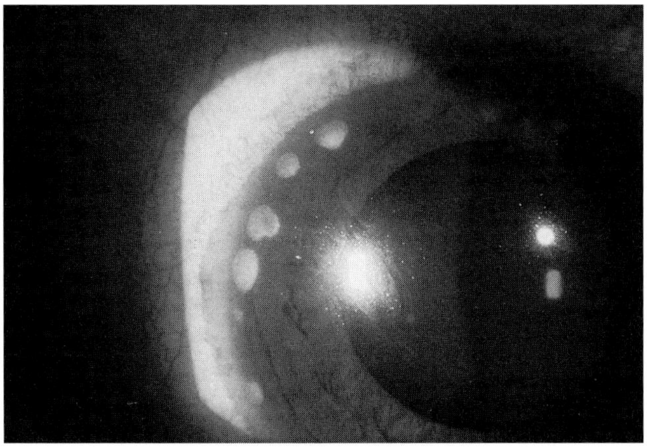

Fig. 5-45 Staphylococcal hypersensitivity keratitis. Multiple peripheral corneal infiltrates are present. Note the clear zone between the limbus and the infiltrate.

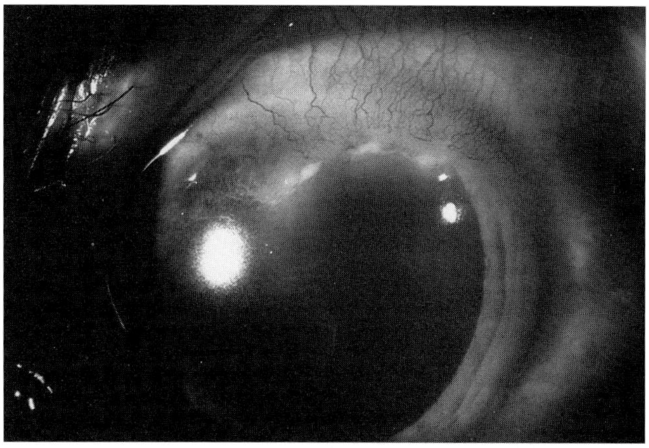

Fig. 5-46 Staphylococcal hypersensitivity keratitis. These active infiltrates, which have begun to coalesce, have small overlying epithelial defects.

Table 5-5 Differential features of staphylococcal hypersensitivity keratitis and infectious keratitis

Feature	Hypersensitivity keratitis	Infectious keratitis
Infiltrate location	Peripheral, oblique meridians most common	Central or peripheral
Number of infiltrates	Multiple infiltrates common	Usually singular infiltrate
Clear zone	Clear zone between limbus and infiltrate	Lucid interval need not be present
Epithelial defect	None (until advanced)	Present
Edema around infiltrate	Minimal to none	Often present
Anterior chamber reaction	Minimal to none	Mild to severe

The differentiation between staphylococcal hypersensitivity keratitis and infectious keratitis can be difficult (Table 5-5). Typically, staphylococcal hypersensitivity keratitis lesions are without epithelial defects until late in their course, appear in multiples, are separated from the limbus by a lucid interval, and have little or no associated anterior chamber reaction. Often slit-lamp examination reveals peripheral corneal scarring from previous episodes in the involved eye, the fellow eye, or both. Infected infiltrates tend to be solitary and to have epithelial defects on presentation. In addition, a significant anterior chamber reaction and surrounding corneal edema may develop. All possibly infected lesions should be treated with antibiotics until infection has been ruled out.

The mainstay of treatment of staphylococcal marginal keratitis is topical corticosteroid administration. These lesions are very responsive to therapy. Topical antibiotic therapy should be included in the regimen if an epithelial defect has developed, and corticosteroids should be withheld until any suspected infection has been ruled out. Treatment of the underlying staphylococcal blepharitis with appropriate eyelid hygiene, antibiotic ointment, and, in some patients, systemic antibiotics such as tetracycline, doxycycline, or erythromycin is also required to help reduce the chance for recurrences.

CORNEAL ALLOGRAFT REJECTION

Corneal allograft rejection is a common cause of corneal graft failure, and it has been reported more than 20 years after transplantation. In general, corneal transplantation is thought to be so successful compared with other types of organ transplantation because of the avascularity of the cornea and because of the anterior chamber-associated immune deviation. These unique features provide an environment largely protected from the host immune system. However, it is now known that this environment is not completely isolated from the host immune response and that the presence of antigen-presenting cells (Langerhans' cells) in the cornea may play an important role in the pathogenesis of corneal allograft rejection.

Risk factors for corneal allograft rejection include young age and those conditions that bring the donor cornea closer to blood vessels (and thus to the host immune system). Conditions that activate the host immune system are also risk factors for rejection (Box 5-14).

The initial symptoms of rejection include redness, diminished vision, photophobia, or generalized eye discomfort. These symptoms are sometimes subtle, and it is important that transplant recipients be appropriately educated to seek prompt medical attention should they experience them. Early graft rejection may be asymptomatic; therefore, periodic routine examinations are required, especially when topical corticosteroids are tapered.

Corneal allograft rejection can produce findings in the epithelium, stroma, or endothelium (Box 5-15). One nonspecific, early sign of rejection is perilimbal conjunctival and episcleral injection. Epithelial rejection is characterized by an elevated, linear, or circumferential infiltrated epithelial lesion that stains with fluorescein and usually advances centrally (Fig. 5-47). The elevated line represents an immune "battleground" between donor and host epithelium, with eventual replacement of the donor epithelium by the host epithelium. Because host epithelium gradually replaces donor epithelium in corneal transplants, usually without producing an epithelial rejection line, this event is not, in itself, a cause of graft failure. It is, however, indicative of increased immune activity directed against the graft, and it may be a precursor to endothelial rejection. As a result epithelial rejection should prompt treatment (e.g., 1% prednisolone acetate every 4 to 6 hours) and close follow-up. Stromal signs of rejection include subepithelial infiltrates similar to those seen in adenoviral keratoconjunctivitis, and may also precede or coincide with endothelial rejection (Fig. 5-48). Their presence should also prompt treatment (e.g., 1% prednisolone acetate every 4 to 6 hours) and close follow-up.

Endothelial rejection results in damage to the endothelial cells, which can ultimately result in the loss of graft clarity and subsequent graft failure. Endothelial rejection is characterized by the presence of keratic precipitates localized to the graft, with or without overlying stromal edema in the graft (Fig. 5-49). These keratic precipitates may line up to produce the classic appearance of an endothelial rejection line (Khodadoust line), typically with edema peripheral to the line (Figs. 5-50, 5-51, and 5-52). The inflammatory reaction is directed against

Box 5-14 Risk Factors for Corneal Graft Rejection

Large graft size
Corneal neovascularization
Young age of patient
Anterior iris synechiae
Loose exposed sutures
Previous graft rejection or failure
Uveitis
Previous surgery
Preexisting ocular inflammation

Box 5-15 Clinical Features of Corneal Graft Rejection

Perilimbal conjunctival injection
Epithelial rejection line
Subepithelial stromal infiltrates
Anterior chamber cell and flare
Keratic precipitates on the graft
Endothelial rejection line
Corneal edema

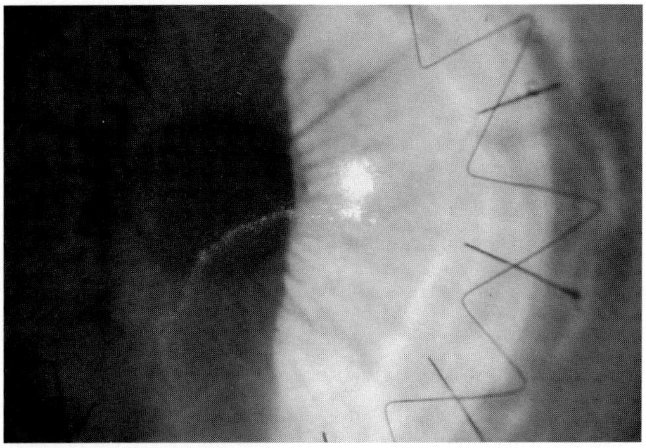

Fig. 5-47 Corneal allograft rejection. An epithelial rejection line is seen extending from the 3 o'clock to the 6 o'clock position 2 months after corneal transplantation.

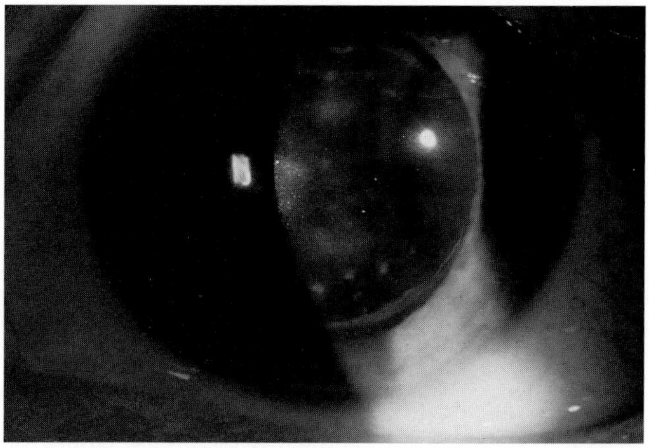

Fig. 5-48 Corneal allograft rejection. Multiple subepithelial infiltrates in this corneal transplant are apparent years after surgery.

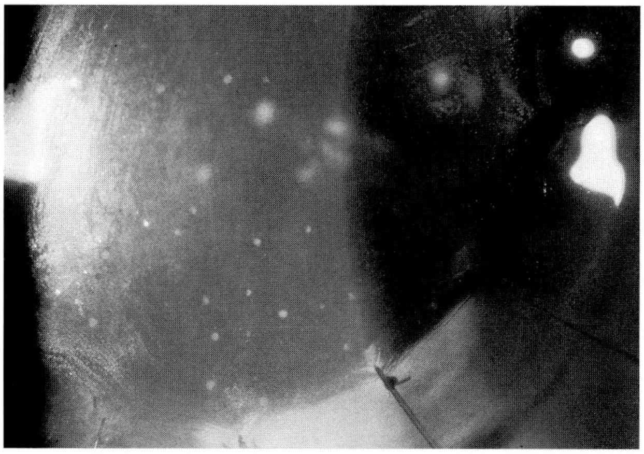

Fig. 5-49 Corneal allograft rejection. Numerous keratic precipitates are seen on the endothelial surface of this corneal graft.

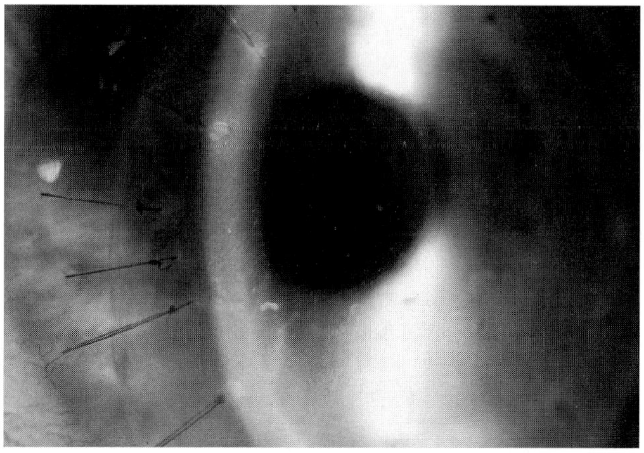

Fig. 5-50 Corneal allograft rejection. An endothelial rejection line is present in this corneal transplant, extending from the 4 o'clock to the 8 o'clock position. Inferior corneal stromal edema is seen on slit-beam examination.

endothelial cells, and their destruction is ultimately responsible for the failure of the graft (Figs. 5-53, 5-54, and 5-55). Prompt recognition (by the patient and the physician) and treatment can help halt the rejection episode, minimize endothelial loss, and preserve graft clarity. In addition, an increased anterior chamber cellular or flare reaction, even in the absence of more specific signs of allograft rejection, should be considered possible evidence of rejection and treated appropriately (e.g., 1% prednisolone acetate every 4 to 6 hours).

The most important factor in the treatment of corneal allograft rejection is early recognition. A large percentage of rejection episodes can be reversed by prompt and aggressive treatment. The mainstay of treatment of endothelial rejection is moderate- to high-dose topical corticosteroids (e.g., 1% prednisolone acetate every hour with edema, every 2 to 4 hours without edema). These

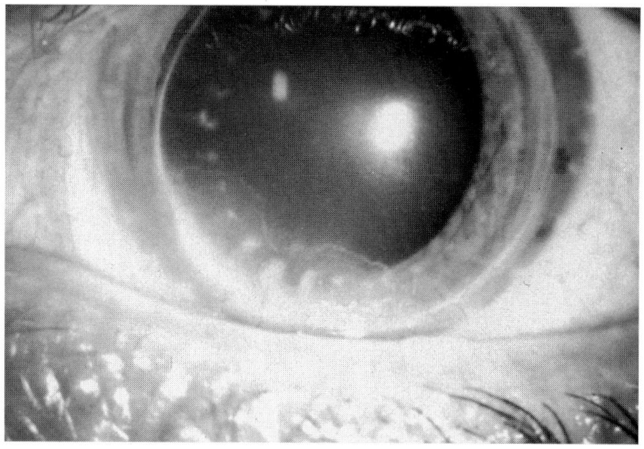

Fig. 5-51 Corneal allograft rejection. A serpiginous endothelial rejection line reaching across the inferior cornea can be seen. Underlying corneal stromal edema develops.

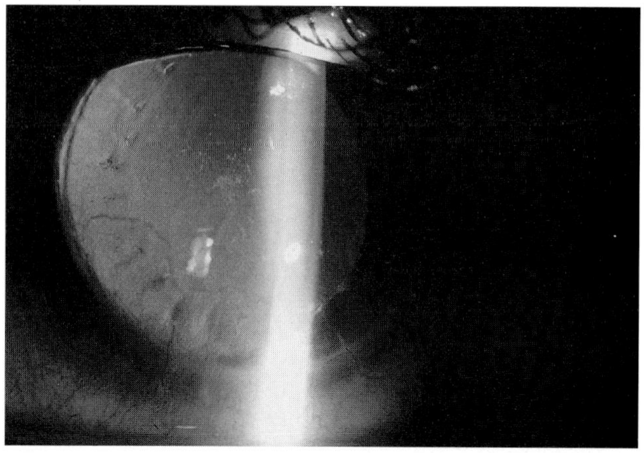

Fig. 5-52 Corneal allograft rejection. Retroillumination off the retina highlights the endothelial rejection line seen in Fig. 5-51. (See color plate.)

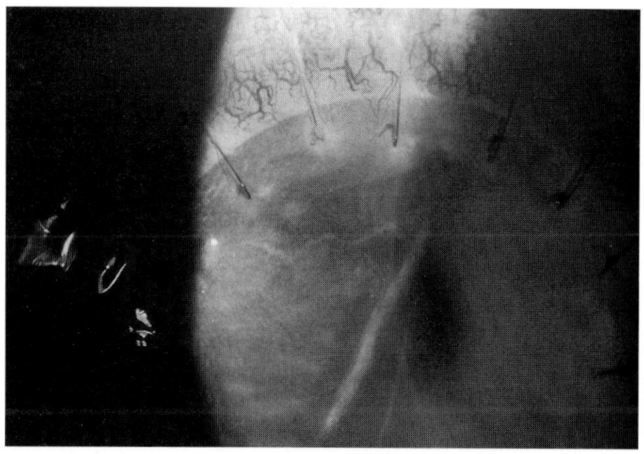

Fig. 5-53 Corneal allograft rejection. In this eye, the endothelial rejection line has traveled inferiorly to superiorly across the cornea. The inferior 80% of the cornea is edematous.

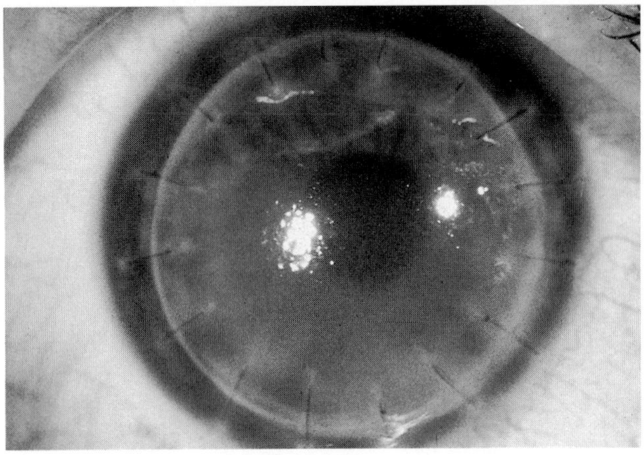

Fig. 5-54 Corneal allograft rejection. Approximately three fourths of the cornea demonstrates epithelial and stromal edema secondary to a recent episode of endothelial rejection.

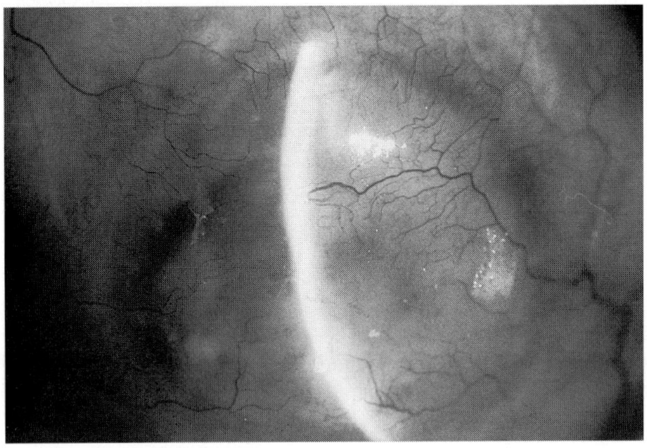

Fig. 5-55 Failed corneal graft. This failed corneal graft reveals edema, scarring, and neovascularization.

agents are usually successful in mild or moderate cases, though severe cases of endothelial rejection may require systemic (oral or pulse intravenous) corticosteroids. Topical cyclosporine is occasionally effective.

CONCLUSION

Systemic diseases can affect the health of the cornea and the anterior segment through various mechanisms. They can produce deposits that can aid in the diagnosis of a specific systemic disorder. Deposition of material can also negatively affect vision. Other systemic conditions are associated with corneal and scleral inflammation and ulceration. Occasionally, the corneal or scleral disease precedes the diagnosis of the systemic disease. In these instances, it is extremely important to diagnose the underlying condition, both to treat the eye and to treat the rest of the patient.

MAJOR POINTS

Of the mucopolysaccharidoses, corneal clouding is not a feature of Hunter syndrome or Sanfilippo syndrome.

The early onset of xanthelasma or corneal arcus may be a sign of systemic hyperlipoproteinemia.

Kayser-Fleischer ring is often an early sign of Wilson's disease and may only be visible gonioscopically in its earliest stages.

Multiple myeloma may produce peripheral crystalline deposits in the cornea.

Thyroid ophthalmopathy may produce exposure keratopathy with or without proptosis.

Thyroid ophthalmopathy may present or progress even after patients have been rendered clinically euthyroid or hypothyroid.

As their immune function deteriorates, patients with HIV infection may develop keratoconjunctivitis sicca, and a variety of secondary infections and neoplasms of the anterior segment.

Scleritis and peripheral ulcerative keratitis may be signs of a systemic autoimmune disease and should prompt a systemic workup.

Necrotizing scleritis may be a sign of severe systemic vasculitis and is associated with a significant 5-year mortality rate.

Topical corticosteroids may enhance collagenase activity and thus potentiate corneal melting in inflammatory ulcerative keratitis.

Hypersensitivity to staphylococcal antigens is the most common association with phlyctenulosis in the United States.

Corneal allograft rejection may present at any time after transplantation and may produce findings in the epithelium, stroma, or endothelium. It is most common in the first few years after transplantation, but it may occur many years later.

Major signs of corneal allograft rejection include keratic precipitates on the graft or an endothelial rejection line, subepithelial stromal infiltrates, stromal edema, an epithelial rejection line, and anterior chamber cell and flare.

Prompt recognition of rejection and initiation of intensive topical corticosteroid therapy can reverse most rejection episodes and preserve graft clarity.

SUGGESTED READINGS

Collaborative Corneal Transplantation Studies Research Group: Effectiveness of histocompatibility matching in high risk corneal transplantation, *Arch Ophthalmol* 110:1392-1403, 1992.

Erhardt CC: Factors predicting a poor life prognosis in rheumatoid arthritis: an eight year prospective study, *Ann Rheum Dis* 48:7, 1989.

Foster CS, Forstot SL, Wilson LA: Mortality rate in rheumatoid arthritis patients developing necrotizing scleritis or peripheral ulcerative keratitis: effects of systemic immunosuppression, *Ophthalmology* 91:1253-1262, 1984.

Friedberg DN, Stetson SM, Orenstein JM, et al: Microsporidial keratoconjunctivitis in the acquired immunodeficiency syndrome, *Arch Ophthalmol* 108:504-508, 1990.

Holland EJ, Olsen TW, Ketcham JM, et al: Topical cyclosporine A in the treatment of anterior segment inflammatory disease, *Cornea* 12:413-419, 1993.

Kamp MT, Fink NE, Enger C, et al: Patient reported symptoms associated with graft reactions in high risk patients in the Collaborative Corneal Transplantation Studies, *Cornea* 14: 43-48, 1995.

Krachmer JH, Alldredge OC: Subepithelial infiltrates: a probable sign of corneal transplant rejection, *Arch Ophthalmol* 96: 2234-2237, 1978.

Lucca JA, Farris RL, Bielory L, Caputo AR: Keratoconjunctivitis sicca in male patients infected with human immunodeficiency virus type 1, *Ophthalmology* 97:1008-1010, 1990.

Lucca JA, Kung JS, Farris RL: Keratoconjunctivitis sicca in female patients infected with human immunodeficiency virus, *CLAO J* 20:49-51, 1994.

Maguire MG, Stark WJ, Gottsch JD, et al: Risk factors for corneal graft failure and rejection in the collaborative corneal transplantation studies, *Ophthalmology* 101:1536-1547, 1994.

Werner SC: Classification of the eye changes of Graves' disease, *Am J Ophthalmol* 68:646-649, 1969.

Werner SC: Modification of the classification of the eye changes of Graves' disease, *Am J Ophthalmol* 83:725-727, 1977.

CHAPTER 6

Anterior Sclera

Episcleritis and scleritis are important ocular conditions, which may present with a red, painful eye and which may be difficult to differentiate from each other. Episcleritis is generally an acute, self-limited, and benign condition that is not destructive to the globe, whereas scleritis may be chronic, destructive, vision compromising, and associated with life-threatening systemic disease. These disorders are separate, distinct entities and should not be considered mild or severe forms of the same condition. The distinction between these conditions is important for their proper workup and management.

Arteriovenous fistulas, high-flow carotid-cavernous fistulas, and low-flow dural-sinus fistulas are intracranial abnormalities that exhibit conjunctival, episcleral, and orbital findings. Although high-flow fistulas can present with acute, severe symptoms, low-flow fistulas are often misdiagnosed for months as conjunctivitis.

EPISCLERITIS

Episcleritis is defined as inflammation of the episclera, the vascularized layer of loose connective tissue lining the surface of the poorly vascularized sclera. It is located just posterior to the conjunctiva and Tenon's capsule. Episcleral blood vessels may be distinguished from the overlying conjunctival vasculature because they have a radial pattern with respect to the limbus rather than the irregular pattern of conjunctival vessels. Episcleritis is a relatively common condition that is generally benign but acute in onset. Most patients are under 45 years of age, and it is more prevalent in women. Patients usually present with an acute onset of local or diffuse red eye that can be variably painful and tender, though it is commonly painless. Pain, if it is present, is usually not severe or radiating, which is one of the characteristics that distinguishes episcleritis from scleritis. Some patients have photophobia. Episcleritis is often recurrent and bilateral, though not always at the same time.

Clinically, episcleritis may present in a simple or nodular form (Box 6-1). Simple episcleritis can present in either a diffuse form, in which there is injection of the episclera across the entire bulbar surface (Fig. 6-1), or sectorial form, in which there is only a localized region of injection (Fig. 6-2). In either case the involved areas demonstrate engorgement of the radial episcleral vasculature, which is often greatest in the interpalpebral fissure. Usually the overlying conjunctival vessels are also involved. Nodular episcleritis presents with a localized area of episcleral and conjunctival injection with edema, thus producing the appearance of an elevated nodule (Fig. 6-3). The nodule is often slightly mobile over the underlying sclera. Tenderness, when present, is usually localized to the involved area.

There is often significant diagnostic confusion between episcleritis and scleritis. Although it may be difficult to distinguish between these conditions, several features learned from the history and physical examination may help to differentiate them (Table 6-1). In general, episcleritis presents with diffuse or localized redness that is either painless or mildly to moderately painful or tender. Pain, when present, is usually described as hot, burning, or "prickly." Scleritis, in contrast, almost always presents with a deep, boring pain that may radiate into the orbits, head, or jaw. The pain is usually described as severe and may keep the patient up at night. Ophthalmic examination of a patient with episcleritis reveals a pink or bright red area of engorged conjunctival and radial episcleral vasculature that blanches with the application of topical 10% phenylephrine. In a patient with scleritis, however, the involved areas typically have a violaceous hue (best seen by gross inspection in natural light), and the involved vasculature does not blanch well with 10% phenylephrine.

Box 6-1 Clinical Forms of Episcleritis

SIMPLE
Diffuse
Sectorial

NODULAR

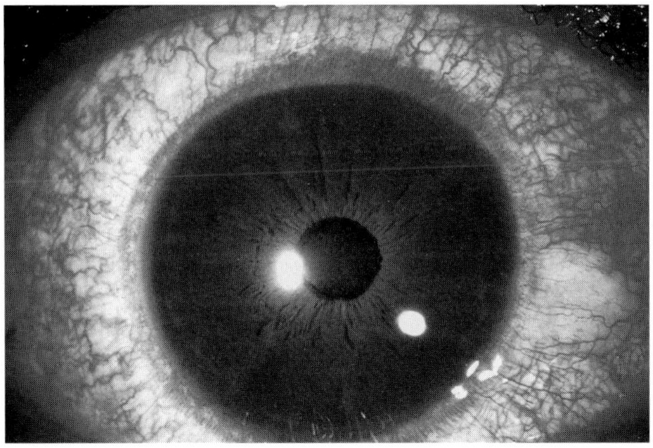

Fig. 6-1 Diffuse episcleritis. In patients with diffuse episcleritis, the entire bulbar surface is involved with episcleral injection. Note the engorgement of these radial episcleral vessels. (See color plate.)

Although most cases of episcleritis are idiopathic, occasionally these are associated with systemic inflammatory or infectious conditions (Box 6-2). It is therefore important to ensure that a thorough medical history and a review of systems are obtained from the patient. Although a systemic workup is generally not indicated for episodes of episcleritis, multiple recurrences, an atypical or a prolonged course, or a medical history and review of systems that arouse suspicion for a systemic inflammatory or infectious condition should prompt further investigation. If laboratory values are requested, the workup should include serology tests for syphilis, Lyme disease, and collagen vascular disorders, determination of uric acid level, complete blood count, erythrocyte sedimentation rate, purified protein derivative, and chest radiography (Box 6-3).

Treatment

Most cases of episcleritis are self-limited and resolve spontaneously in 1 to 3 weeks, although multiple recurrences are common. Treatment of any underlying disease is important. Supportive therapy with artificial tears or a topical antihistamine/vasoconstrictor may be helpful for patients with mild episcleritis. Treatment of persistent or painful cases includes the use of nonsteroidal antiinflammatory drugs (NSAIDs) and occasionally corticosteroids. Topical NSAIDs are generally useless, whereas systemic NSAIDs can be extremely effective. These should be administered at a full pain reduction dose and then tapered over weeks to months, depending on the patient's response. Topical corticosteroids are also effective, but are associated with side effects. A mild corticosteroid (e.g., fluorometholone) is often strong enough to improve symptoms rapidly. Systemic corticosteroids, though effective, are rarely required to treat episcleritis. If an as-

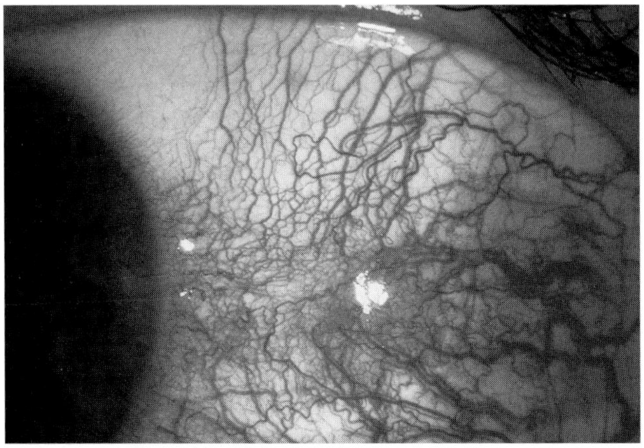

Fig. 6-2 Sectorial episcleritis. In patients with sectorial episcleritis, only one area of the bulbar surface is involved. These radial episcleral vessels are injected, whereas the deeper sclera appears uninflamed. (See color plate.)

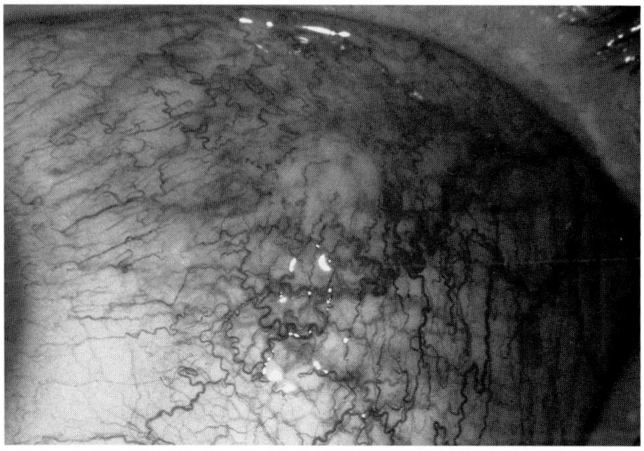

Fig. 6-3 Nodular episcleritis. In patients with nodular episcleritis, an area of localized episcleral edema creates an elevated protrusion. The nodule is often tender and may be slightly mobile over the underlying sclera.

Table 6-1 Major distinguishing clinical features of episcleritis and scleritis

Feature	Episcleritis	Scleritis
Pain	Painless or mildly painful and tender	Very painful
Appearance	Involved areas appear red	May appear bright red or violaceous
Effect of phenylephrine	Usually blanches with 10% topical phenylephrine	Does not blanch with topical 10% phenylephrine
Epithelial defect	No epithelial defect	Epithelial defect with necrotizing scleritis

Box 6-2 Major Systemic Diseases Occasionally Associated with Episcleritis

Rheumatoid arthritis
Systemic lupus erythematosus
Syphilis
Herpes zoster infection
Inflammatory bowel disease
Gout
Acne rosacea
Lyme disease
Atopy

Box 6-3 Laboratory Workup for Recurrent or Atypical Episcleritis

Venereal Disease Research Laboratory (VDRL) or rapid plasma reagin (RPR) test
Fluorescein treponemal antibody (FTA) or microhemagglutination-*Treponema pallidum* test (MHA-TP)
Rheumatoid factor (RF)
Antinuclear antibody (ANA)
Lyme titer
Complete blood count (CBC)
Erythrocyte sedimentation rate (ESR)
Uric acid
Purified protein derivative (PPD)
Chest radiography

sociated systemic condition has developed, appropriate systemic therapy may be indicated for selected patients.

SCLERITIS

In contrast to episcleritis, scleritis is a painful, often destructive inflammatory process involving the sclera. It is associated with systemic inflammatory diseases, some of which have life-threatening complications, and systemic therapy is required to control the inflammation.

Box 6-4 Clinical Forms of Scleritis

ANTERIOR

Diffuse
Nodular
Necrotizing with inflammation
Necrotizing without inflammation (scleromalacia perforans)

POSTERIOR

Patients with scleritis generally present complaining of gradual onset of a diffuse or localized area of redness and tenderness, along with a constant, deep, boring pain that may radiate to the orbit, temple, head, or jaw. They often report that the pain increases in severity in the evening and keeps them up at night. They may also report tearing, photophobia, or diminished vision. Clinically, scleritis presents in anterior and posterior forms (Box 6-4). Anterior scleritis can present in either a diffuse (most common and least severe), nodular, or necrotizing form. Examination reveals diffuse scleral injection and swelling (diffuse form) or localized tender nodules of scleral inflammation (Fig. 6-4). The involved areas can have a violaceous hue (best seen by gross inspection in natural light) and are associated with overlying conjunctival and episcleral injection (Fig. 6-5). It may be difficult to distinguish between episcleritis and scleritis, though patients with scleritis tend to have more severe pain, and the involved areas do not blanch well with topical 10% phenylephrine. Areas of scleral thinning and translucence may be evidence of previous attacks of scleritis.

Necrotizing anterior scleritis is the least common form of anterior scleritis and may present either with inflammation or without inflammation. Necrotizing anterior scleritis *with* inflammation usually presents with severe pain and intense scleritis, and the involved areas exhibit signs of scleral necrosis with an overlying conjunctival epithelial defect. Choroidal pigment may become visible

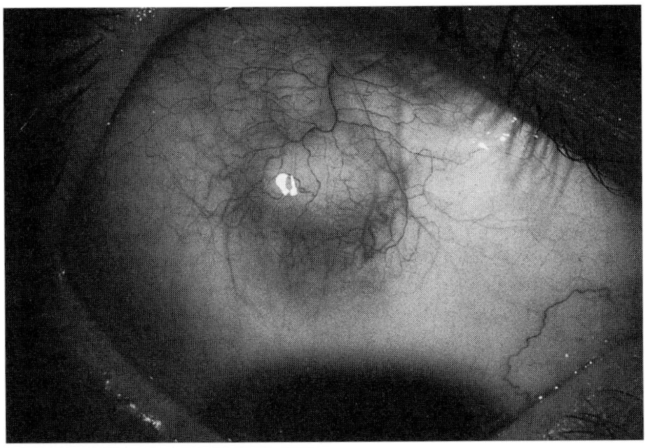

Fig. 6-4 Nodular scleritis. An area of localized scleral nodular inflammation is evident superiorly. Between the nodule and the limbus, the sclera is gray, indicating scleral thinning from previous episodes of scleritis.

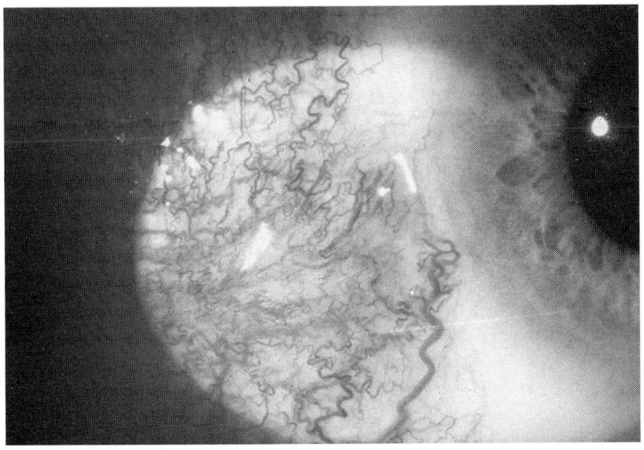

Fig. 6-5 Nodular scleritis. This area of nodular scleritis has a prominent underlying violaceous hue. (See color plate.)

as the sclera thins (Fig. 6-6). Peripheral ulcerative keratitis may develop, which increases the likelihood of underlying Wegener's granulomatosis. Necrotizing anterior scleritis with inflammation is an ominous sign. As many as 40% to 60% of these patients may lose vision, and clinically necrotizing scleritis with inflammation is a marker for life-threatening systemic complications of inflammatory disease. Without adequate systemic immunosuppression, as many as 30% of these patients die within 5 years, and 50% die within 10 years of the onset of scleritis because of the complications of severe systemic vasculitis.

Necrotizing scleritis can also occur after ocular surgery, and it is often termed *surgically induced necrotizing scleritis* (Figs. 6-7, 6-8, and 6-9). It may occur weeks to years after cataract extraction, trabeculectomy, pterygium excision, retinal detachment repair, and even strabismus surgery. Surgically induced necrotizing scleritis is also highly associated with systemic vasculitis.

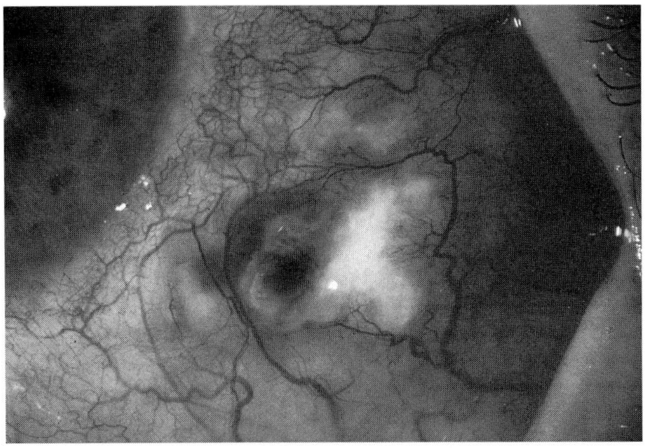

Fig. 6-6 Necrotizing scleritis. An area of necrotizing scleritis with an overlying conjunctival epithelial defect with visible uveal pigment is seen a few millimeters from the limbus.

Necrotizing anterior scleritis *without* inflammation is known as *scleromalacia perforans*. It is generally found in patients with long-standing severe rheumatoid arthritis. In contrast to the other forms of anterior scleritis, it presents as painless necrotic scleral lesions in a relatively quiet eye. These active lesions characteristically produce no notable ocular inflammation or discomfort, and result in areas of severe scleral thinning, often with visible or protruding underlying choroid (Fig. 6-10). Perforation is rare. Patients may present due to a newly noted discoloration of the eye or for diminished vision secondary to induced astigmatism.

Posterior scleritis refers to scleritis involving primarily the posterior segment of the eye, and it may occur alone or in association with contiguous anterior scleritis. It usually presents with pain, occasionally exacerbated by eye movement. Vision is frequently reduced because of inflammatory and exudative changes of the posterior segment. Findings on anterior segment examination may be deceptively normal if no associated anterior scleritis has developed, whereas findings on posterior segment examination reveal choroidal thickening or a mass lesion, choroidal folds, exudative retinal detachments, choroidal detachments, or optic disc edema. B-scan ultrasonography may reveal a *T sign* demonstrating posterior scleral thickening (Fig. 6-11). If the inflammatory process involves posterior Tenon's capsule or adjacent orbital structures, the clinical features may mimic an orbital inflammatory pseudotumor and can include proptosis, significant pain on eye movement, limitation of motility, or ptosis.

The pathogenesis of scleritis may be related to a type III hypersensitivity reaction (immune-complex deposi-

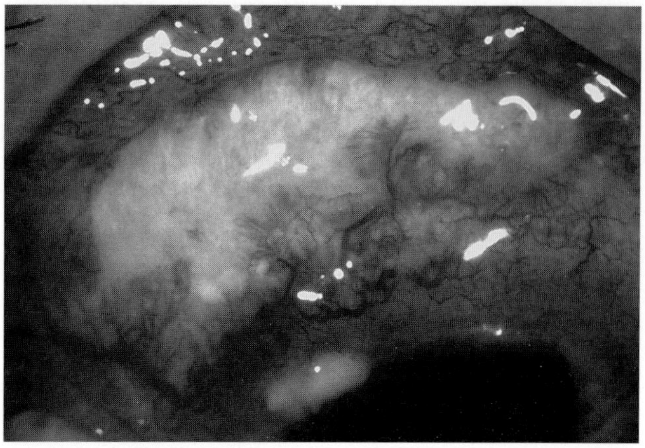

Fig. 6-7 Surgically induced necrotizing scleritis. A large area of necrotizing scleritis is seen at the superior limbus, where extracapsular cataract surgery was performed several months earlier.

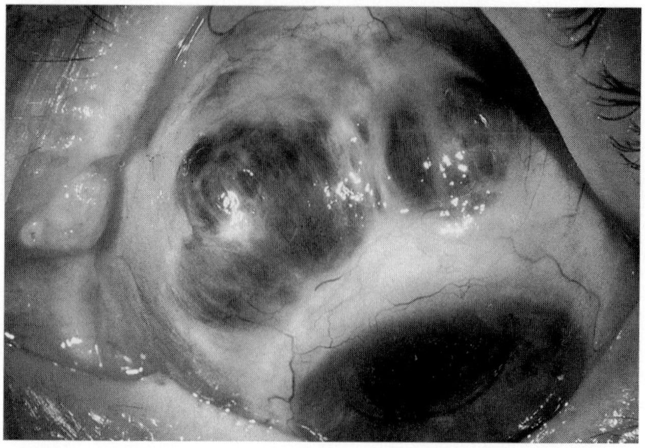

Fig. 6-10 Scleromalacia perforans. A large area of superior scleral thinning, protrusion, and uveal show is seen in this eye with scleromalacia perforans.

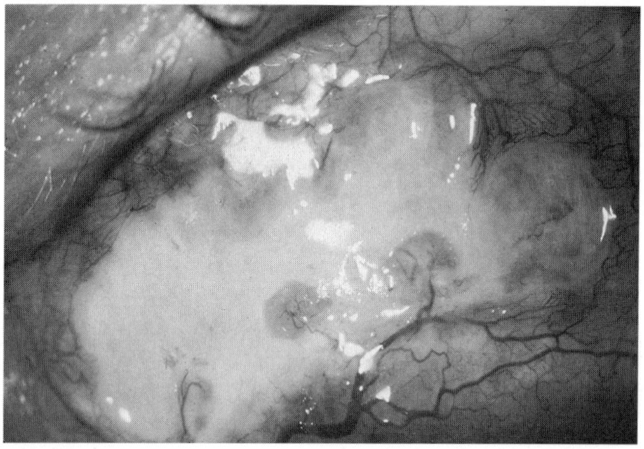

Fig. 6-8 Surgically induced necrotizing scleritis. After 1 month of treatment, the eye seen in Fig. 6-7 is beginning to heal, and new conjunctiva is starting to cover the scleral epithelial defect.

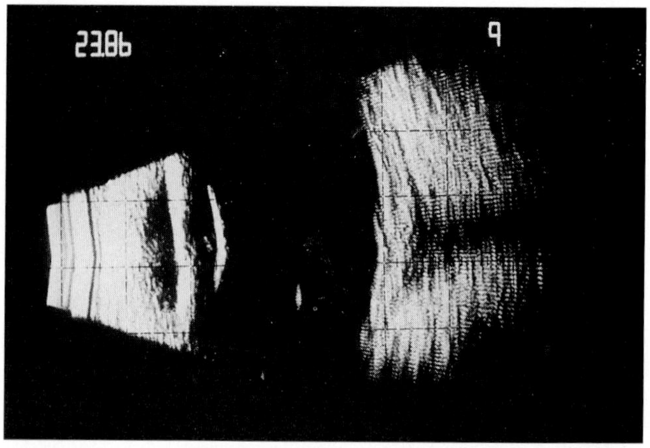

Fig. 6-11 Posterior scleritis. A *T sign* of echolucency behind the sclera and around the optic nerve is visible on B-scan ultrasonography of this eye with posterior scleritis. (Courtesy of Deborah BenArosh, C.O.A.)

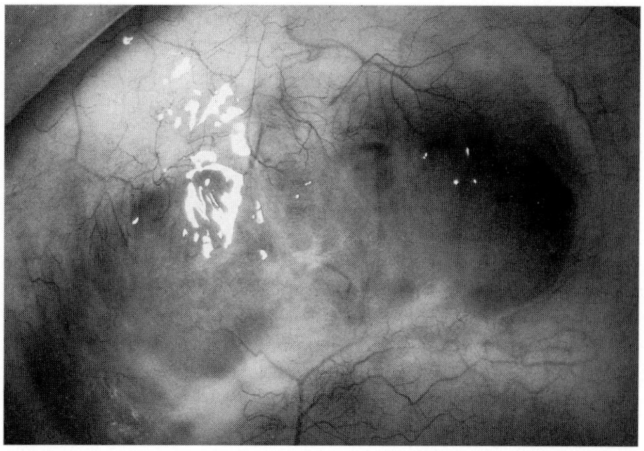

Fig. 6-9 Surgically induced necrotizing scleritis. One year after surgically induced necrotizing scleritis, the eye seen in Figs. 6-7 and 6-8 has healed with significant scleral thinning. Vision returned to baseline after the correction of significant induced astigmatism.

tion). In as many as 50% of patients with scleritis, an underlying systemic inflammatory disease is identified as the cause. The most common associated condition is rheumatoid arthritis, although scleritis is associated with other collagen vascular diseases and vasculitic processes including Wegener's granulomatosis, systemic lupus erythematosus, polyarteritis nodosa, relapsing polychondritis, and inflammatory bowel disease (Box 6-5). It is therefore essential that whenever scleritis is diagnosed and the underlying systemic cause is unknown, the patient undergo a complete workup for associated conditions. The workup should include a complete blood count, erythrocyte sedimentation rate, and serology testing for collagen vascular disorders including rheumatoid arthritis, systemic lupus erythematosus, Wegener's granulomatosis, and polyarteritis nodosa, as well as for syphilis and medical clearance for systemic corticosteroids. Skin testing for tuberculosis, serology

Box 6-5 Major Systemic Diseases Associated with Scleritis

Rheumatoid arthritis
Wegener's granulomatosis
Polyarteritis nodosa
Relapsing polychondritis
Inflammatory bowel disease
Systemic lupus erythematosus
Syphilis
Lyme disease
Tuberculosis
Reiter's syndrome
Behçet's disease
Sarcoidosis
Gout

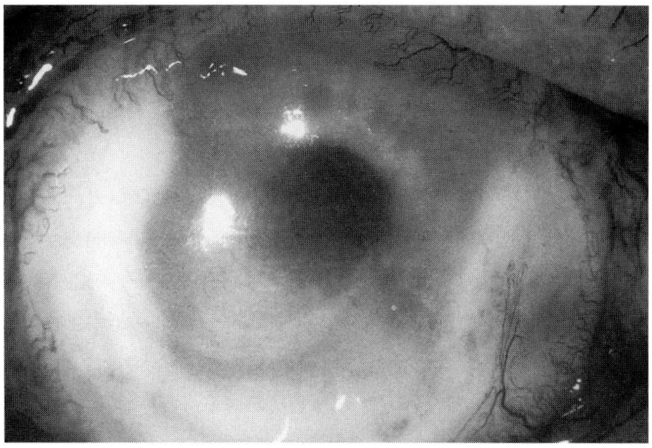

Fig. 6-12 Infectious scleritis. A large inferior *Pseudomonas aeruginosa* corneal ulcer involves the sclera.

Box 6-6 Systemic Workup for Scleritis

Venereal Disease Research Laboratory (VDRL) or rapid plasma reagin (RPR) test
Fluorescein treponemal antibody (FTA) or microhemagglutination-*Treponema pallidum* test (MHA-TP)
Rheumatoid factor (RF)
Antinuclear antibody (ANA)
C and P antineutrophil cytoplasmic antibodies (ANCA)
Angiotensin-converting enzyme (ACE)
Lyme titer
Purified protein derivative (PPD)
Chest radiography
Uric acid
Urinalysis
Complete blood count (CBC)
Erythrocyte sedimentation rate (ESR)

testing for sarcoidosis, human leukocyte antigen typing, and chest and sacroiliac radiography may also be considered (Box 6-6).

Treatment

The treatment of scleritis involves systemic therapy because topical treatment with either NSAIDs or corticosteroids is typically ineffective. Initial therapy with oral NSAIDs, such as ibuprofen, naproxen, or indomethacin, may be effective for milder cases; if one agent is ineffective, another may be tried. Once the scleritis is under control and in remission for several weeks, therapy may be slowly tapered and stopped. Severe cases or those unresponsive to NSAIDs may require systemic corticosteroids. The usual initial starting dose is approximately 1 mg/kg per day prednisone. This dose may be tapered after a clinical response is demonstrated, but a maintenance level is often required for several months after the remission of scleritis. Corticosteroids can then be tapered off over 4 to 12 weeks. Concurrent treatment with systemic NSAIDs can facilitate the reduction and discontinuation of systemic corticosteroids. Periocular corticosteroids are generally contraindicated and may increase the risk for scleral melting or perforation. Patients with severe necrotizing scleritis and systemic vasculitis, or patients whose disease is not well controlled on prolonged systemic corticosteroids, may require more potent immunosuppression with cytotoxic agents such as methotrexate, cyclophosphamide, azathioprine, cyclosporine, or chlorambucil. These medications may be used alone or in combination with systemic corticosteroids, and patients should be under the concurrent care of a rheumatologist or an internist. Surgical therapy is rarely required for patients with scleritis; it is reserved for the rare globe perforation or impending perforation. In these unusual cases, scleral, dural, pericardial, or fascia lata patch grafting may be performed after aggressive preoperative immunosuppressive therapy to prevent melting of the graft. These grafts may be covered with a conjunctival flap or an amniotic membrane graft to aid healing.

Another uncommon form of scleritis is infectious scleritis, which usually results from direct infection of the sclera after surgery or trauma or from direct extension of the infection through a corneal ulcer or panophthalmitis (Fig. 6-12). Endogenous infection through septic emboli is another uncommon mechanism. Many different organisms are associated with infectious scleritis including bacteria, fungi, viruses, and parasites. Therapy for infectious scleritis must be

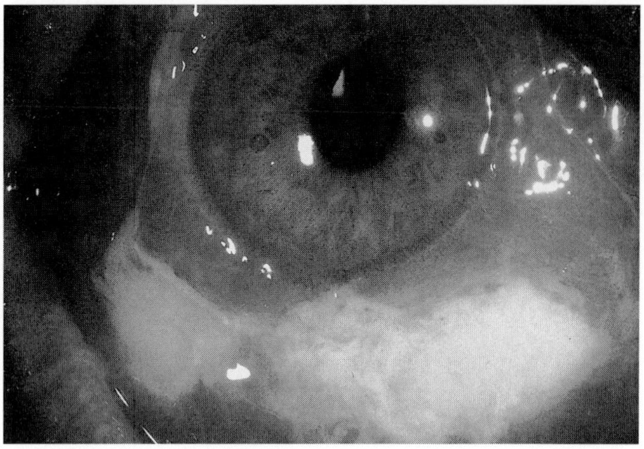

Fig. 6-13 Infectious scleritis. *Proteus mirabilis* scleritis was caused by an infected scleral buckle. The infection resolved with topical and systemic antibiotics after removal of the buckle.

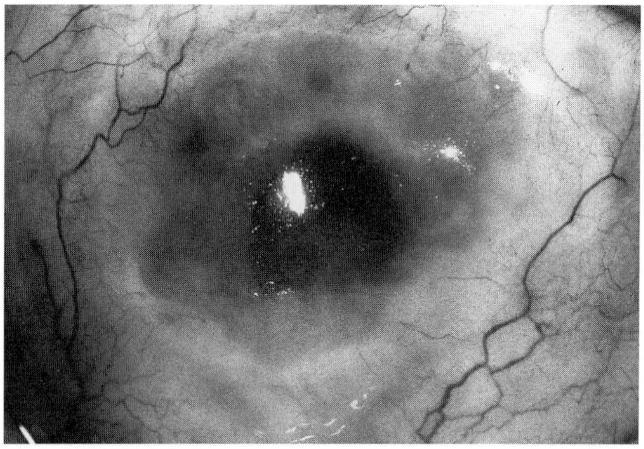

Fig. 6-14 Infectious scleritis. Six months after intensive topical and systemic treatment with fluoroquinolones for the *Pseudomonas aeruginosa* sclerokeratitis seen in Fig. 6-12, the infection resolves with moderate scarring and neovascularization.

tailored to the causative organism, which is determined by culture or by an examination of abnormal tissue. Any foreign bodies (including scleral buckling components) associated with the infection should be removed (Fig. 6-13). Although the visual prognosis is guarded, medical therapy with topical and systemic antibiotics (especially fluoroquinolones, which have good intraocular penetration) is often successful in eradicating the infection (Fig. 6-14). Surgical debridement of necrotic tissue may be helpful in some patients.

CAROTID-CAVERNOUS SINUS FISTULA

Carotid-cavernous sinus fistulas (CC fistulas) and dural-sinus fistulas are two examples of arteriovenous fistulas. A CC fistula is a high-flow communication between the internal carotid artery and the cavernous sinus, and a dural-sinus fistula is a low-flow communication between meningeal branches of the internal or external carotid artery and the cavernous sinus. Either condition may produce red eye with conjunctival injection and chemosis, and either may be an unrecognized cause of chronic conjunctivitis.

CC fistulas arise most commonly secondary to head trauma, surgery, or angiography, but they may develop spontaneously after the rupture of an aneurysm. The resultant arteriovenous shunt increases pressure within the cavernous sinus system, which is transmitted along the superior ophthalmic vein to the orbit and globe. Clinically, the elevated venous pressure can produce marked conjunctival vascular engorgement with chemosis, eyelid swelling, pulsating exophthalmos, elevated intraocular pressure, dilated retinal veins, and retinal hemorrhage or ischemia. Auscultation of the globe may reveal a bruit, and the patient may report pulsatile rushing or the sound of roaring on the affected side. At times third, fourth, sixth, or seventh cranial nerve palsy is part of the findings. Traumatic CC fistulas are usually accompanied by the appropriate clinical history of trauma, though a latent period may ensue between the traumatic event and the onset of symptoms. Chronically, arterialization of the conjunctival veins may occur, producing a characteristic corkscrew appearance. Visual loss can result from chronic ocular ischemia or secondary glaucoma.

Angiography reveals the shunt and confirms the diagnosis of CC fistula. Computed tomography, magnetic resonance imaging, or ultrasonography of the orbits may also reveal a dilated superior ophthalmic vein or enlarged (engorged) extraocular muscles. The treatment of CC fistulas involves closure of the fistula through an endoarterial balloon, embolization, or surgery.

DURAL-SINUS FISTULA

Dural-sinus fistulas are indirect means of communication between meningeal branches of the external or internal carotid artery and the cavernous sinus. These low-flow fistulas may produce some similar, though less dramatic, findings of CC fistulas including conjunctival and episcleral engorgement, secondary glaucoma, and occasionally mild proptosis (Table 6-2). Orbital bruits are usually absent. Chronic fistulas can cause arterialization of the conjunctival blood vessels, resulting in a corkscrew pattern (Fig. 6-15). These fistulas usually occur spontaneously in middle-aged and elderly women, and they often resolve spontaneously. Chronic red eye in this condition is sometimes mistaken for chronic conjunctivitis (Fig. 6-16).

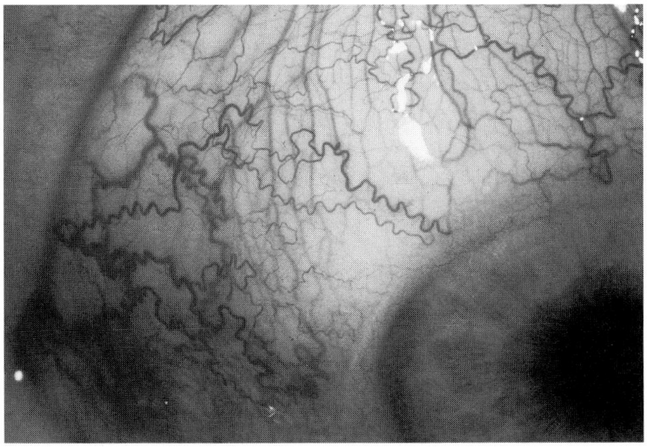

Fig. 6-15 Dural-sinus fistula. This low-flow dural-sinus fistula causes arterialization of the conjunctival blood vessels, producing a corkscrew pattern.

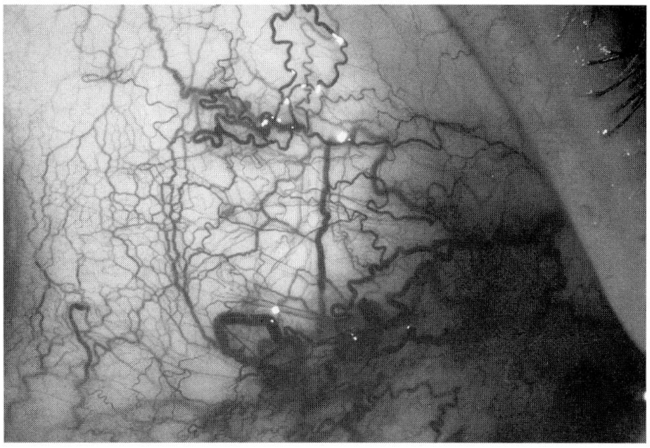

Fig. 6-16 Dural-sinus fistula. Engorgement of the conjunctival blood vessels mimics chronic conjunctivitis, but no discharge occurs.

Table 6-2 Differential features of carotid-cavernous sinus fistulas and dural-sinus fistulas

Feature	Carotid-cavernous sinus fistula	Dural-sinus fistula
Type of flow	High flow	Low flow
Cause	Usually posttraumatic	Usually spontaneous
Proptosis	Usually present, may be pulsating	Proptosis mild or absent
Vasculature	Marked engorgement, chemosis	Mild engorgement
Secondary glaucoma	May be associated with secondary glaucoma	May be associated with secondary glaucoma
Orbital bruit	Present	Absent
Resolution	Does not resolve spontaneously; requires repair	Often resolves spontaneously or after angiography

As with CC fistulas, the diagnosis of dural-sinus fistulas may be confirmed by angiography. Because most of these fistulas resolve spontaneously, however, the initial evaluation may be deferred in favor of less invasive diagnostic techniques such as orbital ultrasonography, computed tomography, or magnetic resonance imaging, which may reveal a dilated superior ophthalmic vein. Color Doppler studies can reveal a reversal of blood flow through the superior ophthalmic vein. Treatment of dural-sinus fistulas that do not resolve spontaneously may be indicated for proptosis, diplopia, or secondary glaucoma. Embolization of the external carotid artery feeder vessels is the most common treatment method, though spontaneous closure after angiography is not uncommon.

CONCLUSION

It is important to distinguish episcleritis and scleritis from each other because of their different workups, treatments, and prognoses. Although episcleritis is usually a benign, self-limited disorder that does not cause loss of vision, scleritis is associated with severe, potentially life-threatening diseases and with visual loss. With the proper workup and treatment, the ophthalmologist not only can greatly improve the patient's visual outcome, but can save the patient's life. High-flow CC and low-flow dural-sinus fistulas can also cause mild to severe ocular disease. They must be identified correctly to provide the patient the appropriate management and follow-up.

MAJOR POINTS

Episcleritis is generally a benign, self-limited, nondestructive ocular inflammatory condition.

Episcleral vasculature may be differentiated from the overlying conjunctival vessels because of its radial orientation with respect to the limbus.

Episcleral vessels blanch with topical 10% phenylephrine, which may aid in distinguishing episcleritis from scleritis.

Episcleritis is infrequently associated with systemic disease. When treatment is required, it usually responds well to oral NSAIDs, topical corticosteroids, or both.

Scleritis is a chronic, painful, progressive, and often destructive ocular inflammatory condition.

Scleral vasculature does not blanch well with topical 10% phenylephrine.

Half the patients with scleritis also have systemic inflammatory disease.

Scleritis is usually unresponsive to topical therapy and generally requires systemic treatment with NSAIDs, corticosteroids, or other immunosuppressive agents.

Without adequate systemic immunosuppression, necrotizing scleritis *with* inflammation is associated with a 30% to 50%, 5- to 10-year mortality rate because of the complications of systemic vasculitis.

Carotid-cavernous fistulas, usually the result of trauma, are a form of high-flow communication between the internal carotid artery and the cavernous sinus. Symptoms are pulsating proptosis, marked conjunctival chemosis, and a rushing sound in the head on the side of the fistula.

Dural-sinus fistulas are low-flow fistulas, usually of spontaneous origin, most commonly found in middle-aged to elderly women. They frequently resolve without treatment.

Dural-sinus fistulas often cause a corkscrew pattern to the conjunctival vessels (commonly misdiagnosed as chronic conjunctivitis) and elevated intraocular pressure.

SUGGESTED READINGS

Books

Foster CS, Sainz de la Maza M: *The sclera*, New York, 1994, Springer-Verlag.

McCluskey PJ, Wakefield D: Scleritis and episcleritis. In Pepose JS, Holland GN, Wilhelmus KR, editors: *Ocular infection and immunity*, St Louis, 1996, Mosby.

Schwan BL, Raizman MB: Scleritis. In Krachmer JH, Mannis MJ, Holland EJ, editors: *Cornea*, St Louis, 1997, Mosby.

Watson PG, Hazelman BL: *The sclera and systemic disorders*, Philadelphia, 1976, W.B. Saunders.

Journals

Erhardt CC: Factors predicting a poor life prognosis in rheumatoid arthritis: an eight year prospective study, *Ann Rheum Dis* 48:7-13, 1989.

Foster CS, Forstot SL, Wilson LA: Mortality rate in rheumatoid arthritis patients developing necrotizing scleritis or peripheral ulcerative keratitis, *Ophthalmology* 91:1253-1263, 1984.

McGavin DDM, Williamson J, Forrester JV, et al: Episcleritis and scleritis: a study of their clinical manifestations and association with rheumatoid arthritis, *Br J Ophthalmol* 60:192-226, 1976.

O'Donoghue E, Lightman S, Tuft S, Watson P: Surgically induced necrotising sclerokeratitis (SINS): precipitating factors and response to treatment, *Br J Ophthalmol* 76:17-21, 1992.

Sainz de la Maza M, Foster CS: Necrotizing scleritis after ocular surgery: a clinicopathologic study, *Ophthalmology* 98:1720-1726, 1991.

Sainz de la Maza M, Foster CS, Jabbur NS: Scleritis associated with systemic vasculitic disease, *Ophthalmology* 102:687-692, 1995.

Sainz de la Maza M, Jabbur NS, Foster CS: Severity of scleritis and episcleritis, *Ophthalmology* 101:389-396, 1994.

Watson PG, Hayreh SS: Scleritis and episcleritis, *Br J Ophthalmol* 60:163-191, 1976.

CHAPTER 7

Anterior Uveitis and Diseases of the Iris

The uveal tract essentially lines the entire eye and can manifest with inflammatory and neoplastic disease processes as well as congenital abnormalities. Although the signs and symptoms of anterior uveitis may be generalized, the underlying conditions that produce this inflammatory reaction are numerous and varied. The importance of a directed history and a careful review of systems in the workup of a patient with anterior uveitis cannot be overemphasized. Often the ophthalmologist plays a valuable role in the early identification of a yet undiagnosed and treatable systemic disorder. Although many conditions cause uveal inflammation, those involving primarily the anterior uvea (e.g., the iris, the ciliary body, or both) are discussed in this chapter.

The iris is the most visible part of the uveal tract and gives the eye its distinguishing color. Because of its accessibility to examination, iris lesions, tumors, and structural abnormalities are conspicuous and striking. It is important to identify these lesions properly to determine their malignant potential. The diagnosis may also provide insight into associated ocular and systemic abnormalities.

ANTERIOR UVEITIS

Anatomy

The uveal tract is a heavily pigmented and highly vascular structure composed of three distinct anatomic components: the iris, the ciliary body, and the choroid. The iris is the most anterior portion of the uveal tract and is the only portion directly visible by external or slit-lamp

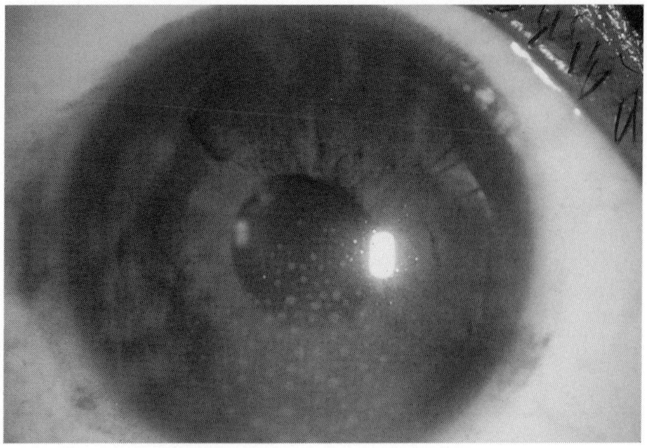

Fig. 7-1 Granulomatous anterior uveitis. Multiple clumps of white blood cells are seen on the posterior corneal surface in this patient with sarcoidosis.

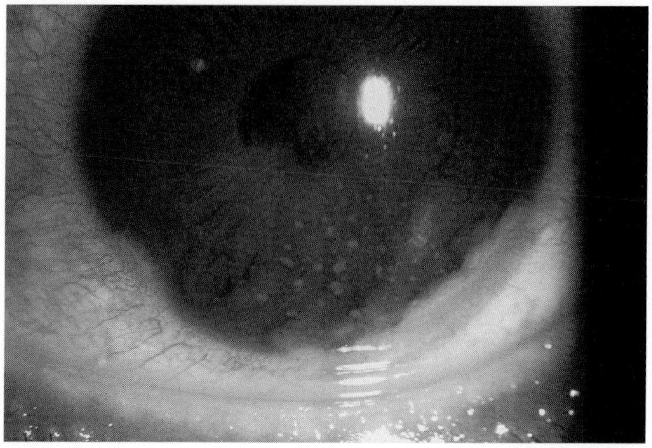

Fig. 7-2 Granulomatous anterior uveitis. Numerous accumulations of white blood cells are seen on the posterior corneal surface and in the inferior anterior chamber angle in this eye with severe anterior uveitis. (Courtesy of Carol L. Shields, M.D.)

examination. The ciliary body is located posterior to the iris root and is responsible for numerous functions, including aqueous humor production and accommodation. The choroid is posterior and lies between the retina and the sclera. Its main role is to provide a blood supply to the outer retina. Together these three components form a continuous uveal lining that can become involved in inflammatory conditions within the eye.

Terminology and Classification

Uveitis is a general term used to describe any inflammatory condition involving the uveal tract. Different terminology and classifications may be used to denote specific sites of the uveal tract primarily involved. For the anterior segment of the eye, the terms *iritis* and *iridocyclitis* are used to describe inflammation of the iris and iris/ciliary body, respectively. The terms *vitritis*, *retinitis*, and *choroiditis* are used to designate inflammation in specific parts of the posterior segment of the eye. The term *anterior uveitis* refers to any inflammation of the iris or the ciliary body, whereas the term *posterior uveitis* refers to any inflammation of the vitreous, retina, or choroid. To formulate a differential diagnosis, workup, and treatment plan, it is useful to distinguish whether uveitis primarily affects the anterior or the posterior segment of the eye. Some disorders present exclusively as anterior or posterior uveitis, though a few (e.g., sarcoidosis, Behçet's disease, syphilis, and tuberculosis) can present in both anterior and posterior segments. It must be remembered that classifying uveitis as anterior or posterior is sometimes difficult because either type may show signs of spillover into its counterpart. For example, severe anterior uveitis may result in anterior vitreous changes, whereas vitritis may manifest with signs in the anterior chamber. When both anterior and posterior segments of the uveal tract are definitely involved, it is called *panuveitis*. The term *endophthalmitis* is reserved for inflammation predominantly centered within the vitreous, and it is considered a special type of posterior uveitis because of its severity and need for prompt diagnostic workup and treatment.

Anterior uveitis can be further classified as either *granulomatous* (Fig. 7-1) or *nongranulomatous*. The former refers to a granulomatous inflammatory reaction with epithelioid and giant cells that forms large mutton-fat keratic precipitates (clumps of white blood cells on the posterior corneal surface) (Fig. 7-2). The latter signifies a nongranulomatous process with lymphocytic and plasma cell infiltration that demonstrates fine keratic precipitates. These characterizations can aid the clinician in suggesting an etiologic disease process.

General Approach

Although there are many different uveitic conditions (Box 7-1), most patients with anterior uveitis have similar signs and symptoms, usually red eye (Fig. 7-3) and photophobia (Boxes 7-2 and 7-3). Once these signs and symptoms are identified, a tailored workup should be formulated based on historical factors and ocular/systemic examination findings. The workup should begin with a careful history, review of systems, and complete ophthalmic examination. A general physical examination should also be performed for possible systemic findings of the suspected underlying disorder. A systemic diagnostic workup including various serologic/radiologic tests can then be initiated, depending on whether the episode of anterior uveitis is unilateral or bilateral, granulomatous or nongranulomatous, and initial or recurrent (Box 7-4).

Box 7-1 Causes of Anterior Uveitis

ARTHRITIS/VASCULITIS ASSOCIATED

HLA-B27-positive anterior uveitis
- Ankylosing spondylitis
- Reiter's syndrome
- Inflammatory bowel disease (ulcerative colitis and Crohn's disease)
- Psoriatic arthritis

Juvenile rheumatoid arthritis (JRA)
Behçet's disease
Sarcoidosis

INFECTIOUS

Syphilis
Tuberculosis
Lyme disease
Herpes simplex virus
Herpes zoster virus

MISCELLANEOUS

Idiopathic
Traumatic
Postoperative
Fuchs' heterochromic iridocyclitis (FHI)
Glaucomatocyclitic crisis (Posner-Schlossman syndrome)
Uveitis-glaucoma-hyphema (UGH) syndrome

MALIGNANCY*

Lymphoma
Leukemia
Retinoblastoma

*These noninflammatory conditions may mimic the clinical findings of anterior uveitis.

Box 7-2 Symptoms of Anterior Uveitis

Sensitivity to light (photophobia), pain
Normal or diminished vision
Acute or insidious onset
Nonocular symptoms (e.g., back pain, joint stiffness, dysuria) from systemic disorders associated with uveitis

Box 7-3 Signs of Anterior Uveitis

Unilateral or bilateral
Conjunctival injection primarily around the cornea (ciliary injection)
Deposits on the posterior surface of the cornea (keratic precipitates or KP) that may vary in size and appearance (fine, whitish KP in nongranulomatous uveitis and large, grayish, "mutton-fat" KP in granulomatous uveitis)
Floating inflammatory cells and protein (flare) in the anterior chamber (usually graded on a qualitative scale of 0 to 4+); if severe enough, these inflammatory cells may form a layer in the anterior chamber (hypopyon)
Fibrin in the anterior chamber
Adhesions of the iris to the front surface of the lens (posterior synechiae), which may cause a small or irregularly shaped pupil
Constricted pupil (even in the absence of posterior synechiae)
Nodules of inflammatory cells on the iris surface (called Koeppe nodules if located on the pupillary margin and Busacca nodules if located on the remainder of iris surface)

Finally, depending on the cause, a treatment plan should be initiated. In general, a cycloplegic agent is used for two reasons: to relieve pain and photophobia by paralyzing the ciliary muscles and to minimize inflammation by stabilizing the blood-aqueous barrier. The other mainstay of treatment is corticosteroids, which are administered in varying doses, frequencies, and delivery routes based on the severity of inflammation. Severe cases may require potent systemic immunosuppressive agents coordinated by a consulting internist or rheumatologist (Box 7-5). However, additional diagnostic tests and therapies are often warranted, depending on the specific diseases being treated. Short- and long-term complications of uveitis (e.g., glaucoma, hypotony, and cataract) must be addressed. Overall the prognosis is excellent for patients with first-time nongranulomatous anterior uveitis and less favorable for those with recurrent granulomatous anterior uveitis.

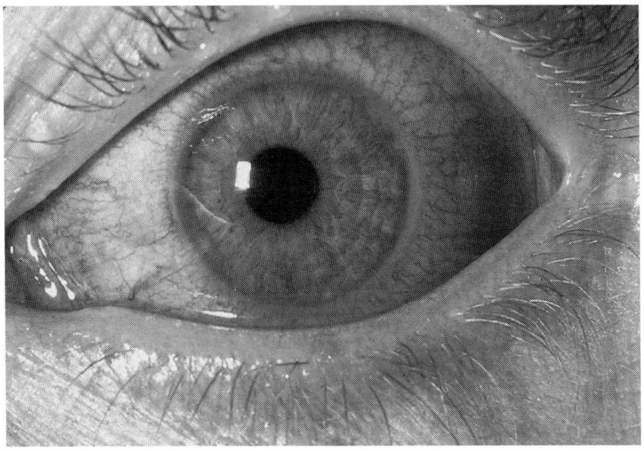

Fig. 7-3 Anterior uveitis. The fine white blood cells in the anterior chamber of this patient with nongranulomatous anterior uveitis cannot be seen. Red eye with perilimbal injection is typically present in eyes with anterior uveitis. (Courtesy of George O. Waring III, M.D.) (See color plate.)

Box 7-4 Workup for Anterior Uveitis

Careful history
Complete ocular examination (especially to rule out posterior segment involvement)
General physical examination (directed at possible systemic findings of the various conditions associated with anterior uveitis)
If the episode is unilateral, appears to be nongranulomatous, and is occurring for the first time and if the patient has an unremarkable history and examination, then no systemic workup is needed
If the episode is bilateral, appears to be granulomatous, or is recurrent and the patient has an unremarkable history and examination, then:
A. Initiate nonspecific diagnostic workup: CBC, ESR (preferably Westergren), ANA, RPR or VDRL, FTA-ABS or MHA-TP, PPD with anergy panel, chest radiography, Lyme titer (if in endemic area and if indicated)
B. Supplement or tailor the diagnostic workup with other tests/subspecialty consults if strongly indicated by symptoms, history, or physical findings (e.g., angiotensin-converting enzyme [ACE] for suspected sarcoidosis, sacroiliac spine radiographs for suspected ankylosing spondylitis, or rheumatology consult for suspected psoriatic arthritis)

Box 7-5 Treatment Guidelines for Anterior Uveitis

Topical cycloplegic (e.g., 1%-2% cyclopentolate, 0.25% scopolamine, or 1% atropine sulfate) 2 to 4 times a day, depending on the severity of inflammation
Corticosteroids:
  Topical (e.g., 1% prednisolone acetate) every 1 to 6 hours for mild to moderately severe inflammation
  Periocular injection (e.g., 40 to 80 mg methylprednisolone subtenons) for persistent or severe inflammation
  Systemic corticosteroid (e.g., 60 to 100 mg prednisone by mouth daily) for severe inflammation
Systemic immunosuppressives (e.g., cyclophosphamide, azathioprine, methotrexate, others), depending on cause and severity (should be coordinated with an internist or a rheumatologist)
Glaucoma treatment (e.g., 0.5% levobunolol or timolol twice a day, brimonidine 2 to 3 times a day, dorzolamide or brinzolamide 2 to 3 times a day, 50 to 75 mg methazolamide by mouth 2 to 3 times a day) as needed

Causes

Some common causes of anterior uveitis are idiopathic, traumatic, and postoperative, and others are more specific disorders such as human leukocyte antigen, locus B27 (HLA-B27)-related conditions, juvenile rheumatoid arthritis (JRA), sarcoidosis, and syphilis. These etiologies can be categorized according to presumed pathogenesis (Table 7-1). These and other important inflammatory conditions are discussed in this chapter.

Idiopathic Idiopathic anterior uveitis is more prevalent than any other type of anterior uveitis. Therefore, a diagnostic workup for a first-time episode of unilateral, nongranulomatous anterior uveitis, with a negative review of systems, is usually not performed. However, for all recurrent attacks or for an initial episode of a bilateral or granulomatous anterior uveitis, a workup should be initiated that includes a careful history and review of systems, complete ocular examination, general physical examination, and serologic/radiologic testing as outlined in Box 7-4.

Traumatic Patients who have had blunt trauma to the eye frequently have accompanying traumatic iritis, which varies in severity depending on the force of the trauma. Sometimes a consensual photophobic reaction is elicited from the traumatic eye when a penlight shines on the opposite normal eye. Although it is important to recognize this condition, perhaps even more crucial is the obligation to rule out any associated ocular injury (e.g., angle recession, retinal tear) with a complete dilated examination (see Chapter 11).

Postoperative Postoperative iritis occurs after almost every intraocular surgical procedure. Varying amounts of cell and flare are seen in the anterior chamber, depending on the surgical procedure and the extent of surgical manipulation. However, disproportionate amounts of inflammation accompanied by excessive pain should be a warning sign for postoperative endophthalmitis (see Chapter 10).

HLA-B27-positive anterior uveitis This category encompasses a group of disorders that is associated with positive results of HLA-B27 testing and that may be present in up to 50% to 60% of patients with anterior uveitis.

Ankylosing spondylitis This can be a crippling disorder affecting young men. Patients have lower back pain or morning stiffness in addition to the symptoms of anterior uveitis. Sacroiliac (*not* lumbosacral) radiographs showing sclerosis and narrowing of the joint space can be diagnostic. Serious complications include pulmonary apical fibrosis and aortitis (in 5% of patients).

Reiter's syndrome This syndrome consists of a triad of nonspecific urethritis, polyarthritis, and conjunctivitis/anterior uveitis. It also affects young men. Organisms such as *Chlamydia, Shigella*, and *Salmonella* have been implicated as triggering episodes of inflammation. Other major diagnostic criteria include keratoderma

Table 7-1 Common causes and clinical features of anterior uveitis

Causes	Clinical signs	Serologic tests	Other diagnostic tests	Systemic treatment
Idiopathic	Cell and flare Ciliary injection	None	None	None
Traumatic	Cell and flare Ciliary injection	None	B-scan ultrasonography or computed tomography as needed	None
Postoperative	Cell and flare Ciliary injection	None	B-scan ultrasonography as needed	None
HLA-B27+:				
Ankylosing spondylitis	Abnormal sacroiliac spine	Elevated erythrocyte sedimentation rate	Abnormal sacroiliac films	Systemic nonsteroidal antiinflammatory drugs
Reiter's syndrome	Urethritis Polyarthritis Conjunctivitis or anterior uveitis	Elevated erythrocyte sedimentation rate	Conjunctival, urethral, prostatic cultures	Tetracycline or erythromycin
Inflammatory bowel disease	Chronic diarrhea alternating with constipation	Per gastrointestinal consultation	Gastrointestinal series	Systemic corticosteroids, sulfadiazine, or both
Psoriatic arthritis	Skin rash Terminal phalanx joint inflammation Nail pitting	Per rheumatology consultation	Joint films	Systemic corticosteroids and other antipsoriatic therapy
Juvenile rheumatoid arthritis	Posterior synechiae and cataract	Positive antinuclear antibody (ANA) Negative rheumatoid factor (RF)	Joint films	Systemic nonsteroidal antiinflammatory drugs and corticosteroids
Behçet's disease	Hypopyon iritis Oral ulcers Genital ulcers	HLA-B27 HLA-B5	Behçet's skin test	Systemic corticosteroids and immunosuppressive agents
Sarcoidosis	"Mutton-fat" keratic precipitates Koeppe and Busacca nodules	Elevated angiotensin-converting enzyme (ACE)	Purified protein derivative (PPD) with anergy Chest radiography Skin/conjunctival biopsy Gallium imaging Bronchial biopsy	Topical, periocular, and systemic corticosteroids
Syphilis	Ghost vessels in cornea (interstitial keratitis) 1′,2′,3′ syphilis	Venereal Disease Research Laboratory (VDRL) or rapid plasma reagin (RPR) test Microhemagglutination-*Treponema pallidum* test (MHA-TP) or fluorescein treponemal antibody (FTA)	Lumbar puncture (if neurosyphilis suspected)	Systemic penicillin

HLA-B27, Human leukocyte antigen, locus B27.

blenorrhagicum (a scaly, erythematous dermatologic disorder involving the palms and soles) and circinate balanitis (a similar rash involving the distal penis). Conjunctival, urethral, and prostatic cultures should be obtained to aid in the diagnosis. Culture findings are often negative, but they may be positive for *Chlamydia* or other organisms, which should then be treated.

Inflammatory bowel diseases Inflammatory bowel diseases (ulcerative colitis more commonly than Crohn's disease) can be associated with acute anterior uveitis.

Patients often experience chronic intermittent diarrhea, which can alternate with bouts of constipation. The bowel disease may be asymptomatic until after the onset of iritis. Patients are often under the simultaneous care of an internist or a gastrointestinal specialist.

Psoriatic arthritis Psoriatic arthritis is another disease in this category that can present with anterior uveitis. However, iritis is not associated with psoriasis without arthritis. Patients typically have an erythematous, hyperkeratotic rash, terminal phalangeal joint inflammation, and nail bed pitting changes. Diagnostic workup and treatment are usually coordinated with a rheumatologist.

Juvenile Rheumatoid Arthritis

Juvenile rheumatoid arthritis (JRA) accompanied by anterior uveitis typically affects young girls with pauciarticular (fewer than five joints) involvement. Ocular inflammation may precede or follow the arthritis. Chronic nongranulomatous anterior uveitis often results in posterior synechiae and cataract formation. Common findings on serologic testing include a negative rheumatoid factor and positive antinuclear antibody. Systemic signs often include fever, rash, and lymphadenopathy. JRA-associated anterior uveitis often requires chronic topical corticosteroid therapy (adjusted by the degree of cell, *not* flare, found in the anterior chamber) and cycloplegia. Consultation with a pediatrician or a rheumatologist is obtained to manage the systemic disease.

Behçet's Disease

Behçet's disease is an idiopathic, occlusive form of vasculitis that typically affects young adults in the Near East and Japan. Classic features include the triad of acute hypopyon iritis, oral ulcers, and genital ulcers. Although the anterior hypopyon iritis may be striking in appearance, it is actually the posterior segment involvement (i.e., retinal hemorrhages, arterial occlusions, periphlebitis, macular edema, ischemic optic neuropathy, and vitritis) that is more prevalent in men. Ophthalmic findings are generally bilateral, recurrent, and chronic. Other characteristic systemic features include ulcerative hemorrhages of the gastrointestinal tract, erythema nodosum of the lower extremities, recurrent arthritis of the wrists and ankles, and central nervous system findings of stroke and cranial nerve palsies.

Diagnosis is based on clinical findings and on positive results of Behçet's skin testing (the skin forms a blister minutes to hours after intradermal puncture with a sterile 25- to 30-gauge needle). Treatment includes the use of systemic corticosteroids or other immunosuppressive agents (e.g., cyclosporine and chlorambucil) and is often coordinated with a rheumatologist.

Sarcoidosis

Sarcoidosis is a multiorgan disease that typically develops with chronic, bilateral granulomatous uveitis. Mutton-fat keratic precipitates, Koeppe nodules (clumps of inflammatory cells on the pupillary border), and Busacca nodules (clumps of inflammatory cells on the iris surface) are classic signs of sarcoidosis (Fig. 7-4). Anterior segment inflammation can be serious enough to result in iris bombé and angle-closure glaucoma because of severe posterior synechiae (Fig. 7-5). Granulomas of the conjunctiva and skin may also develop. Depending on the degree of suspicion, diagnostic tests include serum angiotensin-converting enzyme and lysozyme, purified protein derivative (PPD) with anergy panel, chest radiography, conjunctival or skin nodule biopsy, gallium im-

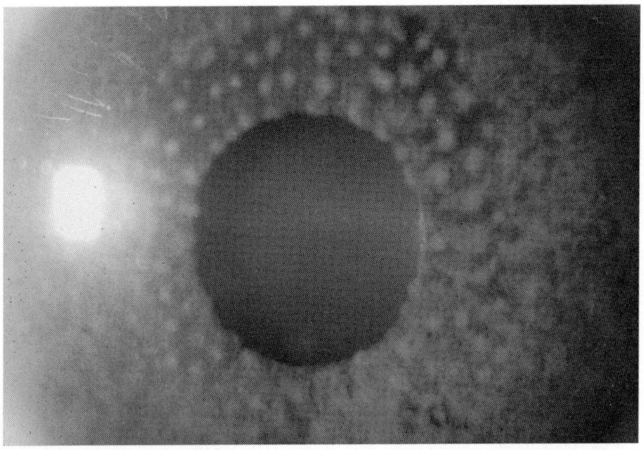

Fig. 7-4 Koeppe and Busacca nodules. Koeppe nodules on the pupillary border and Busacca nodules on the iris surface are obvious in this eye with sarcoid uveitis.

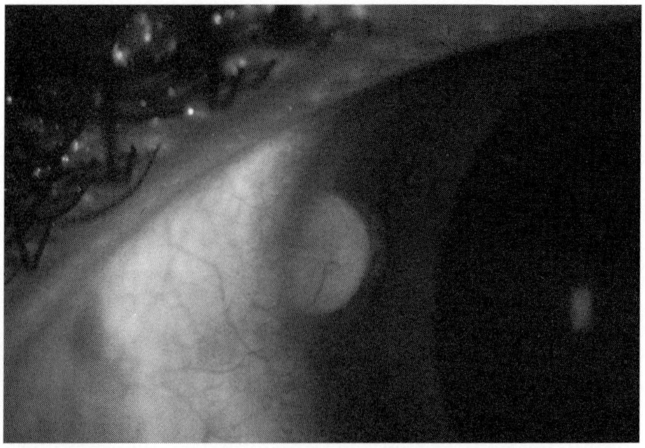

Fig. 7-5 Sarcoid granuloma. A large intraocular sarcoid granuloma in the anterior chamber angle is evident in this eye with sarcoidosis. (Courtesy of Carol L. Shields, M.D.)

aging of the head and neck, and endotracheal transbronchial biopsy. A biopsy specimen of a conjunctival nodule can provide a simple, rapid, and safe histopathologic diagnosis for many patients with suspected sarcoidosis. Nondirected conjunctival biopsy, that is, a biopsy specimen from an apparently normal conjunctiva, has a low yield in the histopathologic diagnosis of sarcoidosis. In addition to topical therapy, periocular and systemic corticosteroids are often necessary. Neurosarcoidosis can cause facial nerve palsy, meningitis, or a space-occupying mass in a small percentage of patients with sarcoidosis. Internal medicine, pulmonary medicine, or neurology specialists should be consulted regarding treatment of the systemic disease.

Syphilis

Syphilis is often referred to as the "great imitator" because its clinical manifestations mimic many disease processes. In the anterior segment, congenital syphilis causes acute interstitial keratitis with accompanying anterior uveitis (keratouveitis) in patients between the ages of 5 and 25 years. Initially the cornea develops a "ground-glass" appearance. Several weeks later significant corneal neovascularization develops. The deep corneal vessels are partially masked by the stromal inflammation, turning the cornea pink (the classic "salmon patch"). Bilateral involvement occurs with congenital disease, whereas unilateral involvement indicates acquired disease, which is generally seen in sexually active adults. Systemic signs such as deafness, Hutchinson's teeth, saddle nose, and frontal bossing often accompany congenital interstitial keratitis. Patients report intense pain and photophobia and can present with systemic signs, including a maculopapular rash of the palms and soles (i.e., secondary syphilis) and central nervous system involvement (i.e., tertiary syphilis or neurosyphilis).

If syphilis is suspected, the workup should include a Venereal Disease Research Laboratory (VDRL) or a rapid plasma reagin (RPR) test and a microhemagglutination–*Treponema pallidum* (MHA-TP) or fluorescent treponemal antibody absorption (FTA-ABS) test. The VDRL and RPR levels decrease and revert to normal with treatment and are used to follow disease activity. The MHA-TP and FTA-ABS levels remain positive. A lumbar puncture should be considered for patients with syphilis who have neurologic or neuroophthalmic signs, posterior uveitis, or papillitis and for patients with concomitant human immunodeficiency virus infection. Definitive treatment involves systemic therapy with penicillin—aqueous crystalline penicillin G 12 to 24 million U/day intravenously for 10 days followed by benzathine penicillin G 2.4 million U each week intramuscularly for 3 weeks. Patients who are allergic to penicillin can receive tetracycline or erythromycin 500 mg by mouth four times a day for 4 weeks, in consultation with an internist, a neurologist, or an infectious disease specialist as needed. It can take months to years for the corneal inflammation to clear. Residual corneal thinning, deep scarring, and visible ghost vessels usually result.

Tuberculosis

Tuberculosis causes chronic granulomatous anterior uveitis with or without posterior segment involvement. Characteristic anterior segment findings include mutton-fat keratic precipitates and iris granulomas. Although rarely found in the United States today, tuberculosis should be suspected in various populations, including patients who are immunocompromised and indigent.

A PPD with anergy panel and a chest radiograph should be obtained to aid in the diagnosis. However, most patients with positive PPD results have subclinical or inactive disease. In fact, many patients have pulmonary tuberculosis without ocular disease; conversely, some patients have ocular tuberculosis without pulmonary disease. Confirming the diagnosis may be difficult. For patients thought to have tuberculosis, a diagnostic trial of isoniazid should be instituted for 2 weeks; if it is beneficial, it should be continued for 6 to 12 months. Multidrug therapy with rifampin and pyrazinamide may be indicated for resistant or severe cases. Therapy should be coordinated with either an infectious disease or a pulmonary specialist.

Lyme Disease

Lyme disease is a spirochetal infection caused by the organism *Borrelia burgdorferi*, and it is transmitted from harboring deer, dogs, cats, and birds to humans by the bite of the vector tick *Ixodes* (*Ixodes dammini* in the eastern United States, *Ixodes pacificus* in the western United States). The most characteristic ophthalmic findings include chronic anterior uveitis and vitritis. Other ocular manifestations include follicular conjunctivitis (early), nummular keratitis, optic neuritis, and panophthalmitis. The classic skin lesion of erythema chronicum migrans occurs at the site of the tick bite and appears as an elevated, erythematous bull's-eye lesion with central clearing. The other clinical features are divided into three stages. Stage 1 comprises skin, eye, and constitutional symptoms, including fever, malaise, myalgias, and arthralgias. Stage 2 comprises neurologic and musculoskeletal abnormalities, including meningitis and arthritis. Stage 3 comprises chronic dermatitis, meningitis, and arthritis.

In addition to clinical symptoms and signs indicative of the disease, diagnosis is aided by checking Lyme immunofluorescent antibody titers or enzyme-linked immunosorbent assay for IgM and IgG (IgM may be negative in the early stages of disease). Unfortunately, these labora-

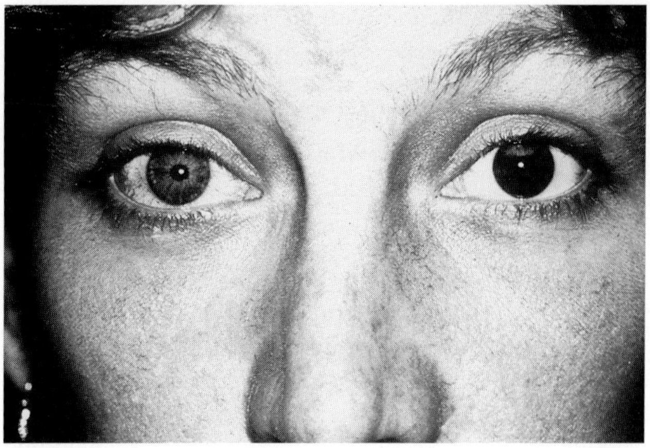

Fig. 7-6 Fuchs' heterochromic iridocyclitis. Numerous flare-ups of Fuchs' heterochromic iridocyclitis have occurred in this patient's right eye. Note the blue right eye and the brown left eye. (Courtesy of George O. Waring III, M.D.) (See color plate.)

tory test results are positive in only 40% to 60% of patients with Lyme disease. Current treatment recommendations of early disease include a 3- to 4-week course of oral tetracycline, doxycycline, erythromycin, or penicillin. Patients with advanced disease and neurologic involvement are treated with intravenous ceftriaxone or penicillin.

Herpes Simplex/Herpes Zoster

Herpes simplex and herpes zoster infections can cause secondary inflammation of the anterior uvea. Anterior uveitis is frequently accompanied by concomitant corneal inflammation (keratouveitis). The inflammatory infiltrates typically form nongranulomatous stellate keratic precipitates diffusely on the corneal endothelium. Occasionally a granulomatous reaction occurs. Chronic inflammation can lead to characteristic patterns of iris stromal atrophy (peripupillary with herpes simplex and segmental with herpes zoster). Unlike many other inflammatory syndromes, which tend to cause ciliary body shutdown and low intraocular pressure, herpetic uveitis is frequently accompanied by the frustrating complication of glaucoma. Particularly with herpes zoster infections, intraocular pressure can be very difficult to control. Management of anterior uveitis involves systemic treatment with antiviral agents (e.g., acyclovir) when indicated in addition to topical corticosteroids and cycloplegic and antiglaucoma agents. Details of herpes simplex and herpes zoster infections are included in Chapter 4.

Fuchs' Heterochromic Iridocyclitis

Fuchs' heterochromic iridocyclitis is an unusual disorder that causes unilateral nongranulomatous anterior uveitis. This condition is rarely symptomatic because the inflammation is often subtle. Ophthalmic signs include diffuse iris stromal atrophy that gives the iris a lighter color on the involved side (Fig. 7-6). Other characteristic findings consist of fine, stellate keratic precipitates on the entire corneal endothelium and the absence of posterior synechiae. The diagnosis is made on ophthalmic examination with no further testing indicated. Treatment with topical corticosteroids is typically ineffective. Fuchs' heterochromic iridocyclitis is often associated with glaucoma and posterior subcapsular cataract formation, both of which may be exacerbated by topical corticosteroids. Patients generally respond well to cataract surgery if it is needed.

Glaucomatocyclitic Crisis (Posner-Schlossman Syndrome)

Glaucomatocyclitic crisis, or Posner-Schlossman syndrome, is a rare but interesting condition marked by unilateral episodes of significantly elevated intraocular pressure (up to 50 to 70 mm Hg) and resultant corneal microcystic edema with mild, acute anterior uveitis. The anterior chamber shows trace cell and flare with fine keratic precipitates and a fixed, mid-dilated pupil with an open angle on gonioscopy. The episodes last from several hours to several days and recur for many years. Treatment involves the use of topical corticosteroids and antiglaucoma agents (typically aqueous suppressants and carbonic anhydrase inhibitors). Pilocarpine is generally avoided to preserve the blood-aqueous barrier.

Uveitis-Glaucoma-Hyphema Syndrome

Uveitis-glaucoma-hyphema, or UGH syndrome, is an inflammatory condition thought to be caused by mechanical trauma to the iris root by the footplates of a rigid anterior chamber intraocular lens or any poorly situated intraocular lens. This traumatic chafing of the iris presumably leads to a cascade of events involving anterior uveitis, secondary inflammatory glaucoma, and eventual hyphema formation. UGH syndrome is seen less often today because of the advancements in open-loop flexible anterior chamber intraocular lenses.

IRIS CYSTS

Primary Iris Cysts

Iris stromal cysts Of the two major categories of primary iris cysts (i.e., stromal and pigment epithelial), stromal cysts are less common. As indicated by the name, they are located in the iris stroma. They are sometimes referred to as congenital epithelial cysts of the iris

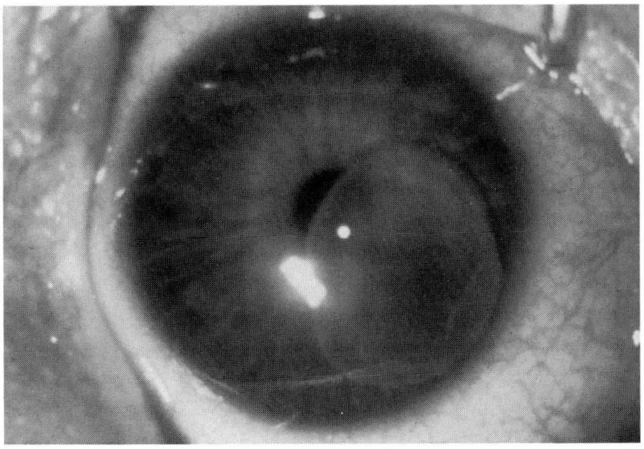

Fig. 7-7 Iris stromal cyst. A large iris stromal cyst partially occludes this patient's pupil. Note its transparent appearance. (Courtesy of Carol L. Shields, M.D.)

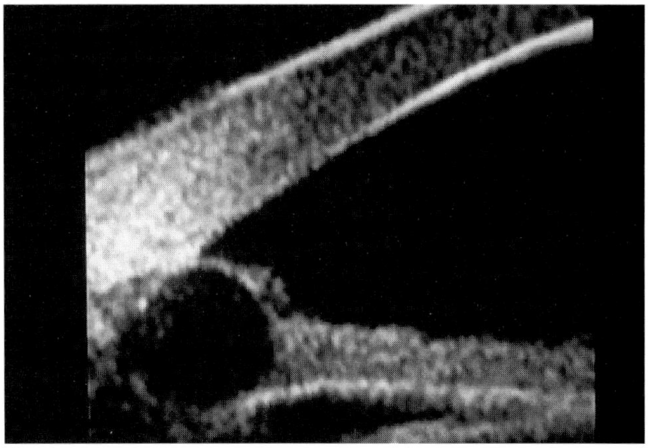

Fig. 7-8 Iris stromal cyst ultrasound biomicroscopy. An ultrasound biomicroscopic photograph of an iris stromal cyst. The cyst originates in the iris stroma, demonstrated by the thin layer of iris on the anterior aspect of the cyst. (Courtesy of Elizabeth L. Affel, M.S.)

because of their developmental nature and their stratified lining of cells, resembling corneal or conjunctival epithelium. These lesions are found in infants and young children, who frequently have no history of surgery or trauma. They are easily distinguished from other malignant iris tumors by their transparent appearance (Figs. 7-7 and 7-8). Although they are benign they may enlarge and occlude the visual axis, and rarely precipitate attacks of angle closure glaucoma. Unless such complications are encountered, observation is recommended.

Iris pigment epithelial cysts Most primary iris cysts arise from the posterior pigment epithelial layer of the iris. They are pigmented, elevated iris lesions that can be mistaken for malignant iris melanoma. These cysts can be unilateral and solitary or present with bilateral involvement, and are usually located in the inferotemporal quadrant of the peripheral iris. Slit-lamp examination reveals a smooth, dome-shaped elevation in the iris, like a ball thrown under a carpet (Fig. 7-9). They may be associated with overlying atrophy of the iris stroma.

Various examination techniques and diagnostic tools can help differentiate iris pigment epithelial cysts from malignant melanoma (Table 7-2). Slit-lamp examination reveals that in contrast to pigment epithelial cysts, malignant melanoma arises from the iris stroma and has an irregular shape and a discrete border. When the peripheral iris is involved, gonioscopy can be useful in delineating angle involvement and further detailing structure. Transillumination is a frequently underused but invaluable technique to distinguish between the two types of lesions: pigment epithelial cysts readily transilluminate whereas malignant melanomas block light. Recently, ultrasound biomicroscopy has proven successful in revealing the underlying cystic or solid structure of the lesion (Fig. 7-10).

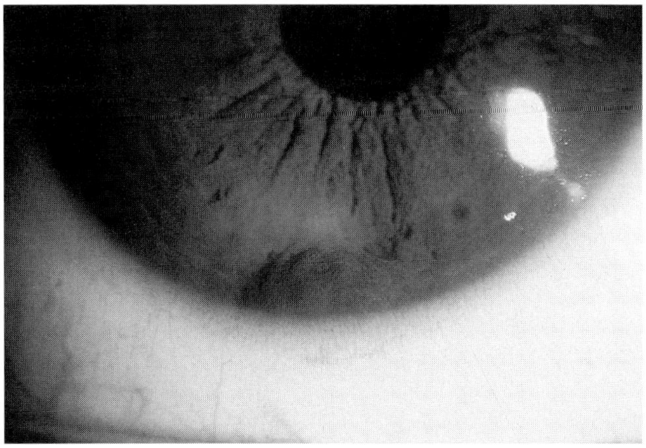

Fig. 7-9 Iris pigment epithelial cyst. An elevated iris mass is visible at the inferior anterior chamber angle. This lesion was smooth and transilluminated, which helped in its differentiation from iris nevus or melanoma.

Pigment epithelial cysts are generally stationary and rarely increase in size. Occasionally, they detach from the iris and float freely in the anterior chamber, potentially causing traumatic damage to the corneal endothelium (Fig. 7-11). In this case, they may be removed by aspiration through a clear corneal incision. Otherwise, no treatment is indicated. It is important to distinguish these lesions from malignant neoplasms of the iris.

Secondary Iris Cysts

Secondary iris cysts result from ingrowth or implantation of surface epithelium in the anterior chamber. Trauma and surgery are the two most common causes

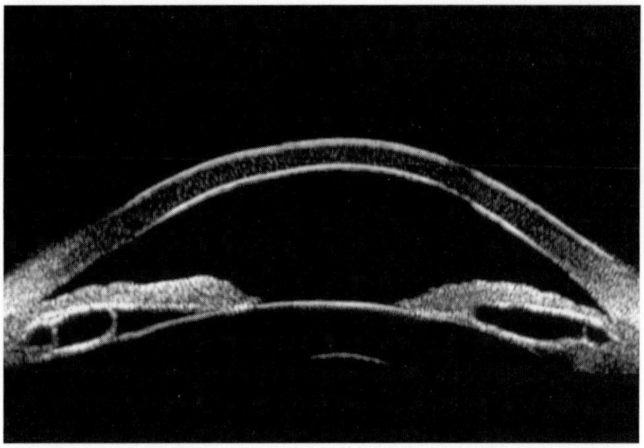

Fig. 7-10 Iris pigment epithelial cyst ultrasound biomicroscopy. This composite ultrasound biomicroscopic photograph demonstrates large pigment epithelial cysts 180° from each other. As these cysts originate in the iris pigment epithelium on the posterior aspect of the iris, they can be seen to push the overlying iris forward. (Courtesy of Elizabeth L. Affel, M.S.)

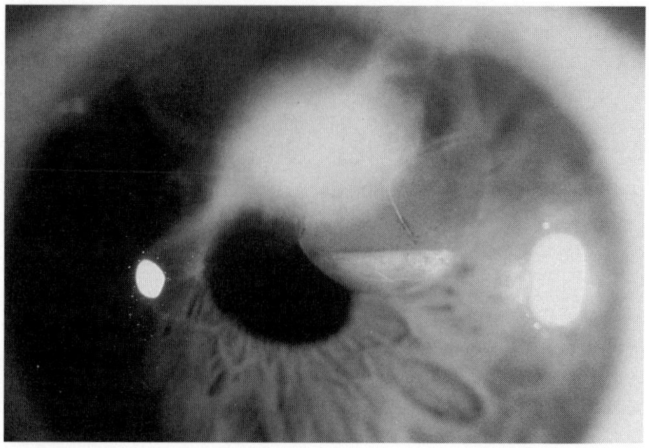

Fig. 7-11 Iris pigment epithelial cyst. This large pigment epithelial cyst of the iris was caused by trauma. It can potentially cause damage to the corneal endothelial surface. (Courtesy of R. Doyle Stulting, M.D., Ph.D.)

Table 7-2 Clinical features of iris pigment epithelial cysts and iris melanomas

Feature	Pigment epithelial cysts	Malignant melanomas
Growth	Minimal to none	Definite growth
Pigmentation	Pigmented	Pigmented (melanotic) or nonpigmented (amelanotic)
Appearance	Smooth, pigmented, and dome shaped	Similar appearance versus a shape with discrete border (depending on localized or diffuse type)
Location	Inferior iris	Inferior iris
Transillumination	Readily transilluminates	Does not transilluminate
Morphology (on ultrasound biomicroscopy)	Cystic structure	Solid structure
Other ocular signs	Secondary glaucoma	Feeder vessels Seeding of tumor to adjacent iris or anterior chamber angle Spontaneous hyphema Secondary glaucoma

(Fig. 7-12). The chronic use of miotic agents (e.g., pilocarpine, echothiophate, physostigmine) is known to cause iris cyst formation.

IRIS TUMORS

Various tumors may present in the iris (Table 7-3).

Nevus

An iris nevus is a benign proliferation of stromal melanocytes that appears clinically as a flat or minimally thickened, hyperpigmented lesion on the iris (Figs. 7-13 and 7-14). These lesions typically appear at puberty and, unlike malignant melanomas, do not grow. They rarely exceed 3 mm in diameter but can be large enough to cause ectropion uveae, sector cataract, and secondary glaucoma (Fig. 7-15). They are usually found in the inferior half of the iris. Recommended therapy includes regular follow-up examinations with serial photographs to document possible growth. Any observed growth or change in appearance warrants concern for malignant transformation.

Malignant Melanoma

Malignant melanoma is a neoplastic proliferation of stromal melanocytes that alters normal iris architecture. Lesions may be localized or diffuse and pigmented

Table 7-3 Clinical features of iris tumors

Feature	Nevus	Melanoma	Metastatic	Inflammatory granuloma
Location	Inferior iris	Inferior iris	Any part of the iris	Any part of the iris
Size	≤3 mm diameter	Variable	Variable	Variable
Pigmentation	Hyperpigmented	Hyperpigmented or hypopigmented	Hypopigmented	Hypopigmented (whitish-gray)
Growth	None	Definite	Definite	Waxes and wanes
Other ocular signs	None	Feeder vessels Seeding of adjacent structures Spontaneous hyphema Secondary glaucoma	Pseudohypopyon Neovascularization of the iris	Ciliary injection Anterior chamber cell and flare "Mutton-fat" keratic precipitates

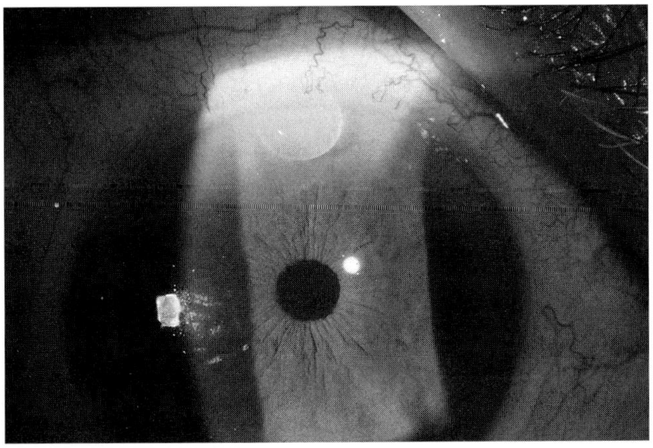

Fig. 7-12 Free-floating anterior chamber cyst. Because this free-floating cyst was causing damage corneal edema with a progressive decline in endothelial cell count, it was removed.

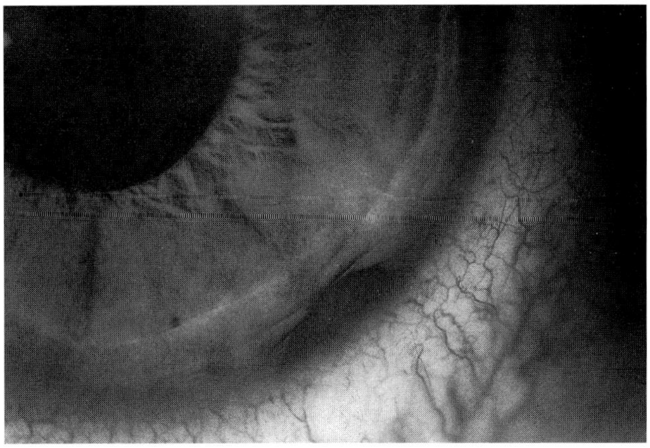

Fig. 7-13 Iris nevus. This darkly pigmented, irregularly shaped, solid-looking mass does not transilluminate light. It is thought to be an iris nevus and is being followed clinically.

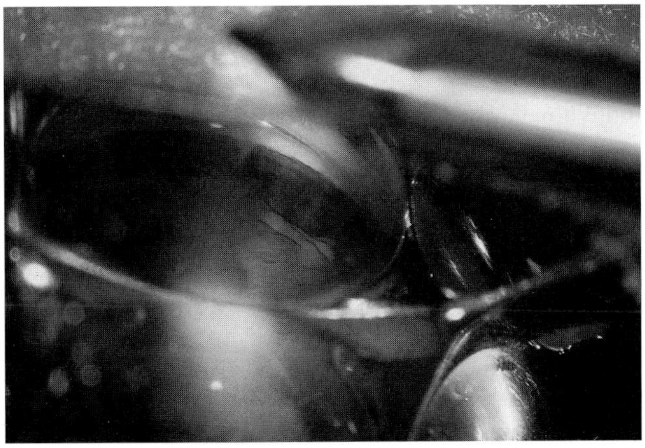

Fig. 7-14 Iris nevus. A gonioscopic view of the iris nevus seen in Fig. 7-13 demonstrates that it does not involve the anterior chamber angle.

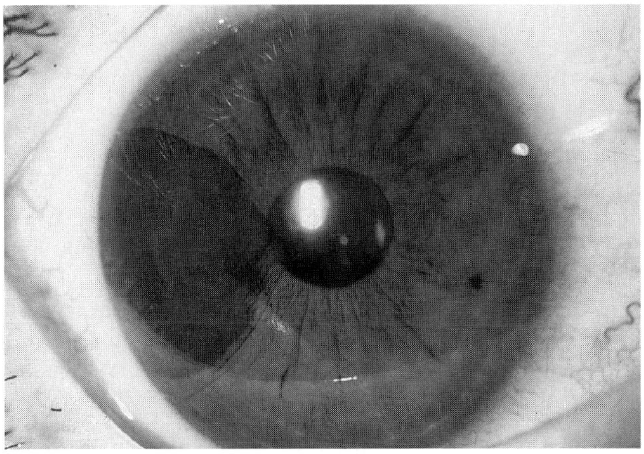

Fig. 7-15 Iris nevus. A large iris nevus measuring approximately 4.5 × 5 mm in this 31-year-old white woman has been followed without documented growth. (Courtesy of Carol L. Shields, M.D.)

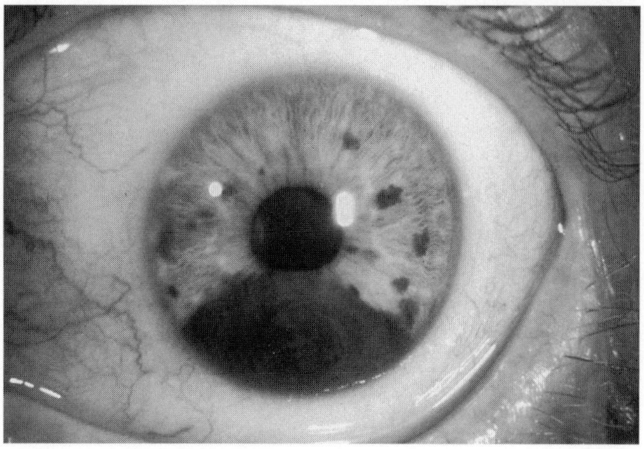

Fig. 7-16 Iris malignant melanoma. This large iris mass was determined histopathologically to be a malignant melanoma. (Courtesy of Carol L. Shields, M.D.)

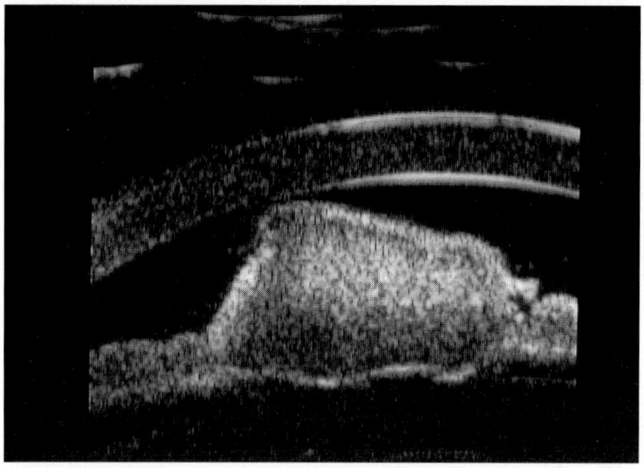

Fig. 7-17 Iris malignant melanoma ultrasound biomicroscopy. Ultrasound biomicroscopic photograph of a large iris malignant melanoma. (Courtesy of Elizabeth L. Affel, M.S.)

(melanotic) (Fig. 7-16) or nonpigmented (amelanotic). Like nevi, they typically occur in the inferior portion of the iris in light-skinned persons. The most important suggestion of malignancy is documented growth. Other signs that may indicate malignancy include large tumor size, prominent feeder vessels, seeding of tumor onto adjacent iris or into the angle, secondary glaucoma, and spontaneous hyphema.

Patients with suspected malignant iris melanoma should be questioned about their history of skin melanoma or other tumors and about constitutional symptoms such as weight loss or anorexia. Evaluation should always include careful slit-lamp examination with gonioscopy, dilated fundus examination, transillumination, and serial photography. Ultrasound biomicroscopy may also be helpful (Fig. 7-17). Suspicious localized lesions require excisional biopsy with iridectomy, iridocyclectomy, or iridogoniocyclectomy, whereas diffuse lesions sometimes require enucleation. Plaque radiotherapy has been used for diffuse iris melanoma. The prognosis for surgically resected focal iris lesions is good but worsens considerably with ciliary body involvement or extraocular extension.

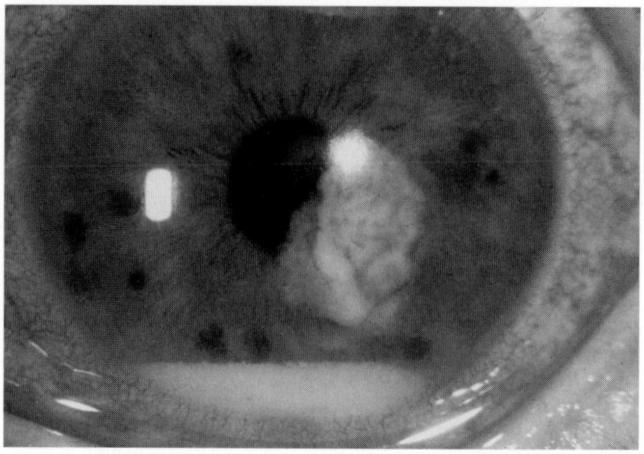

Fig. 7-18 Iris metastasis. A large vascularized metastatic lesion to the iris is seen. A pseudohypopyon consisting of tumor cells is present. (Courtesy of Carol L. Shields, M.D.)

Metastatic Tumors

Metastatic tumors to the uveal tract are the most common form of intraocular malignancy. However, they develop more frequently in the posterior uvea than in the iris. Clinically, they are distinguished by their amelanotic appearance and their tendency to present as multiple nodules on the iris of both eyes. They may also be accompanied by iris neovascularization and cells in the anterior chamber, sometimes mimicking iritis and forming a pseudohypopyon (Fig. 7-18). These tumors involve the superior and inferior portions of the iris and can grow rapidly (Fig. 7-19). The most common sources of primary tumor include lung cancer in males and breast cancer in females.

Metastatic iris tumors are often diagnosed by a history of primary cancer and typical findings on ophthalmic examination. However, they can be the first manifestation of an unknown primary neoplasm. In this case, fine-needle aspiration biopsy can be useful in confirming the diagnosis and directing further workup for the primary lesion. In general, these metastatic tumors respond well to local radiation and systemic chemotherapy.

Inflammatory Granuloma

When examining any iris lesion, the possibility of an inflammatory granuloma, such as those caused by sarcoidosis, tuberculosis, or leprosy, should be included in

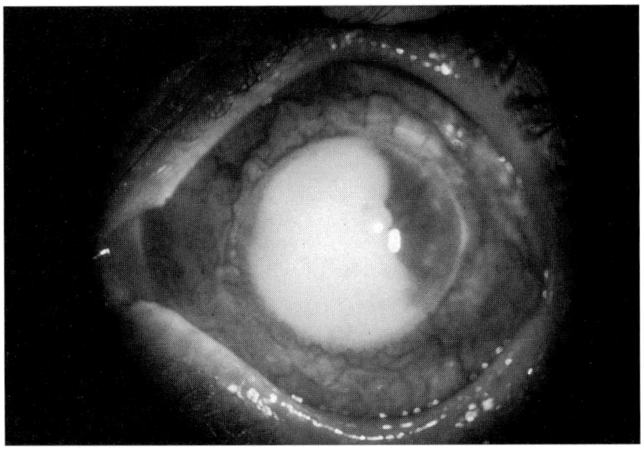

Fig. 7-19 Iris metastasis. Metastatic colon cancer to the eye has almost entirely filled the anterior chamber with tumor cells.

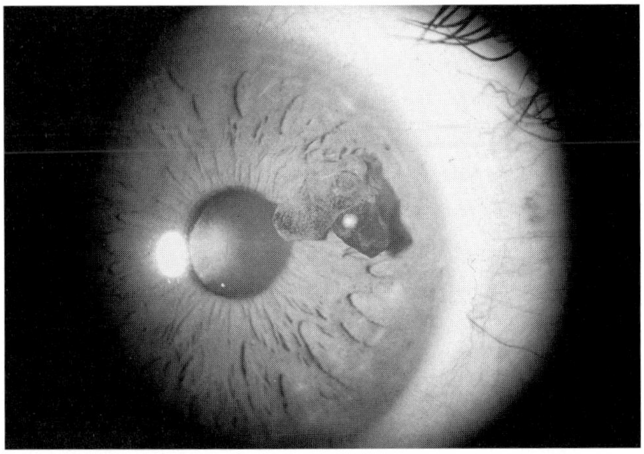

Fig. 7-20 Vascular iris tumor. A large vascular iris tumor is present. It intermittently touched the corneal endothelium and caused corneal edema. (See color plate.)

the differential diagnosis. These whitish-gray lesions are composed of clumps of inflammatory cells and can resemble neoplastic iris lesions. They tend to be multifocal and can be located anywhere on the iris. When present, they are usually accompanied by signs of active inflammation caused by the systemic condition.

Juvenile Xanthogranuloma

Juvenile xanthogranuloma (JXG) is a benign histiocytic inflammatory disease of unknown cause that usually affects infants and children younger than 3 years of age. Most patients have self-limited skin lesions only. They are dome-shaped, elevated nodules that are yellow-reddish-brown in color. They may be few or multiple, and their diameters range from 1 to 20 mm. The number of nodules can increase for the first year or two, but then

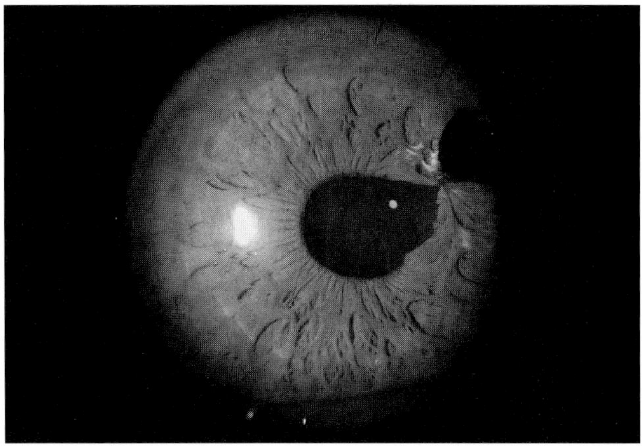

Fig. 7-21 Vascular iris tumor after resection. The iris tumor seen in Fig. 7-20 is shown at 6 weeks after resection. A prolene suture was used to partially close the iridectomy.

the nodules regress and typically disappear in the next 3 to 4 years. The lesions consist of uniform histiocytes, Touton giant cells, and other inflammatory cells.

Similar nodular lesions may develop in the iris and ciliary body. Although often unilateral, they may be bilateral. These lesions can produce serious consequences. The fragile, thin-walled blood vessels of the nodules are prone to bleeding and may cause a hyphema. JXG is important in the differential diagnosis of spontaneous hyphema in a child. Recurrent hyphema can cause glaucoma and corneal blood staining.

Diagnosis is aided by identifying a typical skin lesion from which a biopsy specimen can be taken. Skin lesions can be observed. Ocular lesions require close follow-up to manage sequelae of bleeding. Iris and ciliary body nodules can be treated with topical and systemic corticosteroids, which may induce regression. Other treatment options include radiation and surgical excision.

Vascular Tumors of the Iris

Vascular tumors of the iris are extremely rare (Figs. 7-20 and 7-21).

CONGENITAL ANOMALIES OF THE IRIS

Aniridia

Aniridia is considered a developmental anomaly of the iris and is discussed in detail in Chapter 2.

Coloboma

Coloboma refers to an absence or a defect in any portion of the eye resulting from faulty closure of the embryonic fissure. When the iris is involved, the coloboma

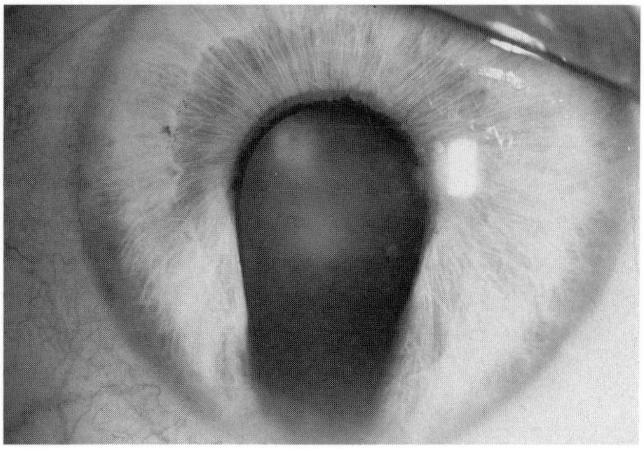

Fig. 7-22 Iris coloboma. A large iris coloboma is present inferiorly, giving the iris a "keyhole" appearance.

is usually located in the inferonasal quadrant where the normal embryonic fissure closes, causing the pupil to be shaped like a keyhole (Fig. 7-22). The lens zonular attachments may also be absent in this area, causing lens defects, sector cataracts, and phacodonesis. Therefore, cataract surgery in these patients should be approached with caution. Iris colobomas may present as an isolated finding or in combination with other ocular defects. Complete ocular examination may reveal the presence of colobomas involving the posterior segment (e.g., retina and optic nerve).

Persistent Pupillary Membrane

The whitish, wispy strands frequently found on the pupillary border are the remnants of the anterior vascular capsule of the tunica vasculosa lentis. These strands are referred to as a *persistent pupillary membrane* and are clinically insignificant.

Iris Heterochromia

Congenital iris heterochromia simply refers to the difference in iris color between the eyes of the same person. This difference in iris pigmentation is frequently detected at birth or in early childhood and is not progressive. Numerous conditions have been noted to cause this strikingly apparent anomaly; either the darker or the lighter iris may be abnormal (Box 7-6).

Box 7-6 Major Causes of Congenital Iris Heterochromia

Hypochromic (involved eye with lighter iris color)
- Congenital Horner's syndrome
- Waardenburg's syndrome
- Fuchs' heterochromic iridocyclitis

Hyperchromic (involved eye with darker iris color)
- Ocular melanocytosis
- Oculodermal melanocytosis (nevus of Ota)

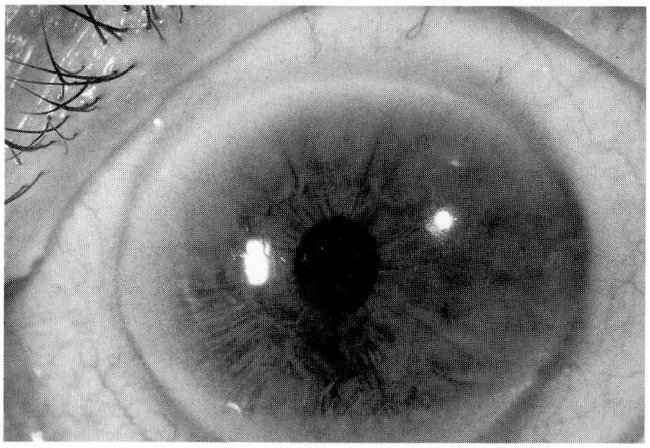

Fig. 7-23 Iridoschisis. The inferior iris appears delaminated in this eye with iridoschisis. The patient has no history of ocular surgery or trauma.

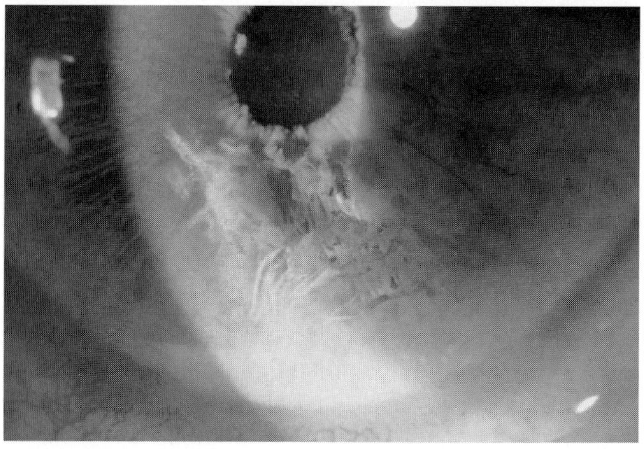

Fig. 7-24 Iridoschisis. A higher magnification view of the eye seen in Fig. 7-23 demonstrates separation of the iris stromal layers seen in iridoschisis.

IRIDOSCHISIS

Iridoschisis is a rare condition that usually appears in the sixth or seventh decade. It is characterized by separation of the layers of the iris stroma, typically in both eyes (Figs. 7-23 and 7-24). Glaucoma develops in approximately half the patients with iridoschisis. Corneal edema may also be seen, perhaps from the iris strands damaging the endothelial cells. The differential diagnosis of iridoschisis includes iridocorneal endothelial syndromes, Axenfeld's anomaly, and Rieger's anomaly. These conditions tend to present much earlier in life. Therapy for iridoschisis is required if glaucoma or corneal edema develops.

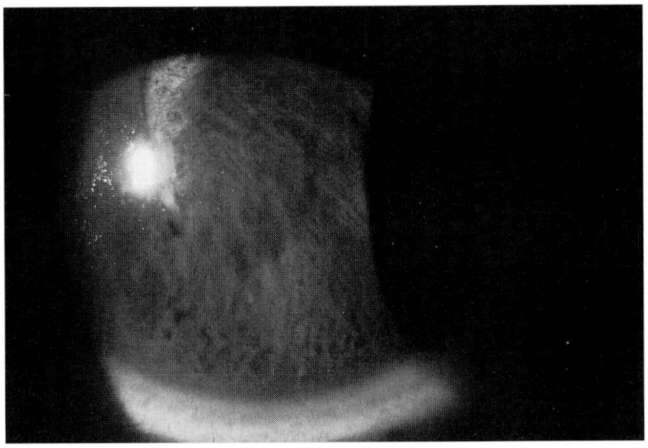

Fig. 7-25 Epithelial downgrowth. One year after a traumatic superior corneoscleral laceration repair was performed, a membrane was noted on the iris covering the pupil, lens, and almost the entire iris, thus causing the iris architecture to flatten. Note the small area of normal iris inferiorly.

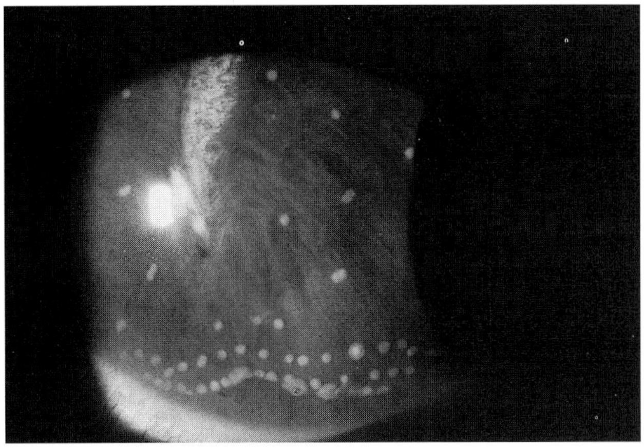

Fig. 7-27 Epithelial downgrowth after application of argon laser. Multiple 100 μm argon laser spots (100 mW, 0.1 second duration) were used to delineate the extent of the epithelial downgrowth membrane. The normal iris inferiorly did not whiten when treated with the laser spots.

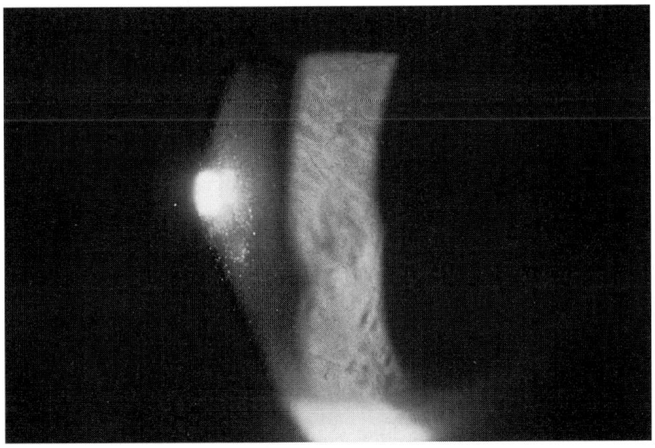

Fig. 7-26 Epithelial downgrowth. Slit-beam examination of the eye seen in Fig. 7-25 demonstrates flattening of the iris surface except for a small area inferiorly. A ridge at the edge of the epithelial downgrowth membrane is evident, and a small degree of vascularization is seen superiorly.

EPITHELIAL DOWNGROWTH

Although rare, surface epithelium can gain access to the inside of the eye through a wound or a fistulous tract. It occurs most commonly after perforating trauma or a poorly closed surgical wound. Predisposing factors include incarceration of intraocular tissue in a wound, wound gape, or the presence of a chronic fistula or bleb. These factors allow corneal or conjunctival epithelium to proceed down the wound and into the eye. The epithelial sheet then grows over the corneal endothelial and iris surfaces.

Symptoms of epithelial downgrowth include ocular pain, photophobia, and diminished vision. Conjunctival injection and an anterior chamber reaction may result. The intraocular pressure may be elevated (from the membrane growing over the angle) or low (from inflammation and damage to the ciliary body). A poorly sealed wound or a fistula may be present. Frequently, a gray-white posterior corneal membrane develops with a slightly elevated, often serpiginous, advancing edge. Corneal edema may overlie the membrane. In many patients a clear or slightly grayish membrane originates at the wound site and grows over the iris surface (Fig. 7-25). The membrane causes flattening of the normal iris crypts and architecture (Fig. 7-26). It can also cause pupillary distortion. In advanced cases the membrane can grow onto the lens, over the ciliary body, and onto the retina. The differential diagnosis includes fibrous ingrowth. This membrane is thicker, grayer and more slowly progressive than an epithelial downgrowth membrane. It occurs much more commonly on the cornea than on the iris. Fibrous ingrowth is often associated with alloplastic tube shunts.

Ocular examination should include a careful Seidel test for a fistulous tract. Specular microscopy may be able to detect a sharp border between the normal corneal endothelial cells and the epithelial cells. Argon laser photocoagulation is useful to confirm the presence of an abnormal iris membrane and to determine its extent. Argon laser spots (100 mW, 0.1 second duration, 100 to 500 μm spot sizes) are focused on areas of suspected epithelial downgrowth. A fluffy white burn spot is created when epithelium is burned (Fig. 7-27). Normal iris does not yield these white spots.

Treatment is extremely difficult, especially for patients with advanced disease. The complete extent of the epithelial downgrowth is delineated by argon laser photocoagulation. The fistulous tract is repaired. All involved iris, ciliary body, lens, and vitreous are excised. Involved cornea is treated with cryotherapy (while air is in the anterior chamber). Involved retina is treated with laser photocoagulation, cryotherapy, or both. A tube shunt is often required to control the intraocular pressure. These eyes do remarkably poorly without treatment, yet such "commando" procedures are unfortunately commonly unsuccessful.

MAJOR POINTS

A systemic workup for patients with a first episode of unilateral nongranulomatous uveitis, in the presence of a negative review of systems, typically yields negative results and is often not undertaken.

A systemic workup is generally indicated for patients with recurrent or bilateral or granulomatous uveitis, or those with a positive review of systems. The workup should be tailored to the most likely underlying conditions.

Sacroiliac (and *not* lumbosacral) radiographs showing sclerosis and narrowing of the joint space can be diagnostic for patients with ankylosing spondylitis. Serious complications of this disorder include pulmonary apical fibrosis and aortitis (in 5% of patients).

Chronic, nongranulomatous anterior uveitis and chronic topical corticosteroid therapy (adjusted by the degree of cell and *not* flare found in the anterior chamber) for JRA often result in posterior synechiae and cataract formation.

Sarcoidosis, though often causing posterior uveitis, is an important cause of bilateral granulomatous anterior uveitis. If a definitive diagnosis of sarcoidosis has not been made, biopsy of a conjunctival nodule often establishes the diagnosis more easily and safely than transbronchial lung biopsy.

Syphilis, tuberculosis, and Lyme disease are three other important causes of anterior uveitis.

It is important to distinguish pigment epithelial cysts of the iris from malignant neoplasms of the iris.

Any observed growth or change in the appearance of an iris nevus warrants concern about malignancy.

Documented growth is the most important sign of possible malignant iris melanoma.

Tumors that have metastasized to the uveal tract are the most common form of intraocular malignancy and are distinguished by their amelanotic appearance and their tendency to present in multiple nodules on the iris of both eyes.

The most common sources of primary neoplasm for tumors that have metastasized to the uveal tract include lung cancer in men and breast cancer in women.

Juvenile xanthogranuloma (JXG) should be considered in the differential diagnosis of spontaneous hyphema in infants and children.

Cataract surgery should be approached with caution in patients with iris colobomas because lens zonular attachments may be absent in this area, causing lens defects, sector cataracts, and phacodonesis, and increasing the risk for vitreous loss during surgery.

CONCLUSION

Anterior uveitis is a common condition that often requires straightforward treatment and no workup. However, certain types of anterior uveitis can signal a serious underlying disease that requires systemic treatment. Recognition of these types of uveitis and appropriate workup by the ophthalmologist can be invaluable in diagnosing such disorders, some of which can be life threatening if not managed properly. Similarly, most iris lesions are benign, but some represent serious ocular or systemic disease that can occasionally be recognized by the ophthalmologist.

SUGGESTED READINGS

Books

Nussenblatt RB, Palestine AG: *Uveitis: fundamentals and clinical practice,* Chicago, 1996, Year Book Medical Publishers.

Journals

Bloch-Michel E, Nussenblatt R: International Uveitis Study Group recommendations for the evaluation of intraocular inflammatory disease, *Am J Ophthalmol* 103:234-235, 1987.

George RK, Chan CC, Whitcup SM, Nussenblatt RB: Ocular immunopathology of Behçet's disease, *Surv Ophthalmol* 42:157-162, 1997.

Helm CJ, Holland GN: Ocular tuberculosis, *Surv Ophthalmol* 38:229-256, 1993.

Moorthy RS, Mermoud A, Baerveldt G, et al: Glaucoma associated with uveitis, *Surv Ophthalmol* 41:361-394, 1997.

Rothova A, van Veenedaal WG, Linssen A, et al: Clinical features of acute anterior uveitis, *Am J Ophthalmol* 103:137-145, 1987.

Wakefield D, Montanaro A, McCluskey P: Acute anterior uveitis and HLA-B27, *Surv Ophthalmol* 36:223-232, 1991.

CHAPTER 8

Lens and Cataract

Lenticular opacification, whether congenital or acquired, remains one of the most common causes of visual reduction. Congenital cataracts are among the leading causes of blindness in children, and early detection and treatment are crucial to minimize amblyopia and to maximize visual recovery.

Age-related or senile cataract is the most prevalent type of cataract and is found in more than 75% of septuagenarians. As the population ages, it is not surprising that the prevalence of cataracts is increasing and that cataract extraction is one of the most frequently performed surgical procedures. No effective medical therapy is available for cataracts; consequently, lens extraction is indicated when the visual impairment caused by the cataract interferes with the patient's normal daily activities. Significant advances in the surgical methods for cataract extraction, from intracapsular to extracapsular and phacoemulsification techniques, have allowed the development of rapid, small-incision surgery and markedly reduced recovery time.

CONGENITAL CATARACTS AND DEVELOPMENTAL LENS ABNORMALITIES

Congenital Cataracts

By definition, *congenital cataracts* are lens opacities that are present at birth. Cataracts that are not present at birth but that develop within the first year of life are referred to as *infantile cataracts*. However, because cataracts that may have been present at birth may not have been detected until later in life, these terms are often used interchangeably. Many ocular and systemic conditions are associated with congenital and infantile cataracts, including infections, developmental and pharmacologic disturbances during gestation, congenital syndromes, and metabolic disorders. Major conditions associated with congenital cataracts are listed in Box 8-1. The incidence of congenital cataracts is reported to be approximately 1 in 250 live births, and approximately one third of them are inherited (usually autosomal dominant), one third are associated with a systemic syndrome or condition, and one third are of unknown cause.

Congenital cataracts may present in several distinct morphologic forms, including anterior polar, posterior polar, nuclear, lamellar (zonular), and sectorial. *Polar cataracts* are characterized by dense central capsular and subcapsular opacification at the anterior or posterior pole of the lens (Fig. 8-1). Opacification is usually smaller than 2 mm in diameter. *Nuclear cataracts* are characterized by focal or complete opacification of the embryonic or fetal nucleus of the lens (Fig. 8-2). Therefore they are usually of intrauterine origin and thus present at birth. The opacity may measure 2 to 4 mm in diameter and may be visually significant. Congenital rubella syndrome is a

Box 8-1 Major Associations with Congenital and Infantile Cataracts

TRAUMA OR CHILD ABUSE

GESTATIONAL

- Prematurity
- Irradiation
- Maternal drug ingestion
  - Corticosteroids
  - Sulfonamides
- TORCH infections

CONGENITAL SYNDROMES

- Primary heredity
- Lowe's syndrome
- Alport's syndrome
- Myotonic dystrophy
- Trisomy 13, 15
- Trisomy 21 (Down's syndrome)

METABOLIC DISORDERS

- Diabetes mellitus
- Galactosemia
- Galactokinase deficiency
- Hypocalcemia

OCULAR DISORDERS

- Anterior segment dysgenesis
- Lenticonus
- Ectopia lentis
- Aniridia
- Microspherophakia
- Persistent hyperplastic primary vitreous

TORCH, Toxoplasmosis, rubella, cytomegalovirus, herpes simplex virus.

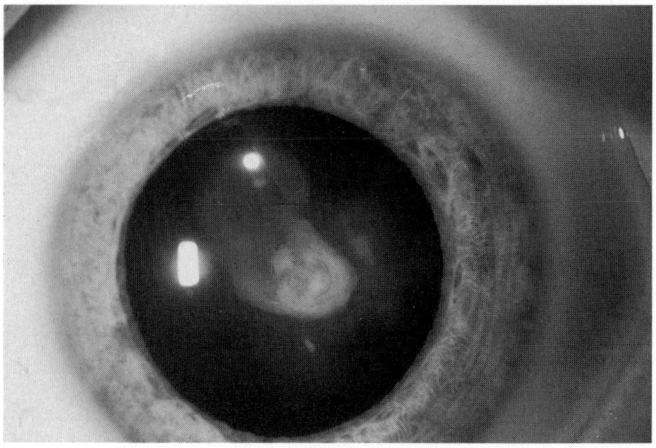

Fig. 8-1 Congenital polar cataract. A central posterior polar cataract is seen. The densest area centrally measures approximately 2 × 2 mm, but an extension has developed superiorly.

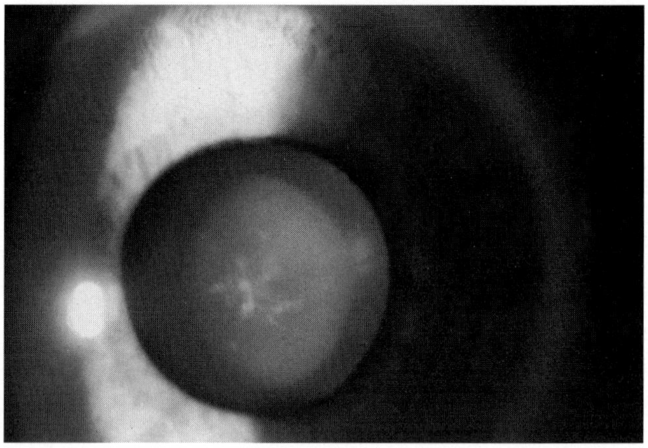

Fig. 8-2 Congenital nuclear cataract. A moderately dense 4 × 4 mm congenital nuclear cataract is present. Because it is larger than 3 mm in diameter, it has an increased risk for significantly affecting vision.

well-known cause of congenital nuclear cataracts. The nucleus of a rubella cataract is characterized by cell nuclei (not normally present in the lens). The lens may also harbor live virus for several years, thus increasing the risk for intraocular viral dissemination and prolonged inflammation after cataract surgery. *Lamellar cataracts* contain opacifications surrounding the Y sutures and the nucleus of the lens, and they may be visually significant. They may also feature riders, which are radial, linear opacities that bend around the equator. In any congenital cataract, if the central opacity is 3 mm or larger, the cataract should be considered visually significant and may require treatment to prevent amblyopia.

The workup of an infant with congenital cataracts entails complete maternal and gestational histories including exposures, infections, and drug ingestions. Any family history of congenital or infantile cataracts should be explored. Ocular examination of the infant should include a careful assessment of the severity of the cataract, size and location of opacification, presence of amblyopia, and presence of any other ocular abnormalities, especially glaucoma. *Sectorial cataracts* (lenticular opacification limited to one peripheral area) may indicate localized mechanical irritation to the lens, such as from a ciliary body mass, and therefore require careful preoperative evaluation. Bilateral cataracts with no associated family history may necessitate a medical evaluation that includes TORCH titers (toxoplasmosis, rubella, cytomegalovirus, herpes simplex virus), urinalysis (blood, protein), serum electrolytes (calcium/phosphorus), serum glucose, and galactokinase level (looking for galactosemia or galactokinase deficiency).

Visually significant congenital cataracts should be treated in a timely fashion to minimize the development of amblyopia. Treatment options include pharmacologic pupillary dilation and surgical cataract extraction. Posterior capsule opacification rapidly follows pediatric cata-

Box 8-2 Major Syndromes Associated with Microspherophakia

Weill-Marchesani syndrome
Alport's syndrome
Lowe's syndrome
Rubella syndrome
Marfan's syndrome
Peter's anomaly

ract extraction, regardless of whether an intraocular lens is implanted. Therefore primary posterior capsulotomy and anterior vitrectomy are usually performed at the time of the initial surgery. Pediatric cataracts are discussed in greater detail in a separate volume in this series.

Microspherophakia

As the name implies, *microspherophakia* refers to a rare developmental anomaly in which the lens of the eye is spherical and small in diameter. Eyes with this condition tend to be highly myopic because of the increased dioptric power of the spherical lens. Although this condition may occur as an isolated phenomenon, it is usually associated with Weill-Marchesani syndrome and occasionally with several other ocular and systemic developmental syndromes (Box 8-2).

Patients with Weill-Marchesani syndrome are short and have broad hands, short fingers, and reduced joint mobility. It is usually inherited as an autosomal recessive condition. The major ocular finding is microspherophakia. Lens zonular attachments tend to be lax and weak. Progressive lens subluxation or even dislocation, occasionally into the anterior chamber, may occur with time. The small, spherical shape of the lens combined with the zonular laxity predisposes to pupillary block and angle-closure glaucoma. In this instance, however, the treatment of choice is cycloplegia, not miosis. Cycloplegics increase zonular tension and consequently aid in flattening the lens centrally and in pulling it posteriorly, thus relieving pupillary block in these rare cases. Miotics relax zonular tension, allowing the lens to remain spherical (maximizing anterior-posterior diameter), and may aggravate anterior displacement of the lens, worsening pupillary block.

Anterior and Posterior Lenticonus

Lenticonus is an uncommon condition in which a localized defect or deformation in the anterior or posterior lens capsule allows the lens to bulge or become ectatic (Fig. 8-3). Consequently, the lens has a different dioptric power in these regions, often producing a characteristic circular "oil droplet" appearance on retinoscopy. Associated lens opacities may also develop. Anterior lenticonus may be associated with Alport's syndrome, whereas posterior lenticonus is usually idiopathic.

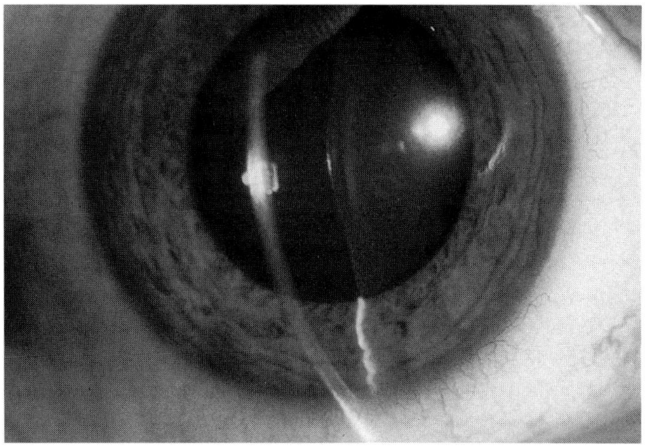

Fig. 8-3 Anterior lenticonus. A small anterior protrusion in the anterior lens capsule, seen during slit-beam examination, indicates anterior lenticonus. This patient has Alport's syndrome.

Box 8-3 Major Syndromes Associated with Ectopia Lentis

SYSTEMIC SYNDROMES

Marfan's syndrome
Homocystinuria
Weill-Marchesani syndrome
Syphilis
Ehlers-Danlos syndrome
Hyperlysinemia
Sulfite oxidase deficiency

OCULAR SYNDROMES

Simple ectopia lentis
Ectopia lentis et pupillae
Congenital glaucoma
Megalocornea
Aniridia

Alport's syndrome is an autosomal dominant condition consisting of hemorrhagic nephritis, progressive nerve deafness, and vestibular dysfunction. Ocular findings may include anterior and posterior polar cataracts and, less often, lenticonus and spherophakia.

Ectopia Lentis

Ectopia lentis refers to a nontraumatic displacement of the lens that may be congenital or acquired. Although trauma is the most common cause of a partially displaced (subluxated) or completely dislocated (luxated) lens, ectopia lentis may occur spontaneously, either in isolation

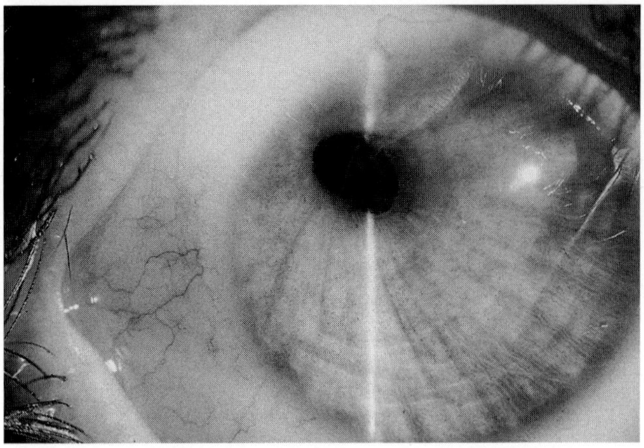

Fig. 8-4 Ectopia lentis et pupillae. Slit-beam examination demonstrates a superotemporal displacement of the pupil and an inferonasal displacement of the lens. The patient has no history of ocular surgery or trauma.

as an inherited condition or associated with several systemic syndromes (Box 8-3). Simple ectopia lentis is usually an autosomal dominant, bilateral condition resulting in progressive superotemporal lens displacement. Lens subluxation may be congenital or, in some cases, delayed until middle age. Initial management of mild cases consists of prescribing the best optical correction possible, whereas advanced cases may benefit from mydriatic therapy or lens extraction. If the lens is displaced out of the visual axis, an aphakic correction may provide the best vision.

Ectopia Lentis et Pupillae

As the name suggests, this condition consists of displacement of both the lens and the pupil. Usually the condition is bilateral but not always symmetric. The pupil may be oval or slit, and it is usually displaced in the opposite direction of the lens (Fig. 8-4). Ectopia lentis et pupillae is usually inherited as an autosomal recessive trait, and it is occasionally associated with glaucoma and cataracts. Significant visual impairment is unusual.

ACQUIRED CATARACTS

Age-Related Cataracts

Age-related cataracts are among the most frequent causes of visual reduction, especially in an aging population, and cataract extraction is the most common ophthalmic surgical procedure performed. In general, age-related cataracts develop after the age of 40 years, and they tend to be progressive. Although the exact pathophysiology of cataract formation is not entirely known, it is thought that some cataracts develop from an acceleration of the conversion of water-soluble lens proteins to water-insoluble lens proteins. In one theory of cataract formation, free radicals, such as those produced by ultraviolet light, may contribute to this process.

Box 8-4 Major Morphologic Varieties of Age-Related Cataracts

NUCLEAR
- Nuclear sclerotic cataract
- Brunescent nuclear sclerotic cataract
- Cataract nigra

CORTICAL
- Cortical cataract
- Mature cataract
- Hypermature cataract
- Morgagnian cataract

SUBCAPSULAR
- Anterior subcapsular cataract
- Posterior subcapsular cataract

MIXED

The three major morphologic classifications of cataract are cortical, nuclear, and subcapsular (Box 8-4). Nuclear cataracts result from progressive opacification or sclerosis of the central nucleus of the lens (Fig. 8-5). Patients may notice a gradual, progressive blurring of vision, more in the distance than at near. Often, as nuclear sclerosis progresses, a myopic shift occurs in the patient's refraction (frequently referred to as "second sight"), and this may be one of the earliest signs of cataract development. Slit-beam examination of the lens reveals that the nucleus is less translucent than the surrounding cortex (Fig. 8-6). The nucleus may also become more pigmented and take on a yellow-brown hue known as *brunescence*. In advanced cases the nucleus may appear brown and sometimes even black (*cataract nigra*) (Fig. 8-7).

Cortical cataracts result from opacification of the lens cortex, and they may be found in isolation or associated with nuclear sclerosis. Different clinical appearances include scattered punctate opacities, small vacuoles, water clefts, and spokelike white opacities. These opacities may be diffusely arranged throughout the cortex or localized to a particular sector. Often patients with cortical cataracts report glare symptoms or monocular diplopia and blurred vision. If the cortical opacification progresses to involve the entire cortex, the lens takes on a diffusely white appearance. Occasionally, the density is so severe it blocks the view of the posterior segment and is called a *mature cataract*. Rarely, the liquefied lens cortex leaks through the lens capsule in these advanced cases (*hypermature cataracts*), producing an inflamma-

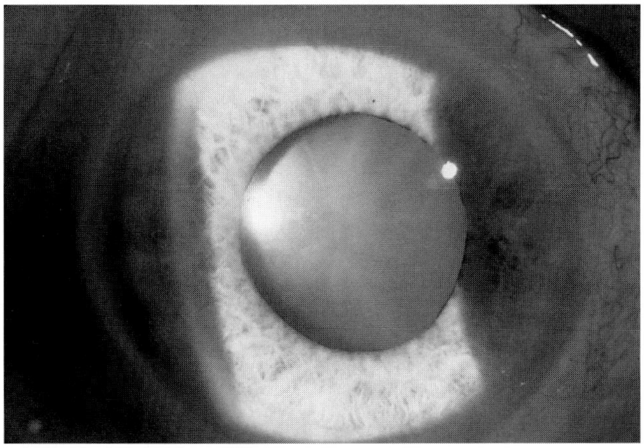

Fig. 8-5 Nuclear sclerosis. This nuclear sclerotic cataract demonstrates a dense yellow-brown discoloration of the lens nucleus. (See color plate.)

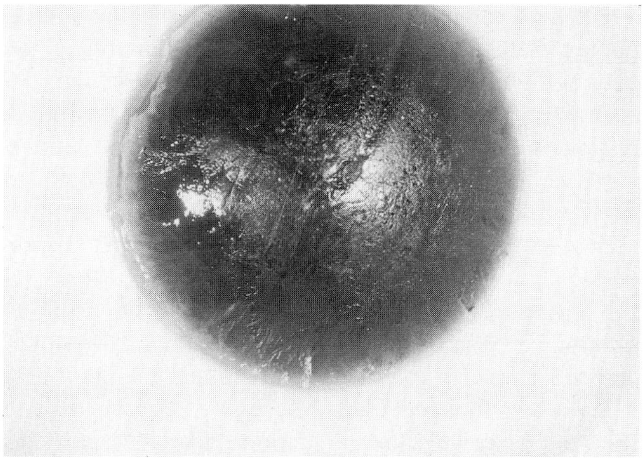

Fig. 8-7 Cataract nigra. An extremely dense brown-black lens after an extracapsular cataract extraction. (See color plate.)

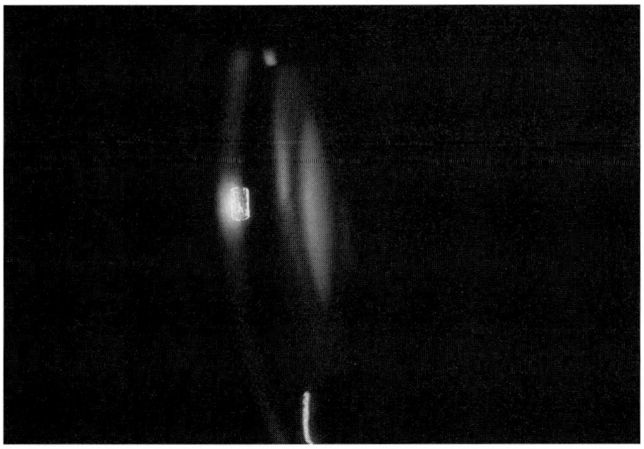

Fig. 8-6 Nuclear sclerosis. Slit-beam examination illustrates the relatively clear lens cortex anterior to the dense nuclear sclerosis.

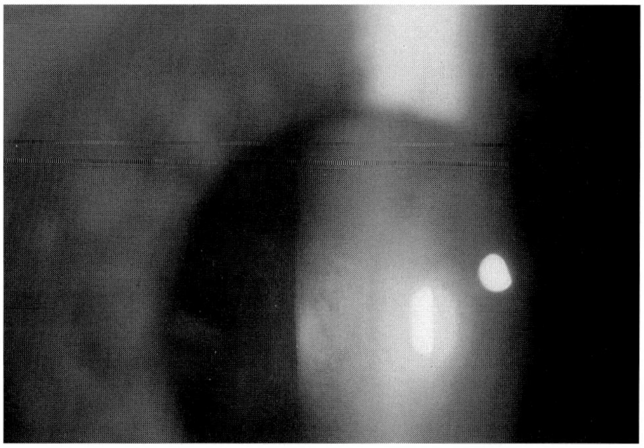

Fig. 8-8 Posterior subcapsular cataract. A thin plaquelike opacity appears against the posterior capsule.

tory reaction and glaucoma known as *phacolytic glaucoma*. If liquefaction of the cortex is complete, the nucleus of the lens may be able to move about freely within the lens capsule, producing what is called a *morgagnian cataract*.

Posterior subcapsular cataracts are caused by posterior migration of the lens epithelium that then produces opacification just beneath the posterior lens capsule, usually centrally (Figs. 8-8 and 8-9). The opacification may be seen as focal subcapsular opacities or a group of opacities that may become confluent with time. This type of cataract is often associated with trauma, uveitis, diabetes, and chronic topical or systemic corticosteroid use. The central location of these opacities often results in impairment of near visual acuity (because of miosis associated with accommodation) more than distance acuity. Disabling glare is frequently associated with subcapsular cataracts because of the light-scattering effect of these opacities. Therefore the testing of visual acuity in

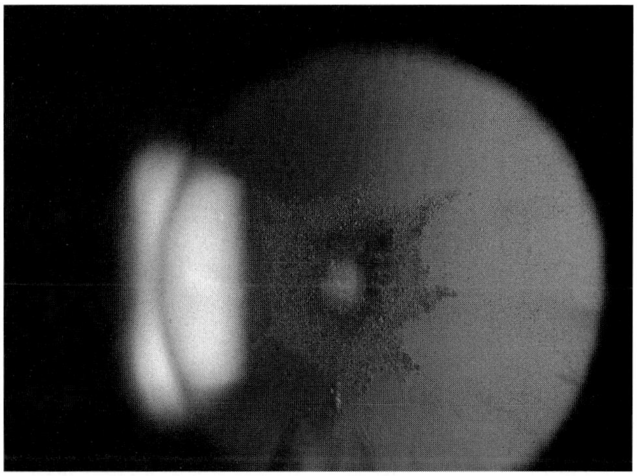

Fig. 8-9 Posterior subcapsular cataract. Retroillumination off the retina highlights the central posterior subcapsular cataract seen in Fig. 8-8.

a darkened room (thus producing pupil dilation and reducing glare) is not an accurate representation of the patient's actual functional visual acuity or disability. Visual acuity testing with room lights on or formal glare testing is a helpful adjunct in the evaluation of these patients.

The goals of the evaluation of the patient with cataract are to establish the degree to which the cataract has impaired the functional ability of the patient and to establish the cataract as the causative agent of the visual reduction and disability. This procedure allows the patient and the physician to develop a treatment plan and realistic expectations regarding progression of visual loss and the options for visual rehabilitation. Elements of the history must therefore include the details and circumstances of visual reduction, such as inability to read, inability to drive, glare symptoms, work-related limitations, or impairment of the ability to perform the activities of daily living. A standardized 14-question inventory, known as the VF-14, has been developed to aid in establishing the degree of functional impairment of the patient with cataract, and it has been shown to be a reliable measure of patients' practical visual limitations.

The ophthalmic examination must be comprehensive, and it must be especially directed to ruling out other causes of reduced vision and to establishing the presence and degree of cataract. External examination should include an evaluation of eyelid position and excursion because exposure may contribute to preoperative visual reduction and complicate the postsurgical healing process. Any evidence of eyelid or conjunctival infection should be appropriately noted and treated before planned surgery to reduce the risk for postoperative endophthalmitis. Corneal examination should be directed to the status of the tear film, surface irregularities, and central opacities that may be contributing to visual reduction. A decreased tear film and punctate keratopathy may suggest dry eye syndrome, which can reduce vision and complicate postsurgical healing. Corneal stromal opacities, edema, or surface irregularities producing irregular astigmatism may also reduce vision and contribute to visual disability in patients who also have cataracts. Preoperative corneal topography and overrefraction with a hard contact lens, as described in Chapter 9, may be helpful in patients in whom the exact cause of decreased vision is not found. Detection of these sometimes subtle corneal abnormalities can be helpful in formulating a treatment plan and in developing realistic expectations for visual recovery. Additionally, the corneal endothelial surface should be examined closely to ensure it is healthy enough to undergo cataract surgery.

Examination of the lens should be thorough and is best accomplished through a dilated pupil. The nature, size, and location of any opacities, including abnormalities of lens shape, position, or movement (phacodonesis) should be noted. The anterior lens capsule should also be closely inspected for evidence of pseudoexfoliation. Retroillumination with the slit lamp or direct ophthalmoscope and streak retinoscopy may be helpful in the detection of subtle yet visually significant disease.

Fundus examination should carefully examine the macula and optic nerve for conditions such as age-related macular degeneration and optic atrophy, which may limit visual recovery. Direct ophthalmoscopy may also allow a comparison between how well the examiner sees into the fundus and how well the patient sees out. Peripheral retinal examination also enables a search for areas of vitreoretinal traction or retinal breaks, which may require attention before surgical intervention.

The evaluation of potential visual function in patients with dense cataracts that preclude detailed fundus examination can be difficult. The presence or absence of an afferent pupillary defect should be carefully assessed. Examination of the fellow eye for posterior segment disease may be helpful if the media are clearer. B-scan ultrasonography is useful to determine whether the retina is attached and whether any gross structural abnormalities or masses of the posterior segment exist. This technology, however, cannot assess the degree of macular functioning. Occasionally, the testing of visual acuity with a potential acuity meter (a device that projects a Snellen vision chart onto the retina) can circumvent lenticular opacities and yield an estimate of potential visual acuity. When an estimate of macular function is not possible based on examination and testing, it is important to communicate to the patient before cataract surgery that, though vision may be expected to improve with surgery, conditions such as macular degeneration, which may limit the degree of visual recovery, cannot be ruled out.

Surgical techniques of cataract extraction have evolved significantly over the years from intracapsular to extracapsular and to small incision phacoemulsification. Intracapsular cataract extraction involves a large incision with enzymatic degradation of the zonular attachments and extraction of the entire lens with its capsule. Planned extracapsular cataract extraction involves a smaller incision, the opening of the anterior lens capsule, expression of the lens nucleus, and aspiration of the cortex. This procedure leaves the capsular "bag" intact for implantation of a posterior chamber intraocular lens. Phacoemulsification is a modification of the extracapsular technique in which the lens nucleus is pulverized ultrasonically by the phacoemulsification handpiece. This technique, combined with foldable intraocular lens technology, has allowed cataract extraction and intraocular lens implantation through wounds smaller than 3 mm (Fig. 8-10). Recently, advances in intraocular lens technology have produced multifocal and astigmatic intraocular lenses. Surgical techniques of cataract extraction are discussed in detail in Chapter 10.

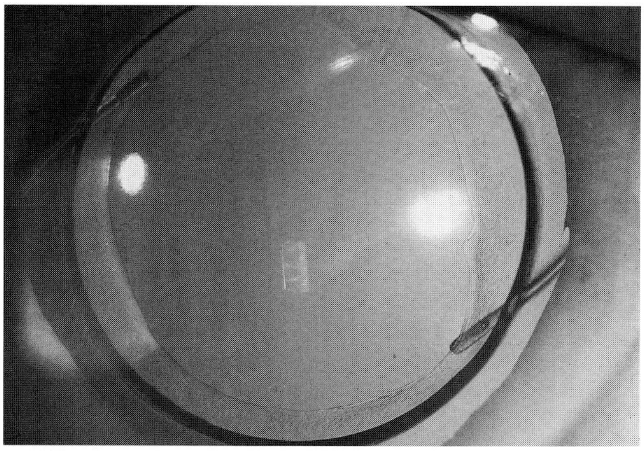

Fig. 8-10 Posterior chamber intraocular lens implant. Retroillumination off the retina of a foldable posterior chamber intraocular lens implant in the capsular bag. The ring outside the edge of the lens is the dilated pupil. The ring just inside the edge of the lens is the continuous circular capsulotomy.

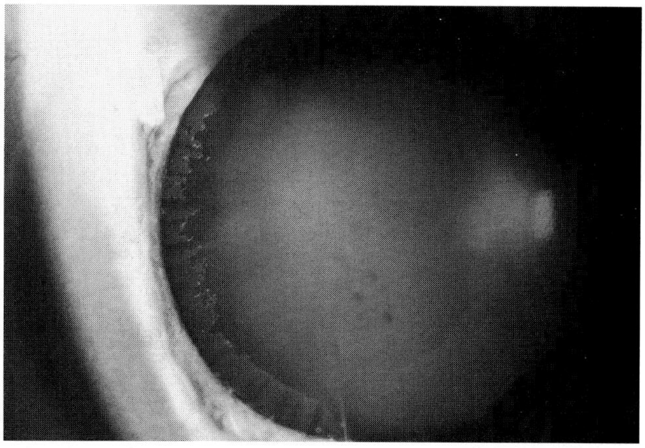

Fig. 8-11 Pseudoexfoliation. In patients with pseudoexfoliation, white fibrillar material is seen on the anterior lens capsule at the edge of the dilated pupil.

Pseudoexfoliation Syndrome

Pseudoexfoliation syndrome is an important condition that may have significant implications regarding cataract surgery. It is characterized by the deposition of an opaque, fibrillar material on the anterior lens capsule, posterior iris, ciliary body, lens zonule, and vitreous face. Accumulation of this whitish material at the pupillary margin suggests the diagnosis of pseudoexfoliation in an undilated patient. Clinically, it may appear as a fine material coating the anterior lens capsule, which may not be well appreciated until pupillary dilation (Figs. 8-11 and 8-12), at which time a midperipheral clear zone may become apparent where the material appears to have been "dusted off" by pupillary movement (Fig. 8-13). This material may also be deposited on the anterior vitreous face in aphakic persons and on the corneal endothelium (Fig. 8-14). The condition may be unilateral or bilateral, and it is associated with the development of open-angle glaucoma in as many as 50% of patients and with decreased endothelial cell density.

The presence of pseudoexfoliation syndrome has great importance with respect to cataract surgery. This condition is associated with weak lens zonular attachments and zonular dehiscence. Additionally, the pupil often dilates poorly. As a result the risk is significantly increased for localized or complete loss of support of the capsular bag because of the lens manipulation required during cataract surgery (Fig. 8-15). Consequently, there are increased risks for vitreous loss and posterior dislocation of nuclear fragments during surgery. Rarely, during expression of the nucleus during planned extracapsular cataract surgery, the entire lens, including the

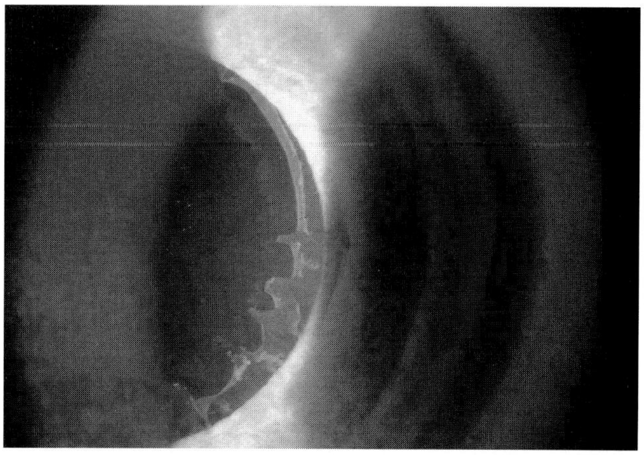

Fig. 8-12 Pseudoexfoliation. The white fibrillar material appears to be "delaminating" off the anterior lens capsule.

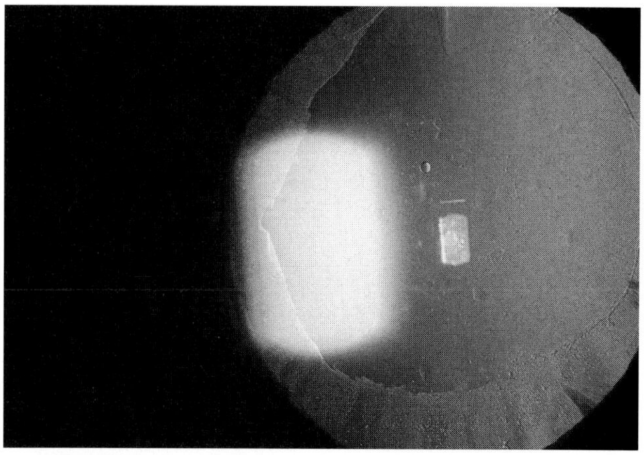

Fig. 8-13 Pseudoexfoliation. Retroillumination off the retina highlights the outer fibrillar opacity. A faint central ring is also seen. The area between the two rings appears to have been "dusted off" by pupillary movement.

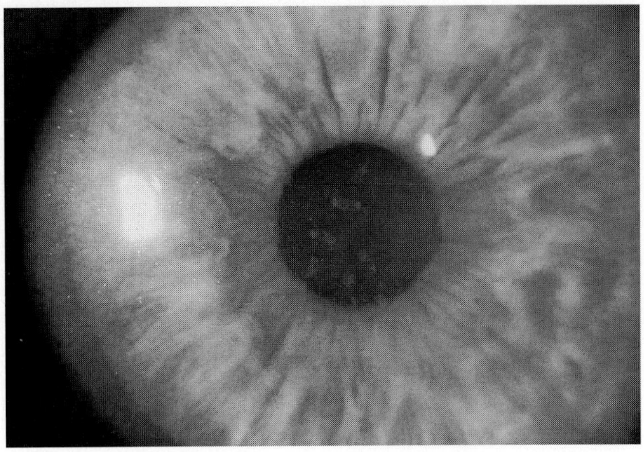

Fig. 8-14 Pseudoexfoliation. This eye demonstrates the white pseudoexfoliation material at the pupillary border and on the corneal endothelial surface.

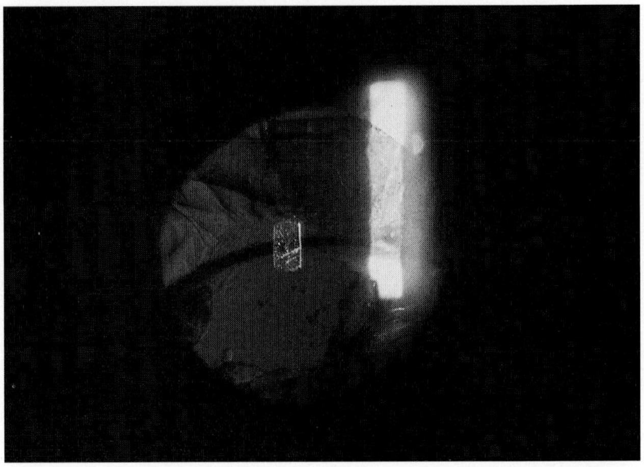

Fig. 8-15 Intraocular lens subluxation in pseudoexfoliation. This posterior chamber intraocular lens has subluxated inferiorly several years after uncomplicated cataract surgery because of poor zonular attachments.

capsular bag, is expressed because of complete zonular dehiscence. Careful preoperative examination to determine the presence of this syndrome and to determine whether any evidence of zonular weakness (suggested by phacodonesis or lens subluxation) exists, combined with careful intraoperative techniques that minimize lens manipulation and zonular stress, can aid in obtaining a successful outcome in these difficult cases. Patients should be informed before surgery that they are at increased risk for surgical complications.

Posterior Capsular Opacity

Posterior capsule opacification, also known as a secondary membrane or an "after cataract," refers to a gradual opacification of the posterior portion of the capsular bag after cataract surgery. This condition results from proliferation and opacification of the remaining lens epithelial cells after a cataract is removed (Fig. 8-16). Some of these cells swell as they attempt to regenerate lens fibers, producing globular masses known as *Elschnig's pearls* (Figs. 8-17 and 8-18). This process may occur over months or years and may affect up to half the patients after extracapsular cataract extraction. As posterior capsule opacification increases, the patient may once again experience progressive glare, halos, and blurred vision and commonly thinks the cataract has returned. When the opacification becomes visually significant, the posterior capsule may be opened noninvasively with the Nd: YAG laser. This technique uses the laser to produce small bursts of energy focused at the level of the posterior capsule. These microscopic "explosions" make small incisions in the capsule and can be arranged so that the central portion of the capsule is "excised" and falls into the vitreous, thus clearing the central visual axis. Complications of this procedure include transient and long-term intraocular pressure rise, pitting of the intraocular lens, intraocular lens dislocation, rupture of the anterior vitreous face and subsequent anterior displacement of vitreous, retinal detachment, and cystoid macular edema. The incidence of retinal detachment after Nd: YAG laser capsulotomy is approximately 1%.

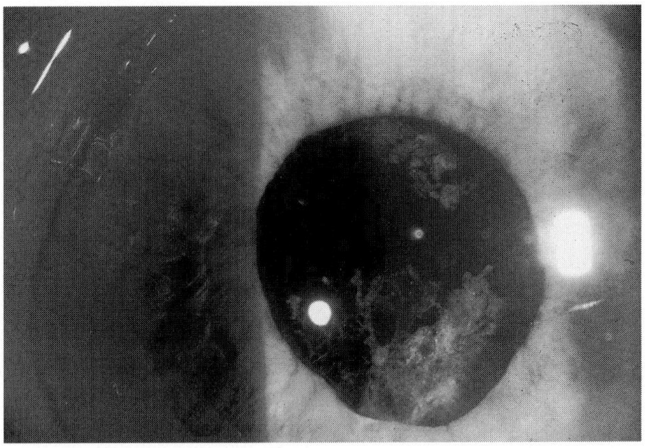

Fig. 8-16 Posterior capsular opacity. Lens epithelial cells that remain in the capsular bag after cataract surgery can migrate toward the center of the posterior capsule and affect vision, termed *posterior capsular opacity.*

Secondary Cataracts

Secondary cataracts may develop as a result of traumatic, inflammatory, toxic, metabolic, or degenerative conditions (Box 8-5). Traumatic cataracts may be caused by blunt injury, thermal and chemical damage, ionizing radiation, or electrical current. Blunt trauma may induce cataract formation, often with a delayed onset, even in the absence of capsular rupture or other significant ocular injury. Typically the opacities develop in the anterior

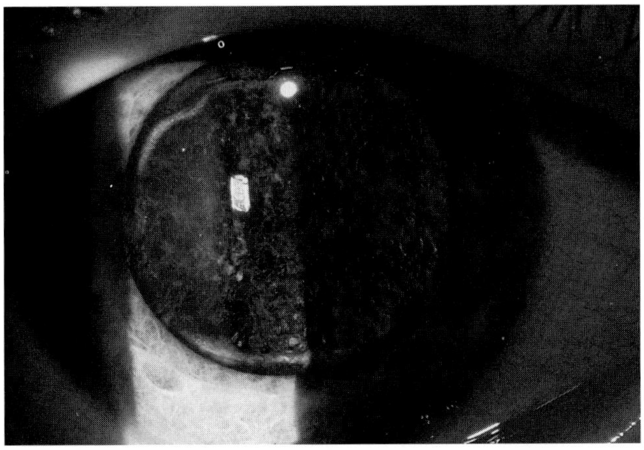

Fig. 8-17 Elschnig's pearls. The lens epithelial cells can swell and produce multiple globular masses, called Elschnig's pearls, along the posterior capsule, which significantly reduces vision.

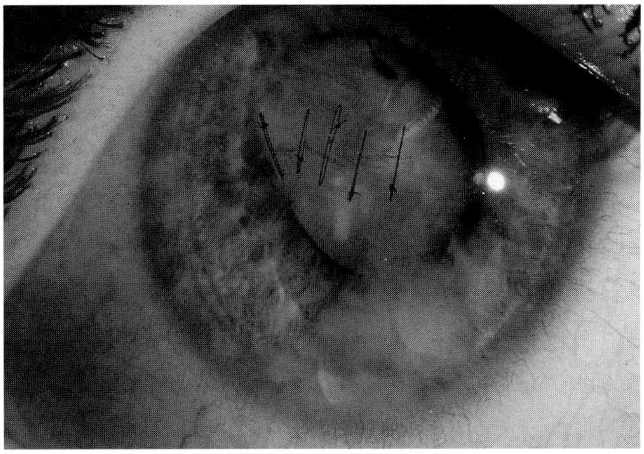

Fig. 8-19 Traumatic cataract. A dense cataract is present several days after a corneal laceration was repaired. At the time of the repair, no lens material was found in the anterior chamber; however, fluffy cortical material is now seen inferiorly.

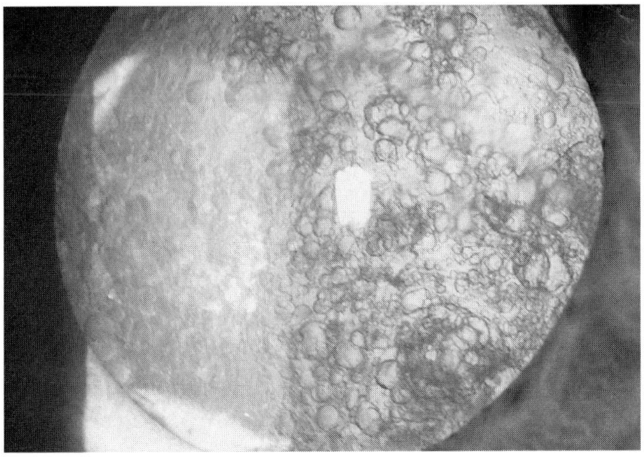

Fig. 8-18 Elschnig's pearls. Retroillumination off the retina highlights the globular Elschnig's pearls seen in Fig. 8-17. (See color plate.)

or posterior subcapsular region, but occasionally they may involve the deeper cortex. Traumatic rupture of the anterior or posterior capsule, whether from blunt or penetrating trauma, may cause a diffuse, white, mature-appearing cataract in a relatively short time after the injury (Fig. 8-19).

Thermal injury (infrared exposure), as seen in persons such as glassblowers who are chronically exposed to intense heat, may also induce cataracts or a true exfoliation of the lens capsule. Although rare, thermal energy absorbed by a highly pigmented lens during posterior segment laser treatment may also induce cataract formation. Continuous exposure to ionizing radiation can induce cataracts that may be stationary or progressive and that are typically located in the anterior or posterior subcapsular regions. The latency period after radiation exposure until cataract formation may be months or years.

Box 8-5 Major Conditions Associated with Secondary Cataracts

TRAUMATIC

- Blunt trauma
- Penetrating trauma
- Thermal injury
- Ionizing radiation
- Electrical shock

METABOLIC

- Diabetes mellitus
- Galactosemia
- Hypocalcemia
- Wilson's disease

MEDICATIONS

- Corticosteroids (topical or systemic)
- Phenothiazines
- Cholinesterase inhibitors

INFLAMMATORY

- Chronic uveitis

DEGENERATIVE

- Retinitis pigmentosa
- Gyrate atrophy
- Usher's syndrome

Electric shock can also produce cataracts by coagulation of lens proteins should the electrical current pass through the lens. Electric cataracts have been reported after accidental electrocution, lightning strike, and electroconvulsive shock therapy. They are typically anterior or posterior subcapsular cataracts that may have a distinctive fernlike or starburst appearance.

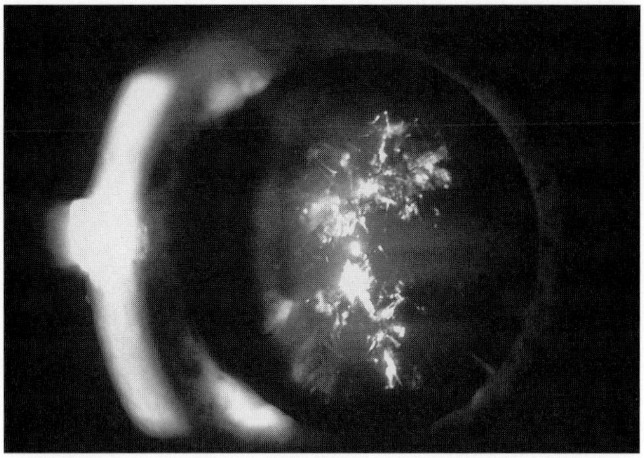

Fig. 8-20 Myotonic dystrophy cataract. Multicolored opacities behind the anterior lens capsule causing a "Christmas tree" cataract are seen in this patient with myotonic dystrophy. (Courtesy of Matthew B. Goren, M.D.) (See color plate.)

The most common metabolic condition associated with secondary cataract formation is diabetes mellitus. Elevated glucose levels within the lens, associated with diabetes, allow the metabolic conversion of excess glucose to sorbitol by the enzyme aldose reductase. Sorbitol is not metabolized by the lens, and its accumulation results in a shift of the osmotic balance, thus drawing water into the lens and producing a reversible lens opacity, as well as a myopic shift in refractive error. Eventually the overall increased water content of the lens contributes to irreversible cataract formation.

Galactosemia and galactokinase deficiencies are autosomal recessive metabolic disorders that can produce cataracts in infants (oil droplet cataract). A deficiency in the metabolic pathway for galactose allows it to accumulate in the serum and enter the lens. Excess galactose is converted to galactitol (dulcitol) by aldose reductase, thus altering the osmotic balance of the lens and drawing in water. Reversal of these cataracts may occur if galactose is eliminated from the diet.

Other metabolic conditions associated with cataract formation include hypocalcemia, which can produce small white cortical opacities, and Wilson's disease, which can produce a characteristic stellate or sunflower cataract.

The most common medications associated with cataract formation include topical and systemic corticosteroids, phenothiazines, and long-term use of anticholinesterases such as phospholine iodide. Prolonged corticosteroid use, whether topical or systemic, is commonly associated with anterior and especially posterior subcapsular cataract formation. Phenothiazine derivatives, such as chlorpromazine, may produce axial pigmentation of the anterior lens capsule and cortex, but it is usually not visually significant.

Prolonged intraocular inflammation, as in chronic uveitis, causes secondary cataract formation. Chronic uveitis produces posterior subcapsular cataract, though a fibrous anterior capsular opacity may develop with significant posterior synechia formation. Additionally, secondary cataracts may be associated with degenerative ocular conditions, such as retinitis pigmentosa, and ocular ischemic syndromes. Myotonic dystrophy, one of the muscular dystrophies, is associated with multicolored lens opacities and causes a "Christmas tree" cataract just posterior to the anterior capsule (Fig. 8-20).

ACQUIRED LENS SUBLUXATION OR DISLOCATION

Although trauma remains the most common cause of lens subluxation (Figs. 8-21 and 8-22), several inherited conditions are associated with acquired lens subluxation or dislocation including Marfan's syndrome, homocystinuria, and Weill-Marchesani syndrome (Box 8-3).

Marfan's syndrome is an autosomal dominant condition characterized by tall stature, long limbs, long fingers (arachnodactyly), flexible joints, and skeletal abnormalities. Connective tissue abnormalities that may affect the cardiovascular system are also found and can produce aortic dilation, dissecting aortic aneurysms, and aortic insufficiency. Zonular abnormalities produce lens subluxation or dislocation in as many as 80% of patients. The subluxation is typically superotemporal and bilateral (Fig. 8-23). The subluxated lens may also become cataractous. Myopia, astigmatism, and retinal tears and detachments are also associated with this condition. Management initially includes optimizing the patient's refractive correction, though as subluxation progresses, surgical lens extraction may be required. Occasionally, aphakic correction without lens extraction may provide good vision.

Homocystinuria is an uncommon autosomal recessive condition also associated with lens subluxation. It is characterized by tall stature, skeletal abnormalities, osteoporosis, and vascular thrombosis. The thrombotic complications of this condition particularly increase the risk for surgical anesthesia. Ocular findings include blue irides (often) and progressive, bilateral lens subluxation in as many as 90% of patients, usually inferonasally. Retinal vascular occlusions have also been associated with this condition. The diagnosis of homocystinuria is confirmed by a sodium nitroprusside test of the urine for homocystine. The ophthalmic management of this condition does not differ from that of other conditions involving lens subluxation, but surgery should be delayed or avoided, if possible, because of the increased risk associated with anesthesia. Systemic management of homocystinuria includes vitamin B-6 supplements and dietary management.

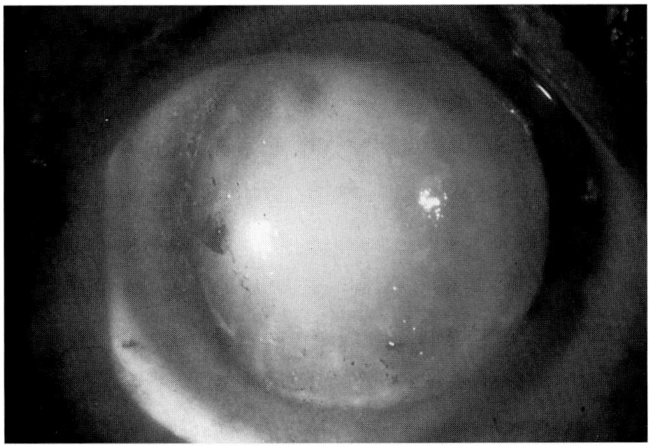

Fig. 8-21 Traumatic lens dislocation. This dense cataract became dislocated into the anterior chamber as a result of blunt trauma.

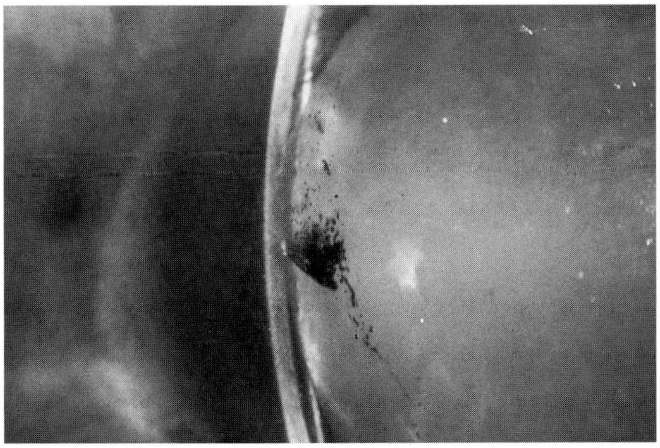

Fig. 8-22 Traumatic lens dislocation. Slit-beam view of the lens dislocated by trauma, seen in Fig. 8-21. Note its position anterior to the iris.

Weill-Marchesani syndrome is another autosomal recessive disorder associated with lens subluxation and is described in greater detail earlier in this chapter. Rare cases of lens subluxation have been reported in association with hyperlysinemia and sulfite oxidase deficiency.

CONCLUSION

Although cataracts in older adults are a common condition not requiring an extensive etiologic investigation, cataracts in infants and children are uncommon and require a workup. It is important to identify the systemic conditions responsible for the cataract. Mild cataracts can often be managed without surgery, but, when required, cataract extraction and intraocular lens placement are successful in most patients.

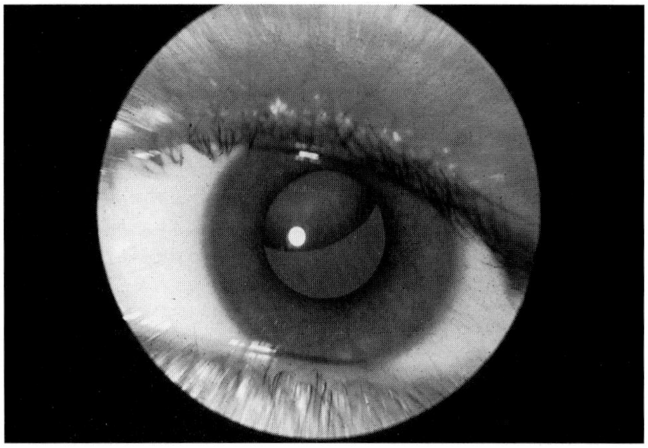

Fig. 8-23 Marfan's syndrome lens dislocation. Because of zonular abnormalities lens dislocation is frequently seen in patients with Marfan's syndrome. Movement is typically superotemporal, as it is in this patient's right eye.

MAJOR POINTS

One third of congenital cataracts are inherited, one third are associated with a systemic syndrome or condition, and one third are of unknown cause.

Congenital cataracts with central opacities 3 mm or larger in diameter should be considered visually significant and may require treatment.

Posterior capsule opacification rapidly follows pediatric cataract extraction, and therefore primary posterior capsulotomy and anterior vitrectomy are generally recommended at the time of cataract extraction.

Cycloplegia, not miosis, is the treatment of choice for pupillary block induced by microspherophakia.

Anterior lenticonus may be associated with Alport's syndrome.

In Marfan's syndrome, the lens subluxation is usually superotemporal. Patients should undergo a cardiac evaluation.

In homocystinuria, the lens subluxation is usually inferonasal. Patients require systemic workup and treatment.

Snellen visual acuity, measured under the favorable lighting conditions of an office examination, may not yield an accurate representation of the patient's functional visual disability caused by the cataract. Check the vision with the lights on if the patient's visual complaints are greater than expected given the Snellen visual acuity.

The presence of a cataract is not an indication for lens extraction. It is important to document the degree of functional limitation the patient is experiencing at distance and at near.

SUGGESTED READINGS

Books

Datiles MB: Clinical evaluation of cataracts. In Tasman W, Jaeger EA, editors: *Duane's clinical ophthalmology,* Philadelphia, 1998, Lippincott-Williams & Wilkins.

Datiles MB, Magno BV: Cataract: clinical types. In Tasman W, Jaeger EA, editors: *Duane's clinical ophthalmology,* Philadelphia, 1998, Lippincott-Williams & Wilkins.

Jaffe NS, Jaffe MS, Jaffe GF: *Cataract surgery and its complications*, St Louis, 1990, Mosby.

Journals

Cenedella RJ: Cholesterol and cataracts, *Surv Ophthalmol* 40: 320-337, 1996.

Klein BEK, Klein R, Linton KLP: Prevalence of age related lens opacities in a population: the Beaver Dam Eye Study, *Ophthalmology* 99:546-552, 1992.

Lambert SR, Drack AV: Infantile cataracts, *Surv Ophthalmol* 40:427-458, 1996.

McCormack P, Simcock PR, Tullo AB: Management of the anticoagulated patient for ophthalmic surgery, *Eye* 7:749-750, 1993.

Speaker MG, Menikoff JA: Prophylaxis of endophthalmitis with topical povidone-iodine, *Ophthalmology* 98:1769-1775, 1991.

Starr MB, Lally JM: Antimicrobial prophylaxis for ophthalmic surgery, *Surv Ophthalmol* 39: 485-501, 1995.

Steinberg EP, Tielsch JM, Schein OD, et al: The VF-14: an index of functional impairment in patients with cataract, *Arch Ophthalmol* 112:630-638, 1994.

Taylor HR, West SK, Rosenthal FS, et al: Effect of ultraviolet radiation on cataract formation, *N Engl J Med* 319:1429-1433, 1988.

West SK, Valmadrid CT: Epidemiology of risk factors for age-related cataract, *Surv Ophthalmol* 39: 323-334, 1995.

CHAPTER 9

Diagnostic Tools

The eye care physician has a wide variety of diagnostic tools at his or her disposal to aid in examining the anterior segment. Many instruments are used routinely, such as the slit-lamp biomicroscope, phoropter, and keratometer, and are not discussed in this text. Other, more specialized devices can be used to enhance the corneal and anterior segment evaluations. Computed corneal topographers are now available to better analyze the corneal curvature. The measurement of corneal thickness also aids in the diagnosis and treatment of corneal disorders. Specular microscopy is an important tool to evaluate the endothelial cells in a manner far superior to simple slit-lamp examination.

Confocal microscopy is a new noninvasive technique to examine the cornea at the cellular level. It may have applications in the diagnosis of corneal infections, such as differentiating bacterial from fungal from *Acanthamoeba* keratitis before culture results are available. It may also aid in distinguishing between various corneal disorders and following corneal healing patterns, such as after refractive surgery. Ultrasound biomicroscopy is another new noninvasive technology that produces high-resolution images of the anterior 20% of the globe.

Rigid contact lenses are commonly used for the correction of refractive errors, especially in patients with high degrees of regular, and especially irregular, astigmatism. As a diagnostic tool, they can be extremely useful in differentiating visual loss resulting from corneal irregularity (correctable with a rigid contact lens) from visual loss resulting from corneal opacity (not correctable with a rigid contact lens) or posterior segment pathology. Many of these tools and techniques can help not only in establishing a diagnosis but also in selecting the best management option.

COMPUTED VIDEOKERATOGRAPHY

Computed videokeratography, also known as corneal topography, is the general term for the many techniques that have been devised to measure qualitatively and quantitatively the curvature of the cornea. These techniques have become extremely important in the diagnosis and treatment of many corneal disorders. In addition, they are widely used before and after corneal refractive surgery.

Before the use of these computed units, the curvature of the cornea was evaluated qualitatively by slit-lamp examination and quantitatively by keratometry. In addition, analysis of circles reflected off the cornea (Placido disc reflections) helped gain a more complete assessment of corneal curvature than keratometry, which only evaluates a central 3-mm ring of cornea. The development of the photokeratoscope allowed these Placido disc reflections to be photographed and saved for later analysis and comparison. However, these images were not standardized, not at all quantitative, and were difficult to compare with one another. Still, small hand-held devices that reflect rings onto the cornea are often useful to evaluate rapidly but imprecisely corneal curvature in the operating room or at the slit lamp.

Significant advances in two unrelated areas, the computer industry and the field of refractive surgery, led to the advent of computed videokeratography. More powerful, less expensive personal computers allowed the practicing physician to use high-technology image analysis to evaluate corneal curvature. One of the important reasons the clinician was interested in the subtleties of

Box 9-1 Computed Videokeratography Techniques

Placido disc
Rasterstereography
Scanning slit beam
Holography
Interferometry

corneal curvature was the growing interest in keratorefractive surgery. Before performing refractive surgery, the surgeon must make sure that the cornea is regular and that no pathology such as contact lens warpage, early keratoconus, or pellucid marginal degeneration has developed to give the best surgical results. In addition, corneal topography allows keratorefractive surgeons to better evaluate their results and plan for additional corneal surgery when necessary.

Several methods exist to image the cornea and determine its curvature. The first and most commonly used technique is to project circles of light onto the cornea (Placido discs), pick up the reflections of the images with a video camera, and analyze by computer the reflected rings. The reflections of the perfect circles are altered depending on the curvature of the cornea. The computer can analyze these modified rings and determine the corneal curvature, including areas of relative steepening and flattening (astigmatism). One disadvantage to this method is that the corneal surface must be relatively smooth to reflect the circles with enough definition to be analyzable by the computer. Consequently, corneas with poor or absent epithelium cannot be analyzed accurately by this procedure.

Another videokeratographic method that does not rely on a smooth epithelial surface projects a grid of known shape and size onto the cornea and uses a video camera to image the grid (rasterstereography). The computer can then analyze changes in the shape of the grid induced by the cornea. This method can produce a three-dimensional representation of the corneal surface, from which it can calculate corneal curvature. Scanning slit beam and holographic techniques can also achieve similar goals without a smooth epithelium (Box 9-1).

Once analyzed by the computer, corneal curvature data are represented by color "maps." A standardized system using "hot" colors, that is, reds and oranges, for steeper areas of cornea and "cold" colors, that is, purples and blues, for flatter areas of cornea, is used by all topography units (Fig. 9-1). The curvature can be portrayed on a relative or an absolute scale. A relative scale determines the flattest and steepest areas of the particular cornea to be portrayed and divides all the colors between those two numbers. In the absolute scale a certain shade of red always indicates the same steep curvature (e.g., 52 D), and a certain shade of blue always depicts the same flat curvature (e.g., 37 D). The strengths of the relative scale are that it maximizes the colors used to depict each cornea and that the steepest areas are always red and the flattest areas always blue. This constantly changing scale means the physician must carefully examine the scale before interpreting a relative scale corneal map. On the other hand, absolute scales are much easier to compare with each other because the same color always means the same curvature. However, in absolute scales, unusually steep or flat corneal curvatures are poorly represented (Table 9-1). Information such as Placido rings, simulated keratometric readings, difference maps, and ray tracings can also be displayed.

Although the actual colors of a corneal map are of great interest, the pattern of the colors may be even

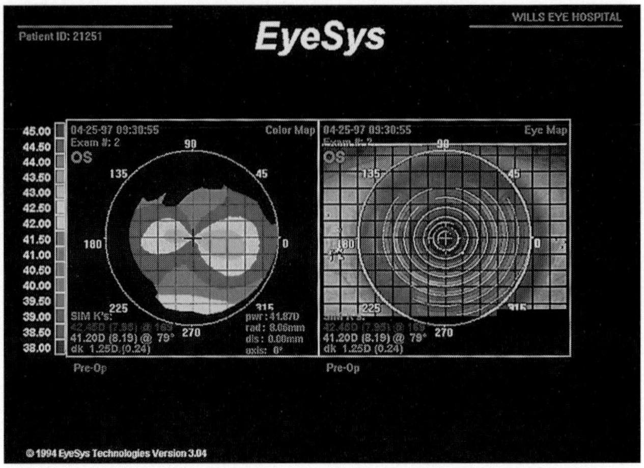

Fig. 9-1 Computed corneal topography. An eye with regular against-the-rule astigmatism. The Placido ring image over a black-and-white image of the eye is on the right. The color-coded display calculated from the Placido rings is on the left. The scale on the far left indicates the dioptric power of each color. Simulated keratometric readings are calculated and displayed at the bottom of both sides. Central corneal power in diopters and radius in millimeters are displayed on the bottom of the color map. (See color plate.)

Table 9-1 Comparison of relative and absolute scales on computed videokeratography

Feature	Relative scale	Absolute scale
Color representation	Different for each cornea	Same for each cornea
Dioptric steps	Different for each cornea	Same for each cornea
Representation of very steep and flat corneas	Good	Fair

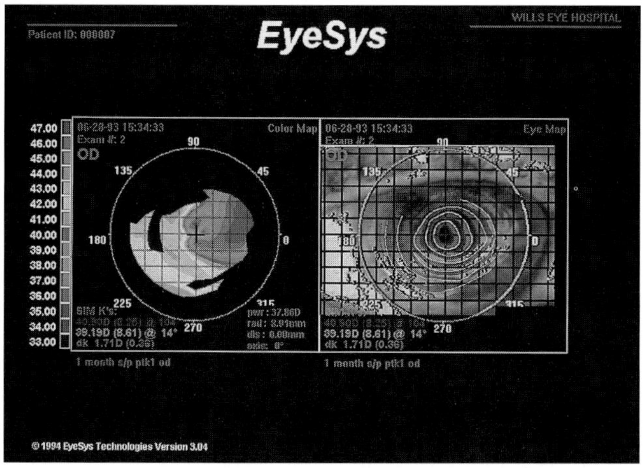

Fig. 9-2 Computed corneal topography. Irregular astigmatism is apparent in the abnormal Placido rings on the right side and the asymmetric colors on the left side. (See color plate.)

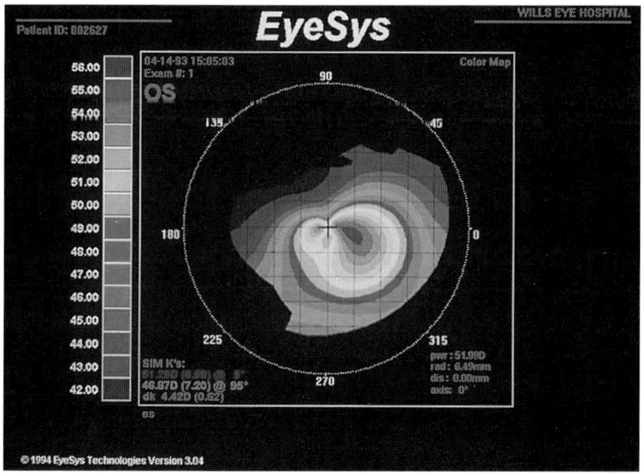

Fig. 9-3 Computed corneal topography. Inferotemporal corneal steepening with superonasal flattening is noted on this color map. The central corneal power is high, measured at 51.90 D. This color map suggests a diagnosis of keratoconus. (See color plate.)

more important. The reproducibility of specific numbers is good, but not great, whereas the reproducibility of color patterns is excellent. Patterns demonstrate areas of relative steepness and flatness and demonstrate their regularity, differentiating between irregular and regular corneal astigmatism (Fig. 9-2). Such information can be extremely helpful in determining causes of diminished vision. Certain patterns are characteristic of certain conditions, such as keratoconus (Fig. 9-3) and pellucid marginal degeneration, whereas other patterns may suggest contact lens warpage. These conditions may be difficult to detect at the slit lamp when mild but are often readily apparent on corneal topography.

The most effective uses of corneal topography include ruling out mild corneal irregularity in eyes with diminished vision of unknown cause. It is also useful in screening patients before keratorefractive surgery to make certain their corneas are regular. It is effective to evaluate results of refractive surgery to determine the regularity and centration of the procedure. The corollary is that it can be helpful in finding the cause of diminished vision after corneal or refractive surgery and also in devising the best corrective treatment. It can also be used to evaluate corneal stability after cataract surgery. Selective suture removal after corneal transplantation can be aided by corneal topography. As software improves, contact lens fitting programs and artificial intelligence diagnostic programs may become more clinically applicable (Box 9-2).

Box 9-2 Uses of Computed Videokeratography

EFFECTIVE

Rule out irregular astigmatism before refractive surgery
Preoperative and postoperative comparisons of corneal curvature
Preoperative refractive surgery reoperation
Evaluation of decreased vision of unknown cause

MODERATELY EFFECTIVE

Often helpful in postkeratoplasty suture removal
Contact lens fitting

POTENTIAL FUTURE APPLICATIONS

"Expert" screening programs to diagnose corneal conditions
Creation of custom-made rigid contact lenses
Real-time guide to corneal therapeutic and refractive surgery

PACHYMETRY

The measurement of corneal thickness is termed *pachymetry*. This measurement was originally accomplished using optical units attached to a slit lamp. However, because of problems with difficulty of use, portability, accuracy, and reproducibility, optical pachymetry has generally been replaced with ultrasound methods. Ultrasound pachymetry measures the corneal thickness from the tear film to the posterior aspect of the endothelium.

Normal corneas are thinnest in the center and thickest in the periphery. Typical central corneal thickness measurements range from approximately 480 μm to 580 μm, with an average of 540 μm, whereas corneal thickness in the periphery can measure upwards of 800 μm. A moderate degree of variability in corneal

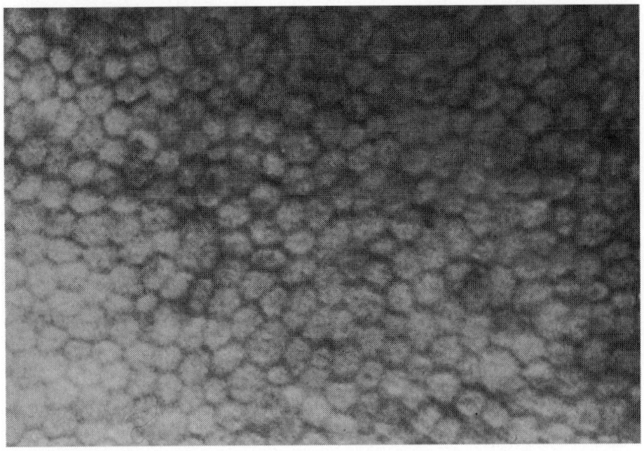

Fig. 9-4 Endothelial specular microscopy. Specular microscopy can image the endothelial cells to evaluate their size and shape. These cells from a normal cornea have a relatively uniform size, and most have the normal hexagonal shape.

thickness measurements exists between different machines and observers; however, less variability occurs centrally than peripherally.

Measurement of corneal thickness is often useful to help determine the health of the corneal endothelium. For example, in eyes with an endothelial dystrophy and cataract, pachymetry can be helpful in judging whether the cornea is healthy enough to undergo cataract surgery. Less often, corneal thickness measurements can also be followed in corneal transplant patients to help detect early graft rejection and in eyes with corneal edema to determine response to treatment. In addition, corneal thickness can be measured in eyes with thinning disorders, such as keratoconus. More recently, with the rise in interest of keratorefractive surgery by which corneas are reshaped by removing tissue, corneal thickness measurements are becoming more important. They are used before surgery to determine whether a cornea is thick enough to undergo a certain procedure and after surgery to evaluate to results of refractive surgery. Additionally, they are often important in evaluating eyes before refractive surgery retreatment.

SPECULAR MICROSCOPY

Corneal specular microscopy is a tool to image reflected light from an optical interface, typically the endothelial-aqueous interface, and less commonly the epithelial-tear interface. Originally, specular microscopy was performed with contact units touching the cornea, but more recently noncontact machines have been developed that can achieve excellent image quality.

Endothelial specular microscopy produces images of the endothelial surface (Fig. 9-4). Endothelial cells can be analyzed in many ways. Endothelial cell size/density (endothelial cell count in cells/mm^2) is the most familiar parameter. Polymegethism (variation of cell size) and pleomorphism (variation of cell shape) are also commonly measured (Box 9-3). The lower the endothelial cell count, the greater the variation in cell size (many small and large cells) and the greater the variation in cell shape (fewer hexagonal cells), the less healthy the endothelium. A normal endothelial cell count is approximately 4000 to 5000 cells/mm^2 at birth, declining with age to approximately 2000 to 3000 cells/mm^2 in late adulthood. A cornea with an endothelial cell count of less than approximately 500 cells/mm^2 is at high risk for corneal decompensation.

Box 9-3 Common Specular Microscopy Parameters

Endothelial cell density (cells/mm^2)
Pleomorphism (variation in cell shape)
Polymegethism (variation in cell size)

Specular microscopy can be helpful in determining the health of the endothelium in endothelial dystrophies, such as Fuchs' dystrophy or posterior polymorphous dystrophy, and in eyes after trauma or surgery. Often this information is useful in deciding whether a particular cornea is likely to do well with cataract surgery or secondary intraocular lens implantation. Specular microscopy may be informative in the evaluation of fellow eyes of patients in whom unexplained corneal edema after cataract surgery develops in the first eye. It can also be used to evaluate the effect of contact lens wear or new surgical techniques, instruments, and intraocular medications on endothelial health. Endothelial specular microscopy is occasionally effective in differentiating various endothelial abnormalities, such as iridocorneal endothelial syndrome from posterior polymorphous dystrophy. It is also used routinely to evaluate the health of the endothelium of donor corneas before corneal transplantation. Epithelial specular microscopy is primarily a research tool to evaluate the effects of new medications and surgical techniques on the epithelium. Specular microscopy is a safe, noninvasive, rapid, easy-to-perform, relatively inexpensive method to evaluate the corneal endothelium (and epithelium) for clinical and research purposes.

CONFOCAL MICROSCOPY

Confocal microscopy is a relatively new imaging technique that uses a contact microscope to evaluate the cornea in vivo. Whereas specular microscopic methods

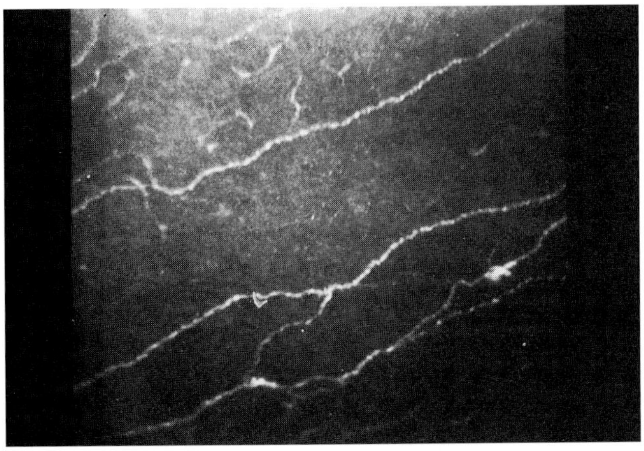

Fig. 9-5 Confocal microscopy. The confocal microscope can image the cornea in vivo. This image demonstrates the basal corneal epithelial nerve plexus. (Courtesy of James D. Auran, M.D.)

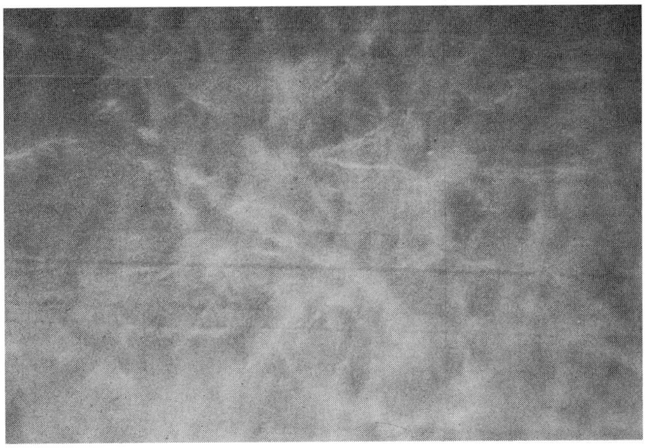

Fig. 9-6 Confocal microscopy. This confocal microscopic image demonstrates multiple *Fusarium* fungal organisms in the superficial stroma. (Courtesy of James D. Auran, M.D.)

only allow for the characterization of endothelial (and less commonly epithelial) surfaces, confocal microscopy permits the visualization of corneal epithelium, stromal keratocytes, and nerves (Fig. 9-5), as well as endothelium.

Confocal microscopic techniques have been used in the diagnosis of corneal ulcers, differentiating *Acanthamoeba*, fungal (Fig. 9-6), and bacterial pathogens. Eyes with herpetic keratitis have also been assessed with this method. Additionally, corneal wound healing (e.g., after incisional and excimer laser refractive surgeries) has been investigated as have effects of contact lens wear and topical medications. Although still in development and not widely available, confocal microscopy may have important clinical and research applications in the future.

ULTRASOUND BIOMICROSCOPY

High-frequency ultrasound is another relatively new method with which to image the cornea and anterior segment in vivo. Ultrasound biomicroscopy (UBM) involves a noncontact fluid bath technique and the use of ultrasound in the ranges of 40 to 100 MHz (typically 50 MHz). UBM can provide a resolution of up to 20 μm with a penetration of up to 5 mm.

UBM is able to image the cornea and other anterior segment structures when the cornea is opacified (Fig. 9-7), looking for iris, anterior chamber angle (Fig. 9-8), and lens pathology. It is also useful to evaluate pathology in the anterior sclera (e.g., differentiating episcleritis from scleritis) and view the ciliary body. The exact position of intraocular lenses can be easily determined using this technique. UBM can be invaluable in searching for small foreign bodies in the anterior segment not visible on slit-lamp examination, perhaps because of

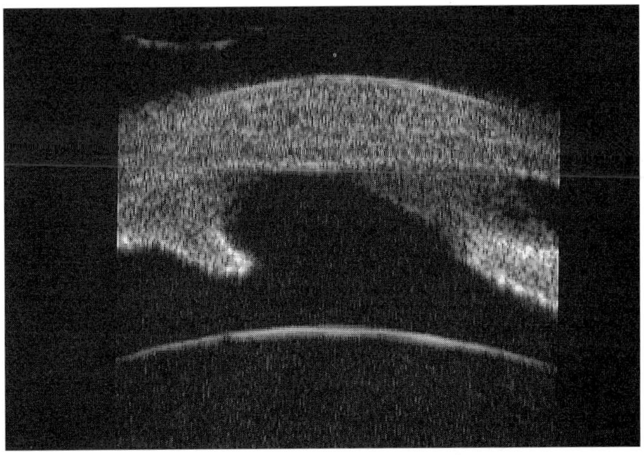

Fig. 9-7 Ultrasound biomicroscopy. This UBM image demonstrates a dense central corneal scar. Significant iridocorneal adhesions are also visible. The anterior lens capsule is evident at the lower part of the figure.

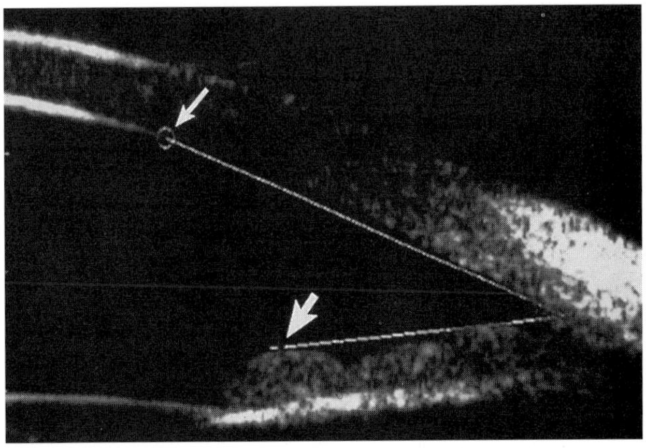

Fig. 9-8 Ultrasound biomicroscopy. UBM can be used to measure the anterior chamber angle. Changes in the angle from before to after surgery can be assessed. (Courtesy of Elizabeth L. Affel, M.S.)

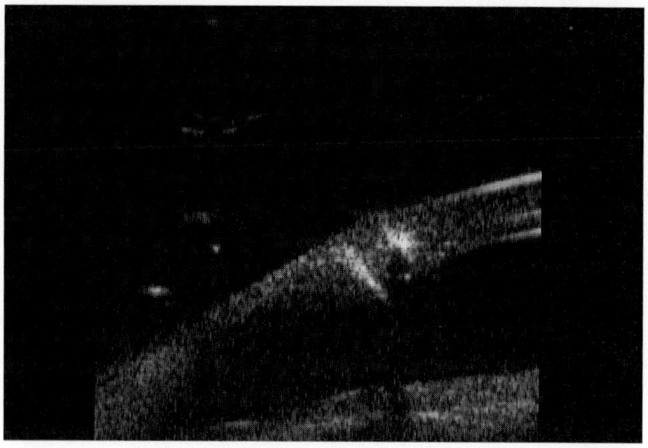

Fig. 9-9 Ultrasound biomicroscopy. A chestnut spike that fell against this patient's eye has perforated the cornea and protruded into the anterior chamber.

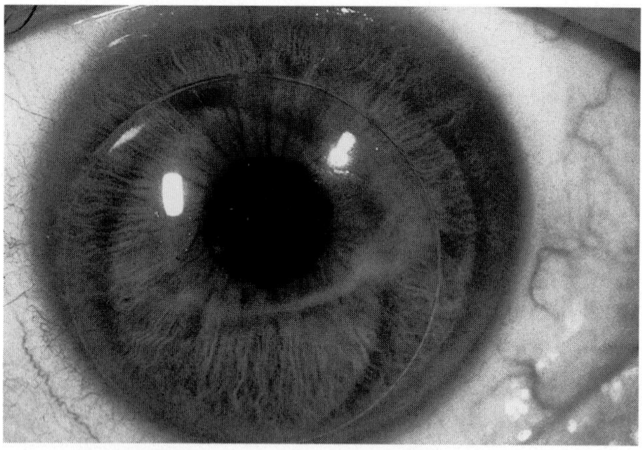

Fig. 9-10 Rigid contact lens. This patient has a large paracentral corneal scar causing significant irregular astigmatism after a large full-thickness corneal laceration repair. A rigid contact lens gives the patient 20/20 visual acuity.

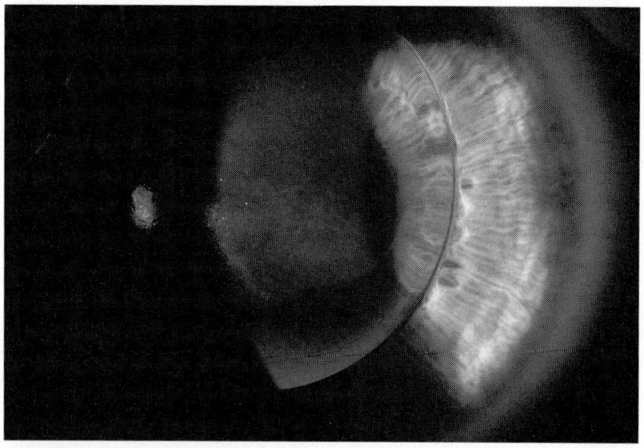

Fig. 9-11 Rigid contact lens overrefraction. This eye has diminished vision from a combination of a moderate corneal scar and corneal irregularity. Rigid contact lens overrefraction neutralizes the corneal irregularity, and the remaining amount of diminished vision is from the corneal scarring.

small size, corneal scarring, corneal edema, or subconjunctival hemorrhage (Fig. 9-9). UBM is rapidly becoming an extremely useful tool in the diagnosis of anterior segment pathology.

RIGID CONTACT LENS OVERREFRACTION

Rigid, typically gas-permeable, contact lenses are used by many people for optical correction. Rigid contact lenses are also an effective tool for treating irregular astigmatism (Fig. 9-10). Often in clinical practice a patient with corneal scarring and irregularity has diminished vision. To best manage the condition, the physician must determine how much of the diminished vision is caused by the corneal irregularity (irregular astigmatism) and how much is caused by the corneal scarring because they are managed differently (Fig. 9-11). A rigid contact lens can be placed on the eye and an overrefraction performed. The rigid contact lens neutralizes any astigmatism (regular and irregular), making only spherical overrefraction necessary. Assuming the contact lens fits reasonably well, the amount that the vision improves with the rigid contact lens overrefraction is the amount of visual disability from the irregular astigmatism. The rest of the diminished vision is from another cause, typically the corneal scarring or the posterior segment.

One technique (Box 9-4) is to obtain keratometry readings from the cornea to be evaluated. The flat keratometry reading is converted to a base curve, and a large (e.g., 9-mm) rigid contact lens is selected and placed in the eye after topical anesthesia. Spherical overrefraction is then performed. If the vision improves significantly compared with manifest refraction, then irregular astigmatism is diagnosed. It can then be managed appropriately with either a rigid gas-permeable contact lens or corneal surgery.

Box 9-4 Technique for Rigid Contact Lens Overrefraction

Obtain approximate flat keratometry readings
Convert keratometric reading to base curve
Select a large (e.g., 9-mm) rigid contact lens in approximate power of patient's refraction
Place a topical anesthetic and then the contact lens in the eye
Perform a spherical overrefraction

CONCLUSION

Many of these diagnostic tools have become integral parts of the anterior segment examination. From the evaluation of subtle changes in corneal curvature or thickness, to microscopic assessment of the various corneal layers, to ultrasonic methods to better analyze the structures in the front of the eye, these techniques can be extremely helpful in the diagnosis and management of corneal and anterior segment pathology. Rigid contact lens overrefraction, though an older technique, is still valuable in the diagnosis and management of corneal pathology. These tools, and others in various stages of development, continue to improve and aid the physician in ophthalmic evaluation and treatment.

SUGGESTED READINGS

Barash D, Goldenberg-Cohen N, Tzadok D, et al: Ultrasound biomicroscopic detection of anterior ocular segment foreign body after trauma, *Am J Ophthalmol* 126:197-202, 1998.

Deramo VA, Shah GK, Baumal CR, et al. Ultrasound biomicroscopy as a tool for detecting and localizing occult foreign bodies after ocular trauma, *Ophthalmology* 106:301-305, 1999.

Karabatsas CH, Cook SD, Figueiredo FC, et al: Surgical control of late postkeratoplasty astigmatism with or without the use of computerized video keratography: a prospective, randomized study, *Ophthalmology* 105:1999-2006, 1998.

Lanzl IM, Augsburger JJ, Hertle RW, et al: The role of ultrasound biomicroscopy in surgical planning for limbal dermoids, *Cornea* 17:604-606, 1998.

Wilson SE, Lin DTC, Klyce SD: Corneal topography of keratoconus, *Cornea* 10:2-8, 1991.

Winchester K, Mathers WD, Sutphin JE, Daley TE: Diagnosis of *Acanthamoeba* keratitis in vivo with confocal microscopy, *Cornea* 14:10-17, 1995.

MAJOR POINTS

Computed corneal topography is useful to rule out mild irregular astigmatism in eyes with diminished vision of unknown cause and to evaluate corneas before and after refractive surgery.

When evaluating corneal topographic "maps," the scale is extremely important.

Corneal topographic patterns are more reproducible than the exact diopter numbers.

Pachymetry and specular microscopy are easy, quick, relatively inexpensive, safe tests to assess the health of the corneal endothelium.

Ultrasound biomicroscopy is an effective tool to image the anterior one fifth of the globe.

Ultrasound biomicroscopy can be extremely useful to evaluate anterior segment structures when the cornea is opacified.

Rigid contact lens overrefraction is an effective technique to help differentiate irregular astigmatism from corneal opacity as a cause of diminished vision.

CHAPTER 10 Anterior Segment Surgery and Complications

Anterior segment surgery ranges from routine cataract extraction and lens implantation, one of the most common surgical operations in the United States, to rarely performed surgery such as permanent keratoprosthesis. It also encompasses surgery first performed centuries ago, such as rudimentary pterygium excision, to the latest in keratorefractive surgery.

CATARACT EXTRACTION AND INTRAOCULAR LENS IMPLANTATION

The many reasons for the development of cataracts are discussed in detail in Chapter 8. Most cataracts are acquired, but they can also be congenital. This section focuses primarily on the treatment of acquired cataracts in adults. Cataracts in adults are generally age related, but some lens opacities may result from other causes such as trauma, inflammation, systemic illness such as diabetes, or medications such as corticosteroids. Cataracts generally advance slowly over years but can advance rapidly over months, or even faster in some patients.

The primary indication for cataract extraction is diminished vision caused by the cataract, significantly affecting the patient's lifestyle. The exact point at which this hardship occurs depends on the patient. Certain patients require little visual function and may delay cataract surgery for years or indefinitely. Other patients with high visual needs seek cataract surgery with much smaller degrees of visual loss. Rarely, a cataract requires removal because it causes inflammation (phacotoxic uveitis) or elevated intraocular pressure (phacolytic glaucoma). Equally as rare, a cataract may expand to a size large enough to block the outflow of aqueous and cause the intraocular pressure to rise dramatically (phacomorphic glaucoma), also requiring surgical removal.

When cataract surgery is performed, preoperative medications are used for antibiotic prophylaxis and pupillary dilatation. Cycloplegic and mydriatic agents are used in combination to achieve maximal dilation. Nonsteroidal antiinflammatory drugs (NSAIDs) can be used to maintain pupil dilatation during surgery by blocking prostaglandin-induced miosis resulting from iris manipulation. Anesthesia may include a peribulbar or retrobulbar block and occasionally a facial block. Newer techniques allow topical and intraocular anesthesia to be used in some patients. Such techniques are especially useful in patients using systemic anticoagulants and those with significant systemic disease. Just before surgery, an antiseptic preparation with povidone-iodine is applied to the eyelids and periocular skin as well as to the conjunctival fornices. The operative eye is then draped in a sterile fashion, and an eyelid speculum is inserted.

The most common method to remove a cataract is with an extracapsular technique. This operation may be

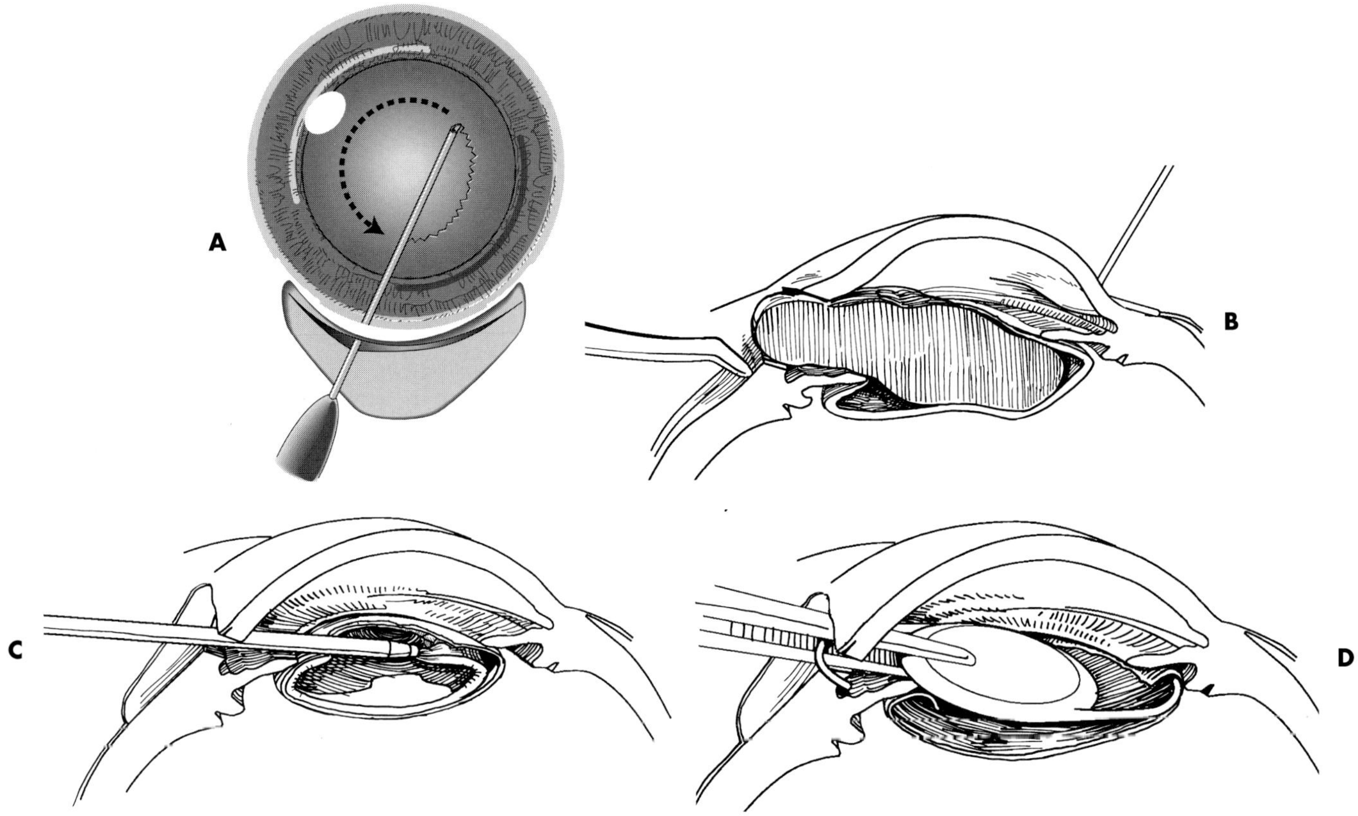

Fig. 10-1 Extracapsular cataract extraction and posterior intraocular lens implant procedure. **A,** After a superior conjunctival peritomy and a limbal incision have been performed, viscoelastic material is placed into the anterior chamber and a can-opener anterior capsulotomy is fashioned with a 25-gauge needle cystotome. **B,** Light pressure is placed posterior to the limbus inferiorly and superiorly to gently express the lens nucleus. **C,** An irrigation/aspiration machine is used to strip residual cortical lens material from the anterior and posterior capsules. **D,** After additional visco-elastic is used to inflate the capsular bag, a posterior chamber intraocular lens is placed in the bag.

performed through large or small incisions. The site of the incision is near the limbus, usually superiorly or temporally, but it can be at any location. The basic steps are to make an incision in the eye, open the capsular bag, remove the cataractous lens, and place an intraocular lens implant in the capsular bag. If required, the incision is then sutured closed.

The planned extracapsular cataract extraction technique using a superior approach will be described (Fig. 10-1 and Box 10-1). It may involve placement of a bridle suture (e.g., 4-0 silk) around the superior rectus muscle to assist with exposure of the surgical wound. A superior limbal conjunctival peritomy is performed for approximately 5 clock hours. Hemostasis is achieved with light cautery. A partial-thickness scleral groove may be created just posterior to the surgical limbus. A small scleral tunnel can be made into peripheral clear cornea. The anterior chamber is entered through the scleral tunnel with a small blade. Viscoelastic is then injected into the anterior chamber to maintain its depth. A cystotome (e.g., a bent 25-gauge needle) is placed in the eye and used to

Box 10-1 Major Steps in Planned Extracapsular Cataract Extraction

- Place a superior rectus bridle suture (optional)
- Perform a superior conjunctival peritomy and obtain hemostasis
- Create a scleral groove for approximately 5 clock hours
- Create a small incision into the anterior chamber
- Fill the anterior chamber with viscoelastic
- Perform an anterior capsulotomy
- Open the wound for approximately 5 clock hours
- Prolapse the lens nucleus
- Partially close the wound
- Remove the residual lens cortex with irrigation and aspiration
- Open the capsular bag with viscoelastic
- Place a posterior chamber intraocular lens in the capsular bag
- Close the wound and remove the viscoelastic

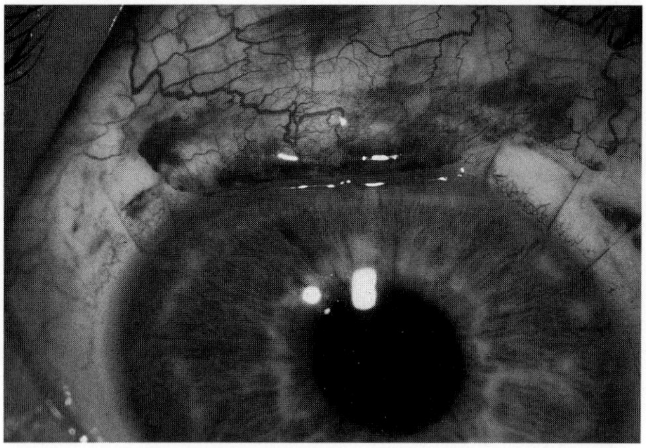

Fig. 10-2 Extracapsular cataract extraction and posterior intraocular lens implant, postoperative day 1. A superior limbal incision was performed and was closed with 10 interrupted 10-0 nylon sutures. The superior conjunctiva partially covers the wound.

create an anterior capsulotomy. The can-opener technique involves using the cystotome to make multiple small punctures in the anterior capsule, near the edge of the pupil, in a circular area measuring approximately 5 to 6 mm in diameter. These punctures must be connected so the central circle of anterior capsule is completely free and can be removed with forceps. The lens nucleus may then be rocked gently with the cystotome to break the nucleus-cortex connections. The cystotome is removed, and corneoscleral scissors or a blade is used to open the wound for approximately 4 to 5 clock hours. Once opened, gentle external pressure is placed a few millimeters behind the limbus inferiorly and superiorly, and the nucleus is slowly expressed from the eye. Once the nucleus is removed, the anterior chamber is reformed with balanced salt solution. The wound is partially closed with sutures (e.g., 10-0 nylon). The residual cortex is removed with irrigation and aspiration. This procedure may be performed using manual or automated techniques. Care must be taken to avoid breaking the posterior capsule, which often results in vitreous prolapse and necessitates anterior vitrectomy. After the cortical material is removed, the capsular bag is filled with viscoelastic, and a posterior chamber lens implant is inserted into the eye and either placed or dialed into the bag. The diameter of the lens optic is generally 6 to 7 mm. The wound is closed with additional sutures as needed, and the viscoelastic is removed with irrigation/aspiration. A miotic may be instilled into the anterior chamber. The bridle suture is removed, and the conjunctiva is brought down to cover the wound. Subconjunctival or topical antibiotics and corticosteroids are typically used at the conclusion of surgery (Fig. 10-2).

An alternative technique to remove the lens nucleus is phacoemulsification (Fig. 10-3). In this method an ultrasonic probe is used to break up the lens nucleus into small fragments and to remove each piece individually. Because the entire nucleus does not have to exit through the capsular opening in one piece, the opening can be small. A tear capsulotomy technique (capsulorhexis) was developed to create a continuous circular opening without breaks; it results in a lower tendency to tear posteriorly than the can-opener technique. In the tear capsulotomy method, a break is created in the anterior capsule with a cystotome, and then the edge of the break is grasped and slowly moved in a circular fashion, connecting at the initial break and creating a 4- to 6-mm diameter opening. The nucleus can then be separated from its epinucleus (hydrodelineation), and the cortex can be separated from the capsule (hydrodissection) by injecting saline through a blunt cannula tip into various portions of the cataractous lens.

Many effective methods to remove the lens nucleus have been developed, including *bowling*, *divide-and-conquer*, *chopping*, *stop-chop*, and *supracapsular* techniques. Whichever technique is used, the phacoemulsification procedure enables the surgeon to remove the cataract through a small (1.5- to 3-mm) incision. Before the advent of foldable intraocular lenses, this small incision had to be enlarged to allow the lens implant to fit into the eye. Currently, small incision intraocular lenses can be inserted through incisions as small as 2 to 3 mm. The optics of such lenses typically enlarge to 5 to 6 mm in diameter. An incision this small is often self-sealing, averting the need for sutures.

Such small incisions have allowed surgeons to move the location of the incision to various clock hours around the eye and also into clear cornea. Many surgeons find that a temporal clear cornea approach works best. With a clear cornea technique, topical anesthetic drops alone can provide sufficient anesthesia for surgery in selected patients. One percent nonpreserved lidocaine (0.75 ml) can be used intracamerally to supplement topical anesthesia (Box 10-2).

Another method to remove cataracts is the intracapsular technique. This operation, popular in the past, is performed infrequently today. It is, however, extremely useful in certain conditions, namely those in which the cataractous lens is subluxed because of broken zonular attachments. In this technique, large (approximately 200°) conjunctival peritomies and limbal incisions are created, typically in the superior quadrant. An enzyme (e.g., alpha-chymotrypsin) is instilled into the anterior chamber to dissolve the zonular adhesions. A suture is placed in the superior lip of the cornea and it is elevated. The superior iris is retracted away from the lens. A cryotherapy probe is placed on the lens, which is frozen and gently extracted from the eye. Ideally, the hyaloid face remains intact and no vitreous prolapses into the anterior chamber. After the wound is partially closed and visco-

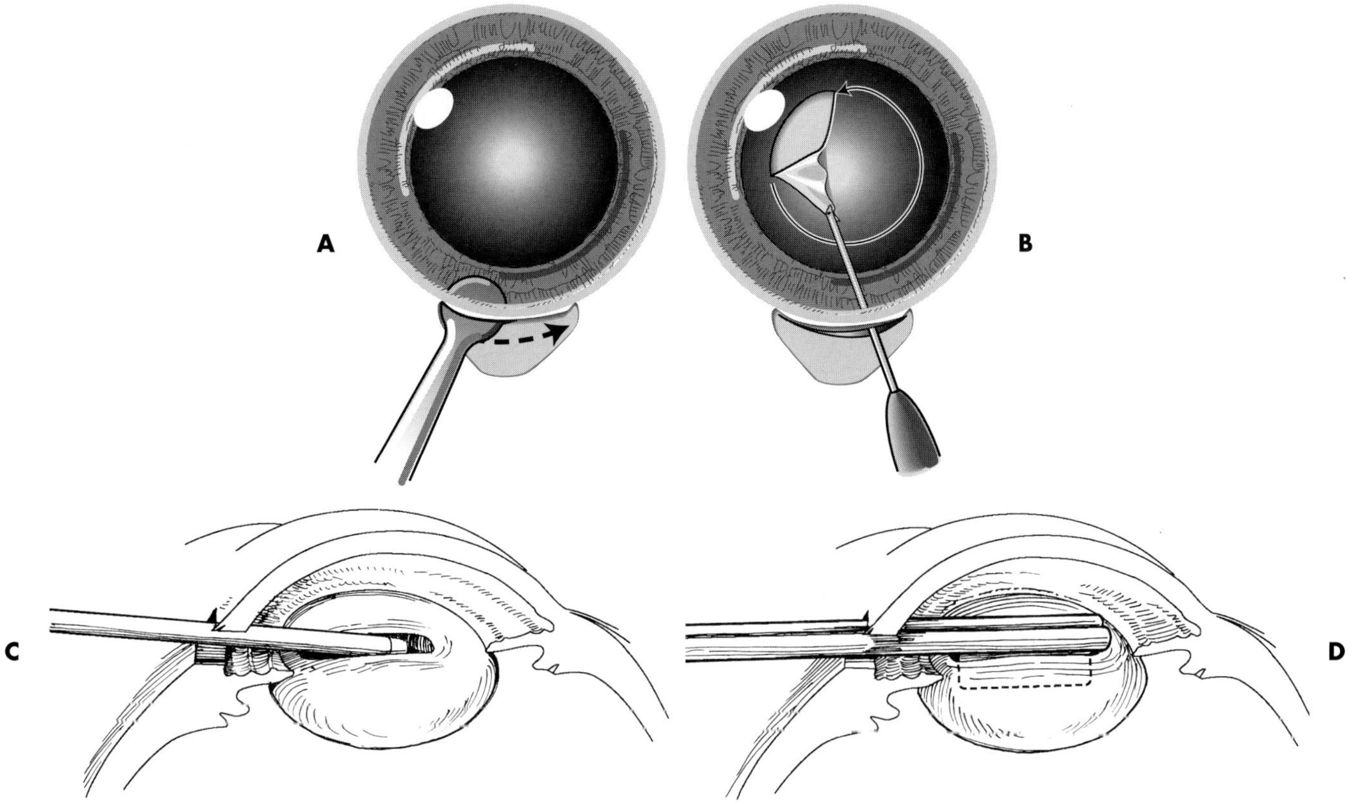

Fig. 10-3 Cataract extraction with phacoemulsification and posterior intraocular lens implant procedure. **A,** After a localized conjunctival peritomy is made, a blade is used to create a small scleral tunnel incision into clear cornea. **B,** After the anterior chamber is entered with a blade and viscoelastic material is injected into the anterior chamber, a continuous circular capsulorhexis is created with a bent 25-gauge needle cystotome. **C,** The phacoemulsification probe is used to remove the lens nucleus. Here a central groove is made. **D,** After a deep central groove is created, a lens cracker is used to fracture the nucleus.

elastic is placed in the anterior chamber, an open-loop anterior chamber intraocular lens implant can be placed in the angle. A peripheral iridectomy is performed, and the wound is sutured closed.

The lack of adequate capsular support does not completely prohibit the insertion of a lens implant in the posterior chamber. A posterior chamber lens can be sutured to the iris or the sclera to secure fixation. A nonabsorbable suture, such as 10-0 prolene, must be used. Additionally, complete anterior vitrectomy, with special attention to removing all the vitreous in the areas of the lens haptics, is required. One advantage of fixation to the iris is no externalized sutures; one disadvantage is significant iris-lens touch with potential increased inflammation. One advantage to scleral fixation is the lack of need for adequate iris; one disadvantage is externalized sutures. Recent scleral fixation techniques require the use of a lens with eyelets in the haptics through which a double-armed 10-0 prolene suture is placed (Fig. 10-4). This newer technique allows the externalized suture knots to be rotated into the globe, minimizing the chance of suture erosion through the conjunctiva (a major problem if the knot is left on the surface or even under a thin scleral flap.)

Postoperative medication regimens after cataract surgery vary but generally include topical antiinflammatory medications (e.g., corticosteroids or NSAIDs) and antibiotics. These medications are continued for days to weeks, depending on the clinical response.

Complications

Retrobulbar local anesthesia can result in a retrobulbar hemorrhage, which, though rare, may require lateral canthotomy and cantholysis if it is severe to reduce intraocular pressure. Deep injections can directly injure the optic nerve or cause an optic nerve sheath hemorrhage. Retrobulbar and peribulbar anesthesia injections are also associated with ocular perforation (Box 10-3).

Pseudoexfoliation, a condition associated with mild to severe compromise of the lens zonule, which holds the

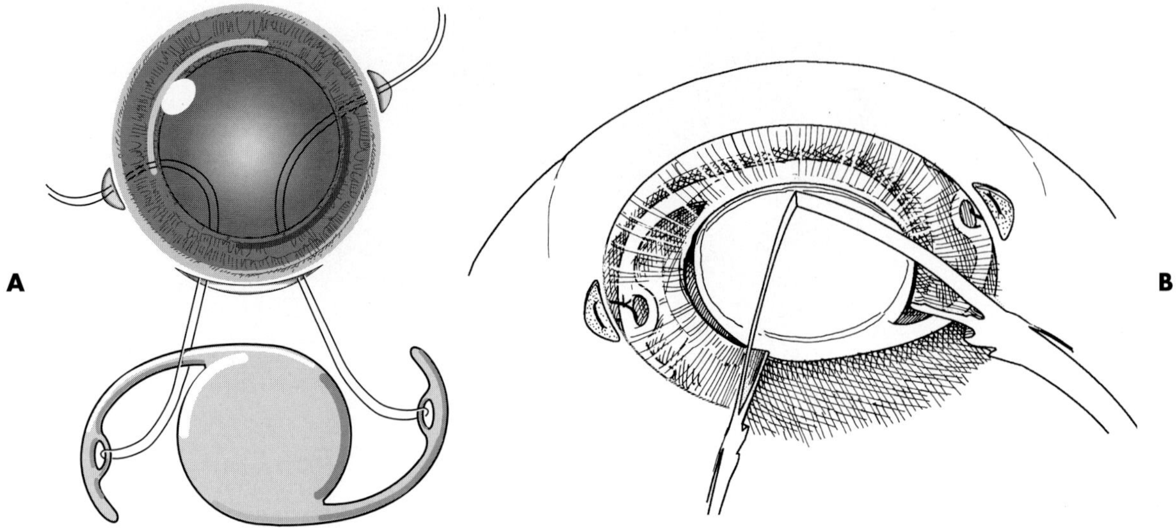

Fig. 10-4 Sulcus sutured posterior chamber intraocular lens procedure. **A,** Two small conjunctival peritomies are performed 180° apart just posterior to the limbus. A superior limbal incision is made. A complete anterior vitrectomy is necessary. A double-armed 10-0 prolene suture is fed through each eyelet of the posterior chamber intraocular lens haptics. The needles from each suture are passed through the wound and under the iris to exit through the sclera just posterior to the limbus in the areas of the conjunctival peritomies. **B,** The lens is inserted into the eye, and the sutures are pulled up and tied with no slack. The knots are rotated into the eye, and the conjunctival peritomies are sutured closed.

Box 10-2 Comparison of Planned Extracapsular Cataract Extraction Versus Phacoemulsification

ADVANTAGES OF PHACOEMULSIFICATION

- Faster surgical technique
- Smaller incision size with:
  - Faster visual recovery
  - Less induced astigmatism
  - Less chance of expulsive hemorrhage
  - Less chance of wound dehiscence after surgery
  - More stable refraction
- Can perform under topical anesthesia
- Can perform using a clear cornea technique

ADVANTAGES OF PLANNED EXTRACAPSULAR CATARACT EXTRACTION

- Technically less difficult
- Can perform with a less clear view through the cornea
- Easier to perform with a small pupil and with a very dense nucleus
- Less chance of capsular rupture and vitreous loss during the learning curve
- Less chance of lens nucleus falling into the vitreous
- No chance of "phacoemulsification burn"
- Less dependence on expensive, high technology equipment

Box 10-3 Complications of Cataract Surgery

MORE COMMON

- Posterior capsular break
- Zonular dehiscence
- Vitreous loss
- Cystoid macular edema
- Elevated intraocular pressure, both short-term and long-term
- Wound leak
- Corneal edema
- Posterior capsular opacification

LESS COMMON

- Retrobulbar hemorrhage
- Phacoemulsification burn
- Iris prolapse
- Endophthalmitis
- Retinal detachment
- Lens nucleus falling into the vitreous
- Anterior capsular phimosis
- Inadvertent intracapsular cataract removal
- Expulsive hemorrhage
- Epithelial downgrowth

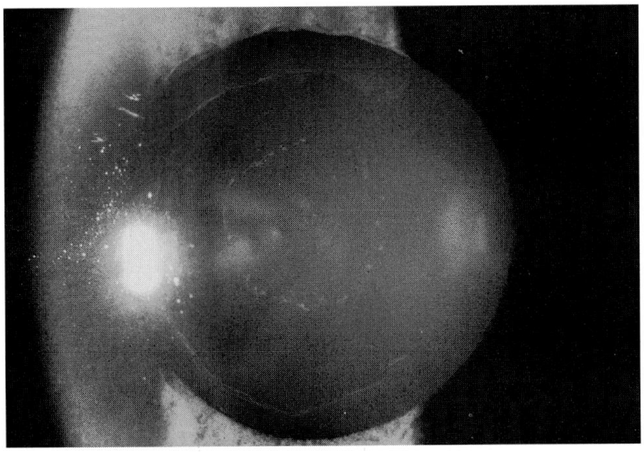

Fig. 10-5 Pseudoexfoliation cataract. Direct illumination of the anterior lens surface after pupillary dilation, demonstrating the classic double ring of pseudoexfoliation. The central clear annulus is where the iris has appeared to rub off the white superficial flaky material on the anterior capsule.

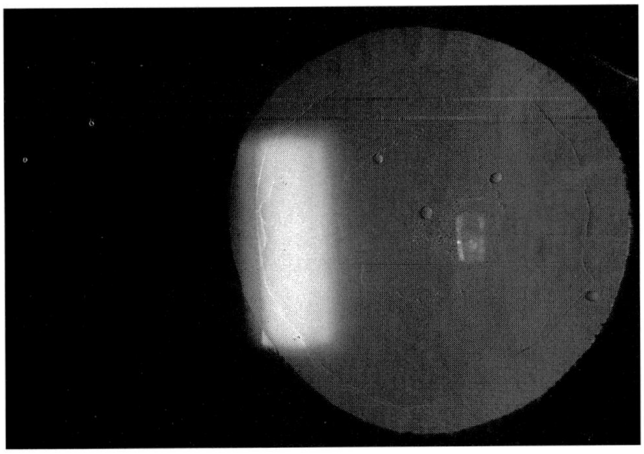

Fig. 10-6 Pseudoexfoliation cataract. Retroillumination off the iris through a dilated pupil highlights the double ring in this condition.

capsular bag in position, is associated with increased complications during cataract surgery (Figs. 10-5 and 10-6). There is a greater likelihood that the zonular fibers will break during surgery, allowing vitreous to prolapse anteriorly and necessitating anterior vitrectomy. Additionally, it is possible that the zonule will disrupt completely, permitting the entire lens and capsular bag to exit the eye inadvertently in an intracapsular cataract extraction fashion.

When the lens zonular attachments break or the posterior capsule develops a rent, the chance is high that the hyaloid face will also rupture and vitreous will enter the anterior chamber and even exit the wound. When such vitreous prolapse does occur, it must be managed with mechanical anterior vitrectomy (Box 10-4). Once vitreous is in the anterior chamber, the phacoemulsification must be stopped immediately. If a significant amount of lens nucleus remains in the eye, the wound must be opened to allow nucleus expression. A lens loop or a thin plastic glide can be extremely helpful in guiding the lens out of the eye and in preventing it from falling into the posterior segment. An automated anterior vitrectomy must be performed to clear the anterior chamber and wound of all vitreous. Peripheral iridectomy is needed to prevent pupillary block. Viscoelastic is then used to keep the vitreous out of the anterior chamber, and a lens implant can usually be inserted. If enough capsule is still present, a posterior chamber lens can be placed. Sometimes it can be placed in the capsular bag, but it is typically placed in the ciliary sulcus for maximal support. When placed in the sulcus, the lens haptics should be oriented perpendicular to the axis of zonular dehiscence or capsular tear. If minimal capsular support remains, an open-loop anterior chamber lens or a sutured posterior chamber intraocular lens can be placed. The need for anterior vitrectomy during cataract surgery increases the chances for postoperative infection (endophthalmitis), glaucoma, retinal detachment, and retinal swelling

Box 10-4 Major Steps in Managing Vitreous Loss During Cataract Extraction

- Stop the phacoemulsification
- If residual nucleus is present, support the lens with viscoelastic, enlarge the wound, and gently deliver the lens remnant(s), often with the aid of a lens glide or lens loop
- Perform an automated anterior vitrectomy to clear the anterior chamber of vitreous
- Remove the bulk of residual cortical material with the vitrector or with manual or automated irrigation/aspiration
- Make sure the wound and anterior chamber are clear of vitreous
- Assess the degree of capsular support
- Use viscoelastic to keep the remaining vitreous back
- If at least two thirds to three fourths of the capsular rim remains, consider placement of a posterior chamber intraocular lens in the ciliary sulcus; once in position, perform a "bounce test" to check lens stability
- If adequate support is not ensured, then consider placement of an anterior chamber or a sutured posterior chamber intraocular lens
- Perform a peripheral iridectomy
- Before closing the wound, again make certain it is free of vitreous

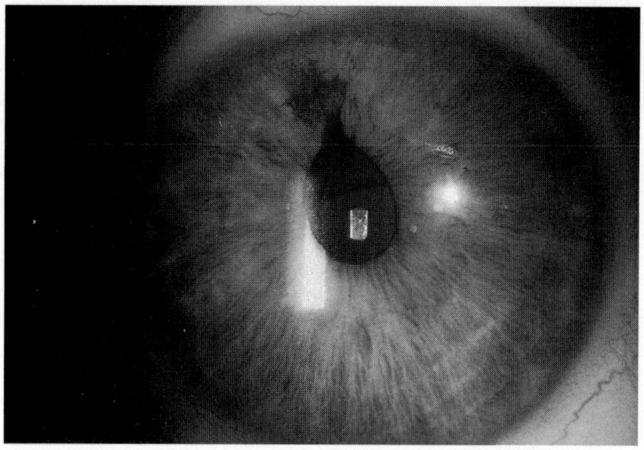

Fig. 10-7 Subluxed intraocular lens. This posterior chamber intraocular lens subluxed inferiorly soon after cataract surgery complicated by a ruptured posterior capsule and vitreous loss. Note the peaked pupil superiorly caused by a vitreous strand to the wound. Such inferior subluxation is often termed *sunset syndrome*.

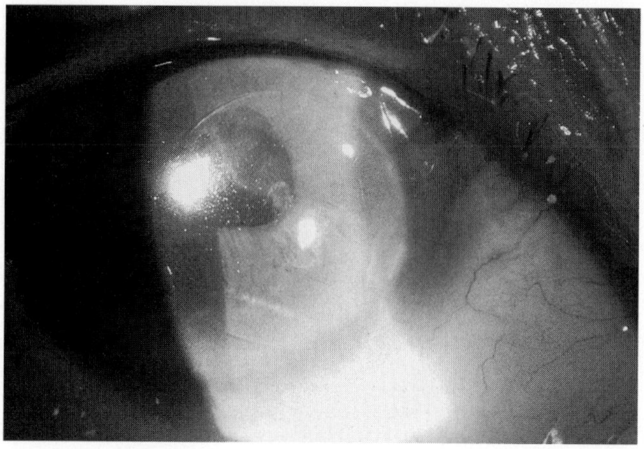

Fig. 10-9 Dislocated posterior intraocular lens. This posterior chamber intraocular lens dislocated into the anterior chamber and caused corneal edema.

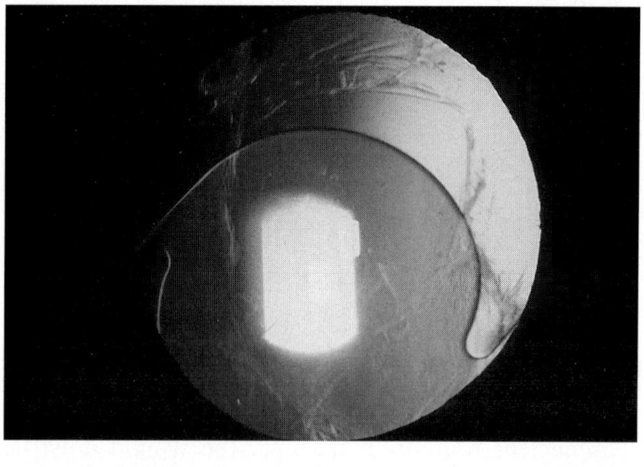

Fig. 10-8 Subluxed intraocular lens. Retroillumination off the retina of a subluxed posterior chamber intraocular lens. Inferior capsular rupture and vitreous loss complicated the cataract surgery. Some posterior capsule is visible. The optic size was only 5.5 mm in diameter.

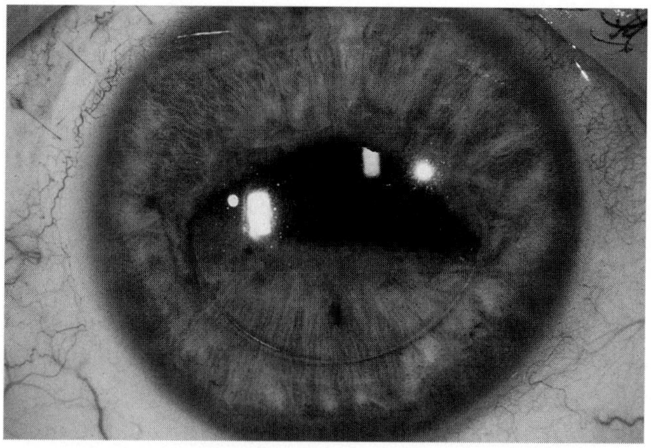

Fig. 10-10 Partial pupillary capture. This posterior chamber intraocular lens subluxed partially through the pupil 1 day after cataract surgery.

(cystoid macular edema). The additional surgery is also associated with increased endothelial cell loss and temporary or permanent corneal edema.

Inadequate capsular support is a common reason for decentered or dislocated posterior chamber intraocular lenses (Figs. 10-7, 10-8, and 10-9). Occasionally, the surgeon who manages a ruptured posterior capsule appropriately with anterior vitrectomy decides inappropriately to place a posterior chamber intraocular lens without sufficient capsular support. In general, a posterior chamber intraocular lens may be placed in the ciliary sulcus if at least 66% to 75% of capsular rim is present. Less than that amount of capsular support significantly increases the risk for lens decentration or dislocation. If the lens is placed in the sulcus, the surgeon can perform a *bounce test* to help verify its stability. The surgeon presses gently and lets go quickly just posterior to the limbus in the areas of the lens haptics to move the lens slightly. If it bounces back to a stable central position, the chance is good that it will remain there after surgery (Fig. 10-10).

During surgery, several additional complications can occur. One is a phacoemulsification burn (Fig. 10-11). This complication results from inadequate cooling of the phacoemulsification tip during surgery, causing a thermal burn of the corneal or scleral entrance wound. It results from insufficient flow of irrigation fluid around the tip during phacoemulsification. It may be caused by a tight wound that crimps the flow or by viscoelastic in the anterior chamber that prevents irrigation flow. Newer sleeves for phacoemulsification handpieces may

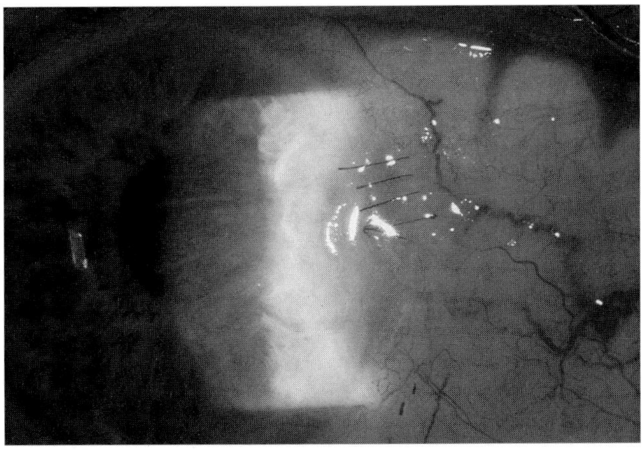

Fig. 10-11 Phacoemulsification burn. Corneal burn from a temporal clear cornea phacoemulsification incision results in corneal whitening and melting. It can be difficult to close with sutures because of tissue loss. Note the corneal striae from multiple tight corneal sutures.

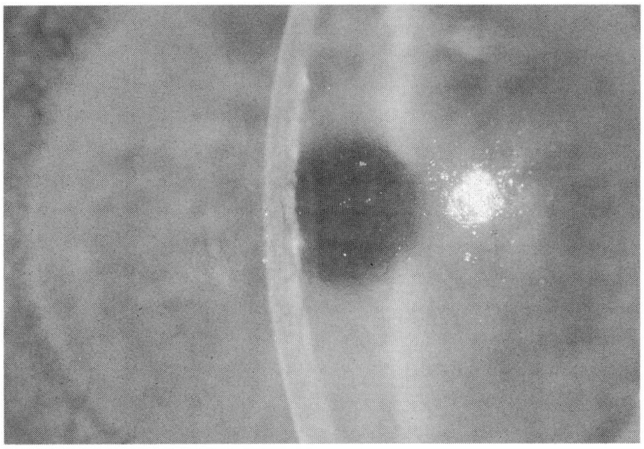

Fig. 10-12 Descemet's detachment. This planar, nonscrolled Descemet's detachment was noted 1 day after cataract surgery. It caused significant corneal edema. Because it was not shredded or scrolled, it was followed up for several months and resolved with clearing of the cornea.

help reduce the chances for this complication. Phacoemulsification burns range from minimal blanching of the wound to severe necrosis and loss of tissue. They are usually managed with multiple sutures to close the wound but may require cyanoacrylate tissue adhesive, or a patch graft with corneal, scleral, or alloplastic tissue, such as pericardium, if the wound cannot be closed primarily. Necrotic tissue is also at higher risk for infection, and these eyes must be carefully monitored after surgery.

When the posterior capsule ruptures during phacoemulsification, the small size of the typical posterior capsule break and the formed vitreous generally keep the lens material from falling posteriorly. However, with large posterior capsular breaks or significant liquefied vitreous, portions of the lens nucleus or the entire lens nucleus can fall posteriorly onto the retina. Should this complication occur, an anterior vitrectomy should be performed, and the residual lens material in the anterior chamber should be cleaned up. If adequate capsular support is present, a posterior chamber intraocular lens may be placed; otherwise, a sulcus sutured posterior chamber lens or an anterior chamber lens is appropriate. The wound should then be closed and the patient referred within days to a vitreoretinal specialist to have the large posteriorly dislocated lens fragments removed through pars plana vitrectomy. The anterior segment surgeon should resist the temptation to remove lens fragments that are deep in the vitreous cavity. Managed appropriately, this major complication can result in an excellent visual outcome.

Small detachments of Descemet's membrane are not uncommon near the cataract surgery entrance wound. Care should be taken not to enlarge these small detachments during surgery. At the end of surgery a small air

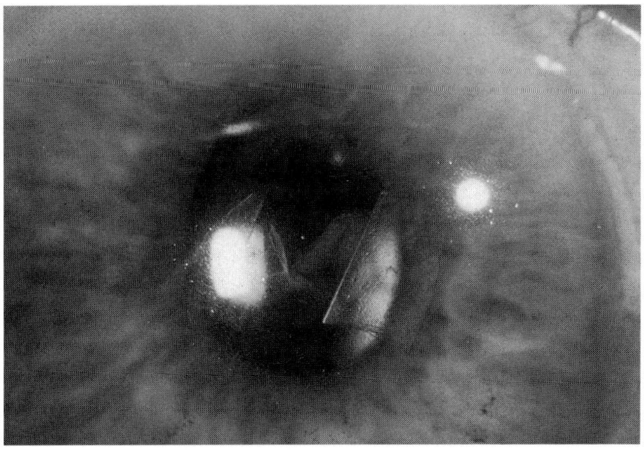

Fig. 10-13 Descemet's detachment. Descemet's membrane was severely damaged during cataract surgery, causing multiple tears and scrolling centrally. These types of detachments, especially when they are large and cause significant edema, generally require surgical repair, which is technically challenging.

bubble can be left in the anterior chamber to push a superior detachment back into position. Rarely large detachments occur. If Descemet's membrane is detached, but not scrolled or shredded, it can be left alone; it often reattaches over several weeks to months without additional surgery (Fig. 10-12). If it does not reattach spontaneously, surgical repair can then be attempted. However, if the detached Descemet's membrane is scrolled, it is best to attempt to unscroll it and reposition it against the posterior cornea (Fig. 10-13). This procedure can be performed using air or a cyclodialysis spatula. The use of viscoelastic is not recommended because if it gets between the detachment and the stroma, it can impede reattachment. Nonexpansile concentrations of intraocu-

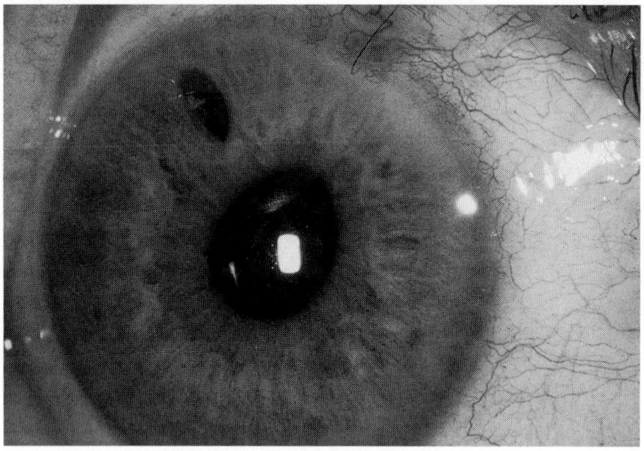

Fig. 10-14 Wound leak. Persistent leak after cataract surgery. An additional suture did not close the leak.

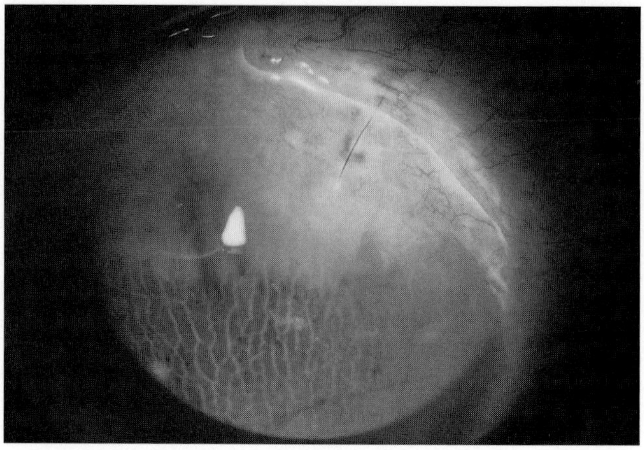

Fig. 10-15 Wound leak. Fluorescein dye demonstrates leakage of aqueous through the wound, termed *Seidel positive,* in the eye seen in Fig. 10-14. (See color plate.)

lar gas, such as SF_6 or C_3F_8, can be used to maintain the detachment in proper position until it reattaches. Rarely, suturing of Descemet's detachments is required to reappose multiple segments, but this procedure often results in severe damage to Descemet's membrane.

In the early postoperative period, the intraocular pressure can be too high or too low. Early elevated intraocular pressure typically results from retained viscoelastic in the anterior chamber, impeding the outflow of aqueous through the trabecular meshwork. It is managed with pressure-lowering medications, especially aqueous suppressants, and generally resolves within a few days as the viscoelastic dissipates. Postoperative hyphema can also elevate intraocular pressure, but it generally resolves over days to weeks. Pupillary block is another cause of elevated intraocular pressure after cataract surgery. It is most common in patients with vitreous loss without a patent peripheral iridectomy. Laser peripheral iridectomy is usually curative.

Abnormally low intraocular pressure is also worrisome. It may be due to a wound leak, through either the primary incision (Figs. 10-14, 10-15, and 10-16) or a paracentesis site. If the anterior chamber is formed and the leak is small, it can be managed medically with aqueous suppressants and a decrease in the antiinflammatory medications. If the anterior chamber is flat or there is iris prolapse, the wound must be resutured. If the wounds are secure, low intraocular pressure may result from a cyclodialysis cleft, choroidal or retinal detachment, or ciliary body shutdown from severe inflammation or aqueous suppressant medication. These conditions must be investigated with gonioscopy and dilated fundus examination and treated appropriately.

The two most dreaded complications of intraocular surgery are intraoperative expulsive hemorrhage and postoperative endophthalmitis. Expulsive hemorrhage results from a broken choroidal blood vessel during sur-

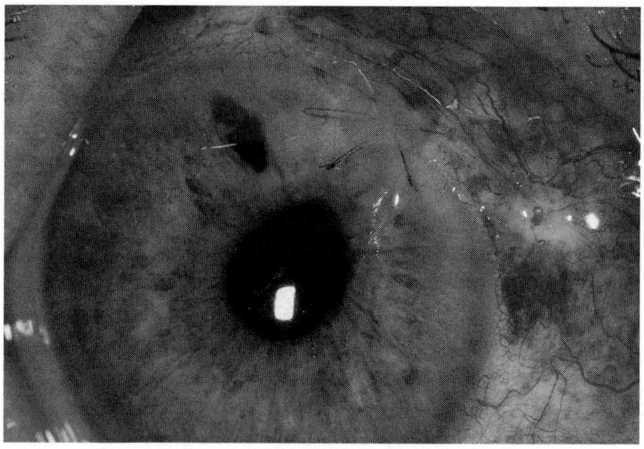

Fig. 10-16 Wound leak repair. A small corneal patch graft was performed 1 day earlier. After debridement of the leaking area to remove any epithelium, a full-thickness graft was performed that sealed the leak in the eye seen in Figs. 10-14 and 10-15.

gery, causing a hemorrhagic choroidal detachment that pushes the intraocular contents out of the surgical wound. Tell-tale signs of an impending expulsive hemorrhage are darkening or loss of the red reflex, shallowing of the anterior chamber, increasing posterior pressure, and firming of the globe. Once suspected, the surgical wound should be closed or at least tamponade should be applied as rapidly as possible. The immediate goal is to prevent loss of intraocular structures. If the wound can be closed, the intraocular pressure will rise to a point to stop the intraocular bleeding. Initially 8-0 silk sutures may be required to close the wound. If the active bleeding stops, an automated vitrectomy can be performed to clear vitreous from the wound and anterior chamber. Often the wound can then be resutured with 9-0 or 10-0 nylon sutures. In general it is best to complete the surgery another day. Risk factors for choroidal hem-

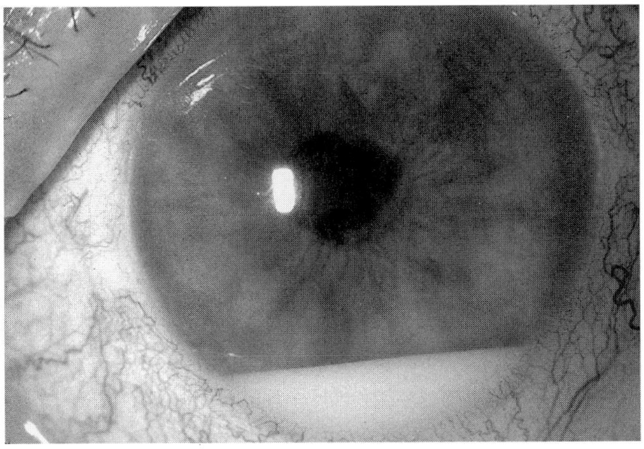

Fig. 10-17 Endophthalmitis. Ten days after cataract surgery, a large hypopyon and fibrin in the anterior chamber are apparent in this patient with endophthalmitis caused by *Staphylococcus epidermidis*.

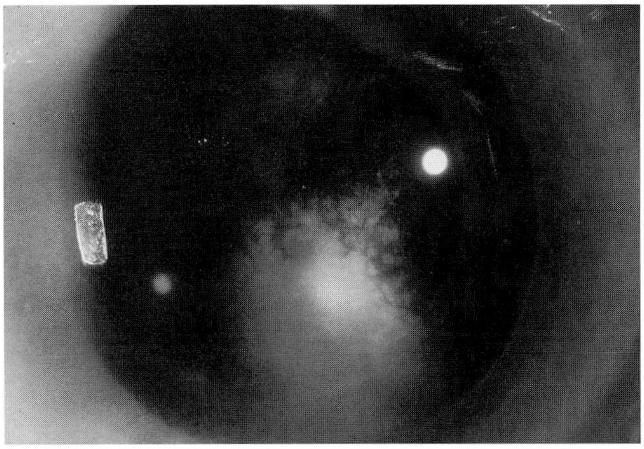

Fig. 10-19 *Propionibacterium acnes* endophthalmitis. A dense gray-white plaque on the lens capsule is frequently found in eyes with *P. acnes* endophthalmitis.

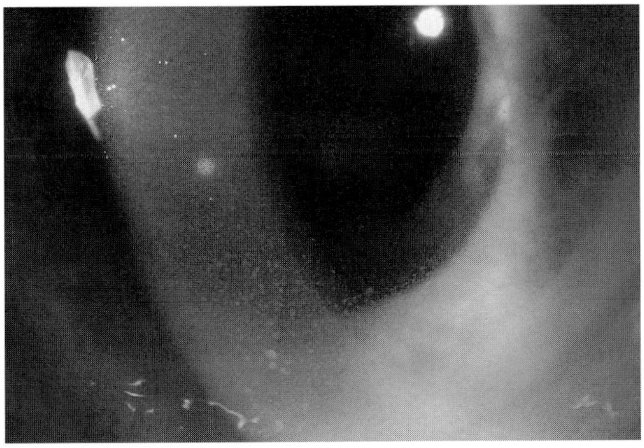

Fig. 10-18 Keratic precipitates. Infection after cataract surgery can be caused by less virulent organisms. The keratic precipitates noted on the inferior corneal endothelium signal a chronic inflammation or infection. This patient had *Propionibacterium acnes* endophthalmitis.

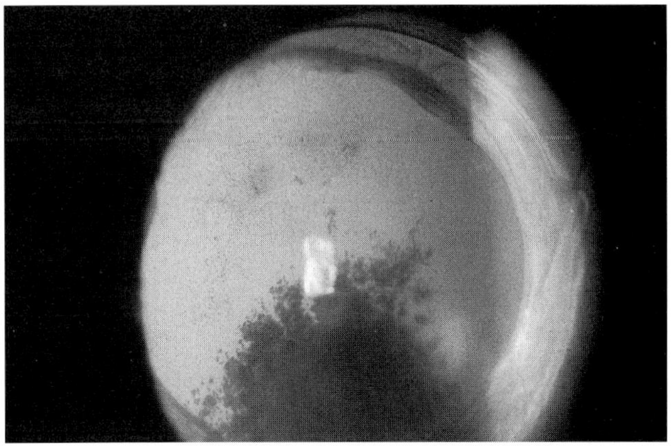

Fig. 10-20 *Propionibacterium acnes* endophthalmitis. Retroillumination off the retina highlights the capsular plaque seen in Fig. 10-19.

orrhage include increased age, systemic hypertension, cardiovascular disease, glaucoma, and preoperative elevated intraocular pressure. Needless to say, the smaller the cataract wound, the easier it is to close and the less likely intraocular contents will be lost. In fact, many small incision cataract surgery wounds are self-sealing, maximally protecting intraocular contents.

Postoperative endophthalmitis can be a devastating complication of any intraocular surgery. It can be caused by less virulent organisms such as *Staphylococcus epidermidis* or more virulent organisms such as *Staphylococcus aureus*, *Streptococcus* spp, and *Pseudomonas aeruginosa*. The typical presentation is acute onset of redness, pain, diminished vision, hypopyon, and vitritis within days of surgery (Fig. 10-17). Once suspected, the immediate workup includes aqueous and vitreous cultures, possible vitrectomy, and treatment with topical and intravitreal antibiotics. The Endophthalmitis Vitrectomy Study found intravenous antibiotics of no use. They did find core vitrectomy beneficial in patients with light perception vision or worse. Endophthalmitis, when diagnosed and treated early, is consistent with a good visual outcome. However, when a virulent organism is responsible, even with rapid treatment, endophthalmitis can result in grave visual loss. Late postoperative endophthalmitis is often caused by less virulent and slower growing organisms such as *Propionibacterium acnes* and fungi. It generally presents with chronic anterior chamber and vitreous inflammation (Fig. 10-18). A gray-white plaque involving the anterior or posterior capsule is often seen with *P. acnes* infections (Figs. 10-19 and 10-20). Although it does not usually result in severe visual loss,

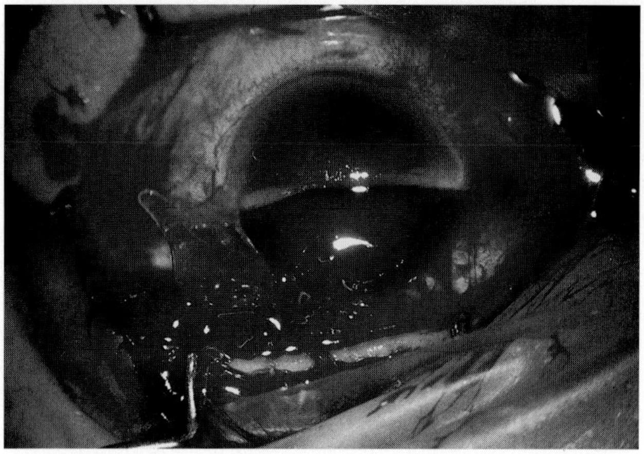

Fig. 10-21 Wound dehiscence. Intraoperative photograph of a large wound dehiscence caused by trauma. The patient had undergone intracapsular cataract surgery many years ago. The anterior chamber intraocular lens is visible at the edge of the wound. The superior cornea is folded under itself, and an expulsive hemorrhage has developed.

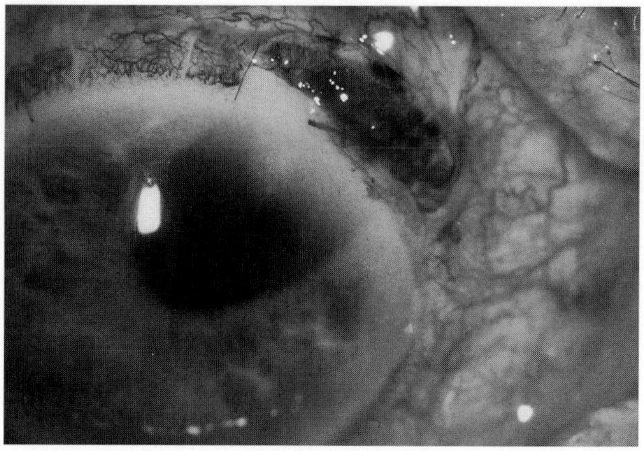

Fig. 10-22 Wound dehiscence. Traumatic wound dehiscence after extracapsular cataract surgery. The iris and the lens haptic protrude from the wound.

such chronic inflammation must be evaluated and treated. An anterior chamber or vitreous tap may be necessary. Topical and systemic antiinfectives are occasionally curative in *P. acnes* and fungal infections, but intraocular medications are often required. If inflammation persists despite aggressive antibiotic treatment, the intraocular lens and capsular bag may have to be removed because the organism may be sequestered in the capsular remnants.

Another dreaded postoperative complication is epithelial downgrowth. It is extremely rare after cataract surgery, but not quite as rare after penetrating trauma. It typically results from a penetrating wound (either surgical or traumatic) that does not heal and seal appropriately, allowing epithelium to grow down the wound and into the eye. The epithelium can grow onto the posterior cornea, iris, and retina, in addition to covering the angle. It is often recognized as a gray-white membrane progressively growing on the posterior surface of the cornea and anterior surface of the iris. It causes the iris to lose its normal crypts, and it can induce ectropion uveae. Although it is often associated with a chronic wound fistula and low intraocular pressure, it can also produce severe glaucoma. When present on the iris, the diagnosis can be confirmed by using an argon laser. On low power, the argon laser produces white laser burns in an epithelial downgrowth membrane but not in normal iris. Once confirmed, epithelial downgrowth must be treated aggressively with laser, cryotherapy, and surgical intervention to save the eye. Unfortunately, even with aggressive treatment, the outcome is often poor.

Even after uncomplicated cataract surgery, eyes are at greater risk for corneal edema, cystoid macular edema, and retinal detachment than they are before surgery. Corneal edema commonly occurs near the wound but can involve the central cornea. It often resolves with medical treatment; if not, penetrating keratoplasty may be required. Cystoid macular edema typically presents 4 to 8 weeks after cataract surgery with diminished vision. It generally responds to medical treatment. When it does not, it can lead to chronic macular damage and diminished vision. Retinal detachment occurs in approximately 1% to 2% of eyes after cataract surgery. Patients with high myopia, lattice retinal degeneration, and a history of a retinal detachment in the fellow eye are at greatest risk.

Traumatic wound dehiscence can also occur after cataract surgery. In general, the larger the cataract wound, the greater the risk for wound dehiscence with trauma. Intracapsular cataract surgery wounds open more readily than extracapsular cataract surgery wounds, and phacoemulsification wounds are even less likely to open with trauma (Figs. 10-21 and 10-22). Emergency surgical repair is necessary.

A common event after cataract surgery is posterior capsular opacification (Fig. 10-23). Approximately 10% to 50% of the time within several years of cataract surgery, lens epithelial cells proliferate on the posterior capsule to such a degree that it interferes with the clarity of vision. The rate of posterior capsular haze may depend on the intraocular lens material used, with acrylic lenses tending to be associated with less haze than silicone or polymethylmethacrylate lenses. Polishing the posterior capsule during cataract surgery may also decrease the risk of haze. When it develops, posterior capsular haze can be rapidly and successfully treated with Nd:YAG laser capsulotomy. The risk is slightly higher for cystoid macular edema, retinal detachment, and glaucoma after posterior capsulotomy. Rarely, after continuous tear capsulotomy, especially in the presence of pseudoexfoliation,

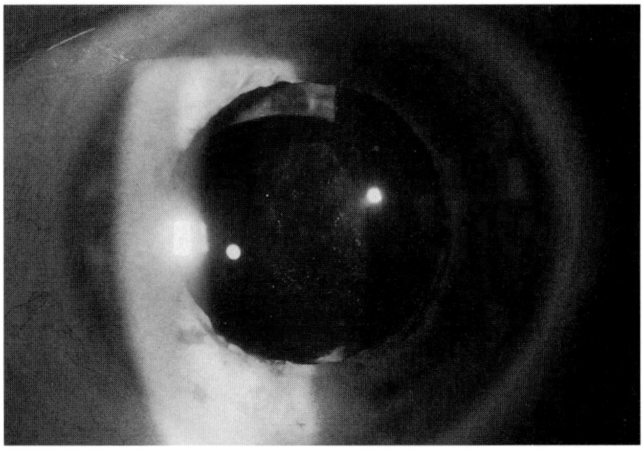

Fig. 10-23 Posterior capsular opacity. The posterior capsule often becomes opacified after cataract surgery, causing decreased visual clarity, glare, and halos. It is typically treatable with Nd:YAG laser posterior capsulotomy.

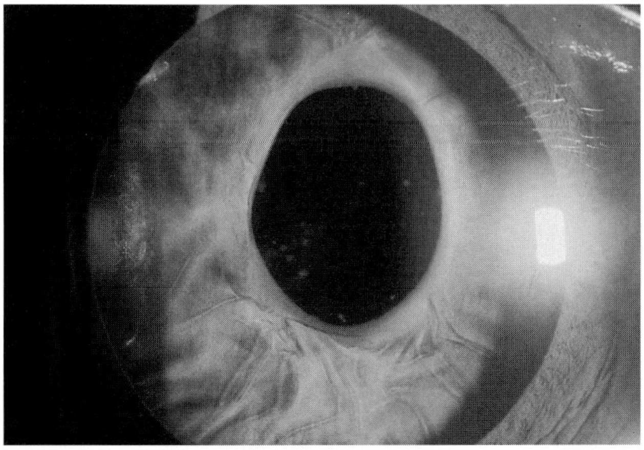

Fig. 10-24 Anterior capsule phimosis. The anterior capsule occasionally becomes fibrotic, causing the anterior capsular opening to shrink. If the opening becomes too small, the vision can be affected. It is treatable with Nd:YAG laser anterior capsulotomy.

the anterior capsular opening shrinks and becomes phimotic (Fig. 10-24). The opacified anterior capsule can then occlude the visual axis, leading to poor vision. Anterior capsule phimosis is best detected early, before complete closure of the opening. An Nd:YAG anterior capsulotomy, creating multiple radial cuts in the capsule, can be curative, though the anterior capsule is often dense and requires significant laser power to open.

PENETRATING KERATOPLASTY

Corneal transplantation, or penetrating keratoplasty, is performed for a wide variety of corneal conditions. The most common reason for corneal transplantation is corneal edema, typically in the forms of pseudophakic or aphakic corneal edema and Fuchs' dystrophy. Two other common indications for corneal transplantation are keratoconus and failed corneal graft, and less common indications include corneal scars and other dystrophies. Most corneal transplants are elective procedures, but emergency corneal transplantation may be required for severe corneal ulcers and perforations.

When it is determined that corneal transplantation is required, donor tissue must be obtained from an eye bank. Donors are routinely screened for dangerous conditions that may be transmitted to recipients, such as hepatitis, human immunodeficiency virus, Creutzfeldt-Jakob disease, rabies, and sepsis. The surgeon should review the donor's paperwork, paying close attention to the endothelial cell count as well as the cause of death, and should examine the tissue personally before surgery.

Anesthesia for corneal transplantation generally consists of a facial block and a peribulbar or retrobulbar block. General anesthesia may be used in selected patients. If the patient has a corneal perforation, general anesthesia is the preferred method to eliminate the possibility of a retrobulbar hemorrhage causing expulsion of intraocular contents through the perforation. Antibiotic prophylaxis, antiseptic prophylaxis, and sterile draping are used before surgery as described for cataract surgery. Intraocular pressure is lowered with digital massage and occasionally intravenous mannitol. Before the eye is entered, all instrumentation and intraocular lenses should be checked to prevent delays during the critical open-sky time of surgery. For example, make certain all the required surgical instruments are ready, the intraocular lens powers are appropriate, and the vitrector or irrigation/aspiration unit functions properly.

The surgical technique begins with an eyelid speculum that places minimal pressure on the globe (Box 10-5). A Flieringa (or equivalent) ring is often placed to aid in maintaining the shape of the globe once the corneal button has been removed. This ring is especially helpful in aphakic eyes, eyes after vitrectomy, and eyes undergoing combined cataract extraction or anterior vitrectomy. Additionally, a ring is mandatory for corneal transplantation in infants and children because their sclera is very contractile and causes significant posterior pressure (Fig. 10-25).

The size of the corneal transplant, which is most effectively determined at the slit lamp before surgery, is checked with calipers. Once selected, the trephine is placed on the cornea, and the epithelium is marked as a final check for size and centration. Typical trephination diameters range from 7.5 to 8.5 mm. The corneal donor button is then trephined, usually 0.25 to 0.50 mm larger in diameter than the recipient trephination. Rarely, same size or 1.0 mm oversize grafts are used. Most commonly, the donor button is trephined from the endothelial side, but artificial anterior chamber systems are available that

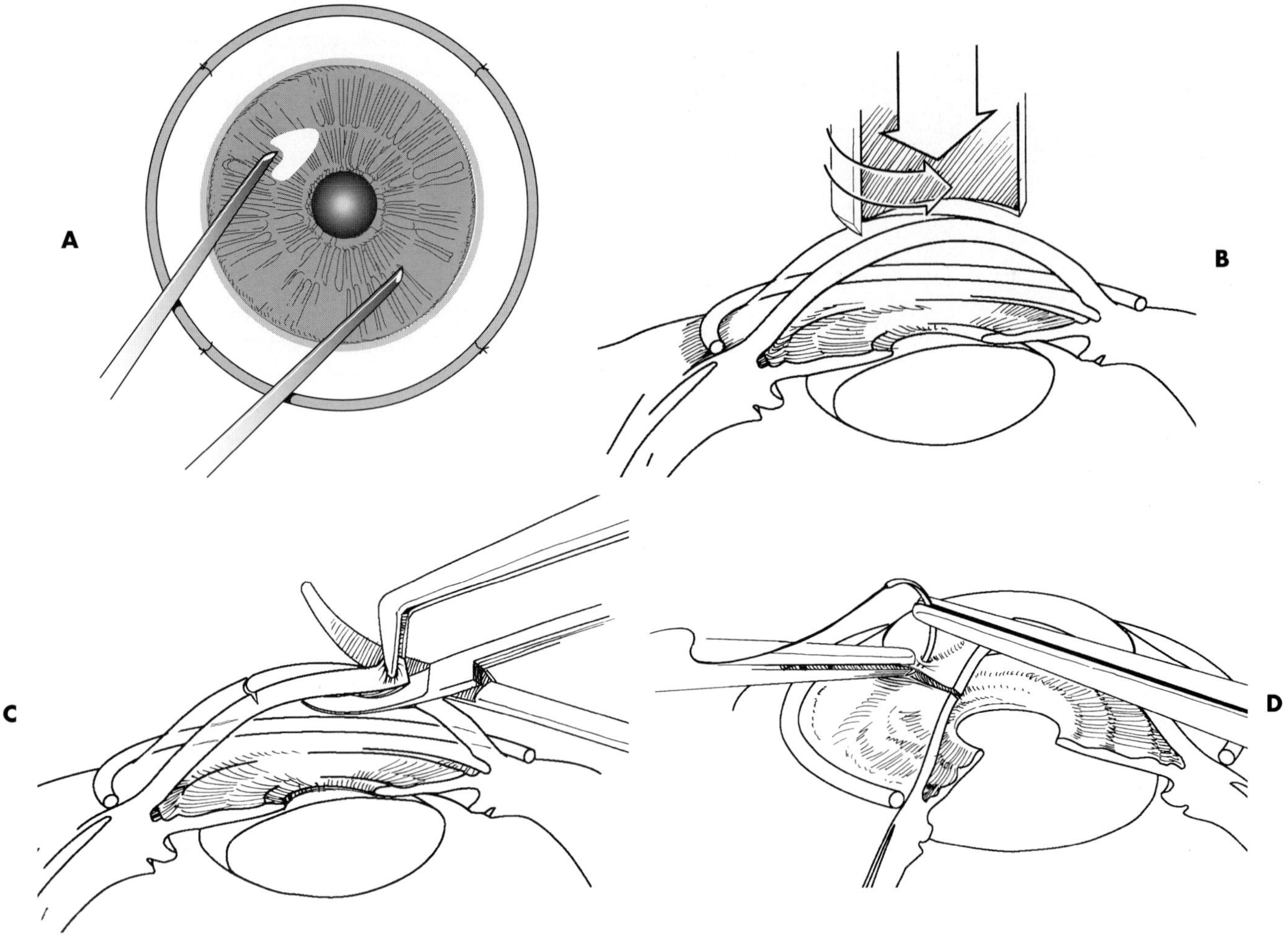

Fig. 10-25 Phakic penetrating keratoplasty procedure. **A,** A Flieringa ring has been placed to stabilize the sclera. Calipers are used to measure the exact size of the graft. **B,** A trephine is placed on the cornea. Using gentle pressure and turning, the cornea is trephined to 70% to 90% depth. **C,** After the anterior chamber is entered with a blade, corneal scissors are used to excise the cornea. **D,** After the cornea is removed and the eye is checked for residual Descemet's membrane, the donor button is placed on the eye and sutured into position with deep (approximately 90% depth) bites.

Box 10-5 Major Steps in the Penetrating Keratoplasty Procedure

- Obtain and examine the donor tissue
- Place an eyelid speculum that minimizes external pressure on the globe
- Place a Flieringa ring (optional)
- Determine the trephine size and mark the epithelium
- Fashion the donor corneal button
- Trephine the recipient cornea
- Enter the anterior chamber
- Remove the recipient corneal button
- Perform intraocular surgery as needed
- Suture the donor cornea in position, intermittently reforming the anterior chamber
- Bury the knots
- Check astigmatism and adjust sutures as necessary
- Inspect the wound and make certain it is watertight

allow trephination from the epithelial side. Once the donor button is prepared, recipient trephination can proceed using one of many techniques. Handheld trephines, with or without a guard, and vacuum trephines (e.g., Barron-Hessburg and Hanna trephines) are available. It is extremely important that the trephine be placed exactly where the surgeon intends (typically centered on the pupil, but occasionally decentered if the pathologic lesion is decentered). The trephination should proceed slowly, allowing the surgeon to stop immediately if the anterior chamber is entered. One technique is to trephine approximately 80% corneal depth and to enter the anterior chamber with a blade; others prefer to enter carefully with the trephine. Once the anterior chamber is entered, corneal scissors are used to remove the button. It is important not to damage the iris and lens during trephination and excision of the corneal button. Care should to be taken to leave an even bevel of

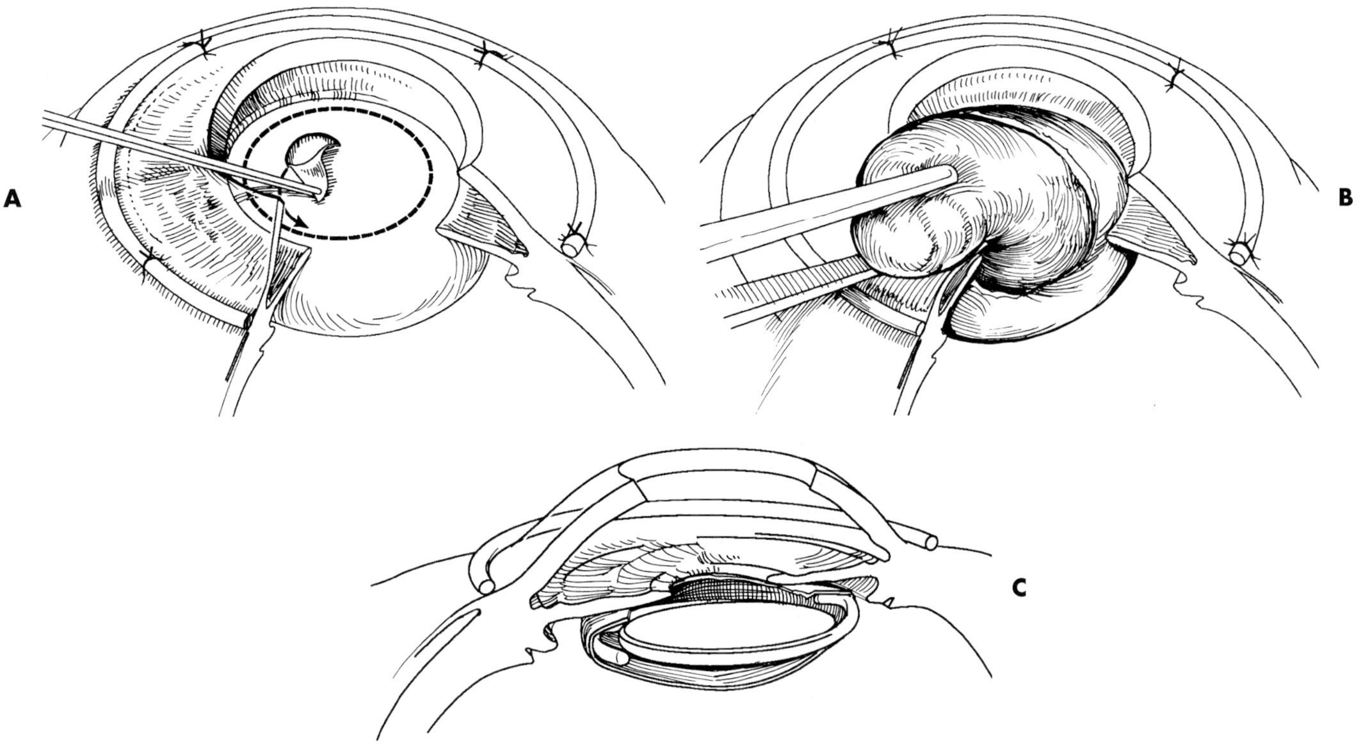

Fig. 10 26 Penetrating keratoplasty, extracapsular cataract extraction, and posterior chamber intraocular lens implant procedure. **A,** After placement of a Flieringa ring, corneal trephination, and removal of the pathologic cornea, continuous circular capsulorhexis is performed. The initial incision can be made with a needle or a cystotome, and the capsulotomy can be performed with a cystotome or fine forceps. Care must be taken so that the elevated posterior vitreous pressure does not force the edge of the capsulotomy to proceed under the iris and into the posterior capsule. When a capsulorhexis cannot be safely performed, can-opener capsulotomy should be performed. **B,** With an intact circular capsulorhexis, hydrodissection with saline around the lens capsule can prolapse the lens nucleus out of the bag, which can then be removed with a cystotome or forceps. Gentle posterior limbal pressure can also be used to express the lens nucleus. **C,** Manual or automated irrigation and aspiration are used to remove the residual lens cortical material. The posterior chamber intraocular lens is placed into the capsular bag, the pupil is constricted with a miotic agent, and the graft is sutured into position.

tissue for 360° because asymmetric bevels tend to create significant astigmatism. Once the button is removed, the surgeon must make certain that Descemet's membrane has not been left behind. Then all necessary planned intraocular surgery, such as cataract extraction, intraocular lens implant, or anterior vitrectomy, should be performed without delay.

When cataract surgery is combined with penetrating keratoplasty, a relatively large (5- to 6-mm diameter) can-opener or continuous circular capsulotomy is performed (Fig. 10-26). The lens nucleus can be hydrodissected with saline, gently rocked out, or both. The cortical material is removed in a fashion similar to routine cataract surgery. The primary difference is that in the open-sky technique, often posterior pressure pushes the posterior capsule forward, increasing the risk for capsular rupture. Once the cortical material is removed, viscoelastic is used to attempt to open the capsular bag, and a posterior chamber intraocular lens is carefully slipped under the anterior capsular flaps. Viscoelastic is placed on the anterior surface of the lens, and the corneal button is sutured in place.

Alternatively, when combined cataract and corneal transplant surgery are required in an eye in which corneal opacity is not severe, cataract extraction and lens implantation can be performed using a standard phacoemulsification technique immediately before corneal transplantation. The advantages are that the cataract surgery is performed in a closed system under more controlled circumstances and open-sky time is reduced. Disadvantages include separate incisions, longer total surgical time, and compromised view of the lens.

A common indication for corneal transplantation is pseudophakic corneal edema. Many of these eyes have older style anterior chamber or iris-fixated intraocular lenses, which are highly associated with progressive cor-

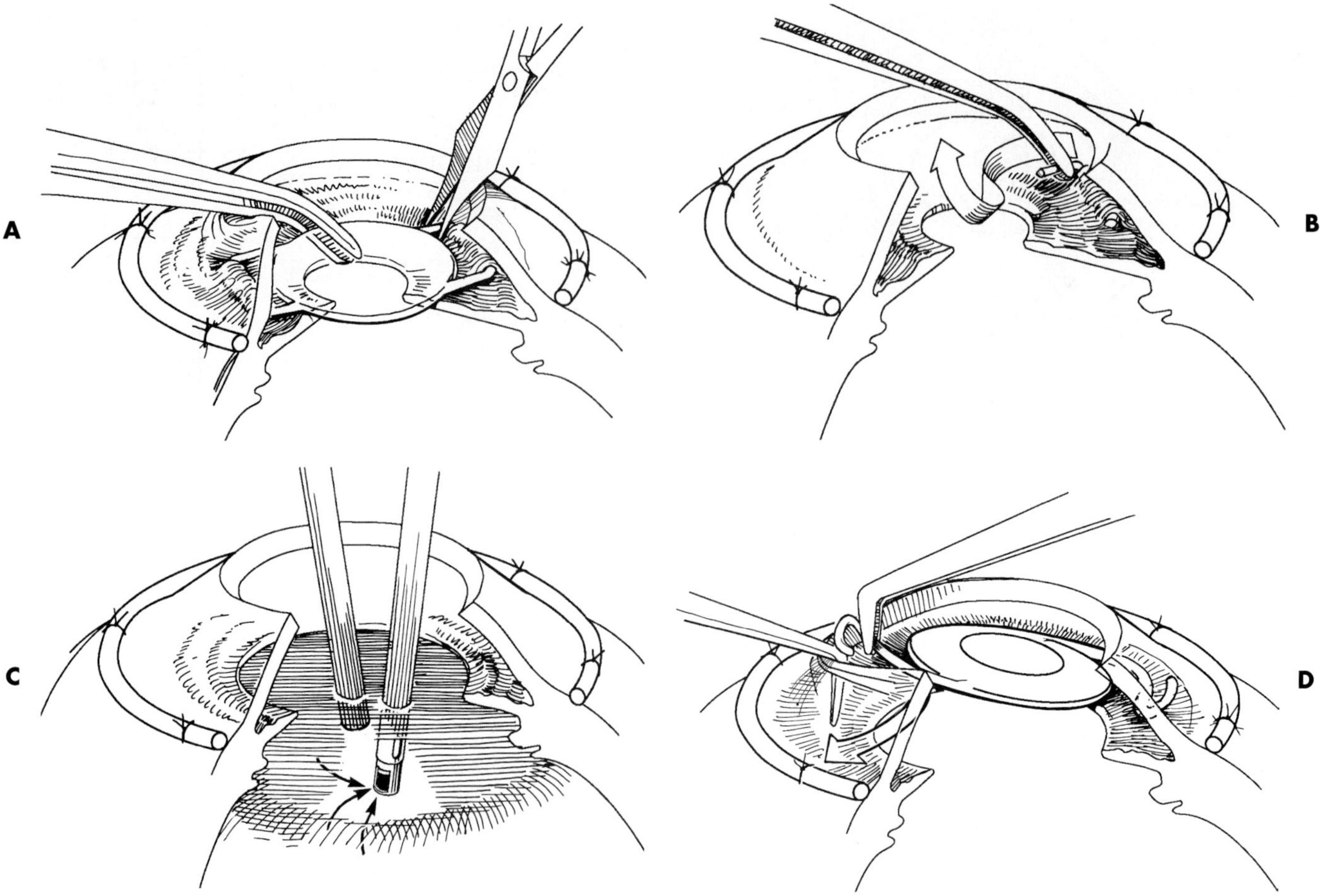

Fig. 10-27 Penetrating keratoplasty, anterior vitrectomy, and anterior chamber intraocular lens exchange procedure. **A,** Closed-loop anterior chamber intraocular lenses can often be embedded in the iris and angle. The haptics are cut, and the optic is removed. **B,** One end of the haptic is cut close to the optic, and the other end is cut near the iris. The longer end is grabbed, and the haptic is gently rotated out of its "cocoon." Care must be taken not to cause bleeding or iridodialysis. **C,** An open-sky core anterior vitrectomy is performed with the aid of a light pipe. It is important to ensure that the peripheral iridectomy is free of vitreous. **D,** An open-loop Kelman-style anterior chamber intraocular lens is placed in the angle while making sure no iris tuck exists.

neal edema. Closed-loop anterior chamber intraocular lenses are especially harmful. When corneal transplantation is performed for pseudophakic corneal edema, all closed-loop and iris-fixated anterior chamber lenses must be removed. Well-positioned open-loop anterior chamber and posterior chamber lenses may be left in place if vitreous does not envelop the lens. Once the lens is removed, the anterior chamber must be examined for evidence of vitreous prolapse. If the hyaloid face is intact, vitrectomy is not necessary, and an open-loop anterior chamber intraocular lens should be placed. If vitreous is present in the anterior chamber, an open-sky anterior vitrectomy should be performed. This procedure is most effectively performed with an automated vitrector and a light pipe. Care should be taken to remove the core vitreous so it does not prolapse through the pupil and to make sure the peripheral iridectomy is free of vitreous. After the vitrectomy, a posterior chamber intraocular lens can be placed if adequate capsular support exists, or an anterior chamber intraocular lens can be situated in the angle (Fig. 10-27). Alternatively, a posterior chamber intraocular lens can be sutured to the sclera or the iris. As briefly described in the section on cataract surgery, a double-armed nonabsorbable suture (e.g., 10-0 prolene) is placed through the eyelet in the haptic of a posterior chamber lens. The two needles are then maneuvered under the iris, through the ciliary sulcus, and out the sclera approximately 1 mm apart. The same procedure is performed 180° away. The lens is placed in the ciliary sulcus, and sutures are tied externally. Because the sutures are single loops around the eyelets in the haptics, the knots can be buried in the globe. Previously created conjunctival peritomies are closed to cover the externalized sutures.

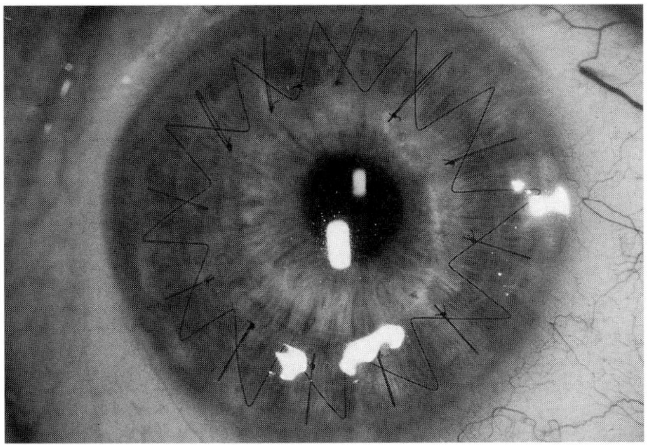

Fig. 10-28 Penetrating keratoplasty. Seven months after penetrating keratoplasty, extracapsular cataract extraction, and posterior chamber intraocular lens implant. The graft was sutured with a combined technique, using 12 interrupted and a 12-bite running 10-0 nylon sutures.

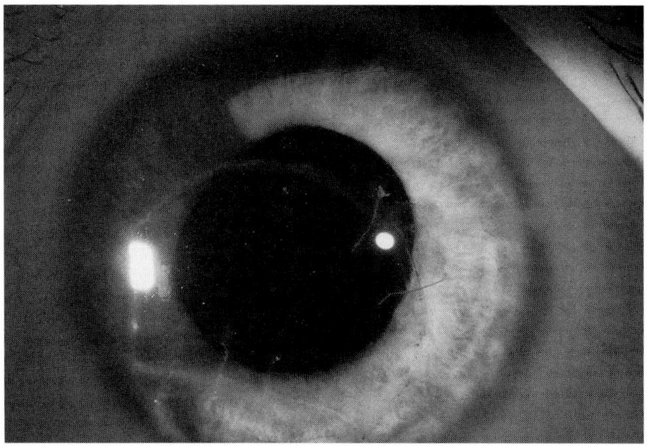

Fig. 10-29 Rotating autograft. Ten years after performing a rotating autograft in a child for a dense linear scar that crossed the visual axis. A noncentral trephination was performed, the corneal button was rotated 180° to move the scar outside the visual axis, and the cornea was sutured back in place. The peripheral scar is visible at the 3 o'clock position. The scar in the graft can be seen inferiorly, far outside the visual axis.

Once all intraocular procedures have been performed, viscoelastic or balanced salt solution is placed in the anterior chamber. The corneal donor button is carefully transferred to the surgical field and sutured into position. The goals of corneal transplant suturing are to secure the wound, to reform the anterior chamber, to create a relatively smooth corneal contour, and to minimize excessive flattening, steepening, and astigmatism. Numerous suturing techniques, including all interrupted sutures, single or double running sutures, and combined interrupted and running sutures, have been used successfully to achieve these goals (Fig. 10-28). The exact number of sutures depends on the size of the graft and the suture technique used. For a typical 8-mm diameter graft, 16 interrupted sutures or approximately a 24-bite running 10-0 nylon suture would generally be used. Running sutures are usually not used if areas of the graft are likely to vascularize or heal before other areas, causing localized areas of suture to loosen. Should differential healing and suture loosening occur with interrupted sutures in place, individual loose sutures can be removed without ill effect. However, should part of a running suture loosen before other areas are well healed, early removal of the running suture risks wound slippage or dehiscence. Such differential healing is more likely in infants and children, in previously vascularized corneas, and in grafts that approach the corneal periphery. Once the sutures are in place, the knots should be buried and the wound carefully checked to be watertight. An attempt should be made to evaluate graft astigmatism at the end of surgery, preferably after the removal of the Flieringa ring. Any gross irregularities should be corrected in the operating room. At the completion of surgery, subconjunctival antibiotics and corticosteroids and topical antibiotics are given, and a pressure patch and protective shield are placed over the eye. In eyes predisposed to postoperative intraocular pressure spikes, such as after combined cataract or anterior vitrectomy surgery and eyes with glaucoma, the intraocular pressure should be checked several hours after surgery.

Relatively central corneal scars affecting vision are, on rare occasions, amenable to treatment with a rotating autograft. This procedure, typically considered in children in whom the chance for graft rejection is greater, involves trephining the cornea in such a way that the scar can be rotated outside the center of vision and the corneal button sutured back into the same eye (Fig. 10-29). Because no donor tissue is involved, there is no chance for graft rejection. Its usefulness is limited because of significant irregular astigmatism.

In eyes with retinal pathology requiring vitreoretinal surgery, in which the corneal opacity is too dense to allow an adequate view of the posterior segment, a temporary keratoprosthesis can be used. This procedure involves trephination of the pathologic cornea and placement of the keratoprosthesis. This small lens is sutured into the graft opening and allows an excellent view of the posterior segment. Polymethylmethacrylate (e.g., Landers-Foulks) (Fig. 10-30) or silicone (e.g., Eckardt) (Fig. 10-31) lenses are available. At the conclusion of the posterior segment repair, the keratoprosthesis is removed and a corneal graft is sutured into position.

After corneal transplantation surgery, subconjunctival and topical antibiotics and corticosteroids are used. Because the corneal epithelium is often compromised in corneal grafts, topical medication toxicity should be minimized. Topical corticosteroids are extremely important in preventing allograft rejection and should be continued

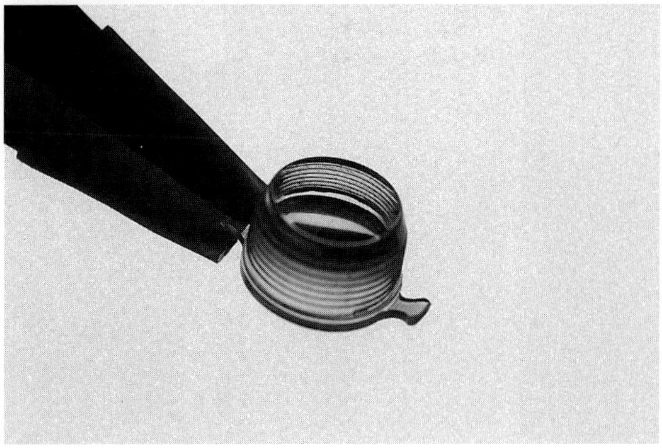

Fig. 10-30 Landers-Foulks temporary keratoprosthesis. This keratoprosthesis is made of polymethylmethacrylate and comes in 6.2-, 7.2-, and 8.2-mm diameter sizes. After removal of the pathologic corneal button, it is rotated into the graft wound with the aid of the threads on the shaft. It is secured by placing 8-0 or 9-0 sutures around the wings and into the peripheral cornea.

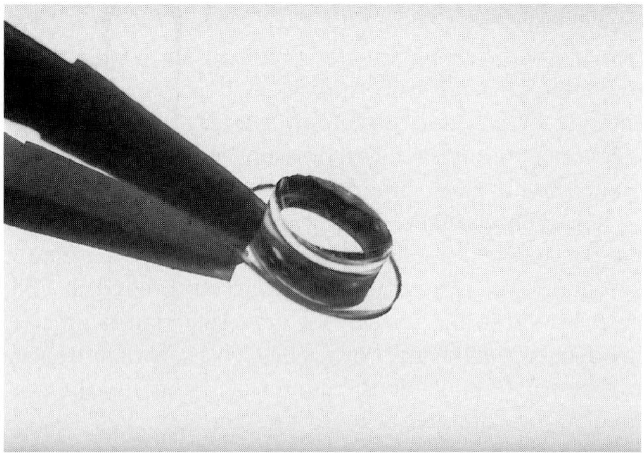

Fig. 10-31 Eckardt temporary keratoprosthesis. This keratoprosthesis is made of silicone rubber and comes in a 7-mm diameter size. It is placed into the graft wound and secured with four interrupted 9-0 or 10-0 nylon sutures in the peripheral cornea. Because of its shorter intraocular cylinder, it gives a better view of the corneal periphery than the Landers-Foulks temporary keratoprosthesis.

for months and often years. In eyes at high risk for graft rejection, high-dose topical corticosteroids and occasionally systemic corticosteroids as well as topical or systemic cyclosporine are used.

Complications

Many postoperative complications, such as endophthalmitis, expulsive hemorrhage, and epithelial downgrowth (Fig. 10-32) are more common after corneal transplantation than after cataract surgery. However, diagnosis and management are similar and are discussed in the section on cataract complications (Table 10-1).

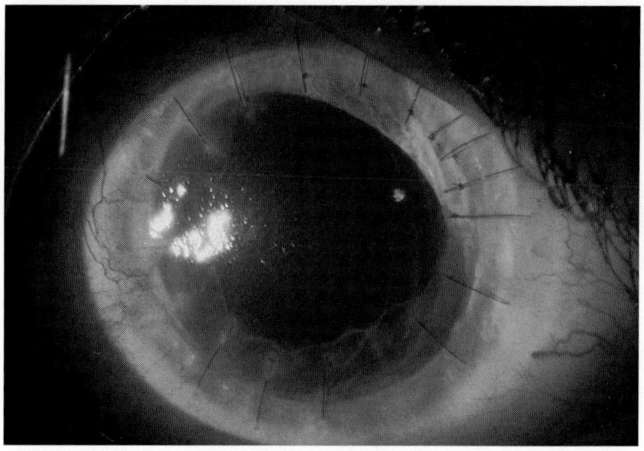

Fig. 10-32 Epithelial downgrowth. An undulating endothelial membrane advancing from the corneal periphery is seen inferiorly, nasally, and temporally.

Table 10-1 General complications of intraocular surgery

Complication	Cataract surgery	Corneal transplant
Increased intraocular pressure	+	++
Wound leak	+	+
Expulsive hemorrhage	+	++
Endophthalmitis	+	++
Epithelial downgrowth	+	++
Retinal detachment	+	++
Cystoid macular edema	+	+

Epithelial defects in the graft are common immediately after penetrating keratoplasty (Fig. 10-33). In eyes without significant ocular surface disease, the epithelial defect typically resolves within a few days to a week or two. Whorl superficial punctate keratopathy is seen commonly after corneal transplant surgery (Figs. 10-34 and 10-35). However, in certain eyes, there is delayed healing of the epithelium (Fig. 10-36). At high risk for this problem include eyes with neurotrophic corneas, significant ocular surface disease, such as from ocular rosacea, and limbal stem cell deficiencies. If delayed healing is suspected, toxic medications (e.g., aminoglycoside antibiotics) should be replaced with less offensive agents (e.g., erythromycin ointment). Topical corticosteroids may need to be decreased temporarily until the epithelial defect heals. Pressure patching and bandage soft contact lenses may be helpful. A temporary lateral tarsorrhaphy is often extremely effective in healing chronic epithelial defects (Fig. 10-37 and Box 10-6).

As with cataract surgery, a wound leak can occur right after surgery. If the anterior chamber is shallow or flat, surgical repair should be performed immediately to min-

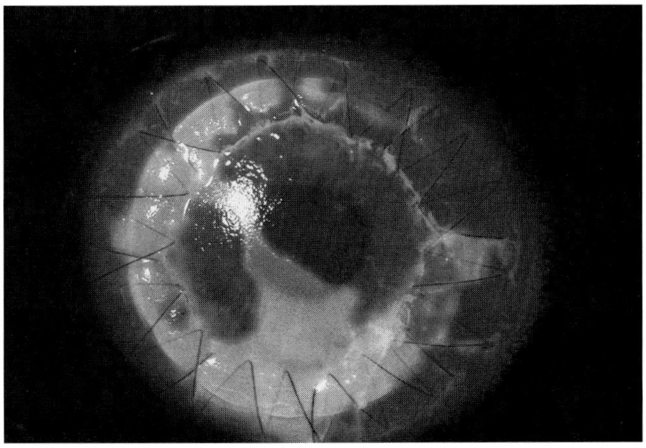

Fig. 10-33 Epithelial defect. Fluorescein staining is used to see a large epithelial defect 1 day after penetrating keratoplasty. The epithelial defect involves the periphery of the graft from the 4 to 12 o'clock positions and the central cornea inferiorly. (See color plate.)

Box 10-6 Complications of Penetrating Keratoplasty

MORE COMMON

Elevated intraocular pressure (short-term and long-term)
Wound leak
Chronic epithelial defect
Broken and loose sutures
Graft rejection
Cystoid macular edema
Cataract
Significant astigmatism
Recurrence of disease
Endothelial decompensation

LESS COMMON

Retrobulbar hemorrhage
Primary graft failure
Suture-related corneal ulcer
Endophthalmitis
Retinal detachment
Expulsive hemorrhage
Wound dehiscence
Epithelial downgrowth

imize trauma to the graft endothelium. If the anterior chamber is well formed, adding aqueous suppressants and decreasing the topical corticosteroids temporarily helps seal the leak. If a suture breaks early in the postoperative period causing the wound to gape or bulge, even with no wound leak, it should be replaced to decrease the chance for severe astigmatism.

Graft rejection and failure are important aspects of corneal transplant management. Primary graft failure occurs when severe graft edema is noted at the end of

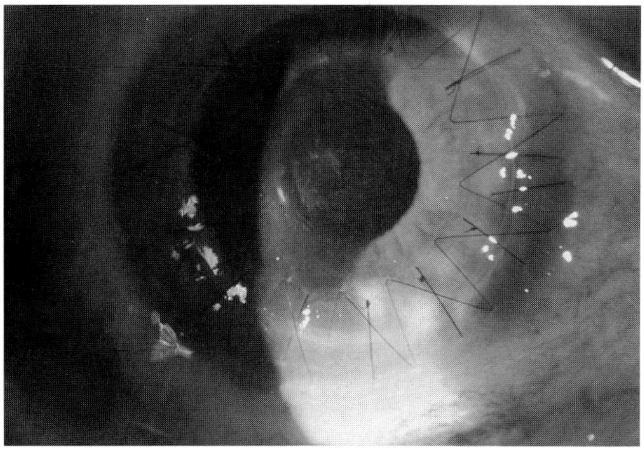

Fig. 10-34 Whorl superficial punctate keratopathy. A gray-white whorl-like pattern is seen in the central epithelium.

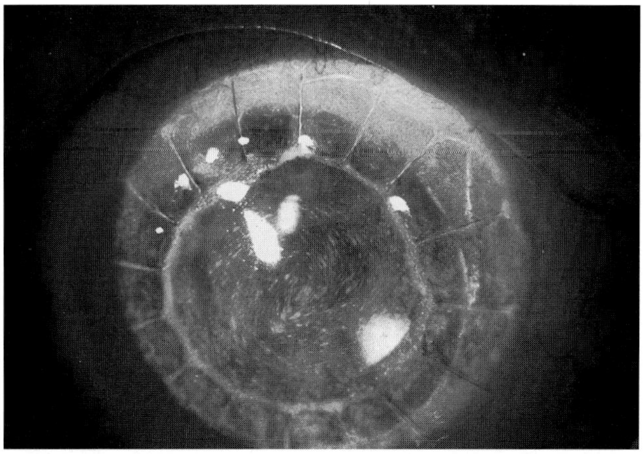

Fig. 10-35 Whorl superficial punctate keratopathy. Fluorescein dye demonstrates a whorl-like epithelial staining pattern, common after penetrating keratoplasty. (See color plate.)

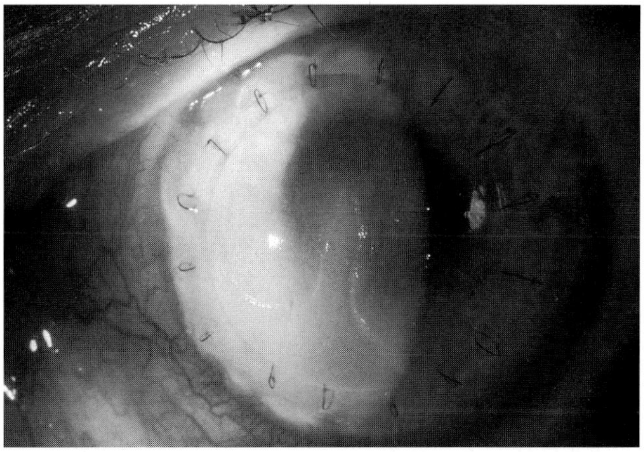

Fig. 10-36 Chronic epithelial defect. Delayed epithelialization in this eye 6 weeks after penetrating keratoplasty results in corneal haze and melting.

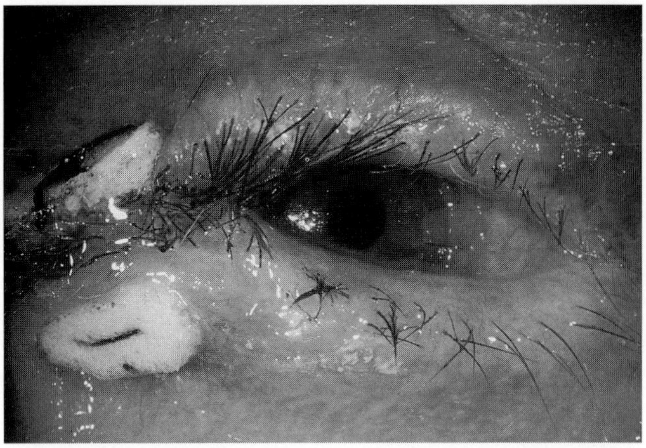

Fig. 10-37 Temporary lateral tarsorrhaphy. A noncutting temporary lateral tarsorrhaphy is an extremely effective procedure to aid in epithelialization after penetrating keratoplasty. It involves local anesthesia to the eyelids and placement of a mattress suture through both tarsal plates. The suture is tied over bolsters to prevent "cheesewiring." It is generally kept in place for 3 to 4 weeks and then removed.

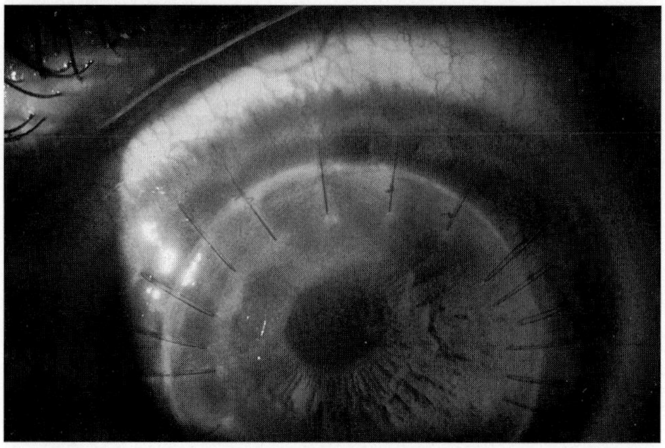

Fig. 10-39 Epithelial graft rejection. An elevated gray-white epithelial line is noted from the 9 to 3 o'clock positions in the peripheral graft area. The superior cornea has significant stromal neovascularization.

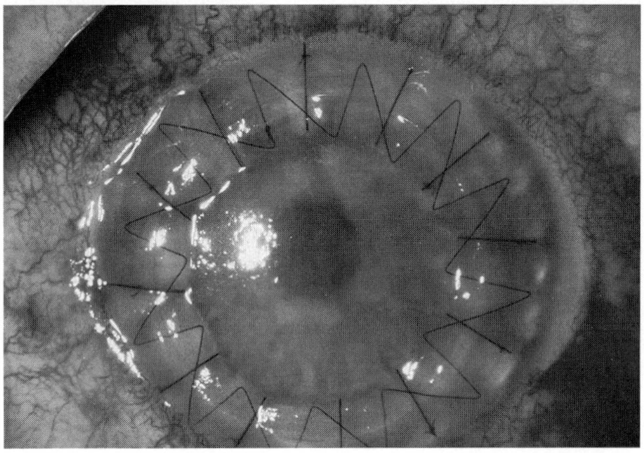

Fig. 10-38 Primary graft failure. Severe corneal edema with a poor view of the iris on postoperative day 1 suggests primary graft failure.

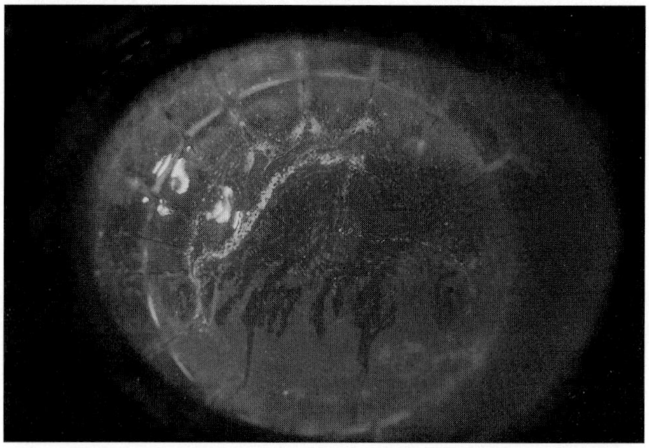

Fig. 10-40 Epithelial graft rejection. Fluorescein dye stains the irregular elevated epithelial rejection line seen in Fig. 10-39. Serial examinations can demonstrate the line to move from the periphery to the central cornea. (See color plate.)

surgery or on the first postoperative day (Fig. 10-38). The graft demonstrates marked thickening and has a gray-white opacified appearance, obscuring the view of the anterior segment structures. Primary graft failure generally results from poor-quality graft tissue or significant endothelial damage at the time of surgery. Occasionally, such grafts clear over 4 to 12 weeks with intensive topical corticosteroids, but if progressive improvement is not noted in that time, corneal transplantation should be repeated to obtain good vision.

Evidence of epithelial and endothelial rejection should be sought on every postoperative visit. Symptoms include redness, discomfort, photophobia, and diminished vision, but some patients are asymptomatic. Eyes with epithelial rejection demonstrate an elevated epithelial ridge on the cornea that stains with fluorescein (Figs. 10-39 and 10-40). Subepithelial infiltrates also signal graft rejection (Fig. 10-41). Signs of endothelial rejection include conjunctival injection, anterior uveitis, keratic precipitates on the endothelium (Fig. 10-42) (occasionally in the form of a line) (Figs. 10-43 and 10-44), and corneal edema. Treatment is with intensive hourly topical corticosteroids and occasionally subconjunctival or systemic corticosteroids. This condition is discussed in detail in Chapter 5.

Grafts may develop corneal edema without signs of endothelial rejection. Newly diagnosed graft edema is typically treated with intensive topical corticosteroids in

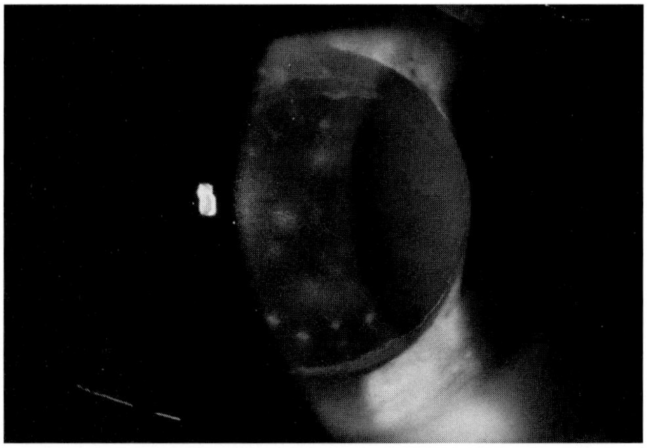

Fig. 10-41 Subepithelial graft rejection. Multiple subepithelial infiltrates are seen in the graft. Although they typically do not cause significantly diminished vision, they signal immune activity. They should be treated and the patient should be followed up closely for the development of endothelial rejection.

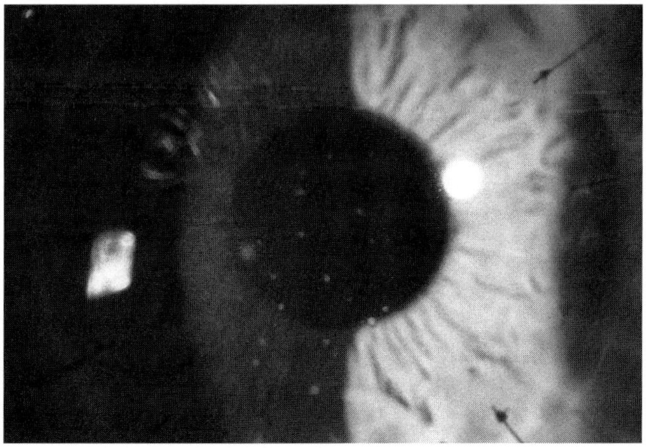

Fig. 10-42 Keratic precipitates. Clumps of white blood cells (keratic precipitates) are apparent on the endothelial surface. They are a sign of early endothelial graft rejection and require treatment.

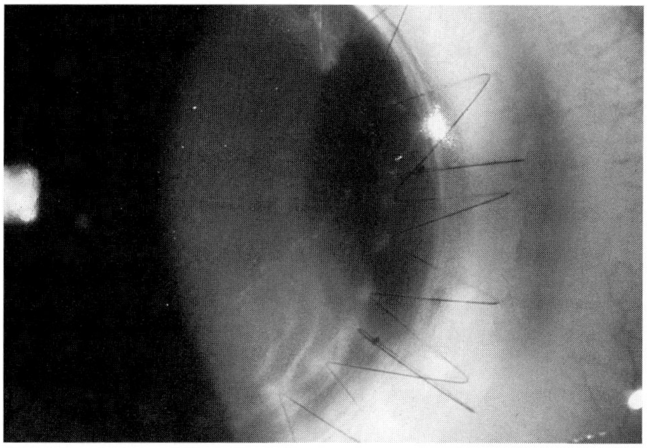

Fig. 10-43 Endothelial graft rejection. An endothelial rejection line (Khodadoust line) can be seen stretching from the 3 to the 6 o'clock positions of the cornea. The central aspect of the line appears slightly elevated, whereas the cornea peripheral to the line is edematous.

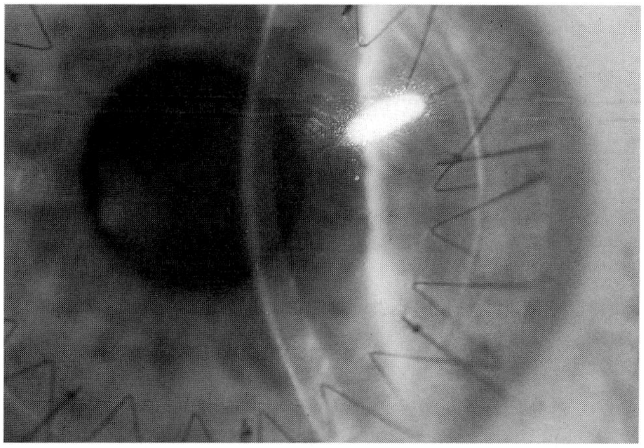

Fig. 10-44 Endothelial graft rejection. The slit beam demonstrates corneal edema peripheral to the endothelial rejection line.

the hope for a reversible inflammatory component. When no improvement is noted, the diagnosis of graft failure is made. It is often unclear whether the graft failure resulted from previous undetected endothelial rejection or nonimmunologic progressive endothelial cell loss. In such eyes, the grafts can often be repeated with good success. Other causes of graft failure include recurrence of the initial condition, such as a corneal dystrophy, infectious keratitis (Fig. 10-45), chronic surface disease causing corneal scarring, and high astigmatism.

Corneal transplant sutures are typically left in place for months to years. They are removed after 3 to 12 months (depending on the surgical technique) if they are thought to be tight, causing astigmatism. Loose and exposed sutures as well as all broken sutures should be removed at the time of discovery. Some surgeons leave in sutures for years if they are not loose or tight and if the eye sees well, whereas others remove all sutures between 1 and 2 years after surgery. The disadvantage to removing all sutures at a set time is that the corneal curvature can shift dramatically and unpredictably, even years after surgery, causing the vision to change for the worse. The disadvantage to leaving sutures in place for extended periods of time is suture loosening and breakage (Figs. 10-46, 10-47, and 10-48).

Exposed sutures cause pain and irritation. Even more important, they can lead to graft rejection, infectious corneal infiltrates (Fig. 10-49), ulcers (suture abscesses) (Fig. 10-50), and rarely endophthalmitis (Fig. 10-51). Exposed sutures should be removed and the eye treated with topical antibiotics, even in the absence of an infiltrate. When an infiltrate or ulcer is present, the removed

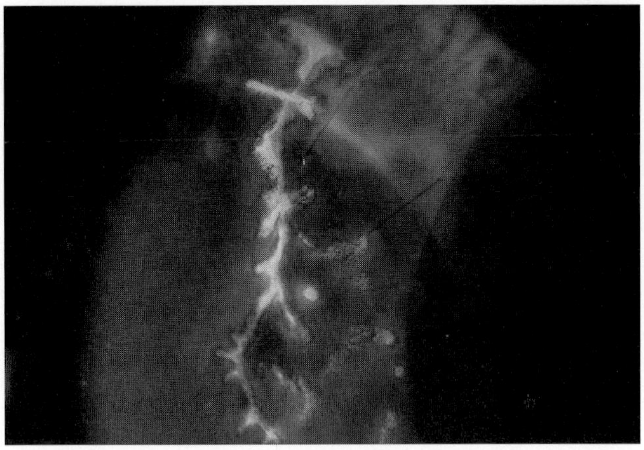

Fig. 10-45 Recurrent herpes simplex keratitis. A herpes simplex virus dendrite can be seen to originate from the host cornea and progress onto the corneal graft. This eye had undergone a corneal transplant for herpes simplex corneal scarring.

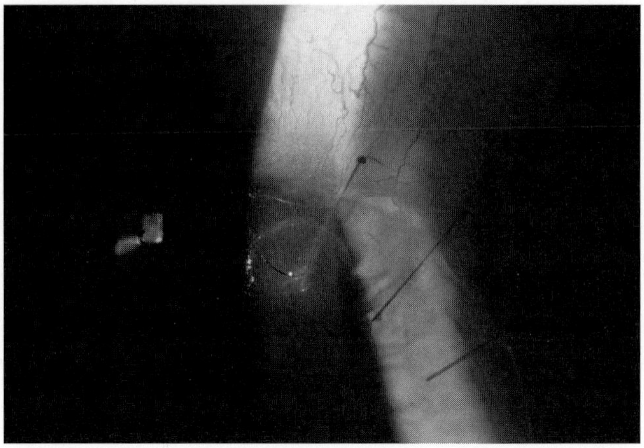

Fig. 10-46 Broken graft suture. A broken, protruding, interrupted 10-0 nylon suture. A windshield wiper effect around the suture can be seen. Such broken, exposed sutures necessitate removal.

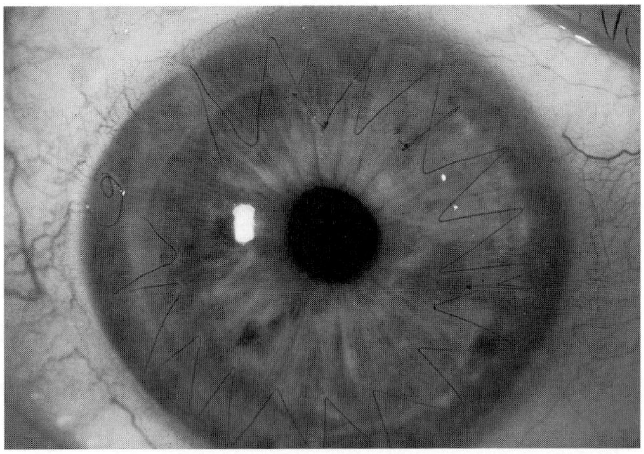

Fig. 10-47 Broken graft suture. A broken, exposed, running 10-0 nylon suture. Assuming the wound is secure, the entire running suture should be removed. If the wound is not entirely secure, the exposed portion of suture can be trimmed, but the remaining running suture will continue to loosen and become exposed.

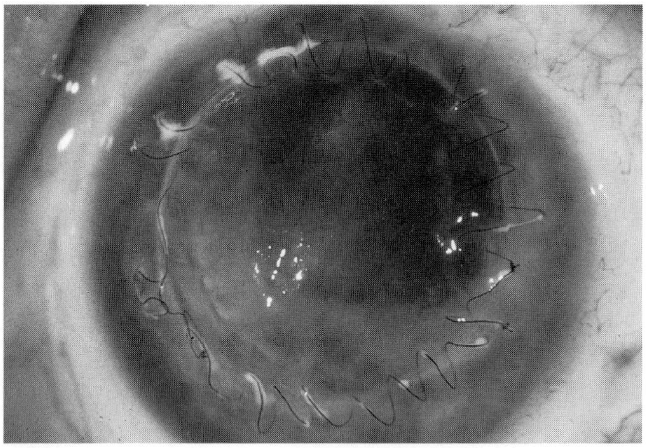

Fig. 10-48 Loose graft suture. This running suture and several interrupted sutures have become severely loosened and exposed to the point of causing corneal infiltration and melting. Removal and close follow-up are required.

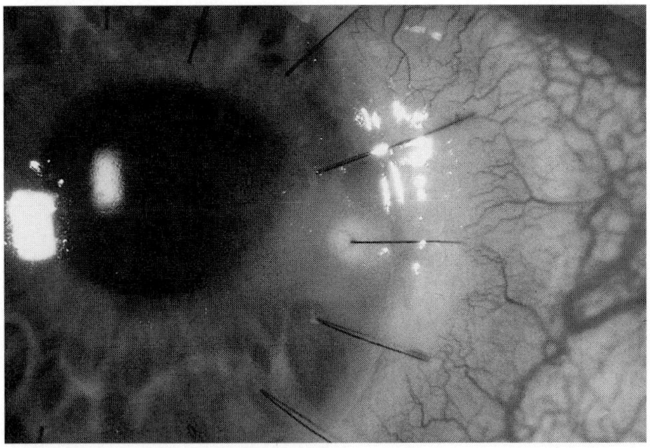

Fig. 10-49 Graft suture infiltrate. A dense corneal infiltrate is present related to a graft suture. Moderate surrounding edema has developed. Suture removal and treatment with intensive topical antibiotics are required.

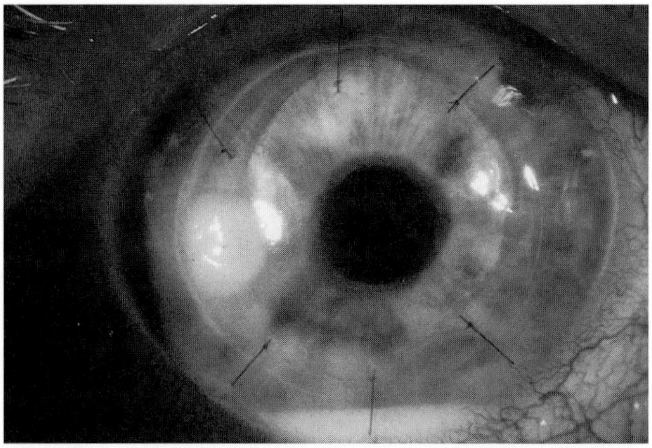

Fig. 10-50 Graft suture abscess. A dense corneal ulcer can be seen at the 9 o'clock position, related to a broken, exposed suture that was removed. A hypopyon is present inferiorly.

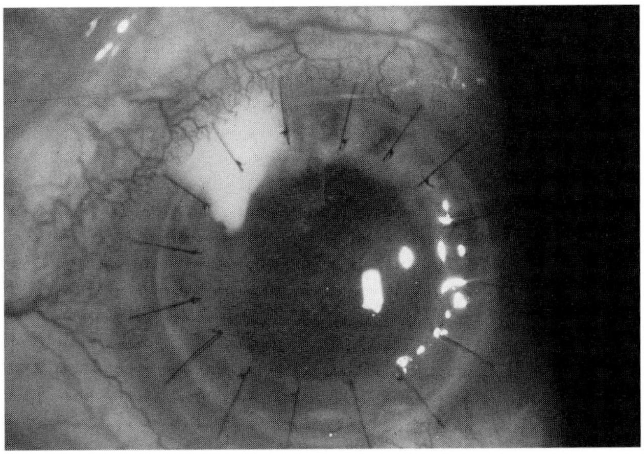

Fig. 10-51 Endophthalmitis. A large clump of fibrin and white blood cells is evident superiorly. Fibrin can also be seen in the anterior chamber covering the posterior chamber intraocular lens. *Staphylococcus aureus* was cultured from the vitreous and anterior chamber.

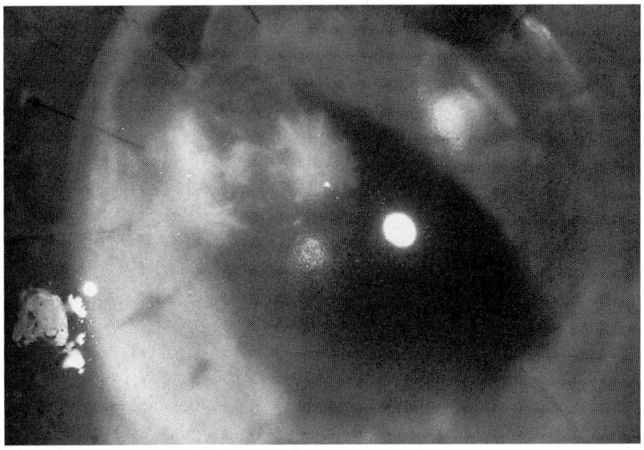

Fig. 10-53 Infectious crystalline keratitis. Multiple areas of patchy infiltrate are noted, one of which is adjacent to a corneal graft suture. The classic crystalline, feathery edges can be seen.

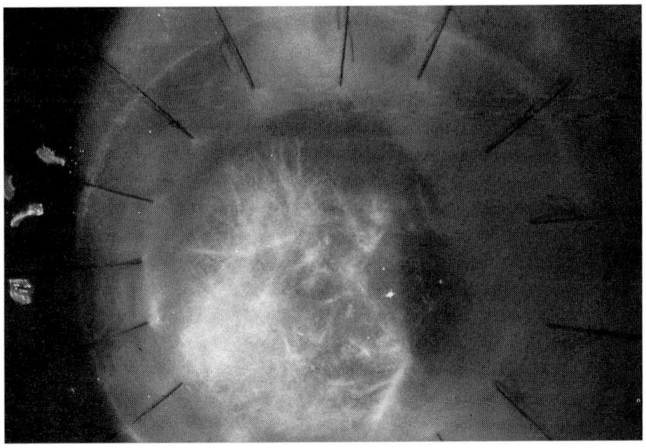

Fig. 10-52 Infectious crystalline keratitis. A large gray-white infiltrate is present in the anterior stroma. It has the typical crystalline projections at the periphery of the infiltrate.

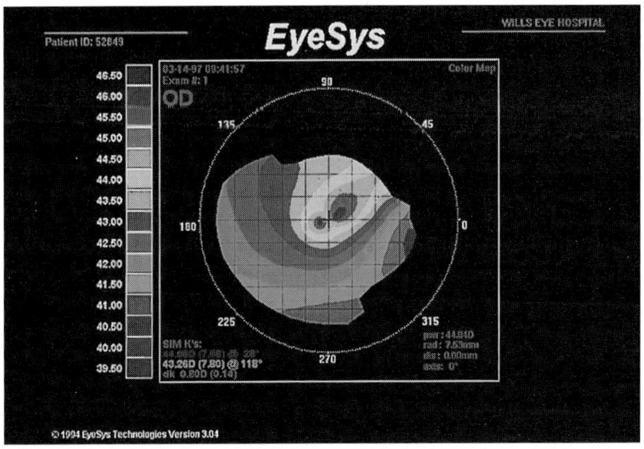

Fig. 10-54 Irregular astigmatism. Computerized corneal topographic analysis of an eye with irregular astigmatism after corneal transplantation. The scale on the left side indicates the dioptric power of each color. The red area in the superonasal aspect of the cornea indicates corneal steepening. The asymmetric aspect of the curvature indicates irregular astigmatism. (See color plate.)

suture should be cultured, and intensive topical antibiotic treatment with close follow-up should be initiated.

An unusual type of corneal infection can occur in patients who undergo corneal transplantation, especially those who have remaining sutures and are still taking topical corticosteroids. Infectious crystalline keratopathy is an indolent infection usually caused by *Streptococcus viridans*, but it can be caused by other streptococcal species, in addition to other organisms, especially gram-positive bacteria and fungi. It usually arises adjacent to a corneal suture, often, but not always, with an epithelial defect. The infiltrate is typically gray-white and is found in the superficial stroma, seeming to track between corneal lamellae (Fig. 10-52). At the edges of the infiltrate is a characteristic crystalline pattern with tiny protruding branches (Fig. 10-53). Because the organisms are intrastromal, they are often difficult to identify on smears and cultures. Treatment is with frequent topical antibiotics, such as fortified vancomycin, until culture results (it is hoped) isolate the precise organism. Patients are often not very symptomatic, and the infection progresses slowly. Unfortunately, it also improves slowly, even with appropriate treatment.

Graft clarity, though important, does not guarantee excellent vision because transplant astigmatism can severely limit visual outcome (Fig. 10-54). Astigmatism can be treated with single running suture adjustment (in the early postoperative period) or selective interrupted suture removal. Mild to moderate astigmatism can be treated successfully with glasses or soft toric contact lenses. Rigid gas-permeable contact lenses can treat higher degrees of astigmatism and provide excellent

Box 10-7 Surgical Correction of Astigmatism after Penetrating Keratoplasty

3-6 D	Relaxing incisions
5-10 D	Relaxing incisions and compression sutures
10-15 D	Wedge resection

Note: For <4 D myopic astigmatism, consider laser in situ keratomileusis (LASIK).

visual acuity. Patients intolerant of contact lenses may be treated with refractive surgery to improve visual outcome.

Correction of Astigmatism in a Corneal Graft

One of the most frustrating problems after corneal transplantation is astigmatism. Selective suture removal is often useful to reduce postoperative astigmatism. Glasses and soft contact lenses can also be helpful with mild to moderate degrees of astigmatism. Rigid contact lenses can correct high degrees of astigmatism but are not well tolerated by some patients. Surgical correction of graft astigmatism can be very effective in selected patients. Relaxing incisions with or without compression sutures and wedge resection are used to treat astigmatism after penetrating keratoplasty. Most recently laser in situ keratomileusis (LASIK) has also been used to treat mild to moderate degrees of myopic astigmatism (Box 10-7).

The preoperative evaluation should include a manifest refraction, standard keratometry readings, and computed corneal topographic analysis. Using this information, the steep axes are identified and marked in the cornea. Regular astigmatism responds best, but asymmetric astigmatism can also be treated successfully. The effect of the procedure can often be monitored during and immediately after surgery to titrate the results using standard keratometry readings, computed corneal topographic analysis, and operating room keratoscopy techniques.

Moderate degrees of astigmatism (typically 3 to 6 D) can be treated with relaxing incisions. Generally 2 to 3 clock hours are incised at each of the steep axes, depending on the degree of astigmatism. These incisions may be performed with a preset diamond blade just central to the graft-host interface; the procedure is identical to the astigmatic keratotomy technique (Fig. 10-55). It is usually performed under an operating microscope, but it can be performed at the slit lamp. Alternatively, a cutdown technique in the graft-host interface can also be used, usually performed at the slit lamp. Here, a metal blade (typically) is used to break the epithelium along the

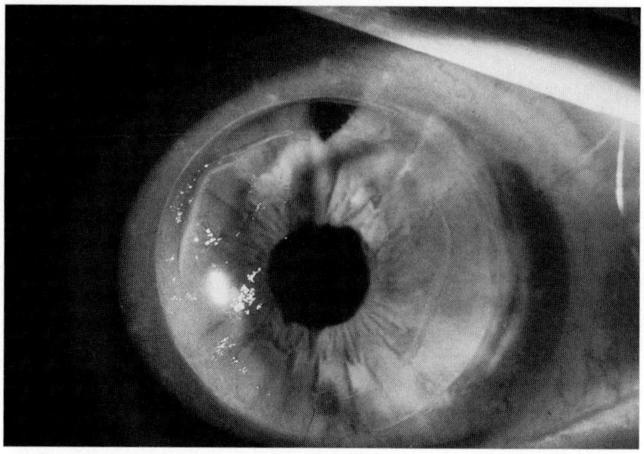

Fig. 10-55 Relaxing incisions. Two arcuate-type relaxing incisions were performed in the body of this corneal transplant at the 4 and 10 o'clock positions. Moderate wound gape, foreign body sensation, and irregular astigmatism have developed.

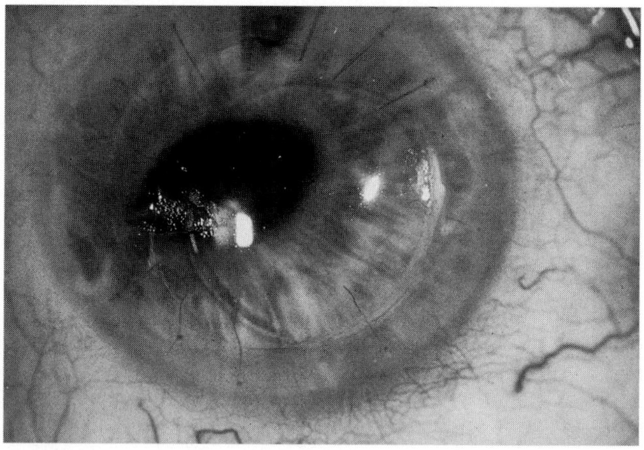

Fig. 10-56 Relaxing incisions. One relaxing incision was placed in the graft-host junction at the 4 o'clock position for approximately 60° to correct asymmetric astigmatism.

intended incisions and cautiously cut into the cornea. The depth of the incision varies, depending on the degree of astigmatism and the configuration of the graft-host interface scar (Fig. 10-56). As a rule, the incision should be approximately 60% to 80% corneal depth. Microperforations and macroperforations can occur, even more commonly than in radial keratotomy (RK), because of the nonuniform interface incised, but they are treated in the same manner. Vision generally improves within 2 to 6 weeks.

Higher degrees of astigmatism (typically 5 to 10 D) can be treated with relaxing incisions and compression sutures. Relaxing incision surgery is identical to that described above. Three to five sutures (e.g., 10-0 nylon or Mersilene) are placed in the graft host interface 90° from the incisions at an operating microscope. These compression sutures are tied tightly, and the knots are buried

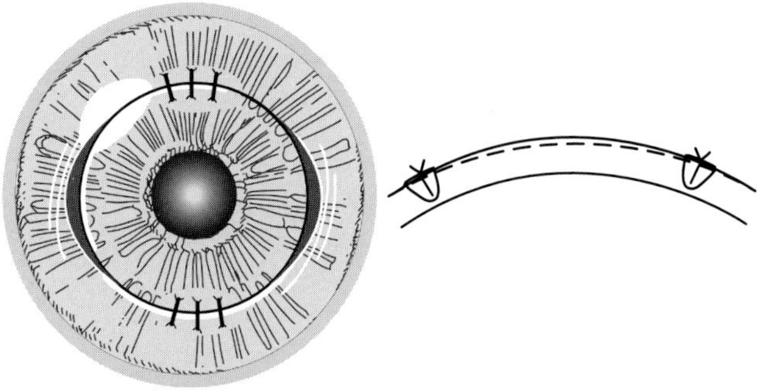

Fig. 10-57 Relaxing incision and compression suture procedure. Relaxing incisions in the graft host junction at the 3 and 9 o'clock positions are combined with compression sutures at the 12 and 6 o'clock positions to correct moderate amounts of against the rule astigmatism. - - - = preoperative corneal curvature.

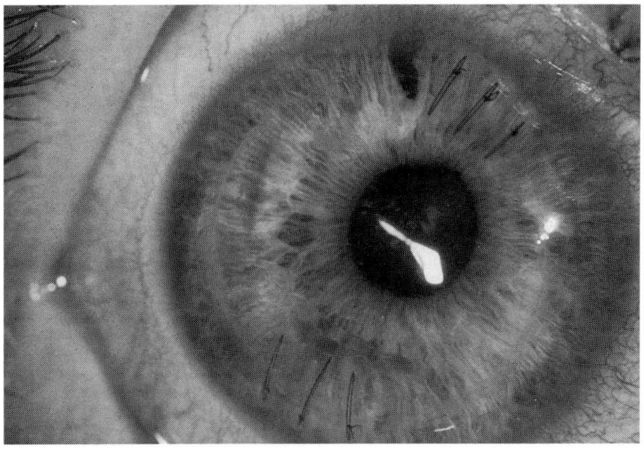

Fig. 10-58 Relaxing incisions and compression sutures. One day after two relaxing incisions in the graft-host junction at the 4 and 7 o'clock positions and 10-0 nylon compression sutures 90° away.

(Fig. 10-57). Immediately after surgery the astigmatism should be 100% overcorrected. These sutures must remain in place for several months and are then removed one at a time, if necessary. It may take several months for vision to improve (Fig. 10-58).

Even higher degrees of astigmatism (approximately 10 to 15 D) can be treated with wedge resection (Fig. 10-59). This procedure is performed on the flat axis using an operating microscope. A crescent 2 to 3 clock hours in length, reaching almost full-thickness cornea, is typically removed. The width of the crescent depends on the amount of astigmatism. The rule of thumb is 0.1 mm per diopter of astigmatism, not to exceed 1.5 mm, but it is approximate. One incision is made in the graft-host interface and the other either from the donor cornea side or the host cornea side. Once the wedge is excised, the wound is closed with five to eight sutures (e.g., 10-0 nylon or Mersilene). A paracentesis to remove a small amount of aqueous can be helpful to close the wound. The sutures must remain in place for 6 to 12 months and are then removed one at a time, if necessary. A common problem after wedge resection is significant irregular astigmatism. Visual recovery is slowest after wedge resection, and it may take 1 year or more for good vision to be restored.

After all these procedures on corneal grafts, postoperative treatment with topical antibiotics and corticosteroids is required. Eyes after penetrating keratoplasty are at greater risk for epithelial healing problems and infections than nongrafted eyes. Additionally, the risk for graft wound problems and graft rejection is always there. Patients should be reminded of the signs and symptoms of rejection (redness, pain, sensitivity to light, and decreased vision) and told to return immediately if they

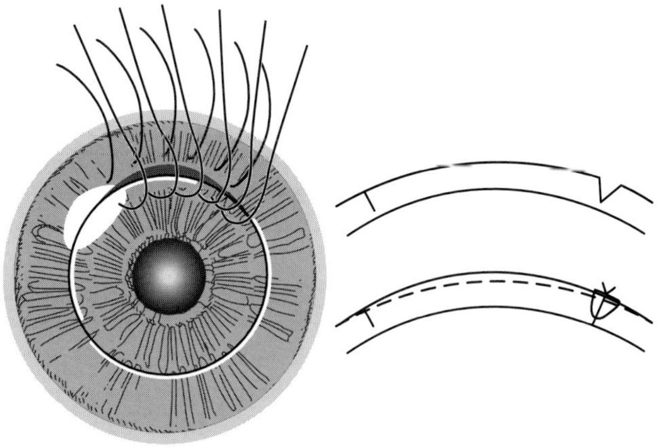

Fig. 10-59 Wedge resection procedure. A wedge of corneal tissue is excised from the flat axis and the area is resutured. An initial overcorrection is desirable. Selective suture removal after several months is often required to titrate the effect of this procedure. - - - = preoperative corneal curvature.

develop. Refractive surgery after corneal transplantation can be extremely rewarding for both the surgeon and the patient as the final step to achieving excellent vision after penetrating keratoplasty.

LAMELLAR KERATOPLASTY

As the success rate for penetrating keratoplasty has improved (because of better tissue quality and availability, surgical techniques, and postoperative management, among other factors), the indications for lamellar keratoplasty have diminished. Lamellar keratoplasty is technically more difficult and time consuming, and often it does not have the same visual potential as penetrating keratoplasty, due to interface opacity. Consequently, it is not frequently performed. However, lamellar kerato-

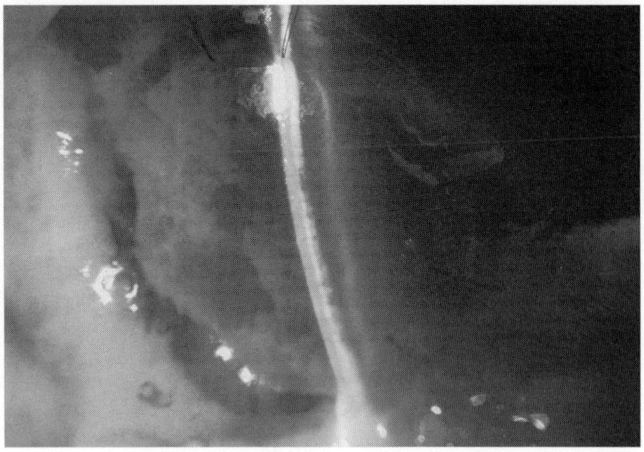

Fig. 10-60 Lamellar keratoplasty. One day after lamellar keratoplasty for a thinned corneal scar after multiple pterygium excisions. A buccal mucosal graft, noted adjacent to the lamellar transplant, is performed to release significant symblepharon.

plasty does have certain advantages over full-thickness corneal transplantation. The anterior chamber is generally not entered, significantly decreasing the risk for glaucoma, cataract, and especially endophthalmitis. Because only the anterior cornea is transplanted, the chance for endothelial rejection does not exist. Currently, lamellar keratoplasty is reserved for middle, and occasionally deep, stromal pathology in which the endothelium is normal. Patients must realize that the best vision after lamellar keratoplasty is in the 20/40 range, not the 20/20 range achieved after successful penetrating keratoplasty. Occasionally, it is also used to prepare an extremely thinned cornea for penetrating keratoplasty. In these cases, a large, often limbus-to-limbus, lamellar graft is performed, and months later a smaller, central penetrating graft is performed for improved vision. Lamellar keratoplasty can also be used when the stroma is thinned, such as after repeated pterygium excision, to stabilize the cornea (Fig. 10-60).

Lamellar keratoplasty is performed using similar anesthesia and preoperative antiseptic prophylaxis as used for penetrating keratoplasty. The eye does not have to be softened as it does before penetrating keratoplasty. Lamellar tissue is most easily fashioned from a whole donor globe; however, whole globes are becoming more and more difficult to obtain. Techniques for creating lamellar grafts from corneoscleral rims (routinely available) can be effective.

The size of the graft must be determined at the slit lamp and checked in the operating room. The trephine guard is set to the appropriate depth for the pathology, as determined before surgery at the slit lamp, often with the aid of pachymetry and ultrasound biomicroscopy. The trephine blade is centered over the pupil or over the area of pathology, and the host cornea is trephined partial

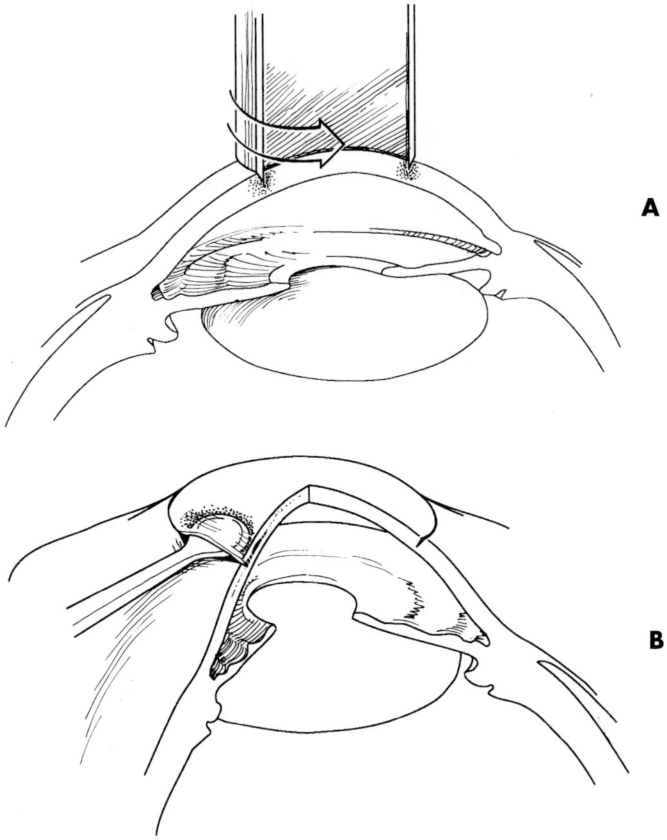

Fig. 10-61 Lamellar keratoplasty procedure. **A,** Using an internal obturator, the corneal trephine is set to a partial-thickness corneal depth. It is used to incise to approximately 50% to 70% corneal thickness. **B,** A "noncutting" spatula is used to dissect the superficial corneal button. A similar technique is used on the donor globe. The donor button is then sutured to the recipient. The smoother the lamellar planes, the less postoperative scarring will result.

thickness. A rounded-end sharp blade is used to begin the lamellar dissection, after which a lamellar spreader (e.g., Martinez dissecting spatula) is used to dissect the lamellar graft. If the plane dissected with the spreader is deeper than the trephination, corneal scissors are used to remove the button (Fig. 10-61). The lamellar dissection should be carried out 0.5 mm peripheral to the trephination to facilitate suturing of the graft. If the lamellar dissection is not deep enough to adequately remove the pathology, a deeper lamellar dissection can be performed. Once the recipient bed is ready, the donor button can be prepared to match the thickness of the bed.

The donor button is typically fashioned from a donor globe. A limbal cutdown is performed with a rounded-end sharp blade or a diamond blade to the desired depth, and 1 to 2 mm of lamellar dissection is begun. Then the lamellar spreader is used in a sweeping motion to create a limbus-to-limbus dissection. A trephine of the same size or 0.25 mm larger is then used to cut out the donor graft.

When only corneoscleral rim tissue is available, it is possible to securely wrap the tissue onto a sphere (such as a sterile ball implant or a hydroxyapatite sphere) and to perform a similar dissection. The lamellar graft is transferred to the recipient and sutured into position using deep bites in the donor and entering the peripheral lamellar dissection on the host. The interface should be carefully cleared of debris with irrigation. Typically 16 interrupted 10-0 nylon sutures are used. The knots are buried. They are usually removed within several months, though they can remain longer. Postoperative medications are similar to those used after penetrating keratoplasty, but less corticosteroid medication is used for a shorter period of time.

Complications of lamellar keratoplasty are similar to full-thickness transplants, with the exception of endothelial rejection. One additional complication is inadvertent entrance into the anterior chamber during the lamellar procedure. This event can lead to aqueous fluid infiltrating the interface between the host cornea and the donor tissue, and ultimately can cause graft failure. If the anterior chamber is entered, the full-thickness wound must be sutured closed to prevent aqueous leakage. Should a large entrance into the anterior chamber be created, it is often best to convert the surgery into full-thickness corneal transplantation. This adverse event is why many surgeons have penetrating keratoplasty tissue available in the operating room.

SUPERFICIAL KERATECTOMY

Anterior corneal pathology, especially elevated conditions, are often treatable with superficial keratectomy. When corneal pathology extends into the middle or deep stroma, lamellar or penetrating keratoplasty is usually a better option. Superficial keratectomy involves surgical excision of abnormal corneal tissue to clear or smooth the cornea, or both. The advantages of this technique include the ability to perform it relatively rapidly, in a minor surgery suite setting, often under topical anesthesia. It is extraocular surgery with no need for donor tissue. Disadvantages include creating an epithelial defect and its limited indication for anterior pathology. Elevated lesions, such as Salzmann's nodular degeneration and keratoconus nodules, respond extremely well to superficial keratectomy (Figs. 10-62 and 10-63).

Sometimes superficial keratectomies are required for diagnostic purposes. In cases of chronic corneal ulceration, in which superficial culture results are negative, a corneal biopsy can be performed; a portion of the specimen is sent for histopathologic examination and a portion is sent for cultures.

The goal of superficial keratectomy is to remove anterior corneal opacity and to leave the remaining cornea with a smooth, clear surface. Nodular lesions can generally be shaved off with a rounded-end sharp blade placed flat against the cornea at the edge of the lesion. The blade is initially pushed forward and backward (*not* side to side) to create a plane between the lesion and the cornea. Often a plane is easily achieved and the lesion can be peeled off, leaving a smooth Bowman's layer underneath (Fig. 10-64). Occasionally, the lesion is strongly adherent to the underlying cornea, and gentle side-to-side cutting is required to remove it. All attempts should be made not to cut deeply into the cornea and to leave it as smooth as possible. At the end of the procedure, the eye is treated as a corneal

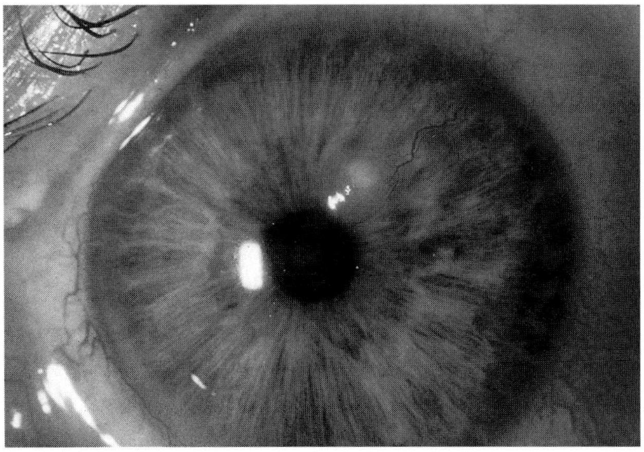

Fig. 10-62 Superficial keratectomy. An elevated gray-white Salzmann's nodule is seen in the paracentral cornea. A small leash of superficial corneal neovascularization develops. It was removed through superficial keratectomy with a blade in a minor surgery setting. A smooth plane was found between the lesion and Bowman's membrane.

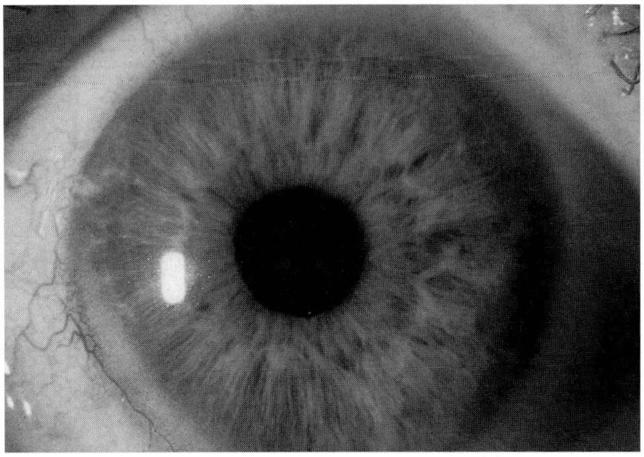

Fig. 10-63 Superficial keratectomy. One month after excision of the Salzmann's nodule seen in Fig. 10-62. No residual nodule or corneal neovascularization is present.

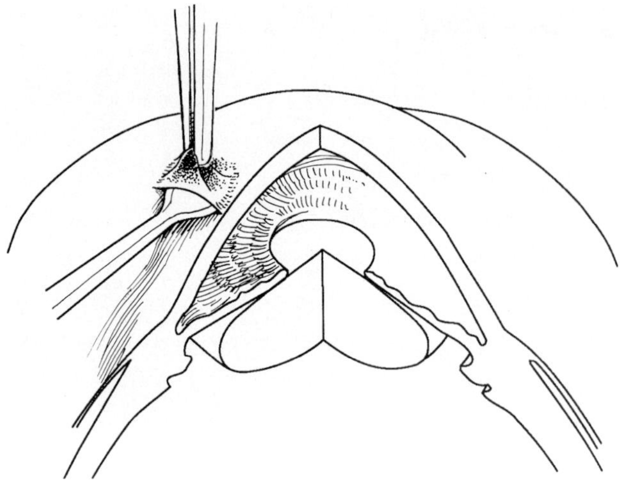

Fig. 10-64 Superficial keratectomy procedure. Elevated corneal pathology can be stabilized with fine-toothed forceps. A flat, sharp blade is used to create a plane under the corneal pathology. Often a front-to-back pushing motion is all that is required to remove the opacity. Occasionally, when side-to-side cutting must be used, care must be taken to create a smooth superficial dissection.

abrasion with antibiotics, cycloplegics, NSAIDs, and occasionally pressure patching. The specimen should be sent for histopathologic examination.

Complications of superficial keratectomy include poor epithelial healing and chronic ulceration, infectious keratitis, irregular astigmatism, scarring, and recurrent pathology. Many of these problems are best avoided by meticulous surgical technique and close follow-up.

EXCIMER LASER PHOTOTHERAPEUTIC KERATECTOMY

Excimer laser phototherapeutic keratectomy (PTK) was approved by the Food and Drug Administration (FDA) in 1995 for the removal of anterior corneal pathology. The laser should not remove greater than one third of the corneal thickness and should leave at least 250 μm of tissue after the procedure. The advantages of PTK over superficial keratectomy with a blade are that it can precisely remove tiny amounts of tissue at a time (0.25 μm per laser pulse) and leave a very smooth surface. The disadvantage is that it does not discriminate between normal and abnormal tissue. When abnormal elevated corneal tissue is easily peeled off the surface, leaving a smooth Bowman's layer, superficial keratectomy is the procedure of choice. When an anterior stromal scar or opacity affects vision and a smooth plane cannot be dissected, excimer laser PTK can be very effective to create a smooth surface. Typical indications for PTK include epithelial, Bowman's, and anterior stromal corneal dystrophies (Figs. 10-65 and 10-66), and anterior corneal scars without significant underlying thinning. Recurrent corneal dystrophies after penetrating keratoplasty can also respond extremely well to PTK (Figs. 10-67, 10-68, 10-69, and 10-70). Elevated lesions that do not readily peel off the cornea are also good candidates for PTK. Additionally, recurrent erosions, though not specifically FDA approved for PTK, respond well to this treatment.

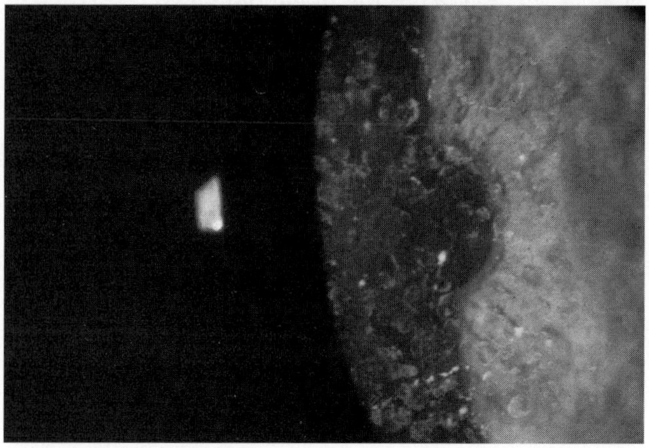

Fig. 10-65 Excimer laser phototherapeutic keratectomy (PTK). Granular dystrophy prior to excimer laser PTK. The pathology in this eye is rather anterior.

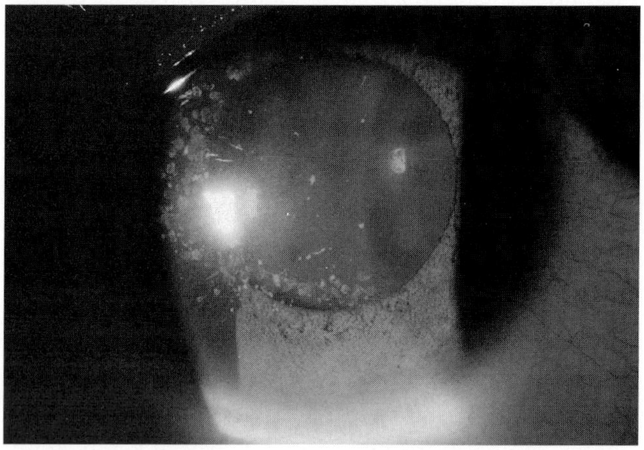

Fig. 10-66 Excimer laser phototherapeutic keratectomy (PTK). Four days after excimer laser PTK for the eye with granular dystrophy shown in Fig. 10-65. The central 6 mm is cleared of almost all of the granular opacities. A few deep granules remain centrally but do not affect vision.

The surgical techniques for the removal of elevated corneal lesions, flat anterior stromal pathology, and recurrent erosions are different (Box 10-8). Some corneas require a combination of techniques for the best results. Elevated corneal lesions are treated by manually removing the epithelium from the tops of the nodules while leaving the epithelium between. The epithelium acts as a protective layer and does not allow the laser to ablate

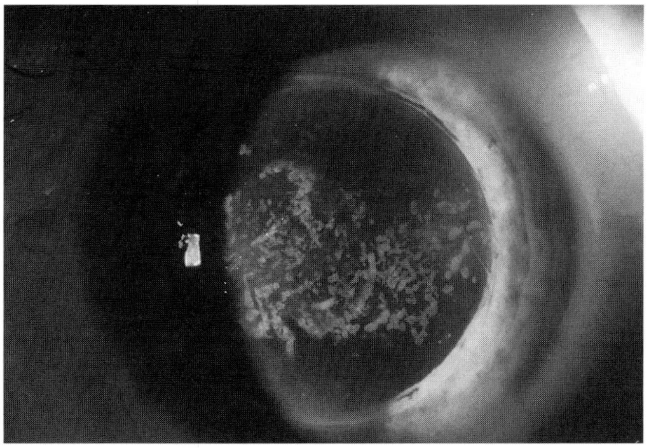

Fig. 10-67 Excimer laser phototherapeutic keratectomy (PTK). Recurrent granular dystrophy in a corneal graft prior to excimer laser PTK. Recurrent dystrophies tend to be superficial.

Box 10-8 Major Steps in Phototherapeutic Keratectomy

TREATMENT OF ELEVATED CORNEAL LESIONS

Debride epithelium from the elevated areas
Apply masking agents to the "valleys"
Use varying size ablation spots to shave down the "mountain tops," leaving the valleys untouched
Check at the slit lamp frequently and reablate as needed

TREATMENT OF ANTERIOR STROMAL PATHOLOGY

For regular epithelium, use a large laser spot to ablate through the epithelium into the stroma
For irregular epithelium, remove the epithelium manually and ablate the stroma directly
Ablate approximately 60% to 75% intended depth
Check at the slit lamp frequently and reablate as needed
Consider an antihyperopia treatment if a deep stromal ablation is performed

TREATMENT OF RECURRENT EROSIONS

Manually debride all loose epithelium
Ablate all exposed Bowman's membrane for 5 μm, taking care not to overlap ablations

the underlying stroma (Fig. 10-71). Masking agents, in the form of artificial tears of varying viscosities, are extremely useful adjuncts in PTK. The masking agent is applied in the "valleys," leaving the "mountain tops" bare. Excimer laser ablation is applied to the mountain tops. Laser spot sizes smaller than the nodules are used and moved around the lesions to flatten them. Masking

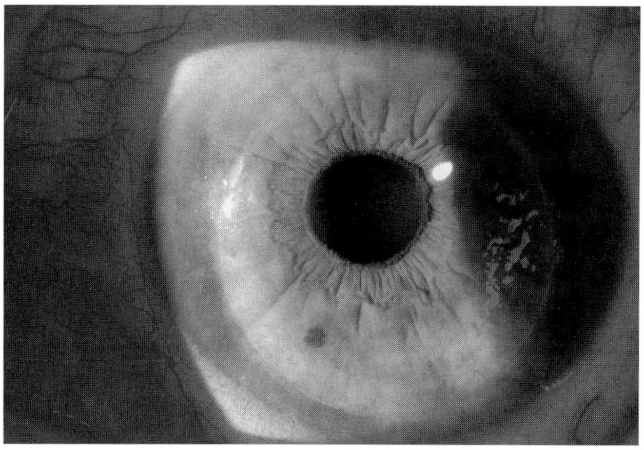

Fig. 10-68 Excimer laser phototherapeutic keratectomy (PTK). Two weeks after excimer laser PTK for recurrent granular dystrophy in the graft seen in Fig. 10-67. The central cornea is crystal clear. Residual granular opacities in the periphery of the graft do not affect vision.

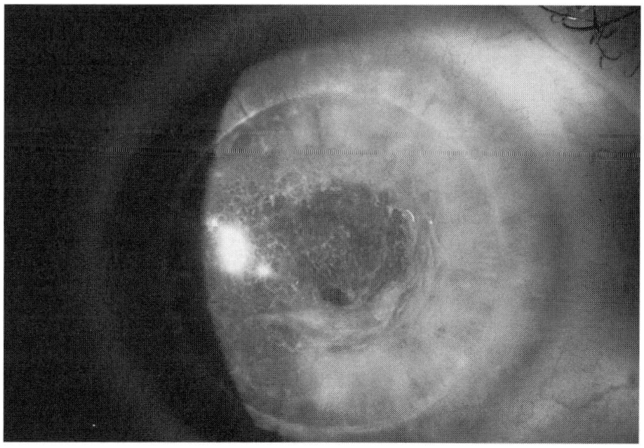

Fig. 10-69 Excimer laser phototherapeutic keratectomy (PTK). Recurrent Reis-Bücklers' dystrophy after corneal transplantation. This advanced recurrence involved deeper stroma than typical with recurrent dystrophies.

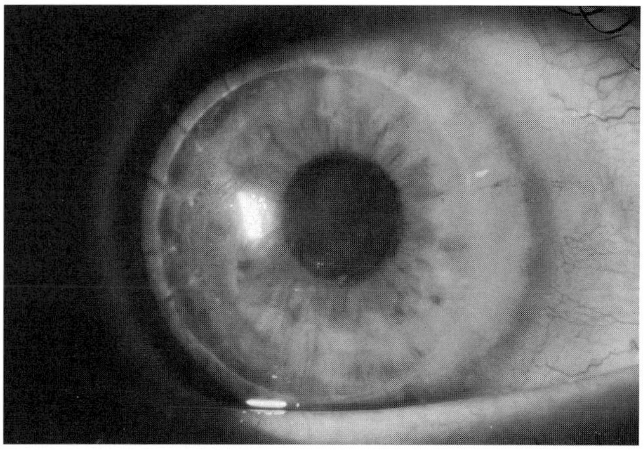

Fig. 10-70 Excimer laser phototherapeutic keratectomy (PTK). One month after excimer laser PTK for the eye with recurrent Reis-Bücklers' dystrophy after corneal transplantation shown in Fig. 10-69. Although the cornea is much clearer, mild residual corneal opacity in the inferocentral cornea can be seen.

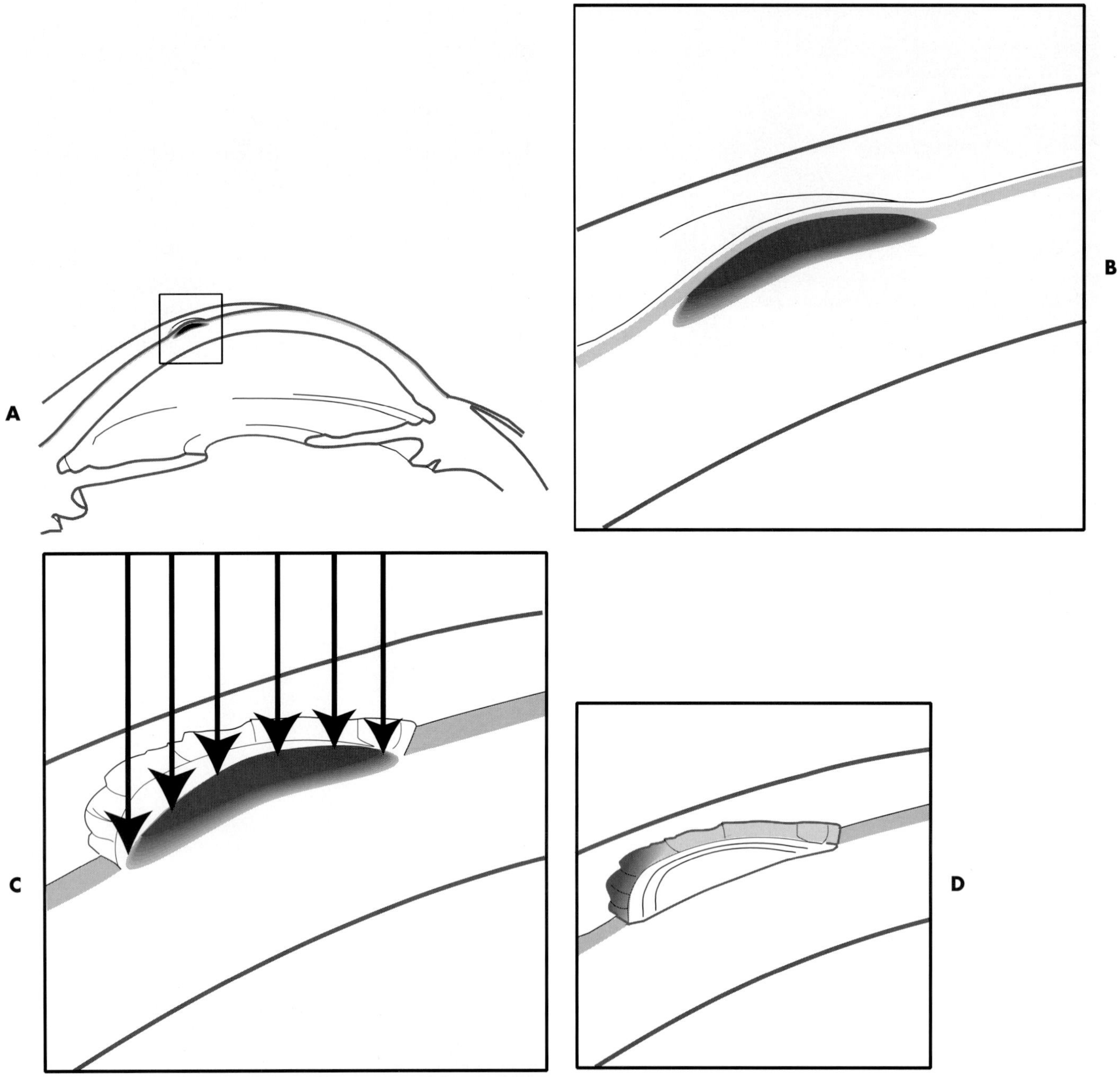

Fig. 10-71 Excimer laser phototherapeutic keratectomy (PTK) for a corneal nodule. **A** and **B,** An elevated corneal nodule that does not respond to superficial keratectomy may be treated with excimer laser PTK. **C,** The epithelium is removed from the elevated nodule. After the epithelium is removed, the excimer laser is used to "shave" down the nodule. Masking agents can be used to protect normal surrounding corneal tissue. **D,** The result should be a smooth base approximately equal to the level of normal surrounding corneal stroma.

agents are reapplied to the low points as needed. After a certain amount of treatment, the patient is examined at the slit lamp and the surgeon determines how much more treatment is required, if any. This "ablate and check" process is continued until the desired result is achieved (Figs. 10-72 and 10-73). The goal is a smoother, clearer surface, but crystal clarity is not necessary. Often, removing the bulk of the pathology improves vision dramatically without greatly changing the refraction. On the other hand, deep ablation may result in a beautifully clear cornea but with severe corneal flattening and induced hyperopia.

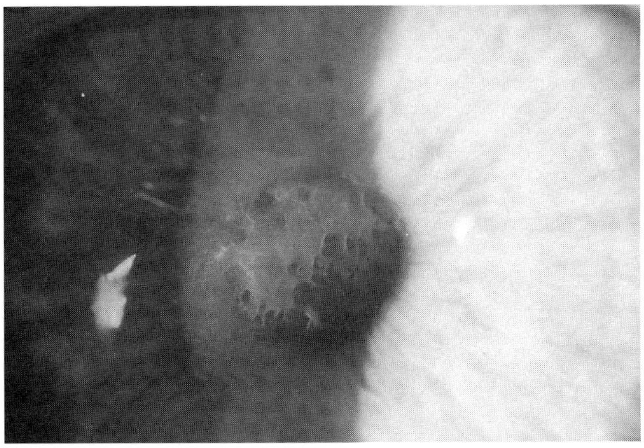

Fig. 10-72 Excimer laser phototherapeutic keratectomy (PTK). This eye with Salzmann's nodular degeneration did not respond to lamellar keratectomy with a blade, so an excimer laser PTK was performed.

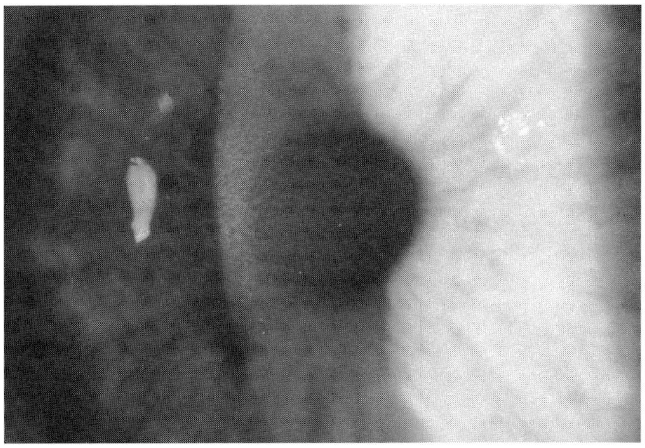

Fig. 10-73 Excimer laser phototherapeutic keratectomy (PTK). Three months after excimer laser PTK for the eye with Salzmann's nodular degeneration shown in Fig. 10-72. The cornea is much smoother and clearer.

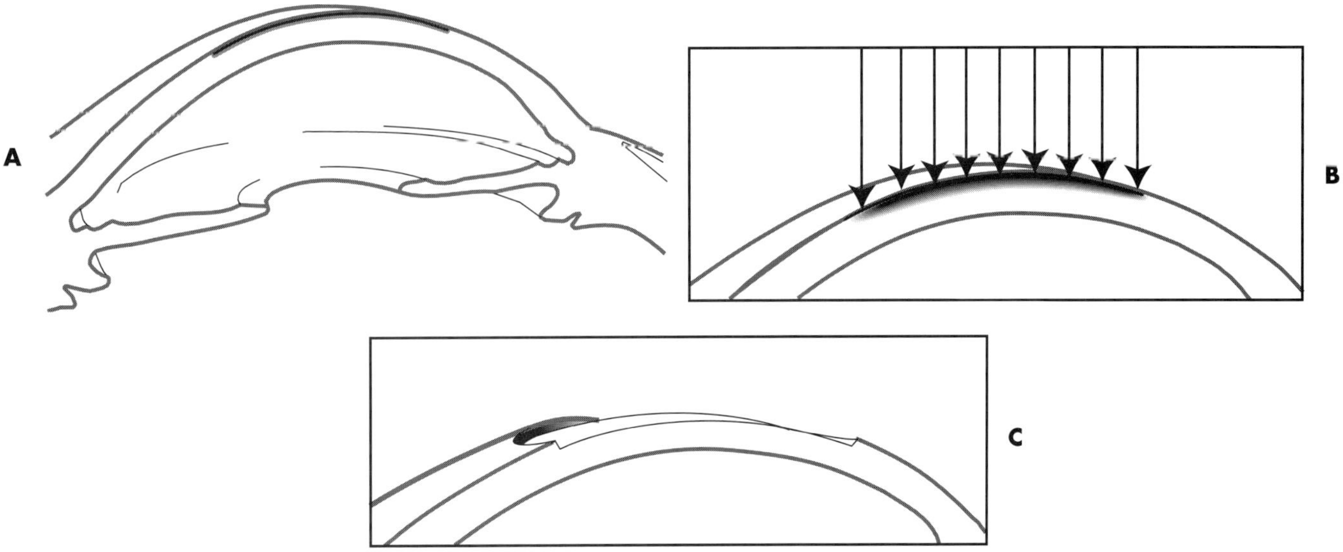

Fig. 10-74 Excimer laser phototherapeutic keratectomy (PTK) procedure for anterior stromal opacities. **A,** Confluent anterior stromal opacities, such as corneal stromal dystrophies, are often amenable to excimer laser PTK. **B,** Because the overlying epithelium is typically smooth, transepithelial treatment is performed through the epithelium and into the anterior stroma. **C,** The result should be a smooth base with the bulk of the stromal opacity removed. Care should be taken not to ablate too deeply because that would result in excessive corneal flattening and induced hyperopia.

Eyes with anterior stromal pathology often have relatively smooth epithelium. In these cases the epithelium is not removed manually but with the laser. A large spot size (e.g., 6 to 6.5 mm in diameter) is selected (Fig. 10-74). The depth of the pathology must be determined before surgery at the slit lamp with the aid of pachymetry and occasionally of ultrasound biomicroscopy. Approximately 60% to 75% of the predetermined depth of treatment is programmed into the laser. Ablation is performed centered over the pupil. The surgeon proceeds with the ablate and check sequence until the desired result is achieved. Here, too, the cornea need not be perfectly clear, but it should be much clearer than before surgery for a good effect (Figs. 10-75 and 10-76). If deep ablation is required to remove most of the opacity, an antihyperopia ablation can be performed. A 2-mm diameter spot is marched around the periphery of the 6- to 6.5-mm central ablation to deepen the periphery, theoretically steepening the central cornea to counteract the flattening effect of the central treatment.

Recurrent erosions can often be successfully treated with medical regimens, anterior stromal micropuncture,

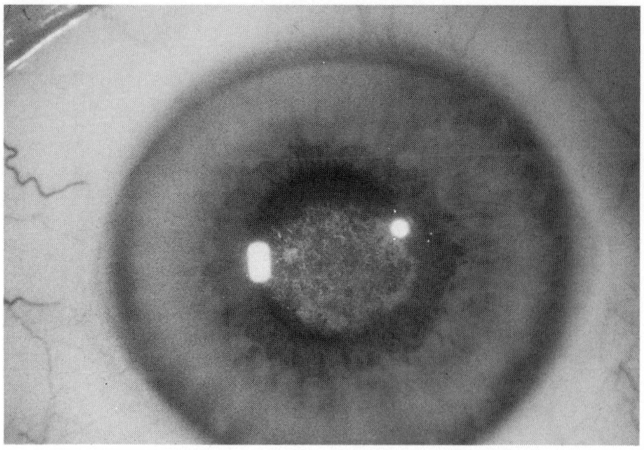

Fig. 10-75 Excimer laser phototherapeutic keratectomy (PTK). Schnyder's crystalline dystrophy with significant central corneal crystals. The patient had severe symptoms of glare before excimer laser PTK.

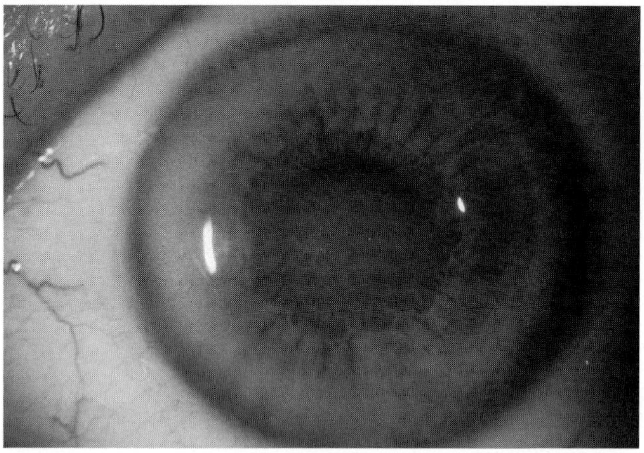

Fig. 10-76 Excimer laser phototherapeutic keratectomy (PTK). Two weeks after excimer laser PTK for Schnyder's crystalline dystrophy. The central crystals are almost, but not entirely, eliminated. The patient's symptoms of severe glare, however, are totally eliminated. The small amount of remaining crystals could have been removed with the excimer laser, but it would have required a significantly deeper ablation and risked causing more induced hyperopia.

and epithelial debridement with or without diamond burr polishing of Bowman's membrane. However, occasionally these treatments are not recommended or they fail, and excimer laser PTK can be attempted. The technique is to debride all loose epithelium mechanically and treat all areas of exposed Bowman's membrane with a 5-µm ablation.

After PTK, the eye should be treated as a corneal abrasion with antibiotics, cycloplegics, NSAIDs, and occasionally pressure patching or a bandage soft contact lens. Complications of PTK are similar to those for superficial keratectomy and include poor epithelial healing, chronic ulceration, infectious keratitis, irregular astigmatism, scarring, and recurrence of pathology. A common problem after PTK is induced hyperopia from deep central ablations. The best way to manage induced hyperopia is to avoid it by ablating as little tissue as possible to achieve the desired effect. Occasionally, a contact lens is required to treat severe induced hyperopia. If significant postexcimer haze occurs after PTK, topical corticosteroids are often helpful. Excimer laser PTK is a promising procedure for a number of superficial corneal problems and often delays or averts more extensive corneal surgery, such as penetrating keratoplasty.

CONJUNCTIVAL FLAP

The conjunctival flap procedure is an extremely effective and generally underutilized operation for the treatment of certain corneal surface abnormalities. Conditions such as chronic sterile corneal ulcerations, painful bullous keratopathy in eyes with poor visual potential, and, uncommonly, indolent corneal infections such as fungal or herpetic keratitis, often respond well to this surgery (Figs. 10-77, 10-78, and 10-79). Contraindications include active infectious ulcers and corneal perforations. The goal of surgery is to stabilize the corneal surface and to improve painful symptoms, but it does not improve vision. The cosmetic appearance is typically good, but it is not the same as that of a normal eye (Fig. 10-80).

The procedure is performed under local, or occasionally general, anesthesia (Fig. 10-81 and Box 10-9). The entire corneal epithelium is debrided with a blunt or sharp instrument. A traction suture (e.g., 6-0 Vicryl or Mersilene) is placed at the superior limbus and is used to pull the globe downward. Local anesthetic is injected into the superior subconjunctival space to separate the conjunctiva from Tenon's fascia, and 12 to 14 mm superior to the limbus, a small conjunctival incision is made. Blunt and sharp dissection between the conjunctiva and Tenon's capsule is then carried down to the limbus superiorly and into the nasal and temporal quadrants. The goal should be a thin conjunctival flap without buttonholes. It is better to have a slightly thicker flap with a small amount of Tenon's tissue than an extremely thin, friable flap at risk for perforations. Once most of the flap has been dissected, the superior conjunctival incision is extended several millimeters nasally and temporally parallel to the limbus.

After the flap is completely undermined, the dissection is carried through the limbal attachments onto the cornea. This peritomy is continued for 360°. The result is a superior conjunctival flap with bridges nasally and temporally. The flap is gently pulled down over the

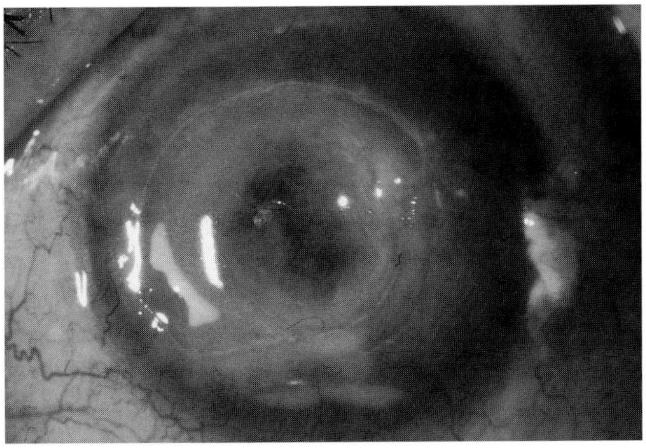

Fig. 10-77 Conjunctival flap. Sterile corneal melt with severe corneal thinning is present in an eye with poor visual potential. Calcific degeneration is present in the cornea from the 8 to 9 o'clock positions, and a hypopyon can be seen inferiorly.

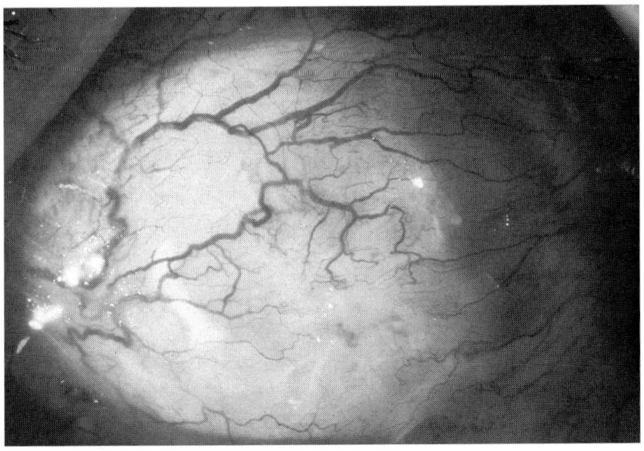

Fig. 10-78 Conjunctival flap. Three weeks after a conjunctival flap in the eye in Fig. 10-77. A few residual Vicryl sutures are still found inferiorly and superiorly.

cornea, and the inferior edge is sutured to the inferior corneal limbus (using episcleral bites) and into the inferior edge of conjunctiva. The superior edge of the flap is sutured to the superior episclera. The flap should lie securely on the cornea without a great degree of tension. Absorbable (e.g., 8-0 Vicryl) or nonabsorbable suture (e.g., 9-0 nylon) can be used. If a buttonhole arises in the flap, it should be closed with a fine suture (e.g., 11-0 nylon). The superior Tenon's/scleral area is left bare to reepithelialize.

Postoperative medications consist of antibiotics and corticosteroids, often in ointment form. Complications

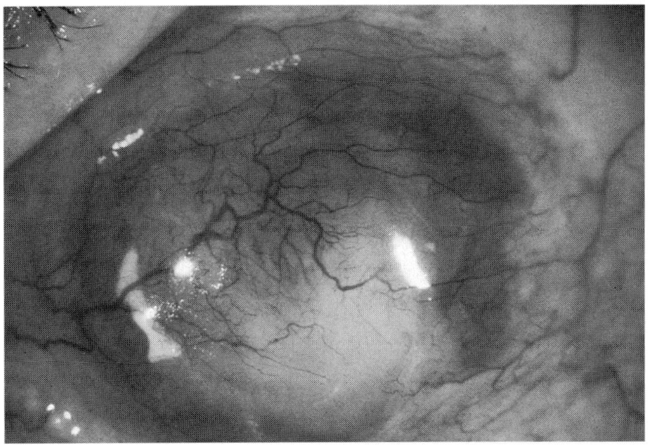

Fig. 10-79 Conjunctival flap. Three months after a conjunctival flap in the eye in Figs. 10-77 and 10-78. Note the gradual thinning and clearing of the flap. The hypopyon is gone, but the calcific degeneration is still present.

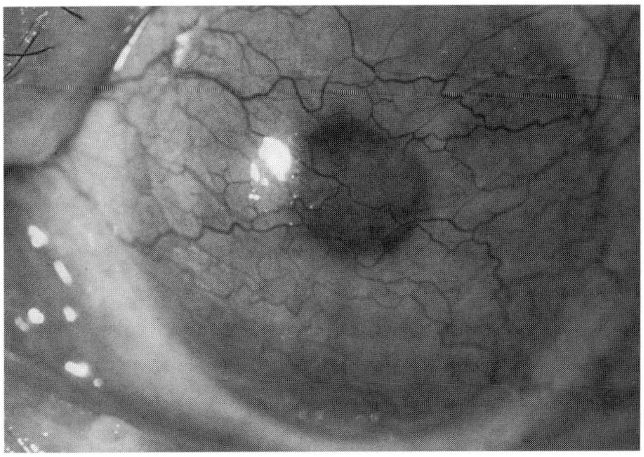

Fig. 10-80 Conjunctival flap. Six months after a conjunctival flap in a different eye. The flap is relatively clear, and the cosmetic result is reasonable.

Box 10-9 Major Steps in the Total Conjunctival Flap Procedure

Manually debride the entire corneal epithelium
Place a superior limbal traction suture
Balloon the superior conjunctiva with local anesthetic
Beginning 12 to 14 mm superior to the limbus, dissect a conjunctival flap
Create a 360° peritomy
Move the conjunctival flap over the cornea and secure it to the inferior and superior limbus

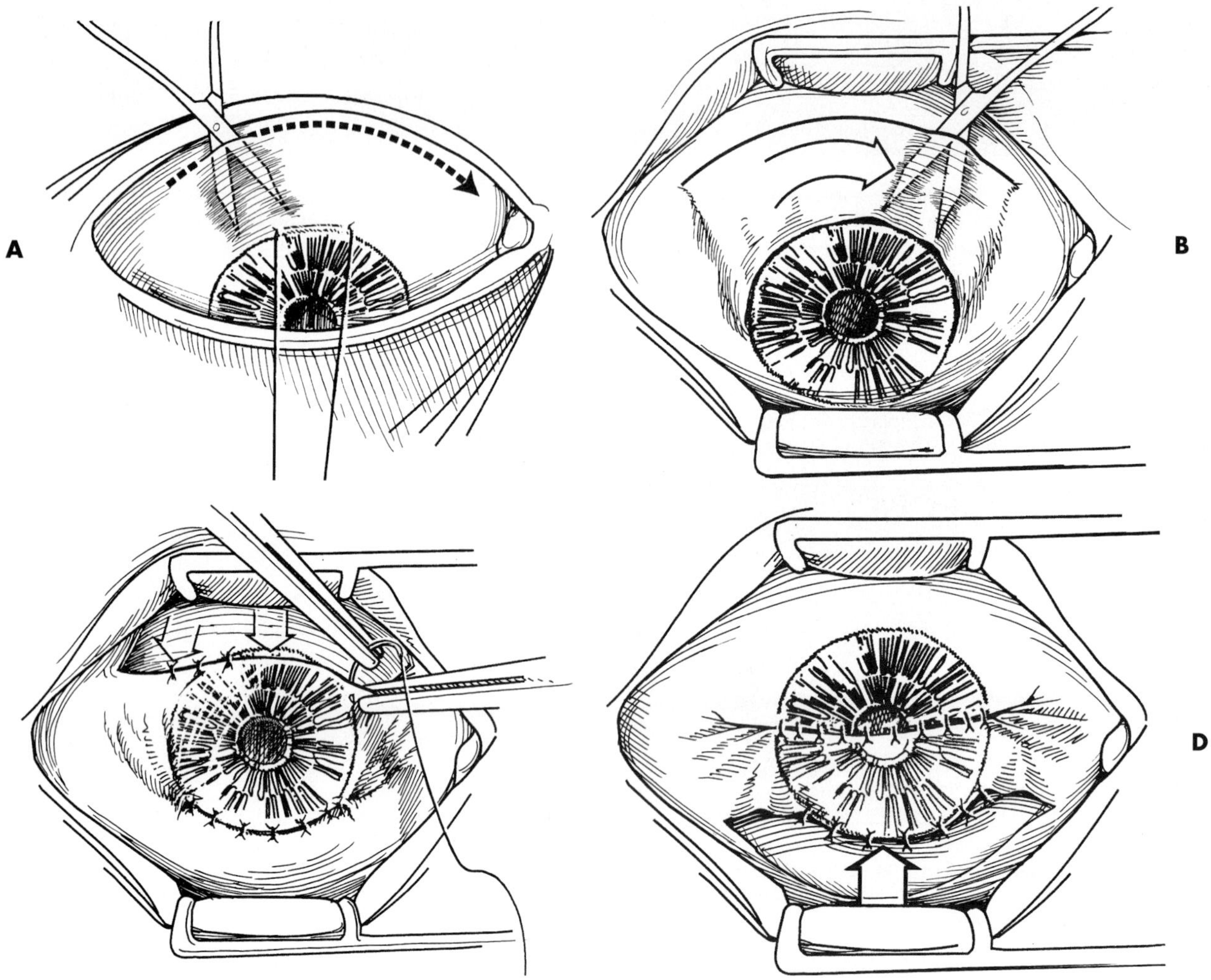

Fig. 10-81 Conjunctival flap procedure **A,** A superior limbal traction suture is placed to pull the eye downward. A conjunctival incision is made approximately 12 to 14 mm superior to the limbus. **B,** The conjunctiva is carefully dissected downward to the limbus. **C,** Once the limbus is reached, a 360° conjunctival peritomy is performed. The conjunctival flap is then moved from the superior sclera to cover the entire cornea. It is sutured to episclera and conjunctiva inferiorly and to episclera superiorly. **D,** When the corneal pathology involves only the inferior cornea, an inferior conjunctival flap can be performed.

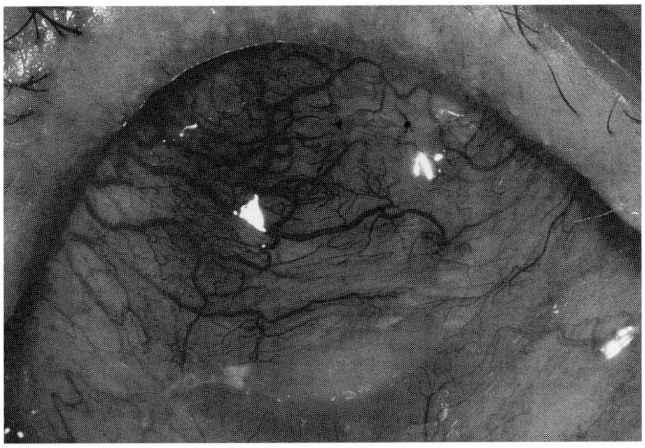

Fig. 10-82 Buttonhole in a conjunctival flap. A conjunctival flap buttonhole, which stains with fluorescein, is present inferiorly. Two 11-0 nylon sutures, which were used to close a buttonhole during surgery, can be seen superiorly.

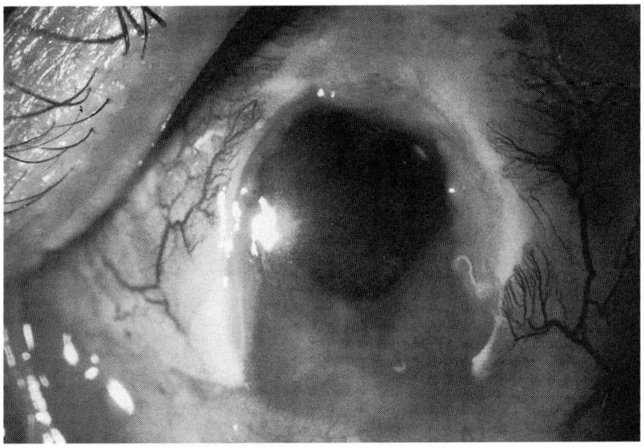

Fig. 10-83 Retraction of a conjunctival flap. The conjunctival flap has retracted and melted, but the central cornea has epithelialized well.

include poorly healing buttonholes (Fig. 10-82) that can lead to chronic epithelial defects and corneal melting or infection. Large buttonholes or extreme tension of the flap can lead to flap retraction (Fig. 10-83). Infection is always a risk, and these compromised eyes require close follow-up. The flap tends to become more transparent, and often cosmetically pleasing, with time.

LIMBAL STEM CELL TRANSPLANTATION

Severe ocular surface disease can result from many conditions. Multiple ocular surgeries, contact lens-induced keratopathy, and aniridia primarily affect the corneal limbal stem cells and cause corneal disease. Ocular cicatricial pemphigoid, Stevens-Johnson syndrome, chronic medication toxicity, and chemical and thermal ocular injuries can affect conjunctival and corneal limbal stem cells, resulting in more widespread ocular damage. Surgical procedures to correct these deficiencies have been developed. They include the transplantation of conjunctiva and limbal tissue as well as corneal and limbal tissue and are obtained from fellow eyes, blood relatives, and cadavers. The terminology for these different procedures is outlined in Table 10-2. Donor material is obtained from the fellow eye in unilateral cases. When a conjunctival deficiency exists and a living related donor is available, a living related conjunctival limbal allograft is performed. When primarily corneal disease exists or a living related donor is unavailable, a keratolimbal allograft is obtained from a cadaver. When allografts are used, systemic immunosuppression is required.

These procedures involve the removal of approximately 2 mm width of limbal conjunctiva for 360° in the recipient. All abnormal corneal epithelium and fibrovascular pannus are excised from the recipient using blunt and sharp dissection. For conjunctival limbal allografts,

Table 10-2 Classification of epithelial transplantation procedures for ocular surface disease

Procedure	Abbreviation	Donor	Transplanted tissue
CONJUNCTIVAL TRANSPLANTATION			
Conjunctival autograft	CAU	Fellow eye	Conjunctiva
Cadaveric conjunctival allograft	c-CAL	Cadaver	Conjunctiva
Living-related conjunctival allograft	lr-CAL	Living relative	Conjunctiva
LIMBAL TRANSPLANTATION			
Conjunctival limbal autograft	CLAU	Fellow eye	Limbus/conjunctiva
Cadaveric conjunctival limbal allograft	c-CLAL	Cadaver	Limbus/conjunctiva
Living-related conjunctival limbal allograft	lr-CLAL	Living relative	Limbus/conjunctiva
Keratolimbal allograft	KLAL	Cadaver	Limbus/cornea

Adapted from Holland EJ, Schwartz GS: The evolution of epithelial transplantation for severe ocular surface disease and a proposed classification system, *Cornea* 15: 549-556, 1996.

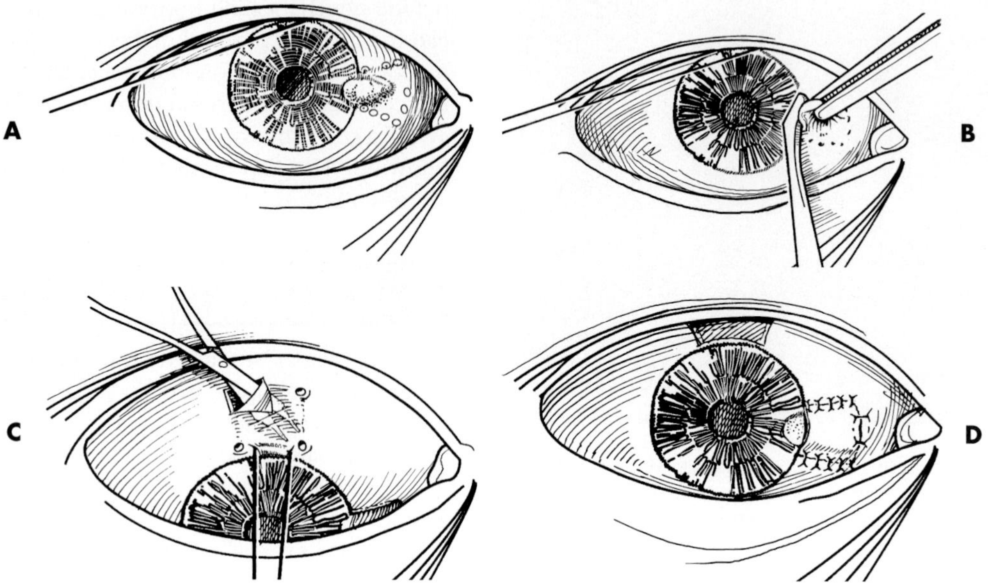

Fig. 10-84 Pterygium excision and conjunctival autograft procedure. **A,** A superior limbal traction suture is placed. The pterygium is outlined with light cautery. **B,** The pterygium is removed from the cornea with a sharp, rounded blade using a front-to-back pushing motion. The pterygium is removed from the scleral side with scissors and blunt-and-sharp dissection. **C,** After the size of the conjunctival defect is measured, the superior conjunctiva is marked with cautery and the conjunctival graft is dissected. **D,** The free conjunctival graft is carefully transferred to the area of pterygium excision, taking care to keep the epithelial side up. It is sutured to episclera at the limbus and conjunctiva elsewhere.

the donor material is fashioned superiorly and inferiorly for 3 clock hours. For keratolimbal allografts, a superficial limbal and corneal specimen with intact epithelium is harvested. It may be obtained in several, typically four, small circular grafts or in fewer large crescentic grafts. These grafts are secured to the sclera and the limbus of the recipient with 10-0 nylon or 8-0 Vicryl sutures, or both.

Complications of these limbal stem cell transplant procedures include poor reepithelialization of the recipient cornea and sterile or infectious keratitis. Most important, rejection can occur in allografts; therefore treatment with topical and systemic immunosuppressive agents for 12 months or longer is required. Once the surface has stabilized, corneal transplantation for vision may be attempted with improved prognosis. Amniotic membrane (the avascular inner tissue of the placenta) transplantation has recently been investigated for ocular surface reconstruction because it appears to promote reepithelialization. It has been used alone and in conjunction with limbal stem cell transplantation for patients with severe ocular surface disease. Recently, amniotic membrane grafts have been used to cover the entire cornea and limbus, on top of which the limbal stem cell transplants are sutured. This technique creates a smooth basement membrane surface for better adherence of the migrating epithelial cells.

PTERYGIUM EXCISION AND CONJUNCTIVAL AUTOGRAFT

Pterygium excision is typically indicated for pterygia that progress centrally and threaten vision and pterygia that cause significant discomfort, difficulty with contact lens wear, or cosmetic problems. These lesions have been surgically excised for centuries with variable success. The primary complication of pterygium surgery is recurrence. Multiple surgical procedures for pterygia have been devised over the years, mainly to decrease the chance for recurrence. The following describes one option, a pterygium excision with a conjunctival autograft. Advantages to this procedure include low recurrence rate, decades of follow-up, and straightforward surgical technique. The main disadvantages are that it is moderately time consuming and that it violates the superior bulbar conjunctiva.

After local (and occasionally topical) anesthesia, a traction suture (e.g., 6-0 Vicryl or Mersilene) is placed at the superior limbus (Fig. 10-84 and Box 10-10). The extent of the pterygium may be demarcated with superficial cautery. Local anesthesia can be used to infiltrate the pterygium to balloon it off the sclera. Westcott scissors are used to excise the conjunctival portion of the pterygium down to bare sclera. Care should be taken to avoid

Box 10-10 Major Steps in the Pterygium Excision and Conjunctival Autograft Procedure

Place a superior limbal traction suture
Mark the extent of the pterygium
Balloon the pterygium with local anesthetic
Dissect the conjunctival and corneal portions of the pterygium, connecting at the limbus, and send for pathologic evaluation
Smooth the cornea and limbus with a diamond burr
Measure the conjunctival defect and mark the superior bulbar conjunctiva
Balloon the superior conjunctiva with local anesthetic
Dissect the conjunctival graft
Slide the graft over the area of pterygium excision and secure in place

cutting the rectus muscle, which is often adherent to recurrent pterygia. The corneal portion of the pterygium is removed with a rounded-end sharp blade. After the head of the pterygium is grasped with forceps, the blade is placed flat against the cornea, just central to the head of the pterygium. Using a forward-backward pushing motion, the pterygium is "peeled" off the cornea. If it is very adherent, some side-to-side cutting is required, but the base should be left as smooth as possible. This dissection is continued to the limbus, to connect with the conjunctival portion, and the pterygium is removed and sent for pathologic evaluation. The cornea should be smoothed with the blade and, if available, a large-tipped (5-mm ball) diamond burr. It is critical that the surface, especially near the limbus, be as smooth as possible to decrease the chances for recurrence.

The conjunctival defect is measured with calipers to determine the size of the conjunctival autograft. The globe is rotated downward, and light cautery or a marking pen is used to mark the four corners of the conjunctival graft on the superior bulbar conjunctiva. Once marked, the superior subconjunctival space can be infiltrated with local anesthesia to aid in creation of the graft. Westcott scissors are used to incise one corner of the graft. Careful blunt-and-sharp dissection are used to create a thin graft (i.e., with minimal Tenon's removal). Although a thin conjunctival graft is ideal, buttonholes should be avoided. Once it is completely undermined, the conjunctival edges are cut, using the cautery marks as a guide. The graft is then slid over to the area of pterygium excision, making certain to keep the epithelial side up. The cautery marks are helpful to establish that the correct side is up. Absorbable (e.g., 8-0 or 9-0 Vicryl) or nonabsorbable (e.g., 10-0 nylon) suture is used to secure the graft. The two

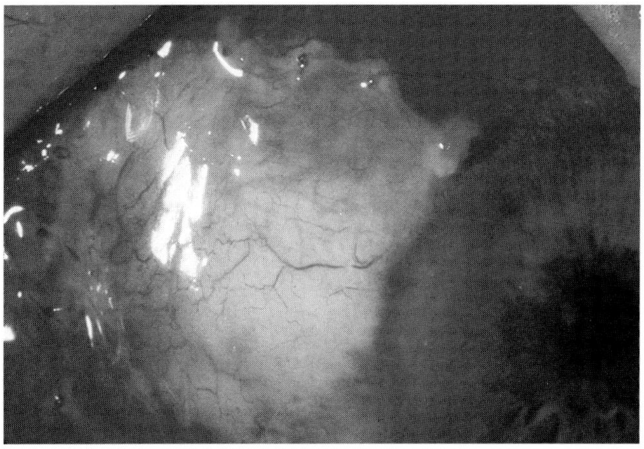

Fig. 10-85 Pterygium excision and conjunctival autograft. One day after pterygium excision and conjunctival autograft. The corneal epithelial defect is healing. The conjunctival autograft is excellently positioned with multiple 8-0 Vicryl sutures.

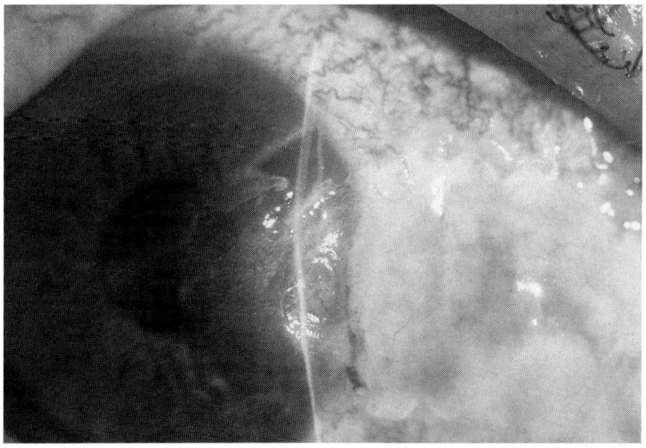

Fig. 10-86 Delle after pterygium excision and conjunctival autograft. A delle, a distinct area of corneal drying and thinning, can be seen adjacent to an elevated conjunctival autograft.

limbal corners are anchored to episclera and conjunctiva while other sutures attach conjunctiva to conjunctiva (Fig. 10-85). All large gapes should be closed. Buttonholes should also be closed with fine suture (e.g., 11-0 nylon).

Postoperative treatment is with topical antibiotics and corticosteroids, often in ointment form. Once the epithelial defects have healed, the antibiotic can be discontinued, but the corticosteroid medication should be continued for several months to prevent recurrence. Intraocular pressure must be monitored while a patient takes corticosteroids.

Complications include delayed healing of the corneal epithelial defect, delle formation (Fig. 10-86), and infection. Flap retraction can occur if the sutures release prematurely. With any large epithelial defect, such as with severe flap retraction or with a bare sclera pterygium

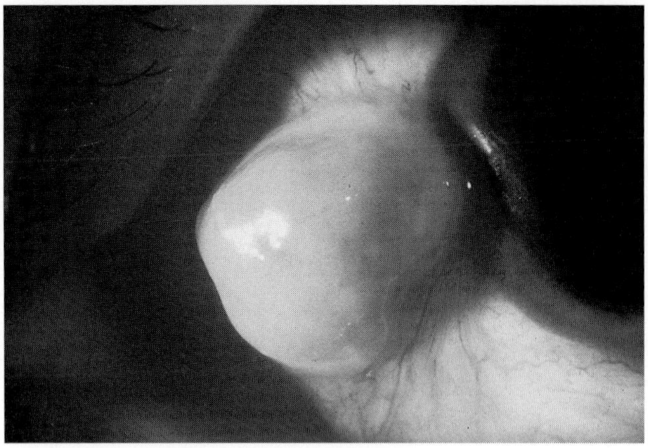

Fig. 10-87 Pyogenic granuloma after pterygium excision with a bare sclera technique. A large elevated nodule of granulation tissue may develop in extensive areas of bare sclera.

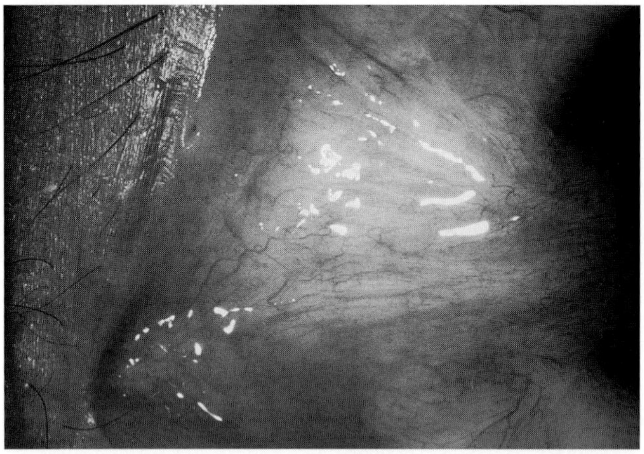

Fig. 10-88 Recurrent pterygium. This pterygium recurred soon after excision. Note the symblepharon formation with conjunctival adhesion to the upper eyelid.

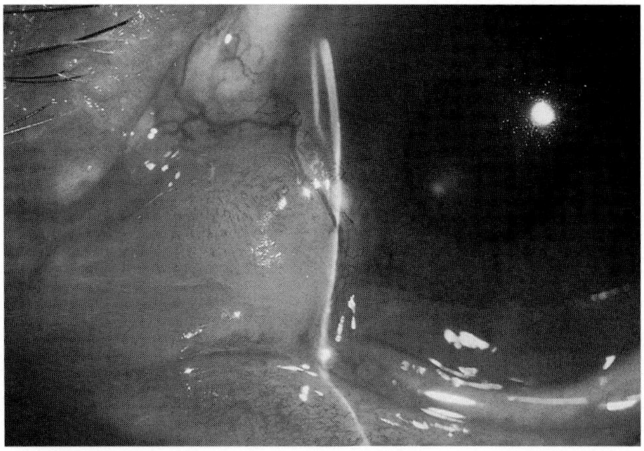

Fig. 10-89 Recurrent pterygium. Significant recurrent pterygium formation after three previous excisions with associated pyogenic granuloma formation and symblepharon. This patient has diplopia on outward gaze in this eye because of restricted ocular motility.

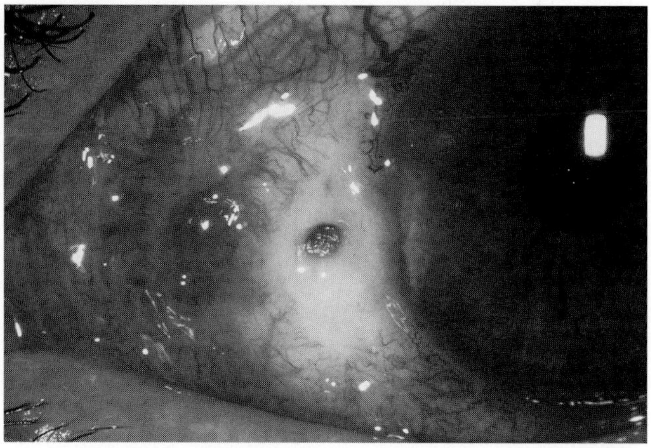

Fig. 10-90 Scleral melting after pterygium surgery. A scleral melt developed 18 days after a bare sclera pterygium excision. This complication, though rare, is more common with the use of topical mitomycin C after pterygium excision.

excision technique, pyogenic granuloma can develop (Fig. 10-87). They generally respond to topical corticosteroids. The most common complication is recurrence of the pterygium that is occasionally worse than the original (Figs. 10-88 and 10-89). Meticulous surgical technique and postoperative corticosteroids are the best ways to avert this complication. Recently, the use of topical mitomycin C to prevent recurrence, especially in reoperations, has been advocated. When used, it should be applied in the operating room, and the area should be covered with conjunctiva. Rare but severe complications including scleritis, scleral melting (Fig. 10-90), and perforation have been reported with the use of mitomycin C for pterygium surgery. Some surgeons have advocated the use of a small subconjunctival injection of mitomycin C into the head of the pterygium several weeks to months before pterygium excision as a method to reduce recurrences.

CONJUNCTIVAL AND CORNEAL TUMOR EXCISION

Most conjunctival tumors are superficial in that they do not involve the corneal stroma, episclera, or sclera. Surgical treatment of squamous cell lesions is relatively straightforward. Conversely, surgeons experienced in melanocytic tumor excision should treat pigmented lesions because these lesions are more difficult to eradicate and they can metastasize.

Squamous cell lesions are treated with excisional biopsy and supplemental cryotherapy. Under local anesthesia, the lesion is excised first from the conjunctival side leaving a wide, approximately 1- to 2-mm, margin.

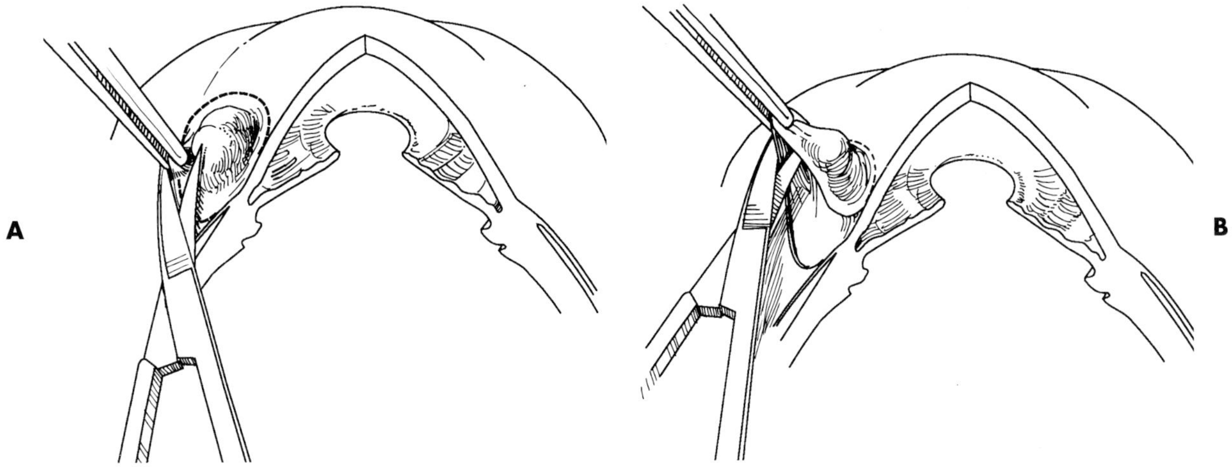

Fig. 10-91 Conjunctival tumor excision procedure. **A,** Conjunctival tumors can extend onto the cornea. A wide excision on both the conjunctival and the corneal sides must be performed. **B,** Scissors are used to excise the conjunctival portion, and blunt dissection with a rounded-end blade is usually adequate to remove the corneal portion. Double freeze-thaw cryotherapy is used to treat the remaining conjunctival edges and occasionally the limbus.

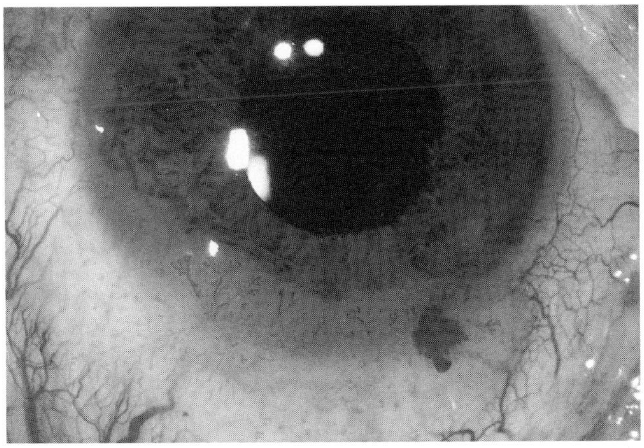

Fig. 10-92 Conjunctival tumor excision. A large limbal conjunctival papillomatous tumor can be seen from the 4 toward the 10 o'clock positions before removal.

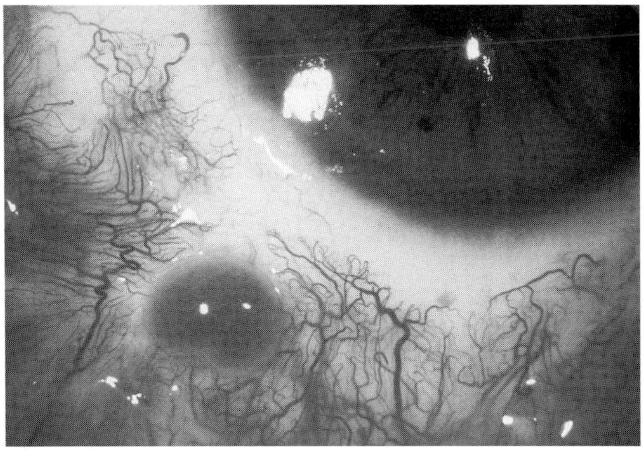

Fig. 10-93 Conjunctival tumor excision. Soon after the surgical excision with supplemental double freeze-thaw cryotherapy of the conjunctival tumor seen in Fig. 10-92, a pyogenic granuloma developed in a large area of bare sclera. It resolved with topical corticosteroids, but recurrent conjunctival tumor must be considered.

The lesion is undermined to the limbus, leaving bare sclera, and then excised. Any abnormal corneal epithelium is removed with debridement with a sharp rounded-end blade, taking care not to incise Bowman's membrane because it is a barrier to invasive tumor (Fig. 10-91). Some surgeons apply absolute alcohol to the involved corneal surface. Double freeze-thaw cryotherapy is then applied to the remaining conjunctival margin and affected limbus, theoretically to eradicate any remaining tumor cells. Large areas of exposed sclera can be partially closed with adjacent conjunctiva using absorbable (e.g., 8-0 Vicryl) sutures.

Postoperative treatment is with antibiotics and corticosteroids. Pyogenic granulomas often develop in large areas of bare sclera (Figs. 10-92 and 10-93). They generally respond to topical corticosteroids and should not be confused with recurrent tumor. The main complication is recurrence of the tumor, which, when it occurs, is typically at the limbus (Figs. 10-94, 10-95, and 10-96). Recurrent tumors occasionally involve the episclera or sclera, and rarely the corneal stroma. Deeper excisions, including sclerectomies and keratectomies, may be required to treat recurrent lesions. Patients must be followed up regularly for recurrence.

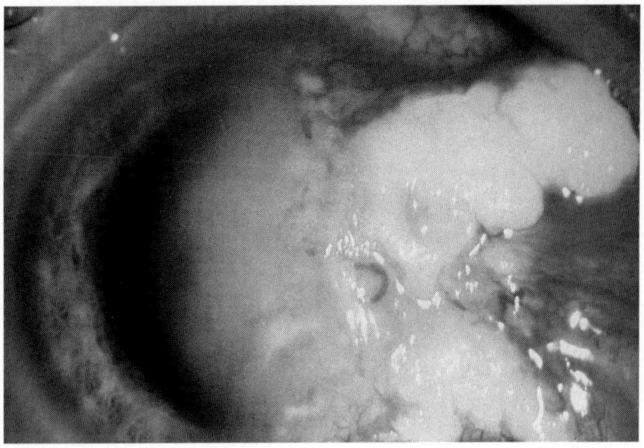

Fig. 10-94 Conjunctival tumor excision. A large leukoplakic, squamous cell carcinoma of the conjunctiva and cornea is seen before excision.

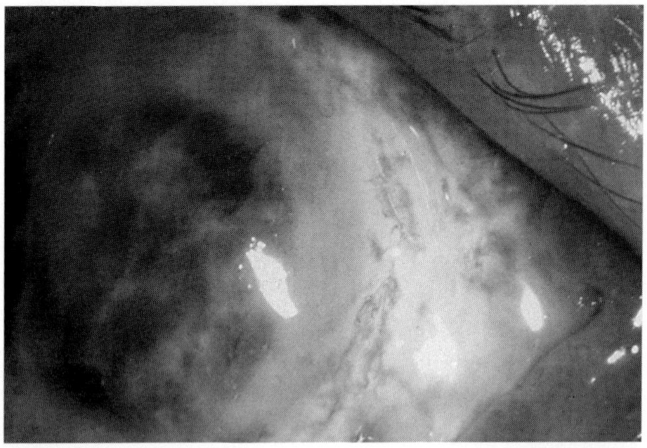

Fig. 10-95 Conjunctival tumor excision. One month after the mass seen in Fig. 10-94 was excised, no apparent residual or recurrent tumor has developed.

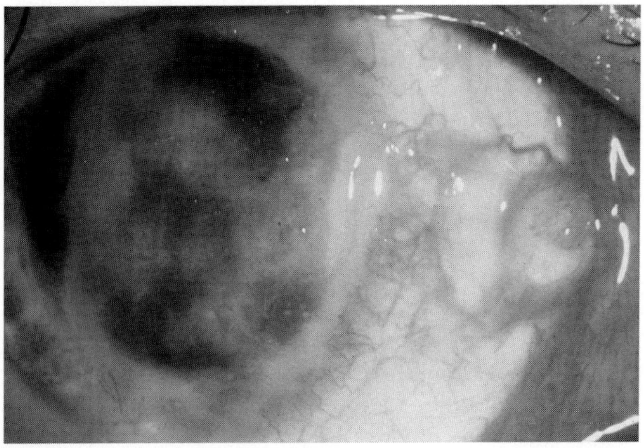

Fig. 10-96 Conjunctival tumor excision. Two months after surgical excision of the mass seen in Figs. 10-94 and 10-95, it has recurred at the limbus, requiring more extensive excision.

CORNEAL PERFORATION SURGERY

The exact type and severity of the corneal perforation determine the mode of treatment. The treatment of traumatic corneal lacerations is covered in Chapter 11. Perforations are generally caused by progressive loss of corneal tissue. This ulcerative process may be infectious or sterile (primarily inflammatory). When an infectious corneal ulcer is suspected, it requires a workup and treatment, as detailed in Chapter 4. The etiology and medical therapy for sterile/inflammatory ulcers or melts are discussed in Chapter 5. The general goal in the treatment of progressive corneal ulceration is to heal the epithelium. Once the epithelial defect is completely healed, the ulcer does not progress. A temporary lateral tarsorrhaphy can be extremely effective is getting the epithelial defect to heal. Severe corneal ulcerations can be followed up closely if the causative process is being adequately treated and the epithelial defect is improving. However, when a corneal perforation is imminent or has occurred, surgical treatment is often indicated.

Various surgical options are available to manage an impending or completed corneal perforation (Box 10-11). Medical-grade cyanoacrylate tissue adhesive (*not* obtained from the local hardware store) is very useful in treating thinned or perforated corneal ulcers. The ulcers must be concave to allow space for the glue to maintain a foothold (Figs. 10-97, 10-98, 10-99, 10-100, and 10-101). Bulging descemetoceles do not respond well to corneal glue. The perforation must be small, ideally smaller than 1 mm. In addition, perforations near the limbus do not do as well with this treatment as do more central ulcers because the glue adheres poorly to conjunctiva. Corneal glue can usually be applied in a minor surgery setting under topical anesthesia. In the rare cases in which a large corneal perforation must be treated with glue, all attempts should be made to keep the glue out of the anterior chamber (Fig. 10-102). A collagen shield trimmed to the size of the base of the corneal perforation can be placed just before gluing to prevent the glue from going into the eye.

Box 10-11 Treatment Options for Corneal Perforations

- Cyanoacrylate corneal glue and bandage soft contact lens
- Lamellar patch graft
- Penetrating corneal graft
- Scleral, dura mater, pericardium, or fascia lata patch graft

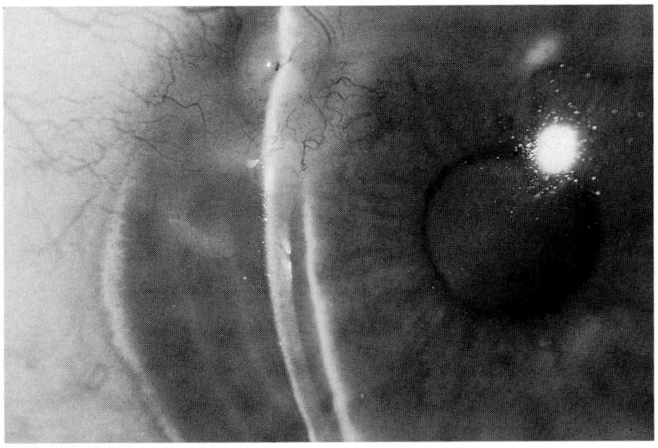

Fig. 10-97 Corneal perforation repair. A full-thickness corneal perforation is seen with a shallow anterior chamber. It was caused by a metallic foreign body that was present for several weeks and then removed.

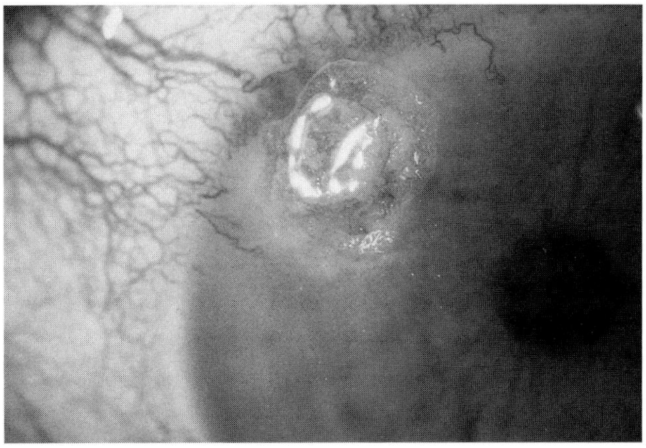

Fig. 10-98 Corneal perforation repair. Cyanoacrylate corneal tissue adhesive was placed to seal the perforation seen in Fig. 10-97. A bandage soft contact lens is used over the glue.

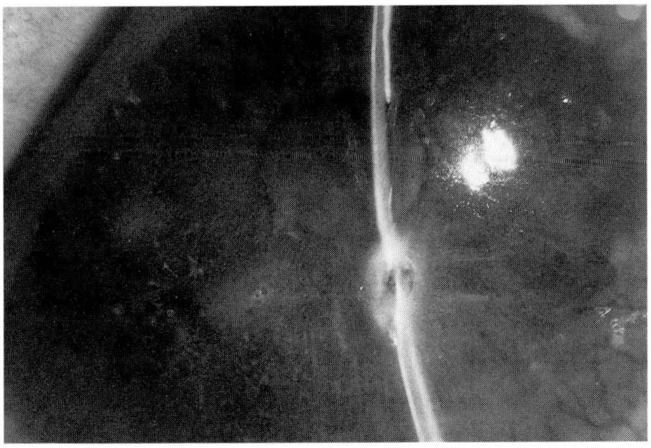

Fig. 10-99 Corneal perforation repair. A full-thickness corneal perforation is seen inferocentrally with a flat anterior chamber. It occurred from a sterile corneal melt in an eye with severe dry eye syndrome.

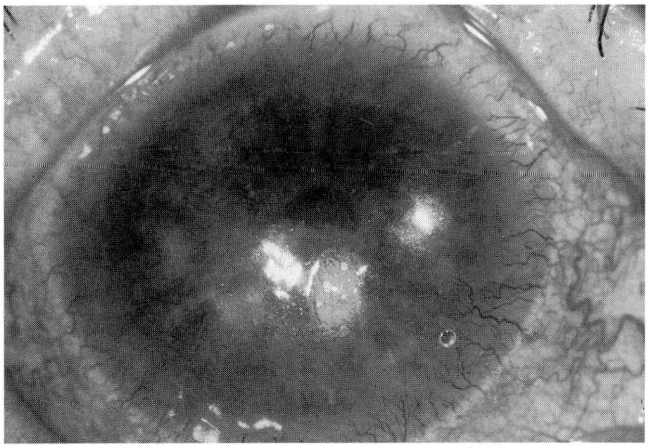

Fig. 10-100 Corneal perforation repair. A small amount of medical-grade corneal glue and a bandage soft contact lens are placed to seal the perforation seen in Fig. 10-99.

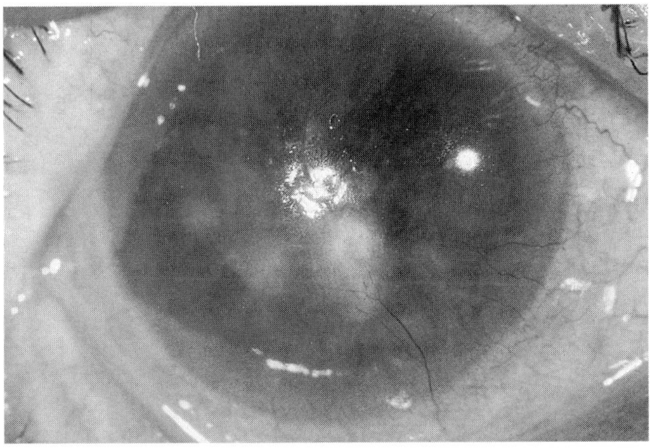

Fig. 10-101 Corneal perforation repair. Two months after the successful gluing of the perforation seen in Figs. 10-99 and 10-100, the glue fell out spontaneously. The perforation was sealed, and the cornea was completely reepithelialized. A moderate localized scar has formed in the area of the old perforation.

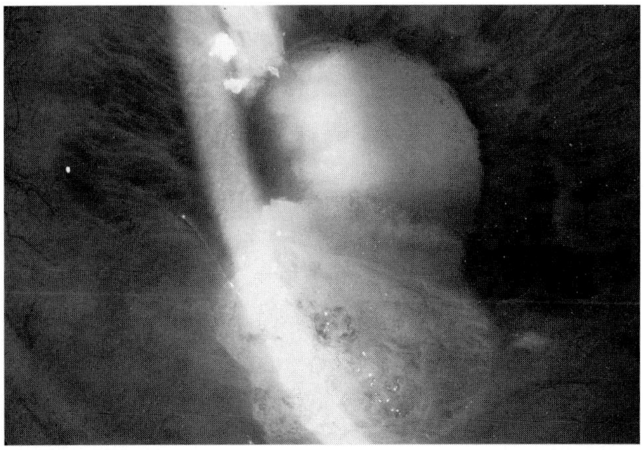

Fig. 10-102 Corneal perforation repair. A large perforation was treated with corneal glue in a patient who could not undergo corneal transplantation. The glue entered the anterior chamber before polymerizing and created a collar-button shape to the glue. A small portion of collagen shield placed at the base of the perforation would likely have prevented this occurrence.

Box 10-12 Major Steps for the Application of Cyanoacrylate Corneal Glue

Insert an eyelid speculum
Debride the epithelium off the area to be glued
Use a cellulose sponge to dry the area to be glued
Apply a small amount of glue to the perforation site
Allow the glue to polymerize
Place a bandage soft contact lens
Remove the eyelid speculum
Check the anterior chamber formation and stability of the glue and the contact lens 1 hour and 1 day later

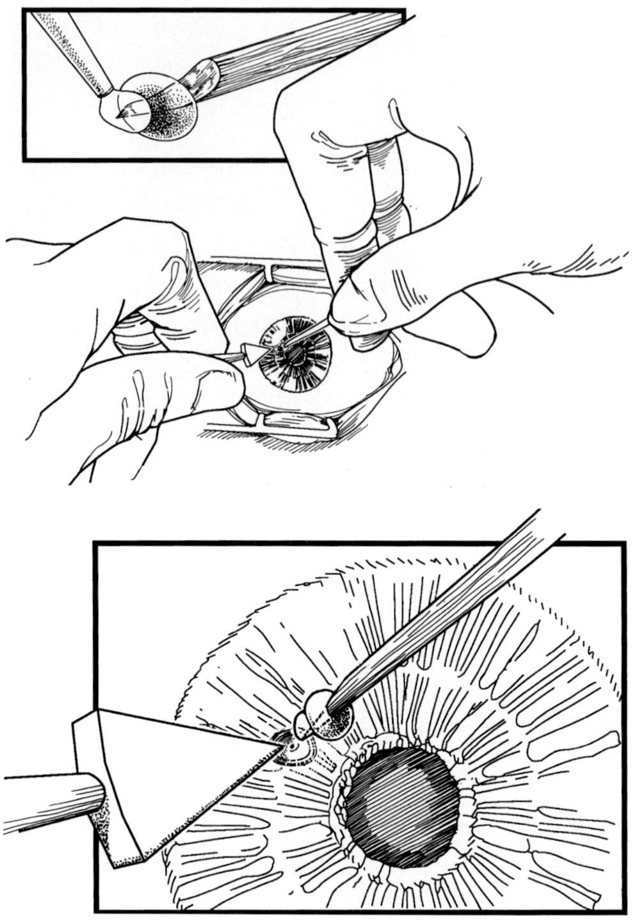

Fig. 10-103 Cyanoacrylate gluing of a corneal perforation procedure. **A,** A cotton-tipped applicator is broken to create a beveled end. Ointment is placed 1 to 2 mm from the end (depending on the amount of glue required to seal the wound). A drop of medical-grade cyanoacrylate glue is placed on the very end of the applicator. Corneal epithelium must be removed from the area to be glued. **B,** A cellulose sponge is used in one hand to dry the perforation site. Once dry, the glue is quickly applied. Just enough glue to seal the perforation should be used. It is allowed to polymerize for several minutes. A bandage soft contact lens is placed over the glue.

Multiple techniques exist for the application of corneal glue (Box 10-12). All require debriding the epithelium from the area to be glued. A small amount of glue is applied to an applicator, the area to be glued is dried with a cellulose sponge, and the glue is placed on the dry ulceration site (Fig. 10-103). Many different applicators have been used, including tiny plastic pipettes, 30-gauge syringes, and the broken flat end of a wooden sterile cotton-tipped applicator. The least amount of glue to seal the perforation and remain securely in place is used. The glue may require several minutes to polymerize before it is solid. A bandage soft contact lens is applied. The patient is examined at the slit lamp 1 hour later and then 1 day later to make certain the contact lens and the glue are in place and that the anterior chamber is forming. Do not expect the contact lens to move much with each blink. Postoperative treatment includes the frequent application of preservative-free artificial tears, topical antibiotic drops, and occasionally aqueous suppressants. The glue tends to remain in place for weeks to months, allowing time for the underlying cornea to heal. Bandage contact lenses require careful replacement with a new lens (using an eyelid speculum to prevent the eyelid from dislodging the glue during the exchange) every 1 to 3 months, depending on the amount of protein buildup on the lens. Once reepithelialization has occurred, the glue falls off on its own.

A perforation too large to glue may require an onlay lamellar patch graft or penetrating keratoplasty. Small peripheral ulcers often do well with lamellar patch grafts because the graft sutures stay outside the visual axis (Figs. 10-104, 10-105, and 10-106). Large peripheral ulcers and central ulcers can be treated similarly; however, the visual result is often poor because of irregularity from the wound edge or sutures centrally. In these cases, a central penetrating graft is often required once the acute inflammation has resolved. It may be best to treat these ulcers initially with larger penetrating grafts so the visual axis remains clear. The disadvantage is that these grafts have a greater tendency to fail because of increased inflammation from the ulceration and may require repeat corneal transplantation. Peribulbar and retrobulbar anesthesia are generally contraindicated in eyes with perforations because of the small chance that a retrobulbar hemorrhage or the mass effect of the local block will cause the expulsion of intraocular contents through the perforation site. Therefore, general anesthesia is typically used.

Corneal tissue is needed for lamellar patch and penetrating grafts. When a lamellar patch graft is performed, the smallest trephine large enough to encompass the entire ulcerated area is selected. The trephine is used to perform trephination of approximately 50% corneal

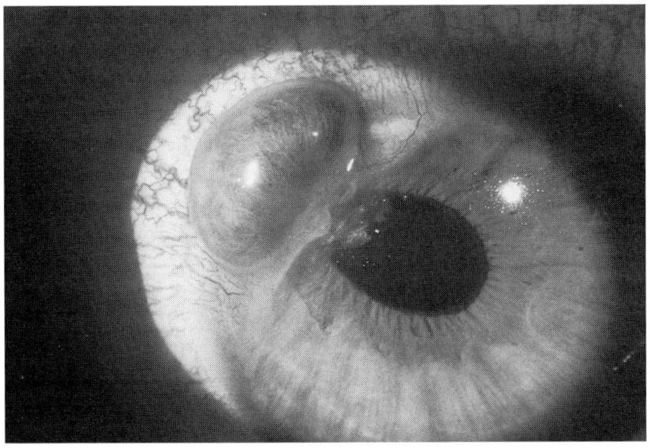

Fig. 10-104 Corneal perforation repair. A large corneal perforation with significant iris prolapse cannot be treated with corneal glue. This eye requires corneal transplantation.

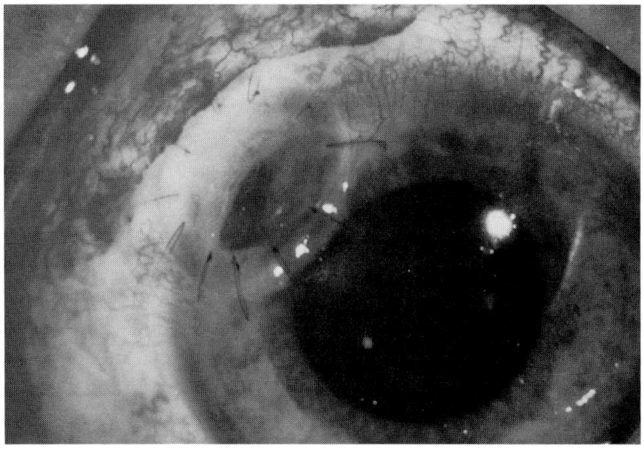

Fig. 10-106 Corneal perforation repair. Ten days after the lamellar corneal patch graft was performed in the eye seen in Figs. 10-104 and 10-105. The corneal graft is healing well, and the conjunctiva is retracting.

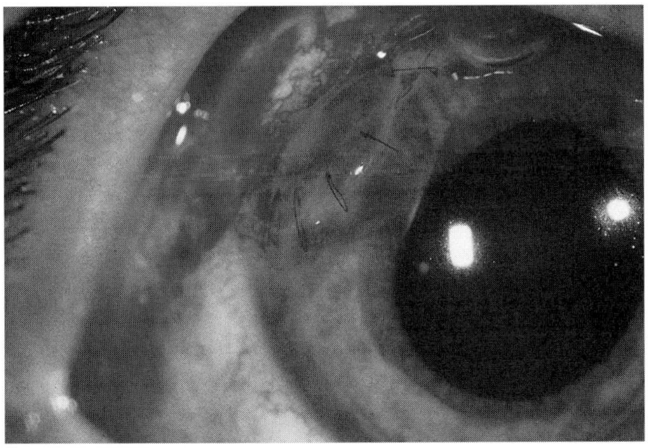

Fig. 10-105 Corneal perforation repair. One day after a lamellar corneal patch graft was performed in the eye seen in Fig. 10-104. The epithelium was carefully peeled from the iris, which was then treated with cryotherapy to prevent epithelial downgrowth. A trephine was placed to encompass the entire lesion, and a partial-thickness corneal and scleral incision was created. A lamellar corneal transplant was placed and partially covered with conjunctiva.

thickness. A sharp blade is then used to slowly deepen the trephination wound to approximately 90% corneal thickness and then to excise the ulcerated corneal button. A trephine of the same size or 0.25 mm larger is used to fashion a donor button from a donor cornea. It is sutured into position with multiple interrupted 10-0 nylon sutures. Wound security is checked after the anterior chamber is reformed through the graft wound or a separate paracentesis. If corneal tissue is unavailable, prepared sclera, pericardium, dura mater, or fascia lata may be used in an emergency.

The technique for central penetrating keratoplasty for a perforated corneal ulcer is similar to that for routine corneal transplantation. Special care must be taken during trephination because the anterior chamber is usually flat and the globe is soft. When a freehand trephination is performed, minimal pressure should be applied and the perforation site monitored to ensure no protrusion of iris or lens occurs. It is extremely important for a 360° mark to be identifiable so that a blade and scissors can complete the excision of the button. A suction trephine (e.g., Barron-Hessburg) may be better than a freehand trephination because less pressure is required for tissue penetration. A shallow incision can be deepened carefully with a sharp blade in a cutdown manner. Once the anterior chamber is entered, the trephination mark is followed with the corneal scissors to complete the excision of the corneal button. Increased inflammation at the time of surgery predisposes to posterior synechiae formation and pupillary block, so at least two surgical peripheral iridectomies should be performed. A corneal donor button 0.5 mm larger than the recipient trephination is sutured in place with multiple interrupted 10-0 nylon sutures.

Postoperative medications and complications are similar to those after routine penetrating keratoplasty. Frequently severe postoperative inflammation requires a higher dose of topical corticosteroids than usual. Nonsteroidal antiinflammatory drops can also be helpful in treating high degrees of inflammation. Additionally, mydriatic/cycloplegic agents can aid in decreasing inflammation and preventing pupillary block. In patients with significant ocular surface disease, punctal occlusion, lateral tarsorrhaphy, or both should be considered to decrease the chance for recurrent corneal melting. Close follow-up is required, especially to evaluate for infection, which is more common after grafts for perforations. Scleral ulcerations and perforations can be treated with

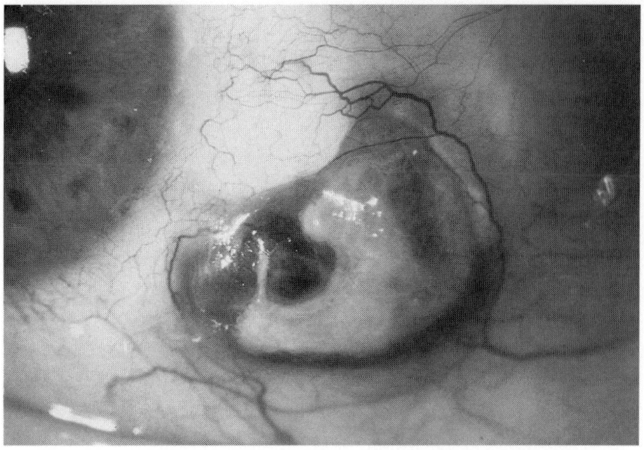

Fig. 10-107 Scleral patch graft. Uveal prolapse is beginning to develop in this eye with progressive necrotizing scleritis. A tectonic graft is required.

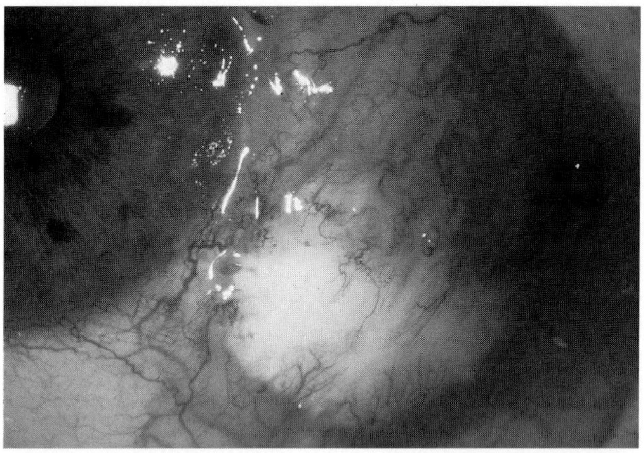

Fig. 10-108 Scleral patch graft. Two weeks after a scleral patch graft for the eye with necrotizing scleritis seen in Fig. 10-107. Adjacent conjunctiva was used to cover the sclera. A small delle is seen at the limbus.

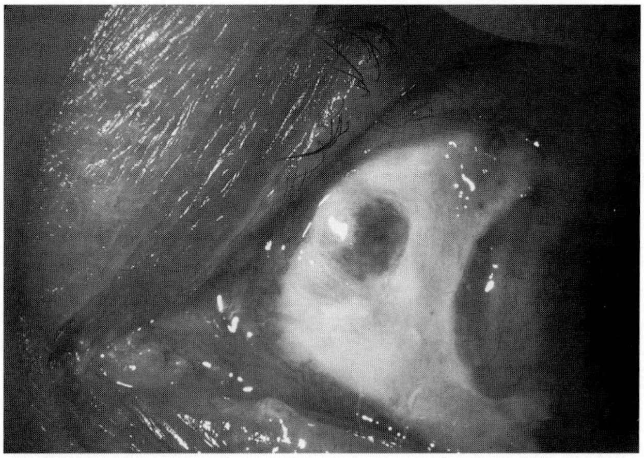

Fig. 10-109 Scleral patch graft. A large area of necrotizing scleritis with early uveal prolapse is seen. No healthy adjacent conjunctiva is present.

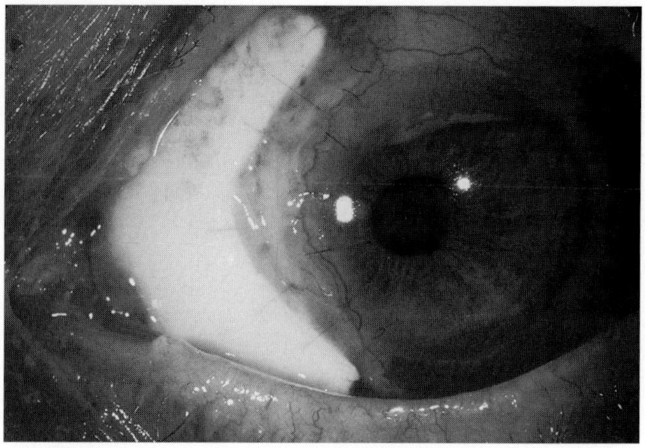

Fig. 10-110 Scleral patch graft. One day after a large scleral patch graft for necrotizing scleritis seen in Fig. 10-109. Because no healthy adjacent conjunctiva was available to cover the graft, an amniotic membrane transplant was used. Two rows of sutures can be seen, one securing the scleral graft and the other securing the amniotic membrane.

scleral or corneal tissue (Figs. 10-107 and 10-108). Tutoplast, preserved dura mater or pericardium, and fascia lata have also been used. If enough adjacent conjunctiva is available, it can be used to cover the graft. Otherwise, an amniotic membrane graft can be used (Figs. 10-109 and 10-110).

PERMANENT KERATOPROSTHESIS

In the rare patient with severe bilateral corneal disease (or unilateral corneal disease with severe visual loss in the fellow eye) not amenable to penetrating keratoplasty, a permanent keratoprosthesis can be considered. This implanted "telescopic lens" can result in very good central visual acuity, but with a severely limited visual field. Before surgery the eye should have good macular and optic nerve function. Typical candidates for permanent keratoprosthesis include patients with bilateral chemical burns, ocular cicatricial pemphigoid, Stevens-Johnson syndrome, and other severe corneal surface diseases.

The many different keratoprostheses and various techniques for implantation are usually performed under general anesthesia. A typical procedure involves securing the keratoprosthesis with autologous tissue, such as periosteum, which must be harvested from the patient at the beginning of the procedure. To minimize eyelid movement and prevent extrusion, the entire bulbar and palpebral conjunctiva is excised, along with the bulk of the superior tarsus, and a permanent tarsorrhaphy is performed at the conclusion of surgery. In addition, to decrease eye movement, the horizontal recti are disinserted. The crystalline lens or pseudophakic lens is

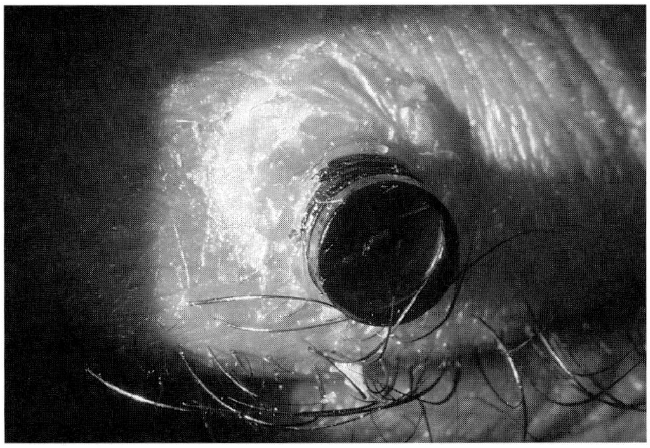

Fig. 10-111 Permanent keratoprosthesis. This permanent keratoprosthesis, in a patient with a bilateral chemical burn, is placed through the upper eyelid. The patient achieved 20/25 central visual acuity with a tunnel visual field.

removed if present. Total iridectomy and core vitrectomy are performed. A small trephine is used to remove a central corneal button, and the keratoprosthesis and its supporting plate are inserted. They are secured with Dacron mesh and periosteum. The outer part of the keratoprosthesis is placed through an incision in the upper eyelid (Fig. 10-111) or the palpebral fissure, and the total permanent tarsorrhaphy is completed.

Postoperative medications include topical antibiotic ointment and systemic antibiotics and corticosteroids. Complications include sterile and infectious endophthalmitis and glaucoma, which can be treated medically or surgically. Retroprosthetic membrane formation can occur. It can be treated with surgical removal or Nd:YAG laser therapy. If the Nd:YAG laser is used, care must be taken not to damage the posterior aspect of the keratoprosthesis. The most common long-term complication is extrusion of the keratoprosthesis, which occurs in many of these eyes within 5 to 10 years.

REFRACTIVE SURGERY

Reducing people's dependence on optical correction, namely glasses and contact lenses, has been a goal of the ophthalmic profession for decades. In the 1970s, modern methods of radial keratotomy (RK) were developed in the Soviet Union and then became popular around the world. This operation involves incisions in the cornea that permanently flatten the central curvature, correcting myopia. More recently, other methods of reshaping the cornea have been devised, among them excimer laser ablation of the corneal surface (photorefractive keratectomy) and creating a lamellar incision and performing the excimer laser ablation in the middle of the cornea (LASIK).

Box 10-13 General Patient Requirements for Refractive Surgery

- Age greater than 18 to 21 years
- Stable manifest and cycloplegic refractions, out of contact lenses
- Complete ocular examination with minimal to no ocular disease
- Normal corneal curvature (typically evaluated by computerized topography)
- Normal corneal thickness (typically evaluated by ultrasound pachymetry and slit-lamp evaluation)
- Normal pupil size
- Complete understanding of various refractive surgery options and their benefits and risks

Other refractive surgery techniques are under investigation, including intracorneal ring implants, intrastromal ablation, and phakic intraocular lens implants, and they may become integral to the refractive surgery arsenal. Recently, LASIK has been used to treat high refractive errors after penetrating keratoplasty.

Although it is important for any surgical procedure, it is imperative that patients undergoing refractive surgery be informed of the different refractive surgery options available and appropriate for their kind of refractive error (Box 10-13). Benefits and risks must be discussed in detail and documented in the medical record. The patient must understand the potential for undercorrection and overcorrection, glare, halos, corneal haze or scarring, corneal irregularity, diminished best-corrected vision, and the need for distance or reading glasses. For surgery to be performed, the patient's refraction must have been stable for several years and the eye free of significant pathology. Before examination the patient should remove contact lenses for a period of time to allow the cornea to stabilize. An evaluation of corneal curvature with computerized corneal topographic analysis should be obtained to make certain the cornea is regular. Cycloplegic and manifest refractions should be performed. Additionally, the pupil size should be assessed in dim and bright illumination because patients with large pupils tend to have more optical symptoms after keratorefractive surgery. Ultrasound pachymetry measurements are important before RK and LASIK.

Radial Keratotomy

Originally, the indications for RK included moderate and high degrees of myopia, and the procedure involved 8, 16, and even 32 radial corneal incisions. It was later determined that more than 8 incisions and incisions that reached very close to the visual axis (closer than a clear

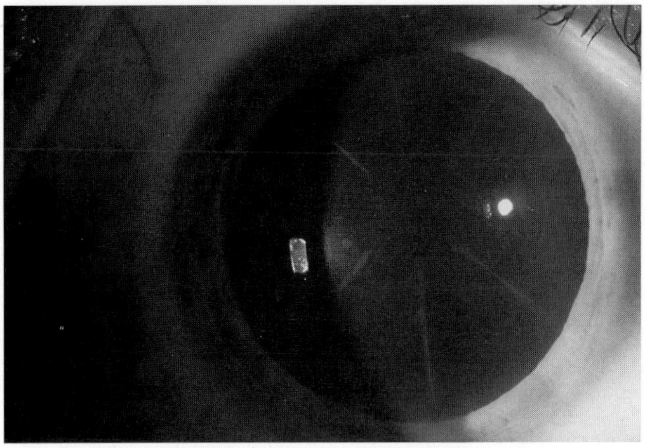

Fig. 10-112 Radial keratotomy (RK). Four years after an eight-incision RK for myopia and a two-incision T-cut for astigmatism.

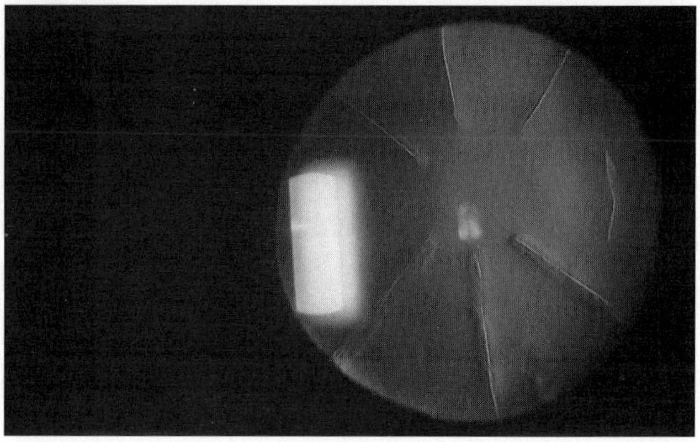

Fig. 10-113 Radial keratotomy (RK). Retroillumination off the retina of the eye seen in Fig. 10-112 of an eight-incision RK coupled with two T-cuts.

zone of 3.5 to 4 mm) were associated with more complications. It was also learned that older patients responded more to the same incisions than younger patients. Consequently, the current indications for RK are low degrees of myopia in young patients (generally <2 to 3 D) and slightly higher degrees of myopia in older patients (generally <4 D). Astigmatic keratotomy can be performed alone or in combination with RK to correct low to moderate degrees of astigmatism (generally <2 to 3 D) (Figs. 10-112 and 10-113).

A patient's age and the amount of intended myopic correction determine the number and lengths of RK incisions. The nomogram for the particular RK technique lets the surgeon know how many incisions to perform and how large a clear central zone to leave. Once all the numbers are double-checked, topical anesthesia and an eyelid speculum are placed in the operative eye, and the fellow eye is covered with an opaque shield (Box 10-14). The operating microscope is used, and ultrasound pachymetry is performed to determine the corneal thickness. The central clear optical zone, centered on the pupil, and the number and placement of the incisions are marked on the epithelium. A diamond blade is set to a percentage of the corneal thickness (typically 90% to 110%, depending on the technique). It is used to incise along the marks, with extreme care taken not to cross into the central clear zone. With the "American" technique the incision is begun at the central clear zone and proceeds peripherally. The main advantage is safety, namely that it is extremely difficult to cross into the central clear zone. The disadvantage is that the incisions are of less uniform depth. With the "Russian" technique the incision begins peripherally and ends at the central clear zone. Although the incisions are of more uniform depth, it is not difficult to extend the incision into the central clear zone or even across the visual axis. A "combined" technique uses a two-sided diamond blade. It is sharp on the entire surface of the American side but only on the deepest 200 μm on the Russian side. The blade is inserted at the central clear zone mark, and the American side of the blade is used to incise peripherally. Once the blade reaches close to the limbus, its direction is reversed and the incision is recut with the deep Russian side of the blade (Fig. 10-114). The blade cannot cut across the central clear zone because only the deep part of the blade is sharp, but the new incision depth is more uniform. This technique combines the safety of the American incision with the efficacy of the Russian incision. Arcuate or tangential astigmatic incisions are performed in a similar manner before the radial incisions. Care should be taken not to cross any incisions because poor healing often results.

Box 10-14 Major Steps in the Radial Keratotomy Procedure

- Check the diamond blade for flaws
- Select the number and length of the incisions from the nomogram
- Mark the 3 and 9 o'clock axes at the slit lamp if astigmatic incisions are planned
- Check the corneal thickness with ultrasound pachymetry
- Set the diamond blade depth
- Mark the central clear zone and the planned radial and astigmatic incisions
- Perform the astigmatic and radial incisions

Surgical complications include microperforations (full-thickness perforations that do not leak spontaneously) and macroperforations (full-thickness perforations that leak spontaneously or with minimal pressure)

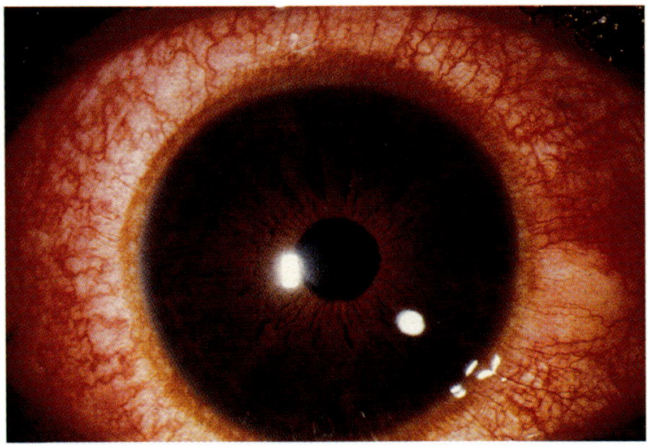

Plate 6-1

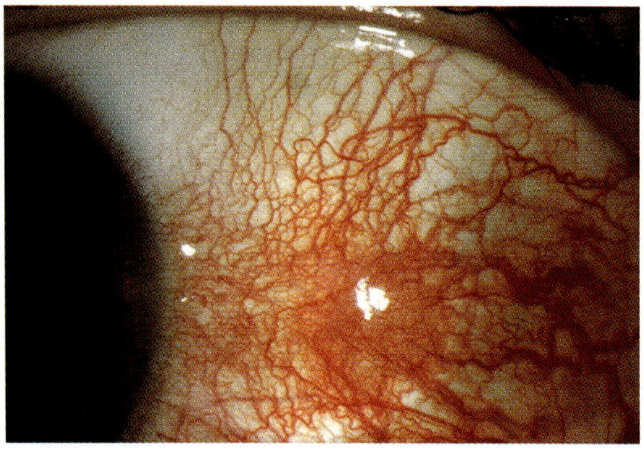

Plate 6-2

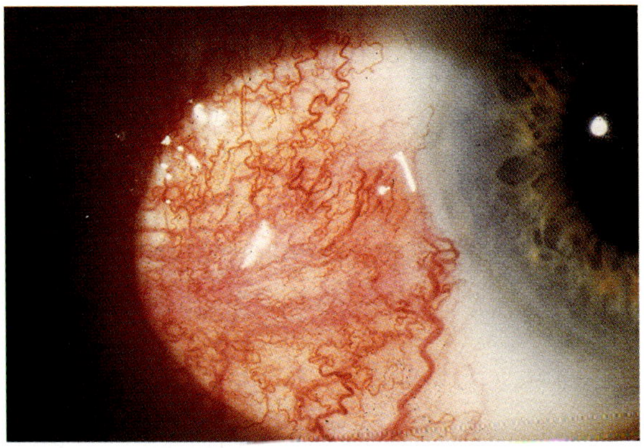

Plate 6-5

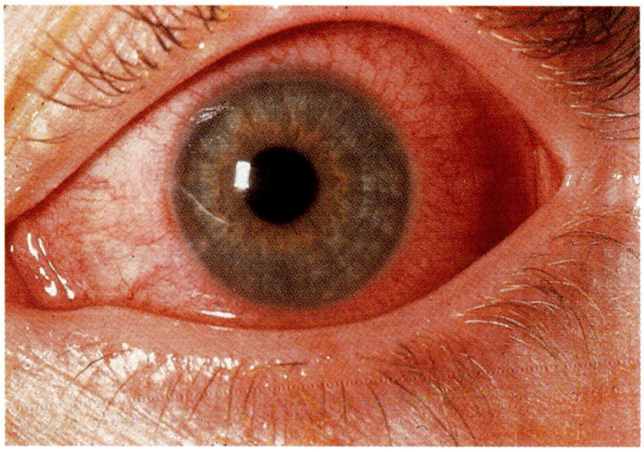

Plate 7-3

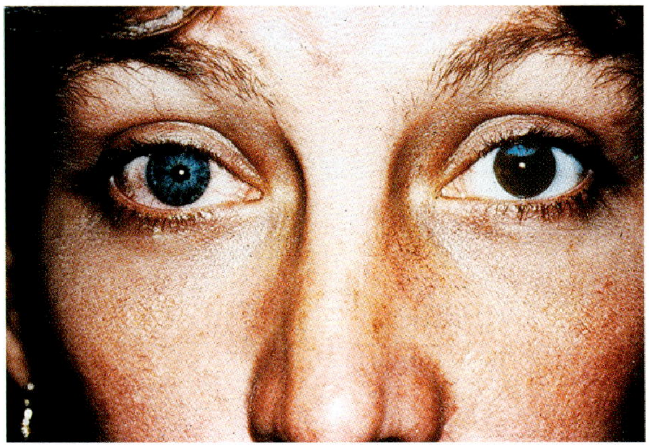

Plate 7-6

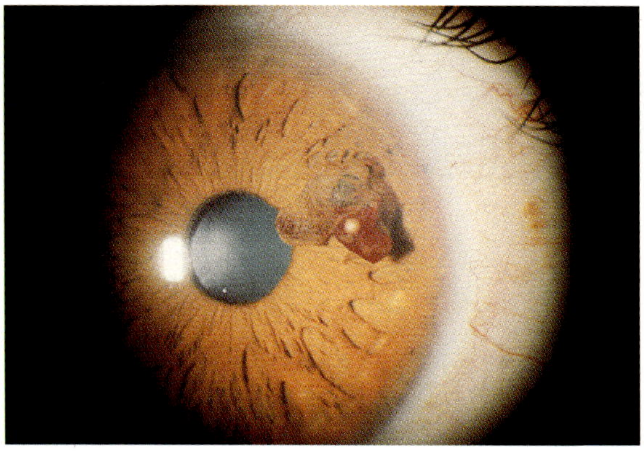

Plate 7-20

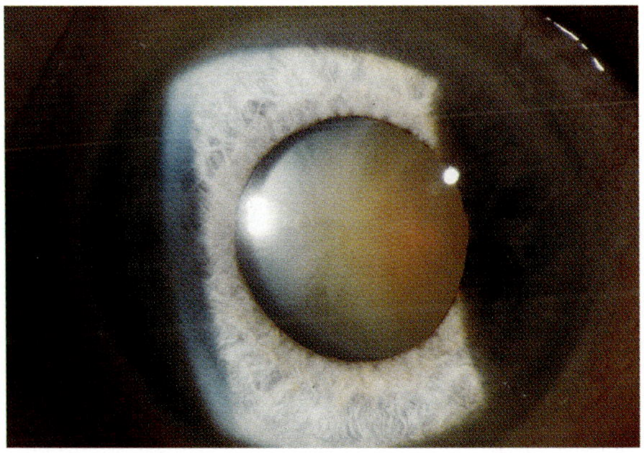

Plate 8-5

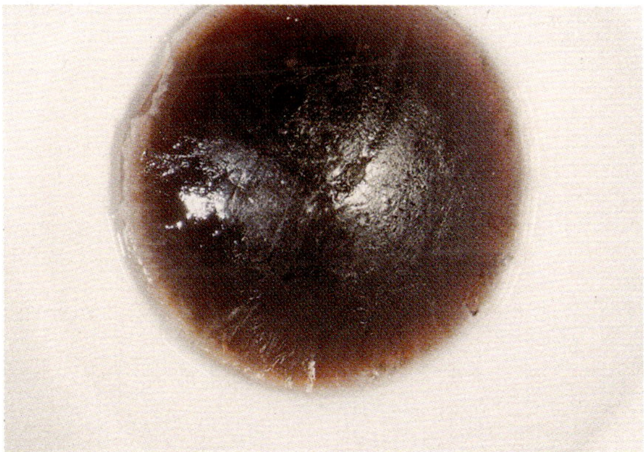

Plate 8-7

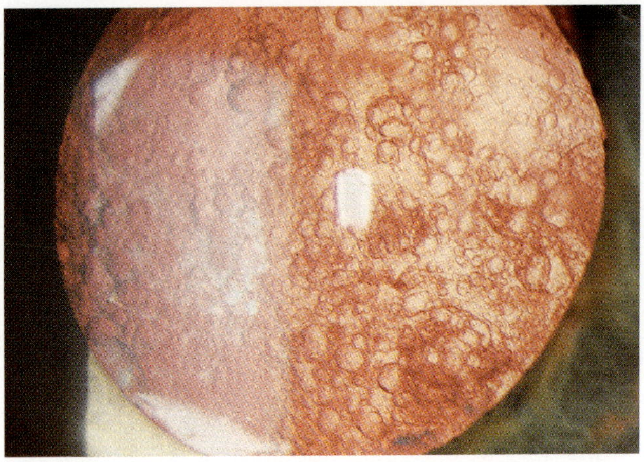

Plate 8-18

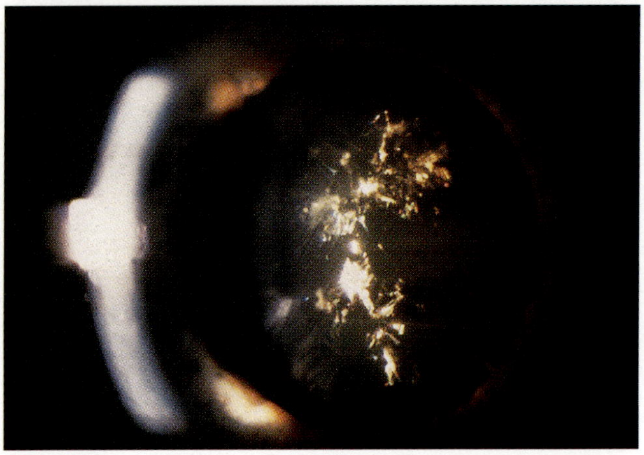

Plate 8-20

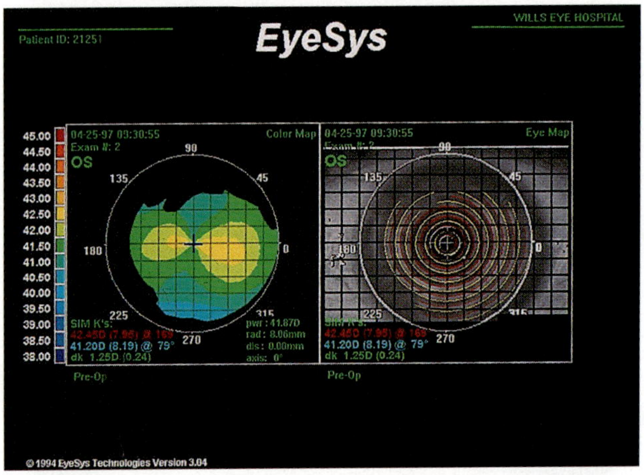

Plate 9-1

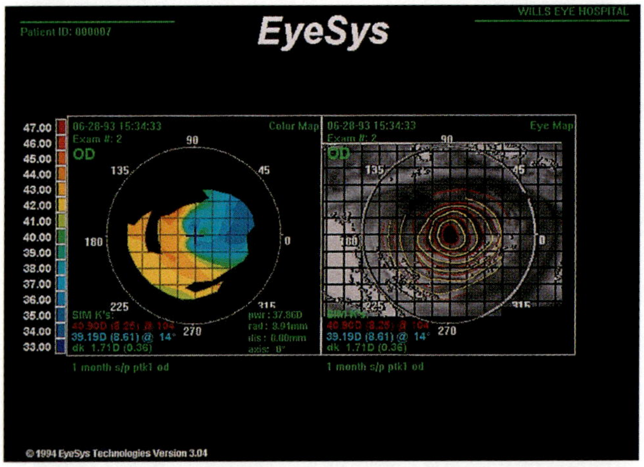

Plate 9-2

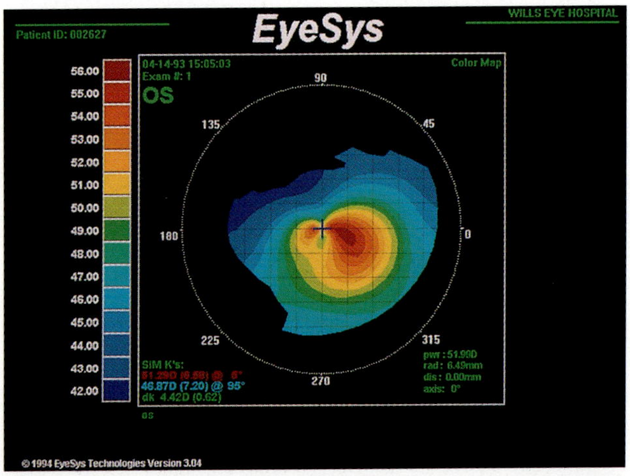

Plate 9-3

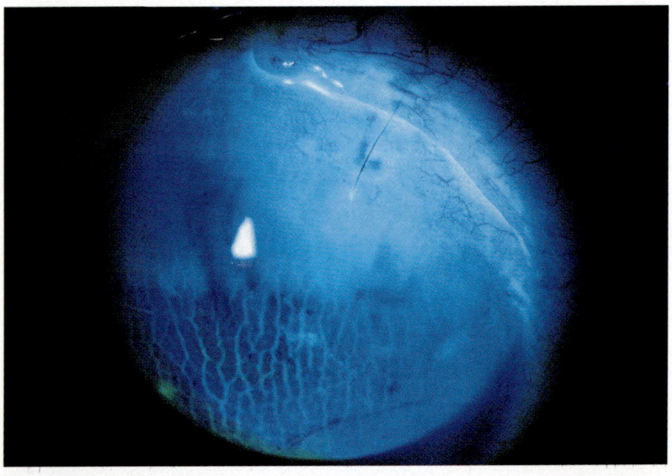

Plate 10-15

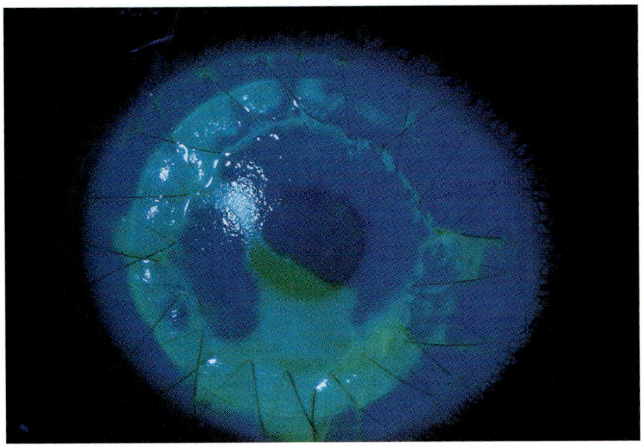

Plate 10-33

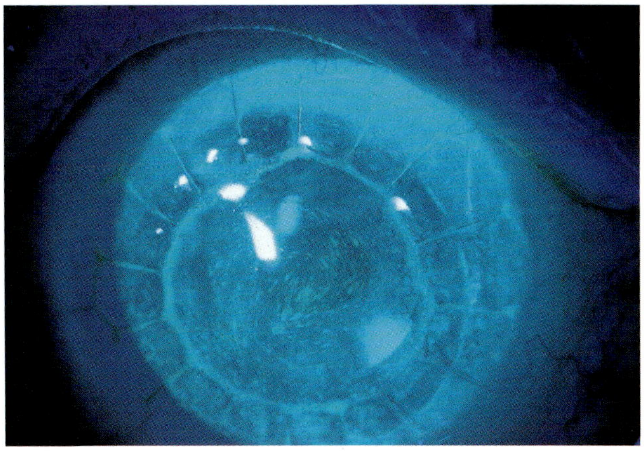

Plate 10-35

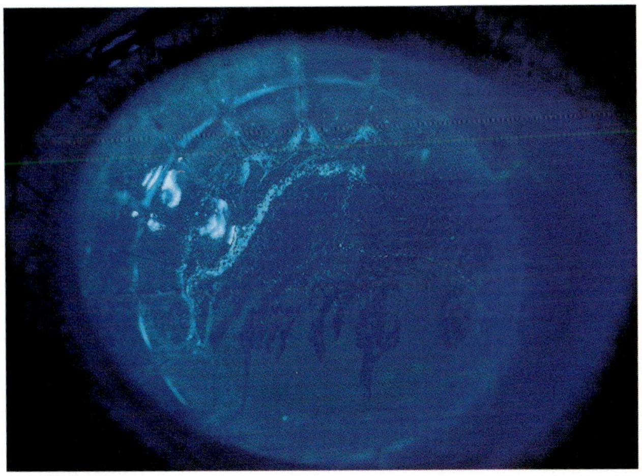

Plate 10-40

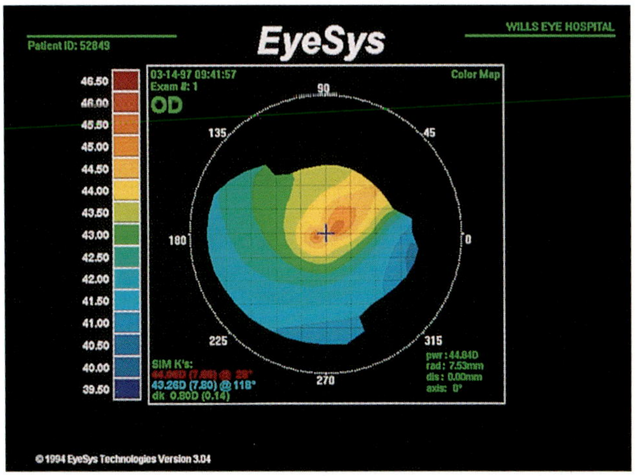

Plate 10-54

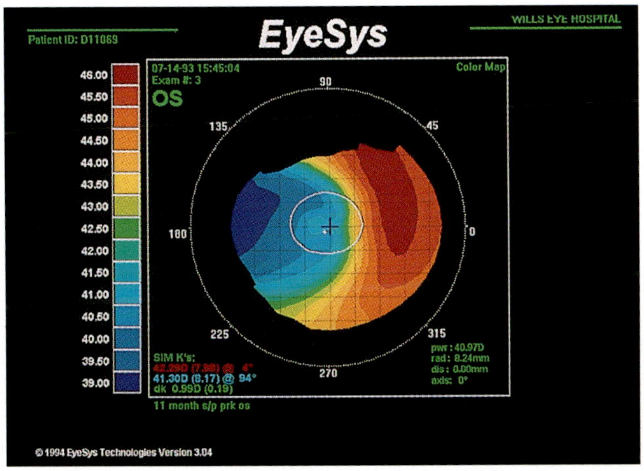

Plate 10-126

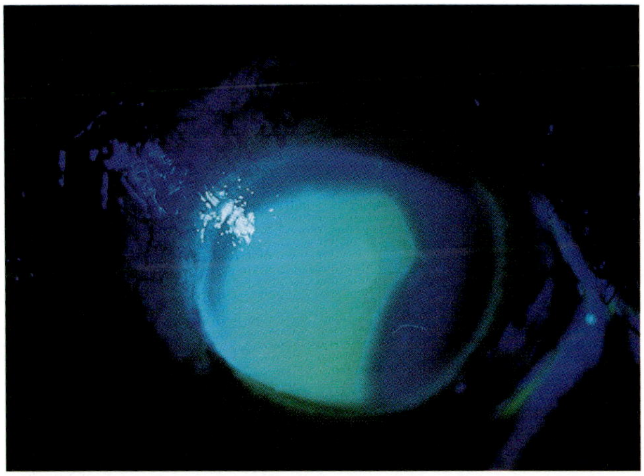

Plate 11-1

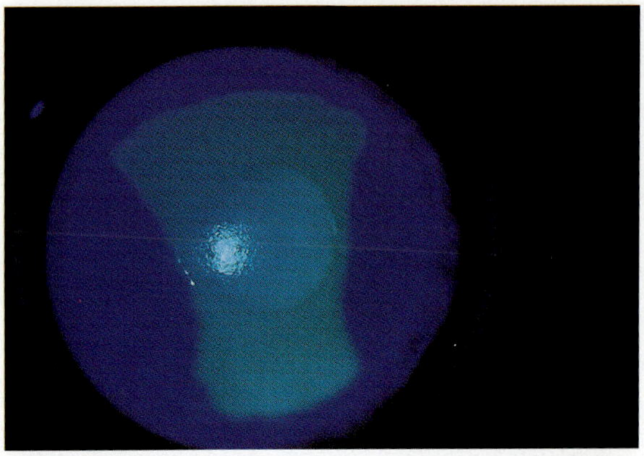

Plate 11-2

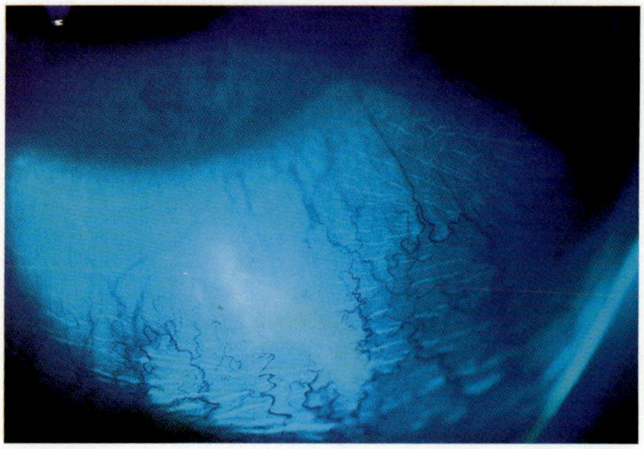

Plate 11-5

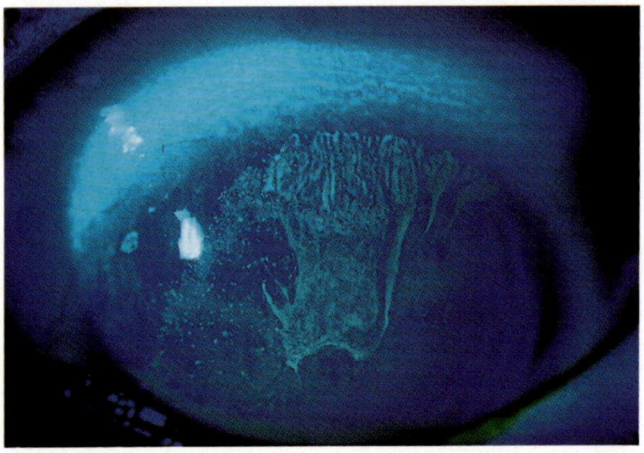

Plate 11-8

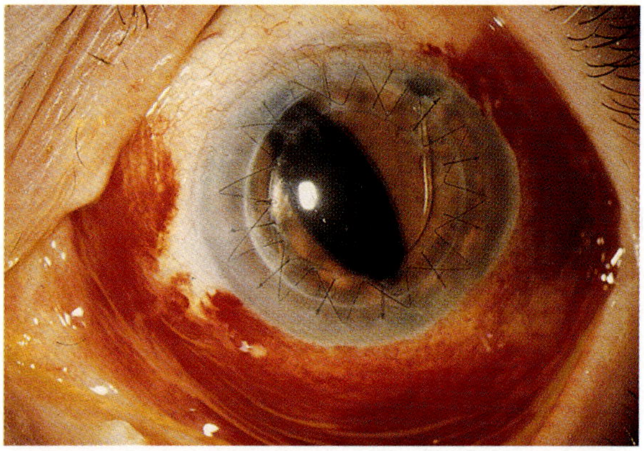

Plate 11-36

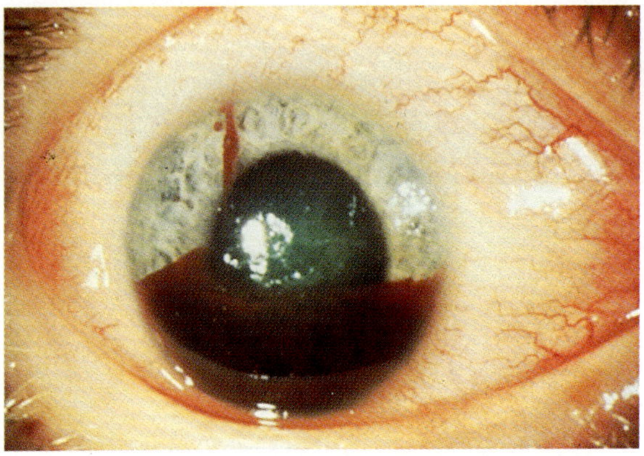

Plate 11-39

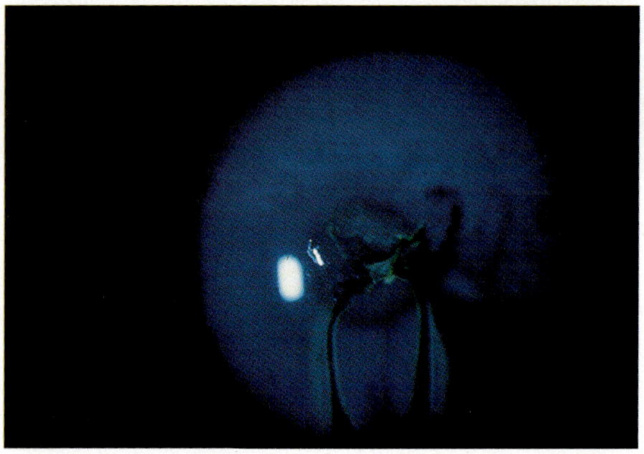

Plate 11-47

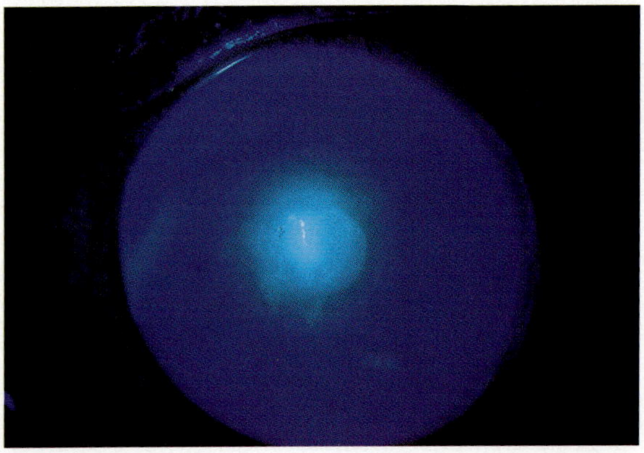

Plate 11-75

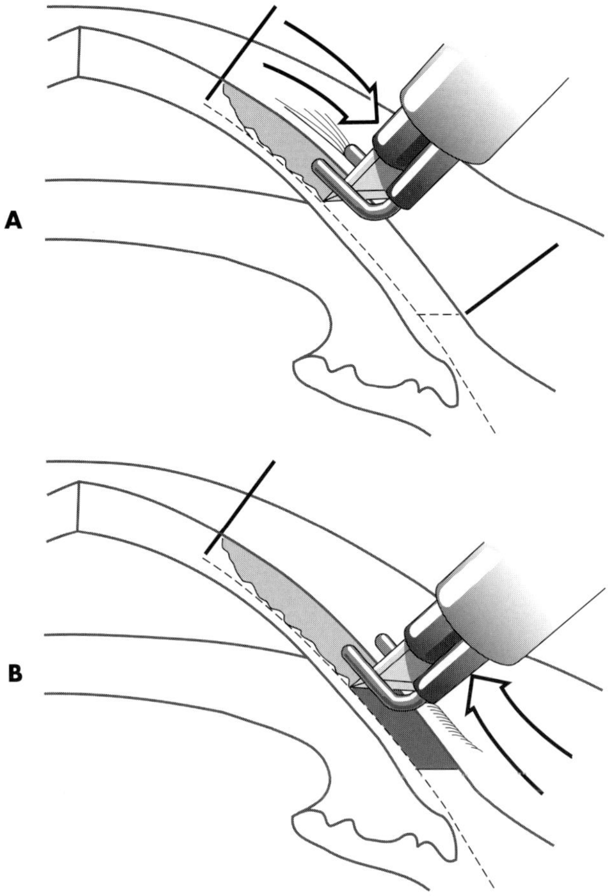

Fig. 10-114 Radial keratotomy. **A,** In the "combined" cutting technique, the initial incision ("American" cut) begins at the optical zone and proceeds toward the limbus. **B,** Without removing the blade from the cornea, the direction is reversed and the incision proceeds toward the optical zone ("Russian" cut). It stops at the optical zone because only the bottom of the blade cuts in this direction.

Box 10-15 Complications of Radial and Astigmatic Keratotomy

- Microperforation
- Macroperforation
- Incision into the clear zone or across the visual axis
- Infection of incisions and, rarely, endophthalmitis
- Traumatic rupture of incisions
- Late hyperopic drift (radial keratotomy)

(Fig. 10-115 and Box 10-15). Microperforations may be observed, but macroperforations require suturing. Incisions that extend into the central clear zone, and certainly those that cross the visual axis, are often associated with significant visual symptoms. It is rare for infections of the incisions (Figs. 10-116 and 10-117), and even more rare for endophthalmitis, to occur. When suspected, incision infections require aggressive treatment because the infection can quickly gain access to the anterior chamber. Crossed incisions can result in significant corneal scarring and surface irregularity (Fig. 10-118). Incisions that reach close to the limbus, especially when coupled with contact lens wear, can induce neovascularization into the RK incisions (Fig. 10-119).

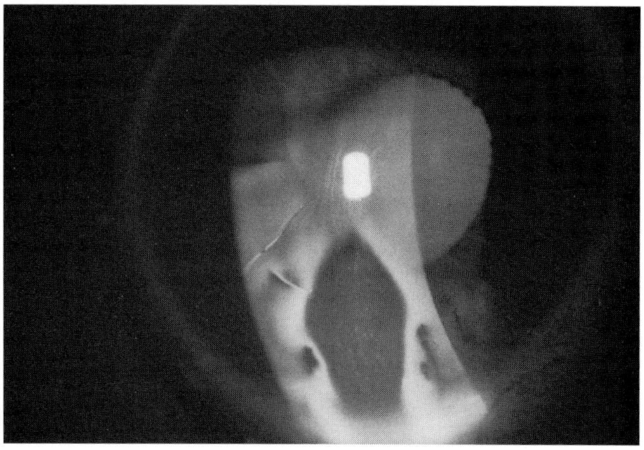

Fig. 10-115 Radial keratotomy macroperforation. Seidel-positive leak from the 6 o'clock radial incision.

The primary long-term problem with RK is refractive instability. Certain patients, especially those with smaller central clear zones, have symptomatic fluctuating vision and hyperopic drift. Patients with fluctuating vision can have vastly different refractions in the morning than in the evening. Long-term follow-up of patients with RK has demonstrated that 43% have at least 1 D of progressive hyperopia from 6 months to 10 years. Remarkably, this hyperopic drift does not seem to abate with time. Rupture of radial and astigmatic keratotomy incisions can also occur with trauma.

Excimer Laser Photorefractive Keratectomy

Another method to treat myopia, astigmatism, and hyperopia is excimer laser photorefractive keratectomy (PRK). In 1995 the FDA approved the excimer laser to treat up to 7 D of myopia at the corneal plane. It has since approved PRK for up to 12 D of myopia and 4 D of astigmatism at the spectacle plane. It recently approved PRK for up to +6 D of hyperopia at the spectacle plane. Advantages of PRK over RK include the wider range of treatable refractive errors, less fluctuating vision, and more stable long-term refraction. Ablation reaches a maximal depth of only approximately 25% corneal thickness (and usually much less) compared with close to 100% corneal thickness for RK, reducing the risk for traumatic

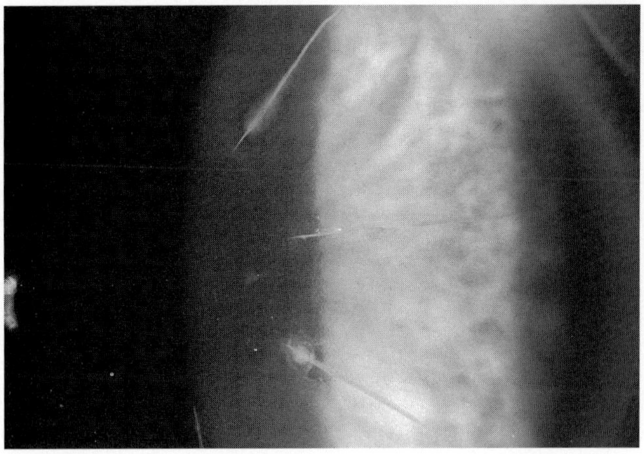

Fig. 10-116 Corneal infiltrates after radial keratotomy (RK). Corneal infiltrates are seen at the central ends of two RK incisions. The special concern is that organisms can easily progress through the incision to deep cornea or even the anterior chamber and cause a vision-threatening infection.

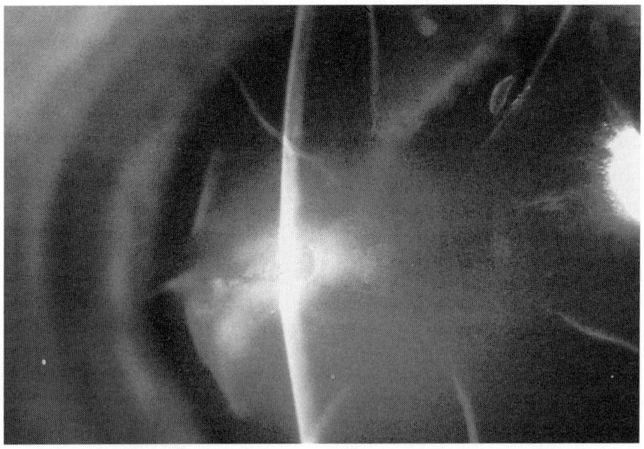

Fig. 10-117 Corneal ulceration after radial keratotomy (RK). Infectious keratitis can develop after RK. The 9 o'clock radial and adjacent T-cuts are both ulcerated with significant adjacent deep corneal infiltration. This infection requires intensive topical antibiotic treatment.

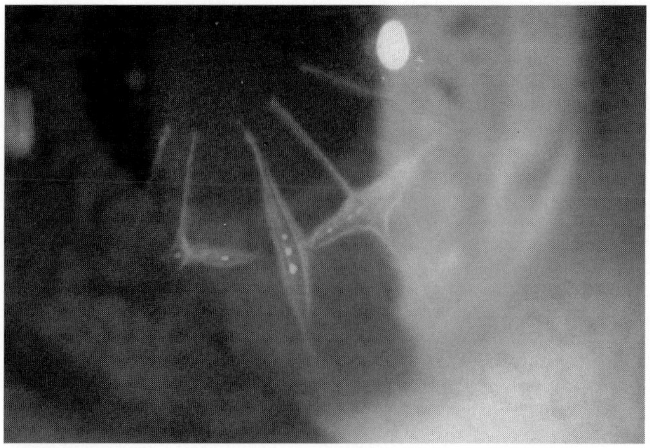

Fig. 10-118 Crossed incisions after radial and astigmatic keratotomy. This eye with 16 radial incisions has several intersecting T-cuts. When corneal incisions intersect, wound gaping and significant scarring often result.

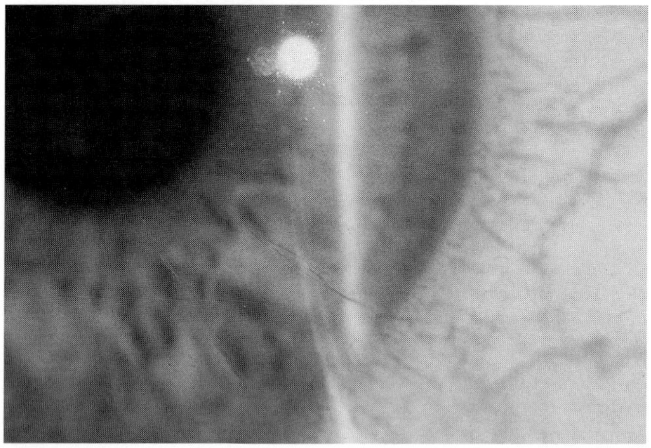

Fig. 10-119 Neovascularization into radial keratotomy (RK) incisions. Corneal neovascularization to multiple peripheral incisions in this eye after a 16-incision RK. This finding is more common in association with contact lens wear. This patient was undercorrected and wore extended wear soft contact lenses.

rupture of the cornea. Disadvantages of PRK compared with RK include more postoperative pain, slower visual recovery, and surgery in the visual axis, with greater potential for central corneal haze and scarring. Additionally, more postoperative topical corticosteroids are generally used after PRK than RK, increasing the risk for corticosteroid response glaucoma.

The exact technique for PRK varies by the specific laser and the surgeon (Box 10-16). The excimer laser machine must be calibrated and the centration checked before use. Anesthetic drops are administered to both of the patient's eyes, and the nonoperative eye is covered with an opaque shield. An eyelid speculum is placed in the operative eye, which is centered under the laser unit's operating microscope. Care should be taken to make sure the eye and the head are level with the floor. An epithelial mark the approximate size of the ablation zone is placed, centered on the pupil. The epithelium is debrided with either sharp or blunt instrumentation. Alternatively, the laser can be used to ablate the epithelium. A smooth Bowman's membrane with no residual epithelial debris in the ablation zone is critical. The laser is then centered over the pupil and the ablation performed (Fig. 10-120). The patient and surgeon must maintain excellent centration during the laser treatment. When astigmatism is being treated, the 3 and 9 o'clock axes are marked at the slit lamp before surgery and lined up appropriately under the laser.

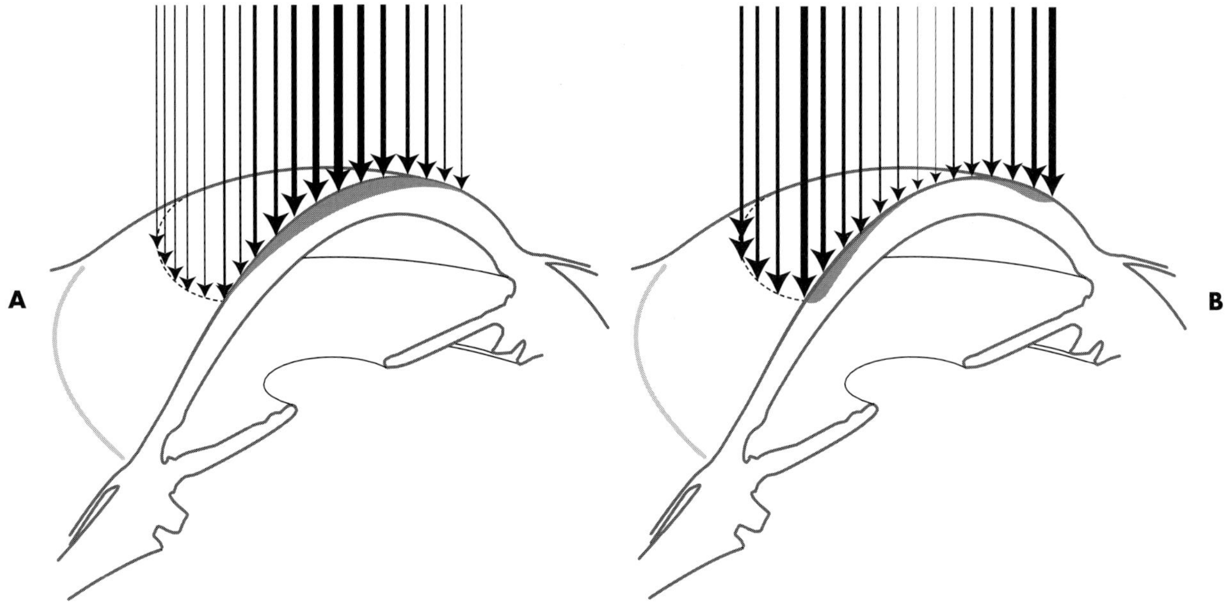

Fig. 10-120 Excimer laser photorefractive keratectomy (PRK) procedure. **A,** PRK for myopia. After epithelial removal, the excimer laser ablates more tissue centrally than peripherally to flatten the central cornea. **B,** PRK for hyperopia. After epithelial removal the excimer laser is used to ablate more tissue peripherally than centrally to steepen the central cornea.

Box 10-16 Major Steps of Excimer Laser Photorefractive Keratectomy

- Check the calibration and centration of the excimer laser unit and amount of refractive error to be treated
- Mark the 3 and 9 o'clock axes at the slit lamp if astigmatism is also being treated
- Make sure the head is level, center the eye under the laser, and tilt the head so the 3 and 9 o'clock axes are lined up with the reticule
- Mark and remove the epithelium over the ablation area
- Make sure all epithelium and debris are off Bowman's layer in the ablation zone
- Center the ablation over the pupil
- Ablate while maintaining centration over the pupil

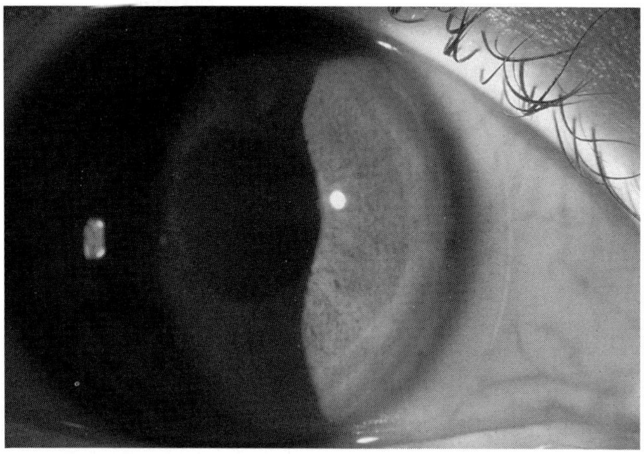

Fig. 10-121 Excimer laser photorefractive keratectomy (PRK). Postoperative day 1 after PRK. An approximately 3 × 4 mm central epithelial defect is covered with a bandage soft contact lens.

The postoperative regimen varies, but typically it includes a bandage soft contact lens and topical antibiotics, corticosteroids, NSAIDs, and preservative-free artificial teardrops. The bandage contact lens, antibiotic drops, and NSAID drops are discontinued after a few days, depending on the healing (Fig. 10-121). The corticosteroid drops are slowly tapered over 1 to 4 months, depending on the refractive results.

Early postoperative complications include delayed reepithelialization and infectious keratitis. Later complications include haze (Figs. 10-122 and 10-123), scarring (Figs. 10-124 and 10-125), irregular astigmatism, and decreased best-corrected vision. Visual side effects include glare and halos, especially in patients with large pupils and those with high degrees of myopia or astigmatism correction, or both. Decentered ablations can cause severe optical aberrations and monocular diplopia (Fig. 10-126). Rarely, the laser ablation is well centered, but asymmetric healing can create a functionally decentered ablation pattern. Consequently, it is recommended that computed corneal topographic analysis be performed approximately 1 month after surgery to assess the surgical

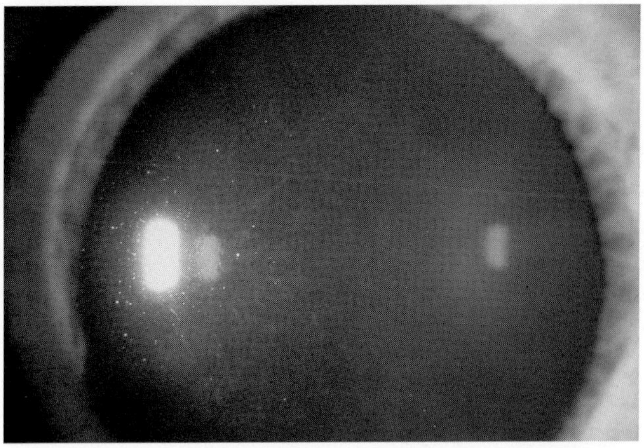

Fig. 10-122 Excimer laser photorefractive keratectomy (PRK) haze. Mild granular anterior stromal haze 1 month after PRK.

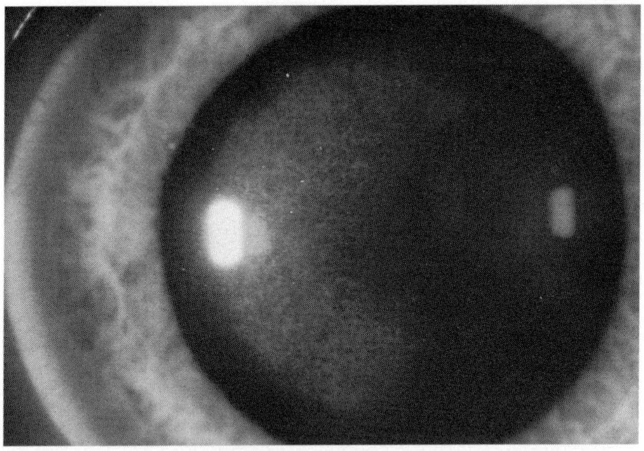

Fig. 10-123 Excimer laser photorefractive keratectomy (PRK) haze. Moderate reticular anterior stromal haze from the 6 to 12 o'clock positions 6 months after PRK. The central cornea is relatively clear, and the patient has excellent uncorrected vision and minimal visual symptoms.

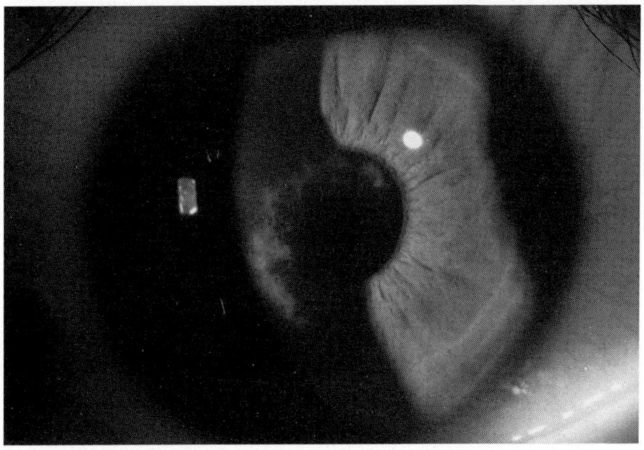

Fig. 10-124 Excimer laser photorefractive keratectomy (PRK) scar. Dense reticular corneal scar in the mid-periphery of the ablation 18 months after PRK. Mild irregular astigmatism is induced.

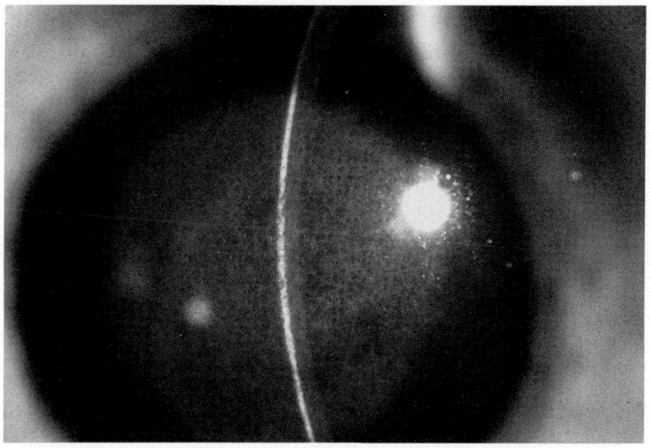

Fig. 10-125 Excimer laser photorefractive keratectomy (PRK) haze. Moderate central corneal haze over the entire 6 mm ablation zone 6 months after PRK. Significant associated regression and decreased uncorrected and best-corrected vision improved moderately with topical corticosteroids.

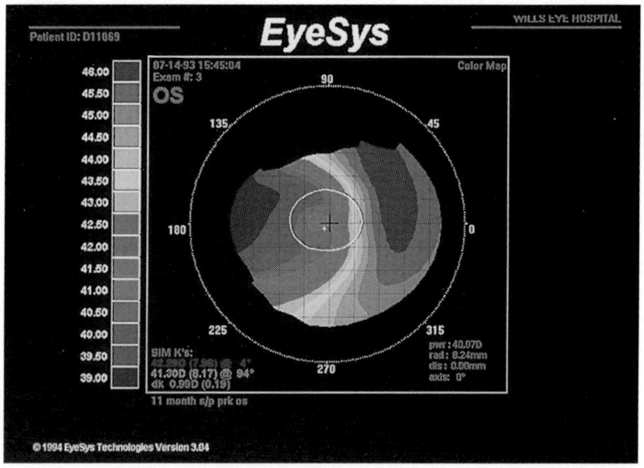

Fig. 10-126 Excimer laser photorefractive keratectomy (PRK) decentered ablation. Computed corneal topographic analysis of an eye after PRK. The scale on the left side indicates the dioptric power of each color. The large circular blue area nasally corresponds to the area of excimer laser ablation. The ablation is significantly decentered. The patient has monocular diplopia and triplopia. (See color plate.)

ablation centration. Intraocular pressure elevations can result from prolonged corticosteroid use. Retreatment for haze, undercorrection, or overcorrection can be performed on eyes with stable refractions 6 months after surgery at the earliest.

Laser In Situ Keratomileusis

Building on the older techniques of myopic keratomileusis with a cryolathe and automated lamellar keratoplasty, LASIK combines the advantages of intrastromal tissue removal with the precision of the excimer laser. In

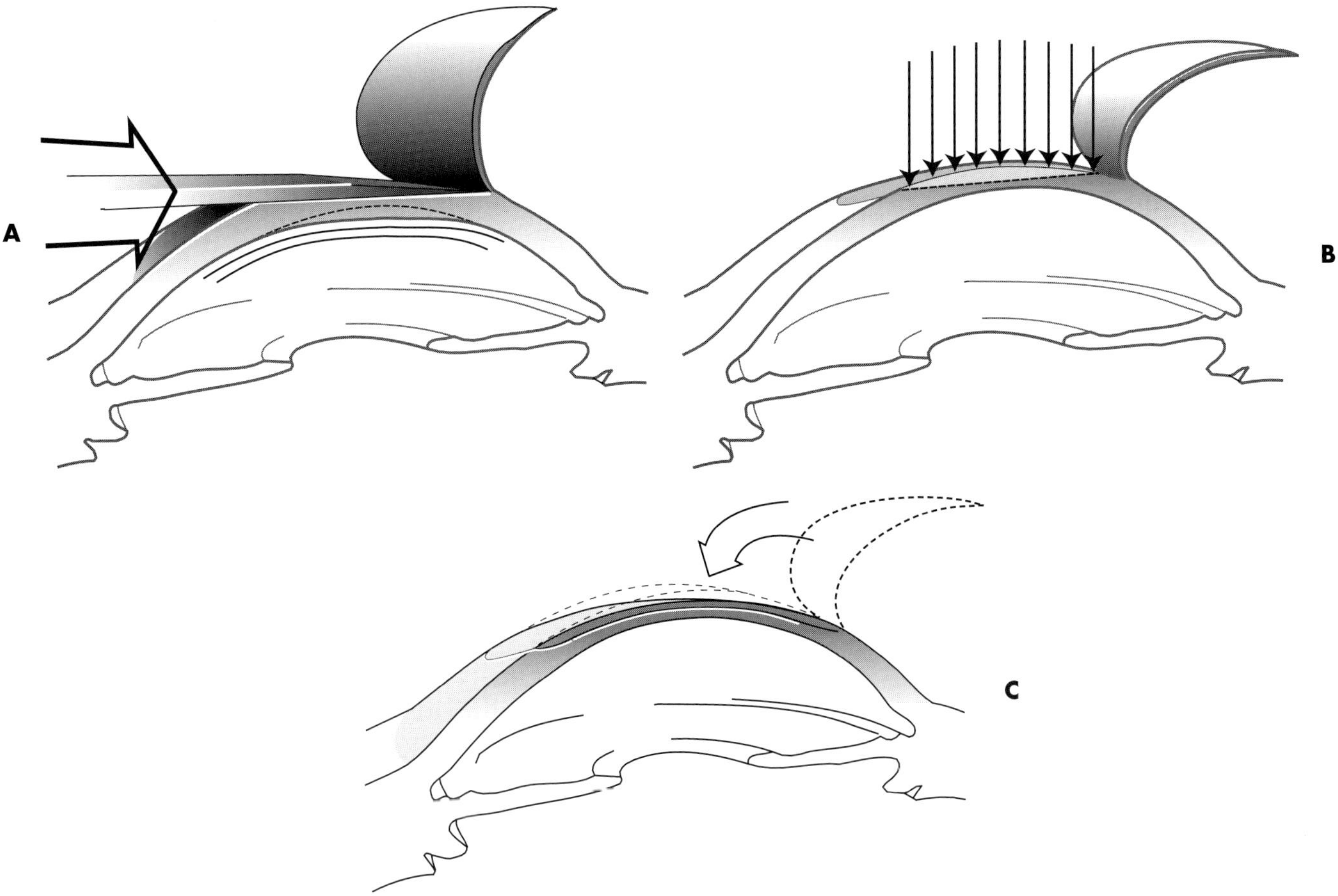

Fig. 10-127 Laser in situ keratomileusis (LASIK) procedure. **A,** After a suction ring is placed to pressurize the eye, a microkeratome is used to fashion a flap of superficial cornea attached by a small hinge. **B,** The flap is reflected, and the excimer laser is used to treat the corneal stroma. **C,** The flap is replaced, the interface irrigated, and the flap is allowed to adhere without sutures.

this surgery, a microkeratome is used to create a lamellar corneal flap, which is moved to the side to allow excimer laser ablation of the stroma. Once the laser ablation is complete, the flap is replaced and allowed to adhere without sutures (Fig. 10-127). The advantages of LASIK over PRK include less postoperative pain and faster visual recovery because of the minimal epithelial defect. Additionally, the risk for corneal haze is smaller, most likely because of the preservation of Bowman's membrane centrally. In general LASIK involves less postoperative medication and fewer follow-up visits. When it is compared with PRK, its disadvantages include the added risk for intraoperative and postoperative flap complications (Table 10-3).

The procedure involves similar laser calibration, patient positioning, and anesthesia to PRK (Box 10-17). The microkeratome must be meticulously maintained and assembled to ensure a good result. Some surgeons

Table 10-3 Comparison of photorefractive keratectomy (PRK) and laser in situ keratomileusis (LASIK)

Feature	PRK	LASIK
Longer follow-up data	++	
Less pain		+++
Faster visual recovery		++
Less postoperative corneal haze		++
Less technically difficult	++	
Less machine dependent	+	
IOP not elevated during procedure	+++	
Less postoperative medication		++
Fewer postoperative visits		++
Less dependent on corneal healing		++
No potential flap complications	+++	
Better results in higher myopes		+

IOP, Intraocular pressure.

drape the eye. The eyelid speculum must create a wide opening to ensure unimpeded movement of the microkeratome. The epithelium in the area of flap incision (temporally with a nasally hinged flap) is marked with dye. This mark allows appropriate replacement of the flap, especially should a free cap occur. A suction ring is placed on the eye, increasing the intraocular pressure to at least 65 to 70 mm Hg. The eye is checked for adequate suction, the microkeratome is engaged in the suction ring, and the flap is created. After the suction ring is removed, the flap is lifted and moved to the side. The stroma is cleared of epithelial debris and excess fluid, and the ablation is performed as in PRK. After the ablation the flap is gently replaced and the interface irrigated. The flap is allowed to adhere for several minutes. Any small epithelial tears should be replaced. If a significant epithelial defect is present, a bandage soft contact lens may be helpful. Once the flap is secure, the eyelid speculum is cautiously removed with care taken to not dislodge the flap. The patient is examined at the slit lamp to make sure the flap is in excellent position and that the interface is clear (Fig. 10-128). If not, the flap must be repositioned or the interface cleared at that time.

Box 10-17 Major Steps of Laser In Situ Keratomileusis (LASIK)

- Laser setup and patient positioning are identical to those for photorefractive keratectomy (PRK)
- Adjust the attempted correction per the LASIK nomogram
- Open the eyelid speculum wide to expose the inferior and superior sclera
- Mark the edge of the cornea where the flap will begin
- Secure the suction ring and check the intraocular pressure
- Engage the microkeratome and create the flap
- Release suction
- Move the flap to the side
- Make sure all epithelium and debris are off the ablation zone
- Ablate as per PRK
- Replace the flap
- Irrigate the interface
- Let the flap adhere
- Carefully remove the eyelid speculum, and check the flap and interface

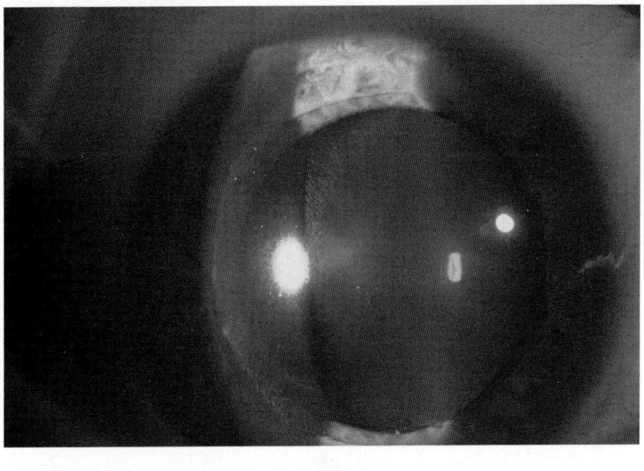

Fig. 10-128 Laser in situ keratomileusis (LASIK). Two weeks after uncomplicated LASIK with a nasal hinge in this right eye. The semicircular edge of the LASIK flap is evident temporally. The flap is in excellent position and is healing well.

Postoperative treatment is typically with antibiotic, corticosteroid, and preservative-free teardrops. The antibiotic and corticosteroid drops are usually discontinued within a week, but the tears are continued for several weeks to months. It is of prime importance that the patient not touch or rub the eye for several days because the flap may become dislodged. The vision is generally good on the first postoperative day and improves over the ensuing several weeks.

Complications of LASIK include many of the complications of PRK (Table 10-4). Specific to LASIK are the flap complications. During creation of the flap, the microkeratome may stop midway, leaving a partial flap, or it can create a flap that is too thin or even buttonholed. In these instances, it is best simply to replace the flap without any laser treatment. A new, slightly thicker flap can generally be created a minimum of 3 months later. The flap hinge can be amputated, leaving a free cap. Laser ablation can proceed, but special attention must be given to cap replacement and adherence. If the microkeratome is not appropriately assembled, the blade may enter the anterior chamber and even damage the iris and lens. New microkeratome designs significantly decrease the risk for this dreadful complication. After surgery the flap may dislodge and require replacement (Fig. 10-129). Infections under the flap are rare but may develop

Table 10-4 General complications of refractive surgery

Complication	RK	PRK	LASIK
Undercorrection	+	+	+
Overcorrection	+	+	+
Glare	+	+	+
Halos	+	+	+
Starburst	+	−	−
Monocular diplopia	+	+	+
Decreased best corrected vision	+	+	+
Fluctuating vision	++	−	−
Progression of effect	++	−	−
Regression	+	+	+
Induced astigmatism	+	+	+
Central corneal haze	−	+	−

(Fig. 10-130). Although mild interface debris is common and causes no symptoms, significant interface opacities can affect vision. Diffuse lamellar keratitis (also called Sands of Sahara Syndrome) is an inflammatory reaction at the level of the flap interface. It generally begins 1 to 5 days after surgery with diminished vision, redness, pain, and photophobia. Slit-lamp examination reveals mild to severe granularity and haziness of the flap interface. Patients with mild to moderate inflammation can be treated with intensive topical corticosteroids (e.g., 1% prednisolone acetate every 1 to 2 hours), but those with severe inflammation may require lifting of the flap and irrigation of the interface in addition to topical corticosteroids.

Prolonged epithelial defects involving the flap can also cause flap melt and scarring, most commonly in eyes with significant anterior basement membrane dystrophy. Epithelial defects at the edge of the flap predispose to epithelial ingrowth, especially after LASIK enhancements. Epithelium may grow under the flap, causing corneal surface irregularity and diminished vision (Fig. 10-131). A thick area of epithelial ingrowth can impede vision and even cause flap necrosis. Large and progressive areas of epithelial ingrowth should be removed by lifting the flap and scraping both the stromal bed and the undersurface of the flap. Microstriae are commonly seen and do not appear to affect visual acuity (Fig. 10-132).

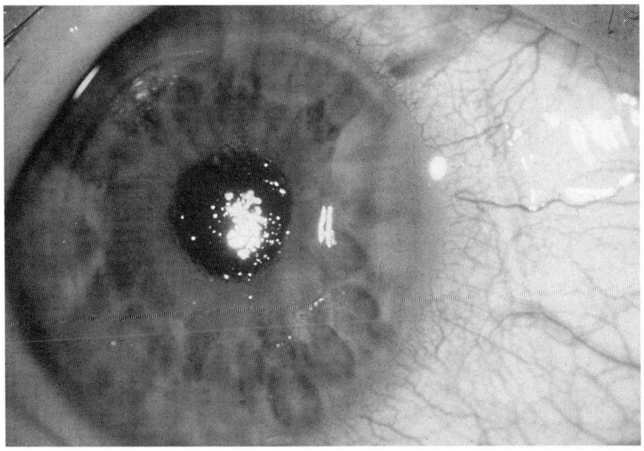

Fig. 10-129 Dislodged laser in situ keratomileusis (LASIK) flap. One day after uncomplicated LASIK, the patient felt pain after rubbing the right eye. A dislodged flap can be seen folded upon itself but still attached at the nasal hinge. The central cornea demonstrates an irregular light reflex. The flap was successfully reapproximated and adhered well.

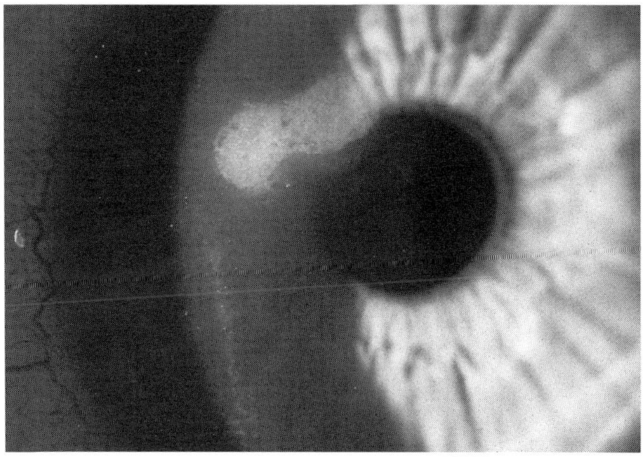

Fig. 10-131 Epithelial ingrowth after laser in situ keratomileusis (LASIK). A gray-white opacity of epithelial ingrowth is seen in the LASIK interface. It slowly enlarged and caused irregular astigmatism. The flap was lifted, and the epithelium was removed from the stromal side and the flap side and did not recur.

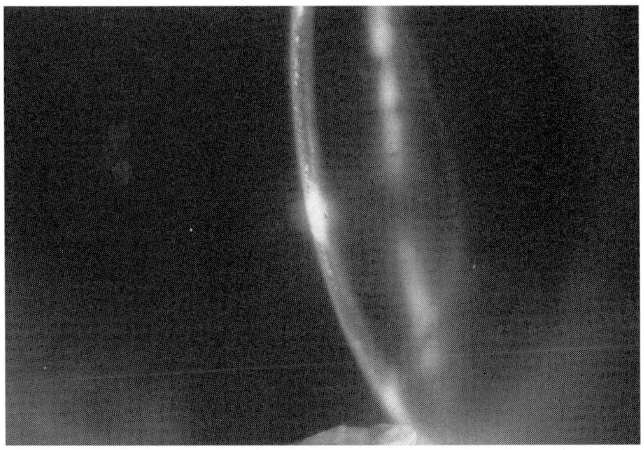

Fig. 10-130 Laser in situ keratomileusis (LASIK) infection. A small corneal ulcer developed after LASIK. Mild surrounding corneal edema was treated with intensive topical antibiotics and resolved.

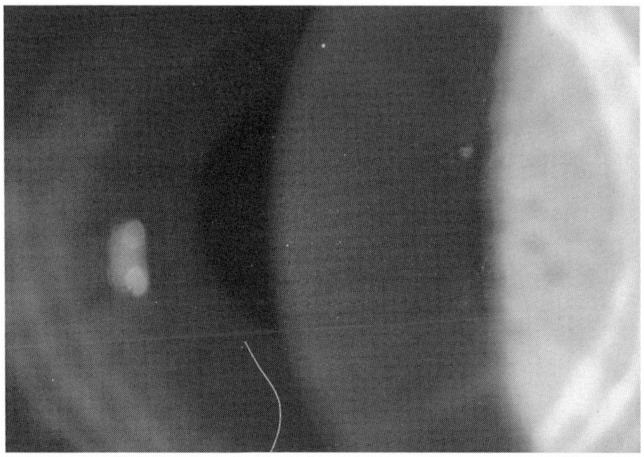

Fig. 10-132 Microstriae after laser in situ keratomileusis (LASIK). Multiple horizontal microstriae are seen in this eye 3 months after uncomplicated LASIK. Microstriae do not appear to affect vision, whereas macrostriae are associated with irregular astigmatism.

Macrostriae and other flap irregularities can cause irregular astigmatism. Reoperations for stable undercorrection or overcorrection can be performed by lifting the flap and reablating. Reoperations ideally take place 2 to 6 months after the original surgery, when the refraction is usually stable and the flap is still easily lifted.

CONCLUSION

Anterior segment surgery encompasses a wide variety of techniques varying from straightforward to complex. The principles of appropriate preoperative evaluation,

MAJOR POINTS

Although cataract surgery is generally extremely successful, it is associated with potentially serious complications.

Certain complications, such as cystoid macular edema or retinal detachment, may develop after uncomplicated cataract surgery.

Cataract surgery (or any intraocular surgery) may rarely result in blindness of the eye if a serious complication such as expulsive hemorrhage or endophthalmitis develops.

A cataractous lens may be removed in toto (intracapsular method) or the lens nucleus may be removed in one piece (planned extracapsular method) or the lens nucleus may be fragmented and removed in small pieces (phacoemulsification technique).

When inadequate capsular support exists for safe routine implantation of a posterior chamber intraocular lens, an anterior chamber intraocular lens or a sutured (to iris or sclera) posterior chamber intraocular lens may alternatively be implanted.

Due to loose zonular attachments, pseudoexfoliation is associated with increased complications during cataract surgery including vitreous loss and inadequate capsular support for a posterior chamber intraocular lens.

When vitreous loss is encountered during cataract surgery, an anterior vitrectomy is required to clear the vitreous from the anterior chamber and wound.

Significant anterior chamber and vitreal inflammation after cataract surgery may signal early endophthalmitis and requires immediate workup and possible treatment.

Corneal donor information needs to be reviewed and the tissue examined preoperatively by the surgeon.

Flieringa ring (or equivalent) placement prior to penetrating keratoplasty is extremely helpful in aphakic eyes, eyes after vitrectomy, and eyes undergoing cataract extraction, and is mandatory in infants and children.

All iris-fixated and closed-loop anterior chamber intraocular lenses and all unstable lenses should be removed during corneal transplantation for bullous keratopathy.

Postoperative epithelial defects in a corneal transplant not responding to medical treatment should undergo a lateral tarsorrhaphy before any stromal melting occurs.

The primary symptoms of corneal graft rejection are redness, discomfort, photophobia, and decreased vision, but patients may be asymptomatic.

Signs of corneal graft rejection, including subepithelial infiltrates, new anterior chamber reaction, keratic precipitates, and corneal edema should be checked for on each postoperative visit.

All exposed corneal transplant sutures should be removed at the time of discovery.

Excimer laser phototherapeutic keratectomy can be extremely effective for elevated and anterior stromal corneal pathology, especially Reis-Bücklers', granular, and lattice corneal dystrophies.

Conjunctival flap surgery is an effective and often underutilized procedure for chronic corneal ulcerations and painful bullous keratopathy in eyes with poor visual potential that have not perforated.

Keys to decreasing the risk of recurrence of pterygia after excision and conjunctival autograft are the creation of a smooth cornea and limbus in the area of excision and the generous use of postoperative topical corticosteroids.

Conjunctival flaps and autografts need to be relatively thin, but without buttonholes, and sutured flat to the surface without excessive tension.

When squamous cell tumors of the conjunctiva recur, it is usually at the limbus.

Cyanoacrylate corneal glue can be extremely effective in the treatment of small impending and completed corneal perforations. A bandage soft contact lens must be used over the glue.

Refractive surgery patients should be out of contact lenses prior to evaluation. They should have stable refractions, essentially normal eyes, and regular corneas. They must have an understanding of the various refractive surgery options and their respective benefits and risks, in addition to realistic expectations regarding the outcomes of surgery.

Prior to PRK and LASIK, the surgeon needs to check the calibration and centration of the excimer laser, and for LASIK, the assembly and function of the microkeratome.

informed consent, sterile preparation, excellent surgical technique, and appropriate postoperative management apply to all of these surgeries. Although not all anterior segment surgeons have to master all these procedures, they should be aware of the benefits and risks to give their patients the best ophthalmic care.

SUGGESTED READINGS

Aldredge OC, Krachmer JH: Clinical types of corneal transplant rejection: Their manifestations, frequency, preoperative correlates and treatment, *Arch Ophthalmol* 99:599-604, 1981.

American Academy of Ophthalmology: Excimer laser photorefractive keratectomy (PRK) for myopia and astigmatism, *Ophthalmology* 106:422-437, 1999.

Chiou AG, Florakis GJ, Kazim M: Management of conjunctival cicatrizing diseases and severe ocular surface dysfunction, *Surv Ophthalmol* 43:19-46, 1998.

Collaborative Corneal Transplantation Studies Research Group (CCTS): Effectiveness of histocompatibility matching in high-risk corneal transplantation, *Arch Ophthalmol* 110: 1392-1403, 1992.

Croasdale CR, Schwartz GS, Malling JV, Holland EJ: Keratolimbal allograft: recommendations for tissue procurement and preparation by eye banks, and for standard surgical procedure, *Cornea* 18:52-58, 1999.

Dinh R, Rapuano CJ, Cohen EJ, Laibson PR: Recurrence of corneal dystrophy after excimer laser phototherapeutic keratectomy, *Ophthalmology* 106:1490-1497, 1999.

Endophthalmitis Vitrectomy Study Group: Results of endophthalmitis vitrectomy study: a randomized trial of immediate vitrectomy and of intravenous antibiotics for the treatment of postoperative bacterial endophthalmitis, *Arch Ophthalmol* 113:1479-1496, 1995.

Gimbel HV, Penno EE, van Westenbrugge JA, et al: Incidence and management of intraoperative and early postoperative complications in 1000 consecutive laser in situ keratomileusis cases, *Ophthalmology* 105:1839-1848, 1998.

Gimbel HV, van Westenbrugge JA, Penno EE, et al: Simultaneous bilateral laser in situ keratomileusis, *Ophthalmology* 106: 1461-1468, 1999.

Holland EJ, Schwartz GS: The evolution of epithelial transplantation for severe ocular surface disease and a proposed classification system, *Cornea* 15:549-556, 1996.

Kenyon KR, Tseng SCG: Limbal autograft transplantation for ocular surface disease/disorders, *Ophthalmology* 96:709-723, 1989.

Musch DC, Farjo AA, Meyer RF, et al: Assessment of health-related quality of life after corneal transplantation, *Am J Ophthalmol* 124:1-8, 1997.

Pérez-Santonja JJ, Sakla HF, Cardona C, et al: Corneal sensitivity after photorefractive keratectomy and laser in situ keratomileusis for low myopia, *Am J Ophthalmol* 127:497-504, 1999.

Rapuano CJ: Excimer laser phototherapeutic keratectomy: long-term results and practical considerations, *Cornea* 16:151-157, 1997.

Rowsey JJ: Ten caveats in keratorefractive surgery, *Ophthalmology* 90:148-155, 1983.

Roy R, Des Marchais B, Bazin R, et al: Role of ABO and Lewis blood group antigens in donor-recipient compatibility of corneal transplantation rejection, *Ophthalmology* 104:508-512, 1997.

Rozsíval P, Feuermannová A: Retreatment after photorefractive keratectomy for low myopia, *Ophthalmology* 105:1189-1193, 1998.

Rubinfeld RS, Pfister RR, Stein RM, et al: Serious complications of topical mitomycin C after pterygium surgery, *Ophthalmology* 99:1647-1654, 1992.

Seiler T, McDonnell PJ: Excimer laser photorefractive keratectomy, *Surv Ophthalmol* 40:89-118, 1995.

Starck T, Kenyon KR, Serrano F: Conjunctival autograft for primary and recurrent pterygia: surgical techniques and problem management, *Cornea* 10:196-202, 1991.

Tseng SCG, Prabhasawat P, Lee SH: Amniotic membrane transplantation for conjunctival surface reconstruction, *Am J Ophthalmol* 124:765-774, 1997.

Waring GO III, Carr JD, Stulting RD, et al: Prospective randomized comparison of simultaneous and sequential bilateral laser in situ keratomileusis for the correction of myopia, *Ophthalmology* 106:732-738, 1999.

Waring GO III, Lynn MJ, McDonnell PJ, PERK Study Group: Results of the prospective evaluation of radial keratotomy (PERK) study 10 years after surgery, *Arch Ophthalmol* 112: 1298-1308, 1994.

CHAPTER 11

Anterior Segment Trauma

Trauma to the anterior segment is a leading cause of emergency department visits and subsequent visual loss. Although traumatic injuries affect persons of all ages, people younger than 18 and older than 70 years are at greatest risk. Additionally males are more likely to experience trauma than females. Injuries can range from mild chemical keratitis and corneal abrasions to devastating ruptured globes and intraocular foreign bodies. Minor trauma usually results in an excellent visual outcome, whereas severe trauma can be blinding. In all patients after ocular trauma, but particularly in children, when an adequate examination cannot be accomplished, an evaluation under anesthesia should be performed.

Anterior segment trauma has numerous causes. Occupational and sports ocular injuries are some of the most frequently encountered in emergency departments. Air guns, BB guns, and physical assault are other common causes of ocular trauma. Motor vehicle accidents are often associated with eye injuries; though air bags can save the head and face from grave injury, they have been associated with significant ocular damage. Falling is another cause of ocular trauma, especially in the elderly, in whom it may cause wound dehiscence after previous intraocular surgery. Many of these injuries, particularly occupational and sports injuries, can be prevented with consistent use of protective eyewear. It is imperative that all physicians educate their patients regarding the prevention of ocular trauma.

CORNEAL ABRASION

Corneal abrasion, among the most prevalent ocular injuries, has many different causes, commonly a fingernail, paper cut, tree branch, or mascara brush. The trauma tears a portion of the epithelial layer from the cornea. It breaks the attachments of the epithelial basal cells to the basement membrane and the underlying Bowman's layer. If Bowman's membrane is not damaged, the abrasion typically heals without scarring, but scarring likely develops if Bowman's layer or the underlying stroma is also damaged.

Corneal abrasion can be suspected by the history. The patient generally knows exactly when the injury occurred and what caused it. Typical symptoms are significant pain, foreign body sensation, photophobia, and tearing. The pain may be so intense that the patient may not be able to open the eye to check the vision. A drop of topical anesthetic can be extremely valuable in obtaining an accurate assessment of visual acuity and a complete ocular examination. Although the patient may simply have a corneal abrasion, the examiner must perform a complete ocular examination to rule out more extensive damage from the trauma, especially because children (and some adults) may not provide the most accurate or complete history of the injury.

Penlight evaluation may reveal an irregular corneal reflex. Slit-lamp examination typically demonstrates an area of epithelial loss. The epithelial defect is best seen with fluorescein staining and a cobalt blue light (Figs. 11-1 and 11-2). Flaps of loose epithelium may be present. The size

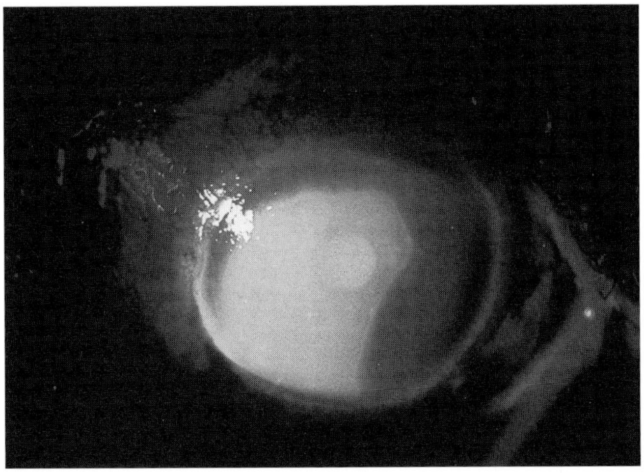

Fig. 11-1 Corneal abrasion. With use of a cobalt blue light, after the instillation of topical fluorescein dye, a large epithelial defect is seen centrally. (See color plate.)

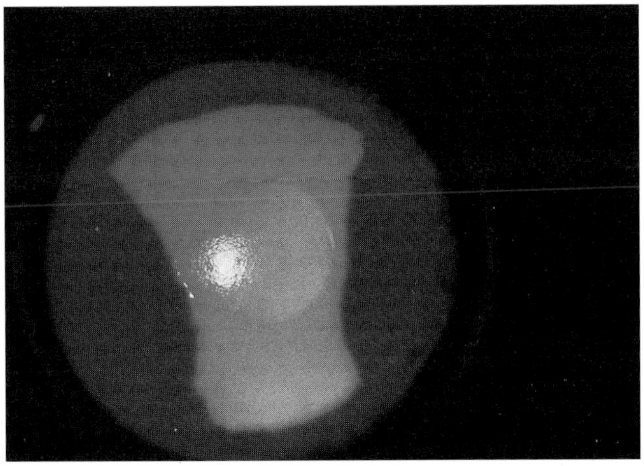

Fig. 11-2 Corneal abrasion. A large central epithelial defect is noted with fluorescein dye and cobalt blue light. Scalloped edges nasally and temporally indicate partial healing of the epithelium. (See color plate.)

and location of the epithelial defect should be documented (Fig. 11-3), and the cornea should be examined for a laceration and for an early infectious corneal infiltrate. The rest of the ocular evaluation should be performed to rule out additional ocular damage, such as a foreign body, traumatic iritis, or hyphema. A conjunctival abrasion may also be found (Figs. 11-4 and 11-5). Occult corneal or scleral perforation can occur, especially from small high-velocity foreign bodies.

Treatment of corneal abrasions generally consists of cycloplegia, antibiotics, and occasionally pressure patching or bandage soft contact lens placement. Topical anesthetics should never be prescribed. Small abrasions may not require cycloplegia. Moderate abrasions can be treated with short-acting cycloplegic agents (e.g., 1% cyclopentolate), whereas large abrasions can be treated with longer-acting medications (e.g., 0.25% scopol-

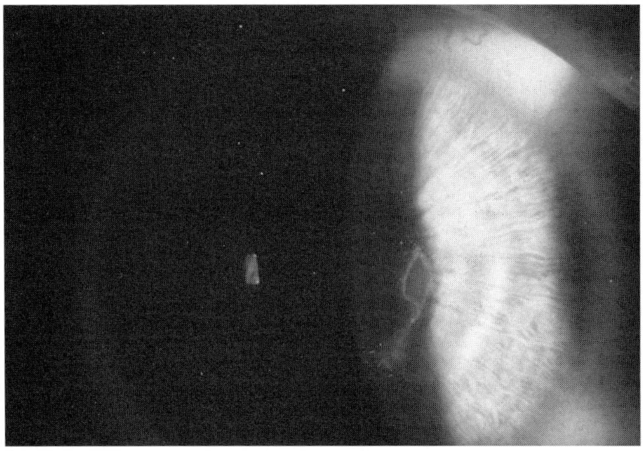

Fig. 11-3 Corneal abrasion. A small corneal abrasion is present. Size and location should be documented.

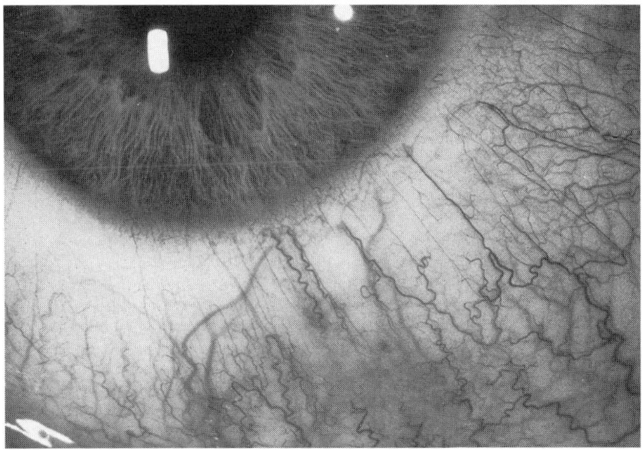

Fig. 11-4 Conjunctival abrasion. A traumatic conjunctival abrasion can be seen inferiorly.

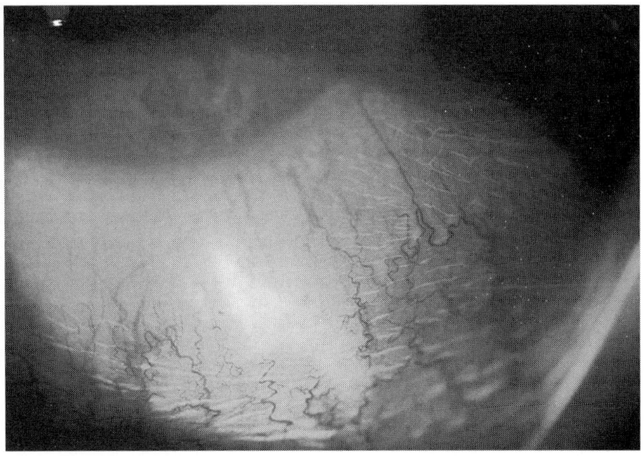

Fig. 11-5 Conjunctival abrasion. With the use of cobalt blue light, after the instillation of topical fluorescein dye, the conjunctival abrasion seen in Fig. 11-4 is highlighted. (See color plate.)

amine). When pressure patching is used, an antibiotic ointment (e.g., erythromycin, bacitracin, polymyxin B/bacitracin, or ciprofloxacin) is placed before firm double patching of the eye. Some patients are uncomfortable with a pressure patch. Alternative therapy can include frequent antibiotic ointment, as often as every 2 hours while the patient is awake. Occasionally, a patient who requires good vision immediately can use a bandage soft contact lens. In this case, an antibiotic drop (e.g., polymyxin B/trimethoprim, ofloxacin, or ciprofloxacin) is used 4 to 6 times a day. In addition a nonsteroidal antiinflammatory drop (e.g., ketorolac, diclofenac, or flurbiprofen) can be used up to 4 times a day (qid) to decrease pain. Bandage soft contact lenses may decrease the pain during the healing phase, but they may also increase the risk for infectious keratitis and are not often used. Contact lens wearers should not be treated with pressure patching or bandage soft contact lenses because of the higher risk for bacterial keratitis. Instead they should be treated with topical antibiotics that are especially effective against *Pseudomonas* spp. Whichever method of treatment is used, patients should be followed up closely until the epithelial defect is completely healed, which typically takes 1 to 4 days. After traumatic corneal abrasions, patients are at higher risk for recurrent erosion syndrome (see Chapter 3).

BLUNT CORNEAL TRAUMA

In addition to an abrasion, blunt trauma to the cornea can cause damage to the endothelium. Typical injuries include a ball or stone hitting the eye and, more recently, air bag trauma. Trauma to the endothelium can result in corneal edema. Associated injuries such as angle recession, traumatic iritis, hyphema, and subluxed, or dislocated, lens may develop (Fig. 11-6).

Endothelial damage can be localized or diffuse. Damage may result if the endothelium is pushed into contact with the lens, the iris, or both. Corneal stretching or shock wave components may accompany the endothelial injury. The result is endothelial dysfunction with subsequent corneal edema. High-speed, nonpenetrating injuries can cause small ring-shaped endothelial lesions. Blunt trauma can rupture Descemet's membrane, similar to what occurs after acute hydrops in keratoconus. Descemet's membrane rupture results in acute severe corneal edema. Such damage can also occur from a forceps injury to the eye during delivery.

Generally, endothelial function returns with time after blunt trauma. Depending on the severity of the damage, it may take days to months for the corneal edema to resolve. Topical corticosteroids and hyperosmotic agents can help decrease inflammation and edema. With no rupture to Descemet's membrane, the cornea may clear completely with no residual opacity or with minimal to moderate haze. After a Descemet's rupture the corneal edema typically clears, but significant residual corneal scarring usually develops.

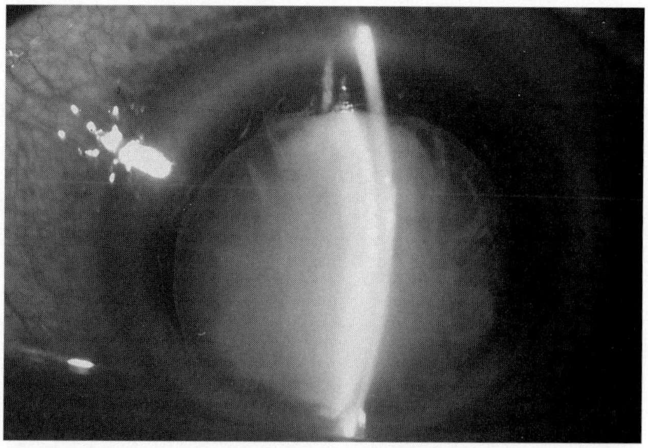

Fig. 11-6 Dislocated lens. The crystalline lens is dislocated into the anterior chamber after blunt trauma.

CHEMICAL BURN

A chemical injury is one of the few ocular emergencies in which minutes count. The prognosis depends on the exact type of chemical, the concentration of the chemical, and the duration of exposure. Initial treatment is copious irrigation to the affected eye or eyes with whatever neutral solution is available, such as water or saline. The more rapidly the irrigation is begun, the better. Chemical injuries are, unfortunately, often bilateral. Most chemical injuries occur in industrial settings and on farms, but they can also occur at home or result from assault. The patient may have associated severe skin burns or other blunt or penetrating trauma, as from a car battery explosion.

Most chemical burns are caused by acid or alkaline material. Acid damage is generally less severe because acid causes a precipitation of corneal proteins that acts as a buffer and a barrier to deeper penetration. Alkali, on the other hand, typically causes more serious injuries. The alkali denatures proteins and saponifies the lipids in corneal cell membranes, allowing alkaline material to quickly penetrate the cornea and enter the eye. Depending on the exact chemical and concentration, the pH in the aqueous rises from seconds to minutes after an alkali injury. A common cause of acid injury is the sulfuric acid in car batteries and industrial cleaners. Common causes of alkali injuries are ammonia (used in cleaning agents and fertilizers), lye (sodium hydroxide, used in drain cleaners), and lime (calcium hydroxide, used in plaster, mortar, and cement). Once the history of a chemical injury is obtained and the pH of the eye is quickly checked with litmus paper (if readily available), the immediate treatment should be irrigation with a neutral solution such as saline, Ringer's lactate, or water. This treatment is begun even before the vision is tested or a complete ocular examination is performed. Irrigation is conducted with topical anesthesia and an eyelid speculum. Automatic irrigating systems using intravenous tubing attached to a contact lens placed in the eye are available but are unnecessary. The pH is periodically rechecked several minutes after stopping the irrigation. Irrigation is continued until a pH of 7 is reached. If a neutral pH is not reached after several liters of slow irrigation, the eye should be examined for retained particulate matter. Using double eversion, the under surface of the upper eyelid should be examined for retained material. If particulate matter is found, it should be removed with a cotton-tipped applicator, forceps, or scraping after topical anesthesia has been administered. Occasionally, surgical excision of conjunctiva embedded with foreign particles is necessary. Once the pH has returned to normal, a complete history can be obtained and the vision should be assessed. The history should contain details regarding the mechanism of injury (including whether it was high-pressure blunt trauma), use of eye protection, exact substance to which the eye was exposed, and the time, type, and duration of treatment before arrival.

Ocular evaluation may be difficult because of severe eyelid swelling. Occasionally, an eyelid retractor may be required to examine the eye even partially. Slit-lamp examination should document epithelial defects of the cornea and conjunctiva, areas of conjunctival blanching, and corneal clarity. Anterior chamber reaction, lens clarity, and intraocular pressure must be assessed. Signs of globe penetration or perforation should be sought. In addition, any evidence of other damage from the trauma, such as to the skin and the eyelids, must be addressed. As previously mentioned, all particulate matter should be removed. Corneas with complete epithelial loss after chemical injuries may not appear to stain immediately with fluorescein, and the examiner may falsely conclude that no epithelial defect has resulted. However, if the cornea is reexamined after additional fluorescein, it demonstrates complete corneal, and often extensive conjunctival, staining.

Minor chemical burns damage the corneal and the conjunctival epithelia (Figs. 11-7 and 11-8), but not the stroma or the conjunctival blood vessels. Severe injuries cause corneal stromal opacification and conjunctival ischemia (Figs. 11-9 and 11-10) and sometimes damage to the sclera, trabecular meshwork, iris, ciliary body, lens, and retina. Because of injury to the trabecular meshwork and from immediate collagen shrinkage, intraocular pressure is often elevated. It may, however, be low because of ciliary body damage. Several grading scales for ocular damage after chemical injury have been developed. Box 11-1 describes Thoft's classification. In general, the greater the corneal stromal opacity and conjunctival ischemia, the worse the prognosis. After severe chemical injuries, the cornea may be only mildly hazy and the patient may have surprisingly good vision. The patient should be told that because of the severity of the injury, the cornea may opacify with time and the vision may deteriorate despite aggressive appropriate treatment.

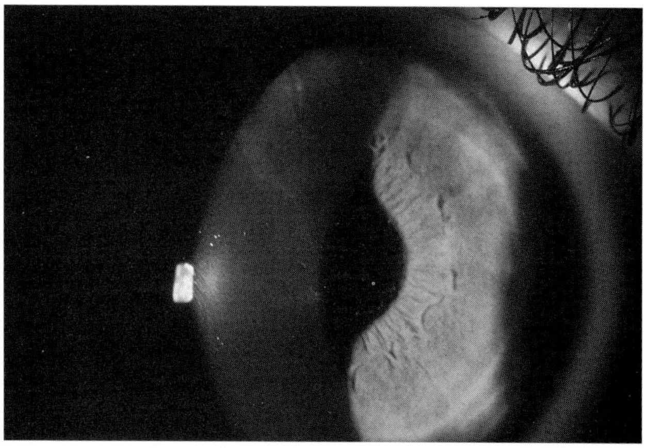

Fig. 11-7 Chemical keratitis. A mild bilateral chemical injury has damaged the corneal epithelium superiorly. Moderate corneal epithelial haze and irregularity have developed.

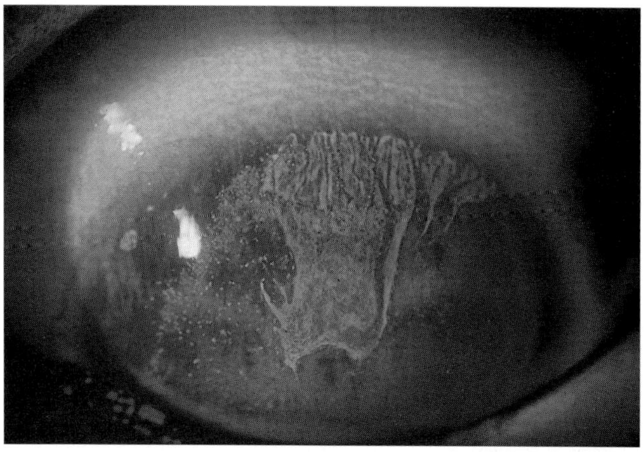

Fig. 11-8 Chemical keratitis. With the use of cobalt blue light, after the instillation of topical fluorescein dye, the fellow eye of the patient in Fig. 11-7 is seen. Note the mild staining and irregularity of the corneal epithelium and the mild staining of the conjunctiva. (See color plate.)

After initial copious irrigation, the management of chemical injuries generally includes medications to decrease inflammation, prevent infection, and aid in reepithelialization. Elevated intraocular pressure must be controlled. Topical corticosteroids and cycloplegic agents are used to decrease the inflammatory response. Vasoconstricting drops, such as phenylephrine, should be avoided. Topical antibiotics are given to prevent infection. In mild injuries, the antibiotics can be used several times a day with or without topical corticosteroids. Typ-

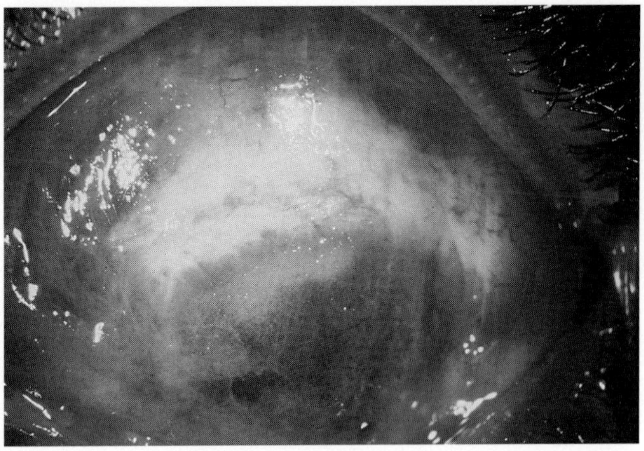

Fig. 11-9 Acid chemical burn. A battery acid injury has severely damaged the cornea and conjunctiva. Significant superior conjunctival ischemia has developed.

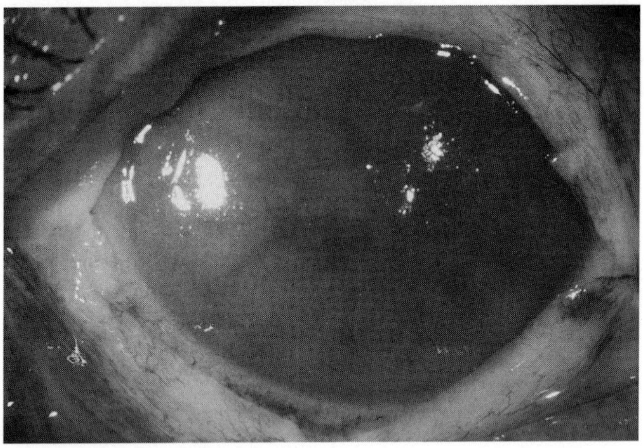

Fig. 11-10 Alkali chemical burn. A strong alkali injury has led to complete corneal epithelial loss with blanching and necrosis of the conjunctiva. Significant corneal edema with a poor view of the anterior chamber can be seen.

ically an antibiotic ointment (e.g., erythromycin) is used every 2 to 4 hours while the patient is awake. In more severe injuries, the corticosteroid and antibiotic can be used as often as every 1 to 2 hours while the patient is awake. These two medications can be given in combination ointment form (e.g., tobramycin/dexamethasone), which has the added benefit of aiding in reepithelialization. Topical corticosteroids can potentiate collagenase activity after the first week or so and promote corneal melting; hence, they should be tapered and discontinued 7 to 10 days after the injury. Elevated intraocular pressure is best managed with aqueous suppressants, such as topical beta-blockers or alpha-agonists, or with topical or systemic carbonic anhydrase inhibitors. Medications that tend to increase inflammation, such as miotics and prostaglandin analogues, should be avoided. Systemic pain medication may be required. Patients with mild injuries

Box 11-1 Thoft's Classification of Chemical Injury

GRADE 1

Epithelial loss only
No conjunctival ischemia
Good prognosis

GRADE 2

Some corneal stromal haze, but iris details seen
Conjunctival ischemia involves less than one third of limbus
Good prognosis, possibly some corneal scarring

GRADE 3

Diffuse corneal haze, iris details blurred
Conjunctival ischemia involves one third to one half of limbus
Guarded prognosis, probable corneal scarring

GRADE 4

Opaque cornea
Conjunctival ischemia involves more than one half of limbus
Poor prognosis, perforation may develop

can be observed closely as outpatients, whereas those with extensive ocular damage should be admitted to the hospital (Box 11-2).

Other medications are often used and may be beneficial after severe chemical injury. Ascorbic acid is a cofactor in collagen synthesis. Systemic sodium ascorbate (1 to 8 g/day) and 10% topical ascorbic acid every 1 to 4 hours have been used. To help decrease polymorphonuclear leukocyte activity, 10% topical sodium citrate may be used every 1 to 4 hours. Oral administration of 250 mg tetracycline qid may decrease collagenase activity. Topical administration of 10% *N*-acetylcysteine every 2 to 6 hours may also reduce collagenase activity. In general, these adjunctive medications are not proven to be effective, but may be of benefit after severe chemical injury to the eye.

The goal of treatment is to achieve corneal and conjunctival reepithelialization with as little permanent damage as possible (Fig. 11-11). If a persistent corneal epithelial defect remains after 2 to 3 weeks, the risk for corneal ulceration increases significantly. Copious preservative-free tear ointment or erythromycin ointment should be applied. A bandage soft contact lens can be tried, but it increases the risk for infectious keratitis. Amniotic membrane transplantation may be helpful in the treatment of persistent epithelial defects. Eyelid surgery may be required to correct entropion, ectropion, or trichiasis, and a lateral tarsorrhaphy may be necessary to

Box 11-2 Treatment of Chemical Injuries

ALL

EMERGENCY IRRIGATION until the pH normalizes
Remove particulate matter, if present
Assess severity of damage

MILD

Cycloplegia (e.g., 1% to 2% cyclopentolate qid, 0.25% scopolamine tid)
Topical antibiotic ointment (e.g., erythromycin, bacitracin, ciprofloxacin every 2 to 4 hours)
Treat elevated intraocular pressure as needed (e.g., 0.5% timolol or 0.5% levobunolol bid, brimonidine bid to tid, 2% dorzolamide or 1% brinzolamide bid to tid, methazolamide 50 to 75 mg po bid to tid)
Pain medication as needed

MODERATE TO SEVERE

In-hospital treatment
Cycloplegia (e.g., 0.25% scopolamine tid)
Topical antibiotic and corticosteroid (e.g., tobramycin/dexamethasone ointment every 1 to 4 hours); topical corticosteroids should be tapered and discontinued at approximately 7 to 10 days
Treat elevated intraocular pressure as needed (as above)
Pain medication as needed
Consider adjunctive therapy
- Sodium ascorbate (e.g., 1 to 8 g/day orally)
- 10% Ascorbic acid drops (e.g., every 1 to 4 hours)
- 10% Sodium citrate drops (e.g., every 1 to 4 hours)
- Tetracycline (e.g., 250 mg qid orally)
- 10% *N*-Acetylcysteine drops (e.g., Mucomyst every 2 to 6 hours)

qid, Four times a day; *tid*, three times a day; *bid*, twice a day.

help achieve reepithelialization. Impending or small frank corneal perforations can be treated with cyanoacrylate corneal tissue glue and a bandage soft contact lens. Larger perforations may be managed with a small patch graft or a large penetrating corneal transplant.

Grades 3 and 4 chemical injuries may result in the extensive loss of limbal stem cells (Fig. 11-12). Long-term visual rehabilitation may require a conjunctival-limbal autograft (for unilateral injuries), keratolimbal allograft (for bilateral injuries), or a mucous membrane transplant from the buccal mucosa. If the corneal surface can be rehabilitated and the eye has good visual potential, corneal transplantation can be attempted, typically at least 18 to 24 months after the injury and at least 6 months after the limbal cell transplant. A permanent keratoprosthesis can be considered as a last resort for bilateral injuries if macular and optic nerve function are good (Fig. 11-13).

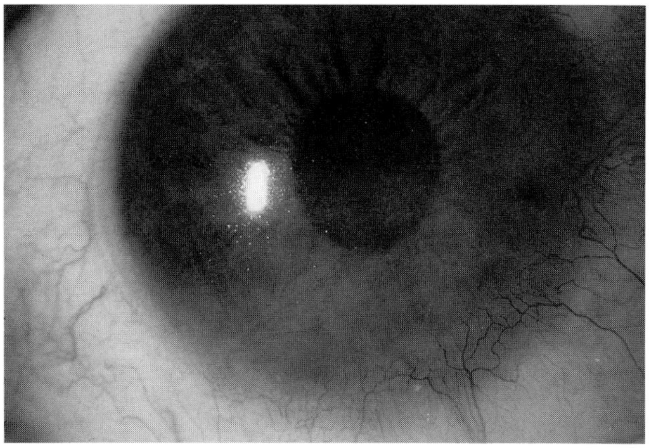

Fig. 11-11 Alkali chemical burn. Superficial and deep stromal blood vessels and moderate corneal scarring are evident inferiorly several years after an alkali injury.

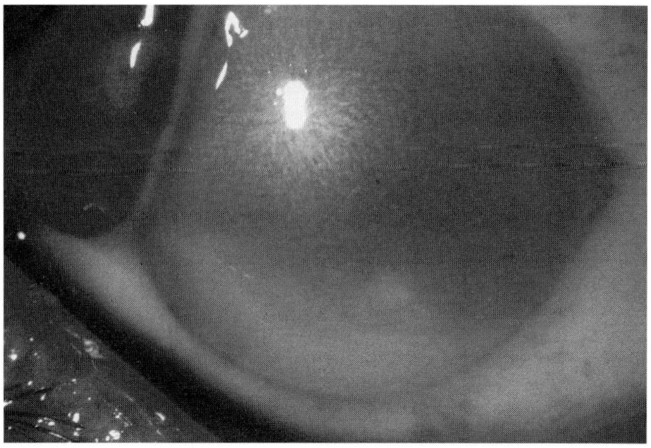

Fig. 11-12 Alkali chemical burn. A severe alkali injury has damaged all the limbal stem cells. No reepithelialization has occurred after 1 month. The relatively smooth corneal surface is Bowman's membrane. Inflammatory debris is seen in the anterior chamber. A pyogenic granuloma is evident at the 9 to 10 o'clock position.

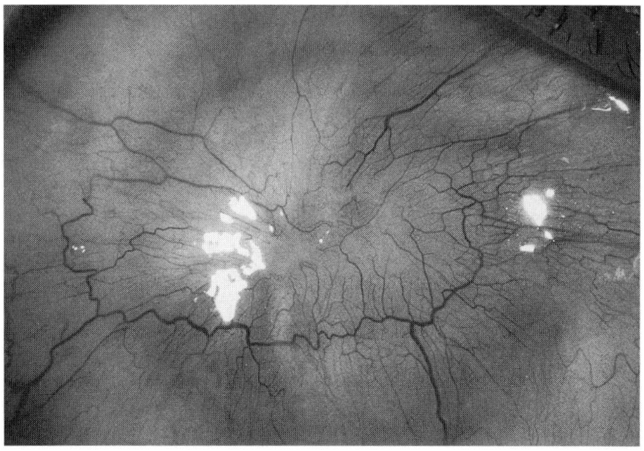

Fig. 11-13 Alkali chemical burn. Severe corneal scarring and neovascularization have developed in this eye years after an alkali injury, resulting in no view of the anterior chamber. In severe bilateral injuries, permanent keratoprosthesis can be considered.

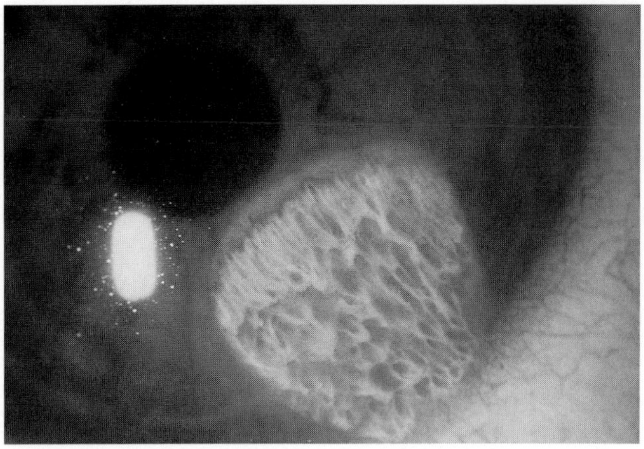

Fig. 11-14 Curling iron injury. Curling iron injuries generally result from extremely rapid contact with the cornea, causing impressive superficial whitening from corneal epithelial necrosis.

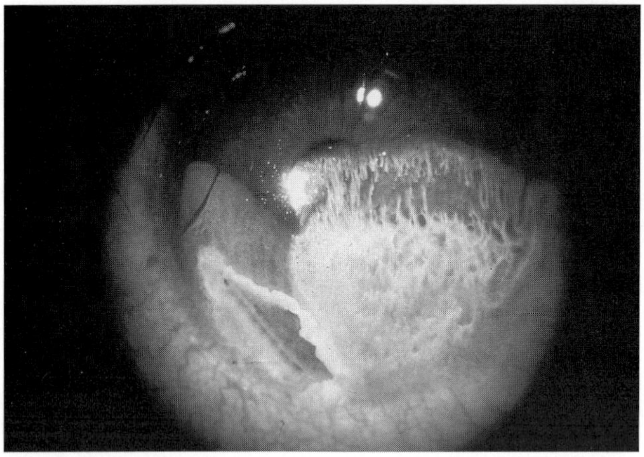

Fig. 11-15 Curling iron injury. The inferior half of a cornea was impacted by the curling iron. Usually, the inferior cornea is involved with this type of injury.

THERMAL BURN

Ocular thermal injuries can be divided into flame burns and contact burns. Flame burns, caused by fire, are relatively common to the face but are less common to the eye because of the rapid closure of the eyelids and the protection they provide. Ocular flame injury generally results when the eyelids are severely damaged from an extensive facial burn. Needless to say, treatment of facial and systemic injuries must be addressed in burn patients. Significant eyelid injury requires treatment simultaneous with eye treatment before the eye can be expected to recover fully.

Contact injury occurs when heated material comes in direct contact with the eye. Typical work-related causes of contact injury are hot metal fragments and drops of molten metal or glass. Home-related causes are droplets of hot grease or oil that splash and hit the eye. Accidental corneal burn can result from contact with a cigarette end (often in toddlers, whose eyes are at the adult waist level). Corneal burns from curling irons are also relatively common (Figs. 11-14 and 11-15).

Severity of the injury depends on the temperature of the agent, the duration of contact, and the size of the area involved. Even small amounts of molten metal or glass can cause significant damage because of the extremely high temperatures and common adherence to the eye on contact (Fig. 11-16). Such injuries can result in deep corneal damage or even perforation. Drops of grease or oil wash out quickly, and a cigarette end or a curling iron is only in contact with the eye momentarily, limiting ocular damage. These injuries may produce an impressive area of corneal

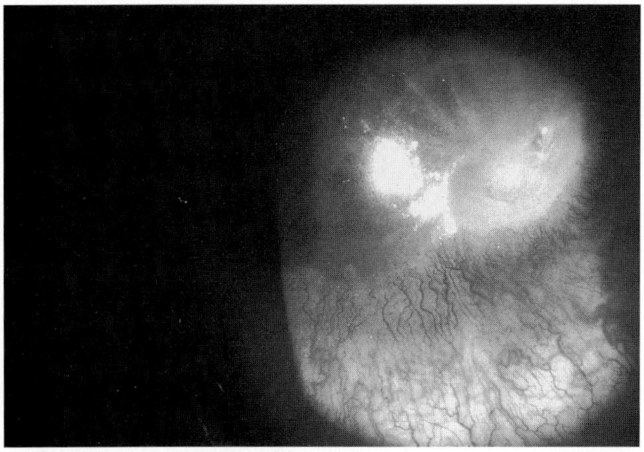

Fig. 11-16 Thermal injury. Molten lead struck this cornea 10 days earlier, causing impressive corneal contraction and melting. Corneal striae can be seen emanating from the site of the trauma.

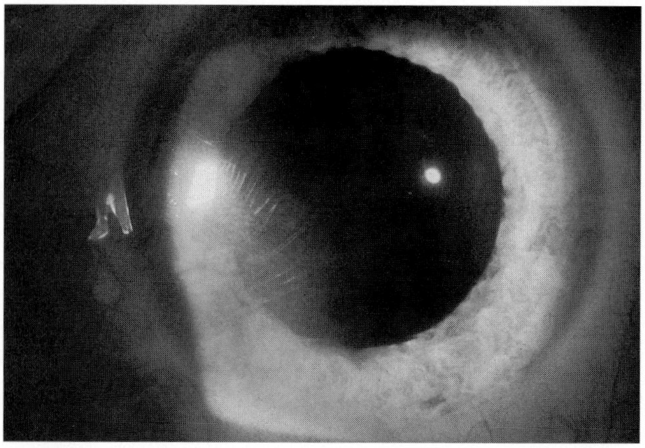

Fig. 11-17 Thermal injury. One month after a hot cement injury to this cornea. This combined chemical and thermal injury healed with residual corneal thinning and flattening. The corneal striae and severe induced astigmatism are in the process of resolving.

epithelial whitening with minimal to no damage to the underlying stroma.

Treatment of severe thermal injuries is similar to that for chemical burns. Areas of stromal heating can demonstrate significant corneal flattening, which tends to resolve over weeks to months (Fig. 11-17). Treatment of superficial burns is similar to that for corneal abrasions. White necrotic corneal epithelium can be left alone or debrided easily at the slit lamp, which may aid in reepithelialization.

ELECTRICAL INJURY

Electrical injury to the eye occurs when an electrical current passes through the ocular area. Extremely high electrical voltage, such as from a lightning strike, and lower voltages, such as from electrical outlets, can cause varying degrees of damage to many different ocular structures. The electrical current typically has separate entrance and exit sites. The severity of the skin burns at these sites is often unrelated to the severity of the internal damage. Significant internal tissue damage can be associated with small entry and exit wounds. Marked systemic injury involving the central nervous and cardiovascular systems may result and require emergency treatment.

The most common ocular manifestation of electrical injury is cataract formation. It is typically unilateral, on the side of the electrical injury, but it may be bilateral. The cataract is classically anterior subcapsular, but it may be posterior subcapsular. If it is severe, it can be removed as a nontraumatic cataract is removed. The face may have mild to severe skin burns. If the eyelids are severely damaged, exposure of the ocular surface can cause significant morbidity. Eyelid reconstruction may be necessary to maintain adequate ocular coverage. Anterior uveitis can develop after electrical injuries. It is treated with cycloplegia and topical corticosteroids, as is traumatic iritis, discussed later in this chapter. Conjunctival, corneal, and scleral necrosis and even perforation can occur in severe injuries (Fig. 11-18). Unfortunately, damage to the skin and the eye is often progressive, despite maximal medical and surgical therapy. The prognosis is guarded for patients with severe electrical injuries.

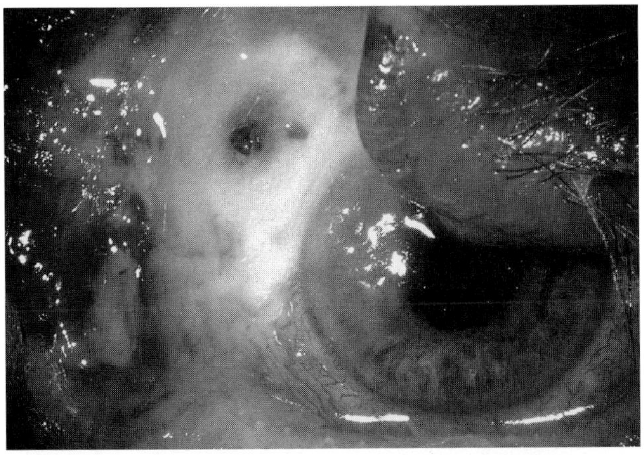

Fig. 11-18 Electrical injury. Eyelid necrosis and scleral melting are evident 1 month after an electrical injury to this side of the head. A small amount of uveal prolapse can be seen. Combined scleral patch graft and eyelid reconstruction were successfully performed.

CORNEAL FOREIGN BODY AND RUST RING

Foreign bodies that embed into the cornea can be composed of various materials, most typically, metal, glass, or vegetable matter. As a general rule, corneal foreign bodies should be removed to improve healing and to decrease the chance for infection and chronic inflammation. The exception is a small, deeply embedded (but not into the anterior chamber), inert (e.g., glass, coal particle) fragment that does not affect the vision and that would result in more damage if removed than if left in place. All vegetable matter must be removed because of the high risk for infection.

As discussed earlier, any significant injury to the eye necessitates complete ocular examination. If a foreign body is found in the cornea, the evaluation should rule out an intraocular foreign body. Computed tomography may be necessary. The conjunctiva and the cornea should be carefully examined for an entrance wound, which may be quite small. Additionally, the iris should be inspected for a peaked pupil or a transillumination defect, which could indicate an intraocular foreign body. The eyelids should be everted to search for additional foreign bodies (Fig. 11-19). Ultrasound biomicroscopy can be very useful in determining the depth of corneal foreign bodies and in searching for subconjunctival and intrascleral foreign material (Figs. 11-20 and 11-21).

Multiple superficial foreign particles can often be irrigated from the cornea and conjunctiva with sterile saline. Most embedded corneal foreign bodies are superficial and are readily removed at the slit lamp (Figs. 11-22, 11-23, and 11-24). This procedure is performed using topical anesthesia. An eyelid speculum is often helpful. Sterile fine forceps or a foreign-body spud is used to shell out the foreign matter. Metallic foreign bodies often leave a rust ring in the underlying stroma after removal of the metal particle (Fig. 11-25). Occasionally the rust ring can be scooped out, but more commonly, a small handheld rust ring drill is required for careful removal of the residual rust (Fig. 11-26). This procedure requires an eyelid speculum and cooperation from the patient. The rust is

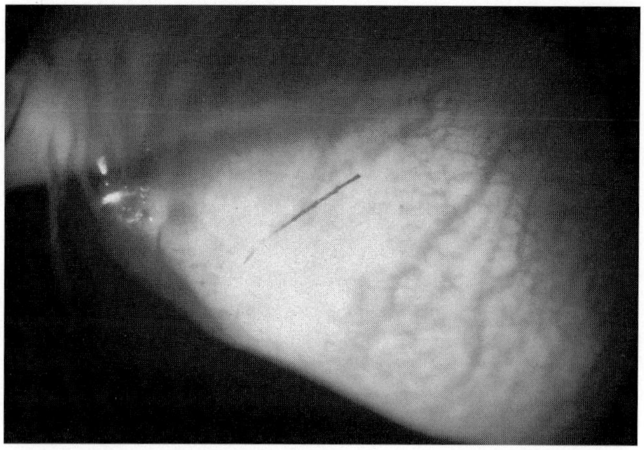

Fig. 11-19 Superficial foreign body. Eversion of the upper eyelid revealed a foreign body (an insect leg) embedded in the palpebral conjunctiva, causing multiple linear corneal abrasions. It was easily removed with fine forceps.

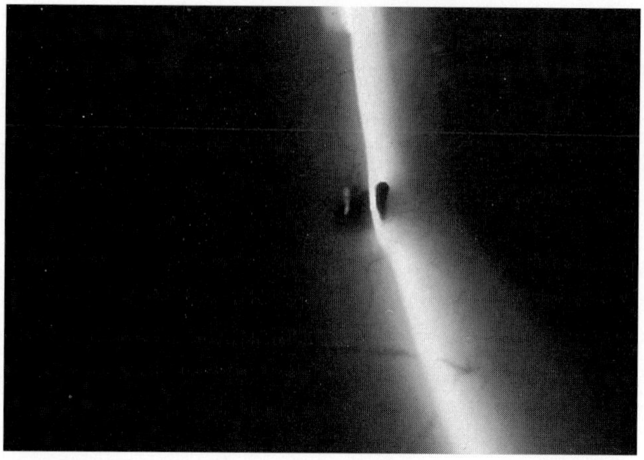

Fig. 11-20 Scleral foreign body. A small metallic foreign body can be seen in the sclera.

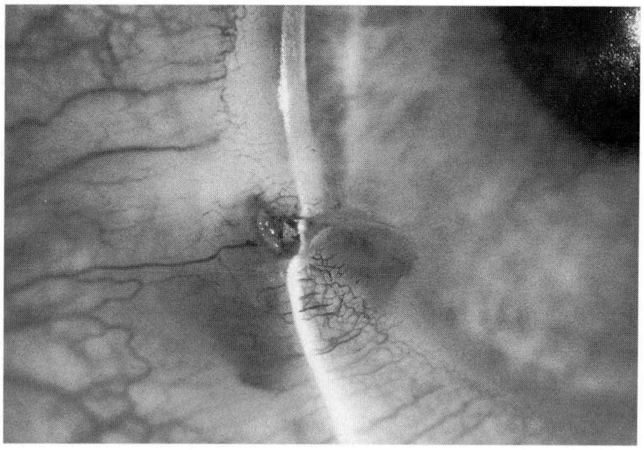

Fig. 11-21 Scleral foreign body. A moderately large metallic foreign body is evident in the cornea and sclera. The slit beam demonstrates its relatively anterior location. It was removed without difficulty with fine forceps at the slit lamp.

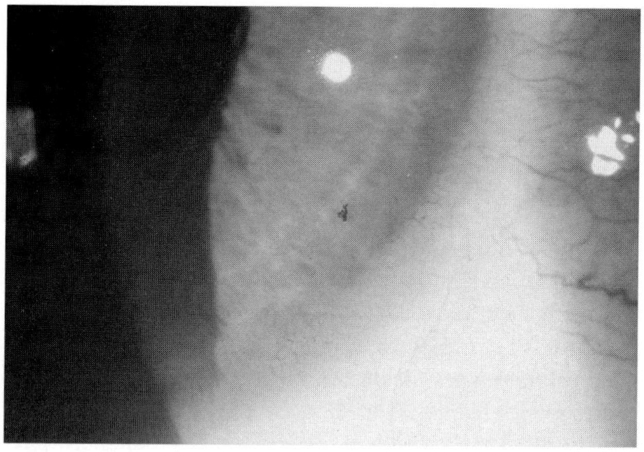

Fig. 11-22 Corneal foreign body. A small peripheral superficial metallic corneal body was easily removed with fine forceps at the slit lamp.

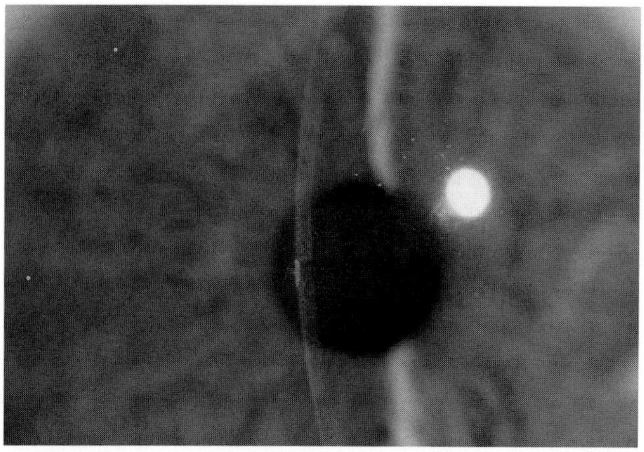

Fig. 11-23 Corneal foreign body. A small superficial corneal foreign body, apparently a thin flat portion of vegetable matter such as from a leaf, is noted in the slit beam centrally. It was easily removed with a foreign-body spud at the slit lamp.

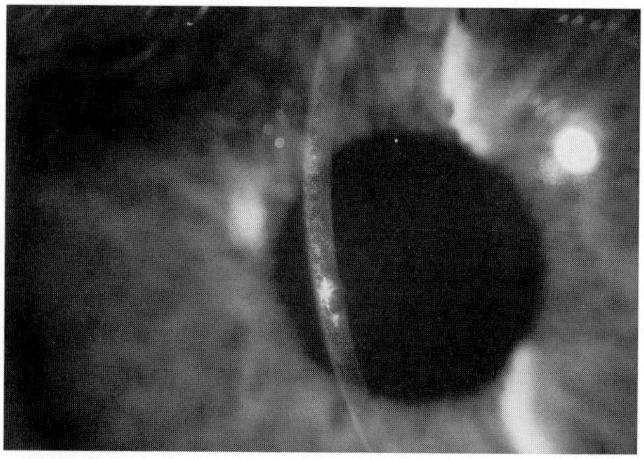

Fig. 11-24 Corneal foreign body. A small, central, metallic foreign body is seen in the slit beam. A small rust ring surrounds the metal, and a faint immune ring approximately 2 mm in diameter surrounds the foreign body.

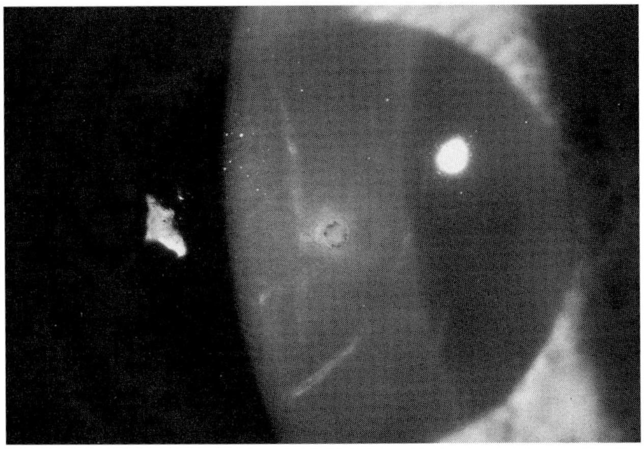

Fig. 11-25 Corneal rust ring. A rust ring can be seen after removal of a small metallic foreign body.

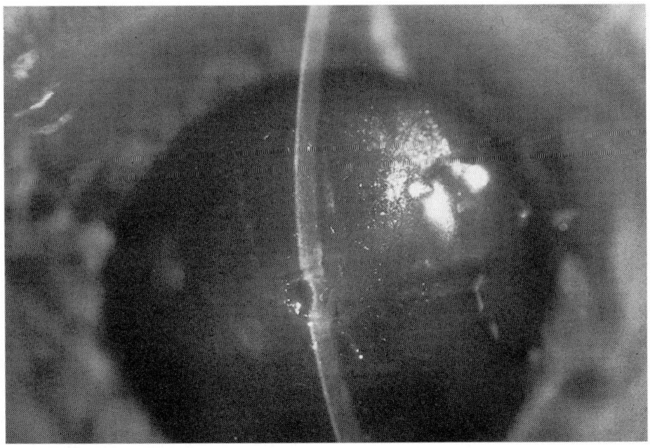

Fig. 11-26 Corneal rust ring. The rust ring seen in Fig. 11-25 has been removed with a small handheld rust ring drill. An epithelial defect and moderate stromal thinning can be observed in the slit beam.

slowly cored out with the drill that is held at an angle to allow good visualization; extreme care must be taken not to penetrate the cornea too deeply. The hand holding the drill should be stabilized on the patient's cheek so that if the patient moves forward, the drill does not enter too deeply. If the rust appears to be extremely deep, it is best to leave it in place. Typically, the cornea heals well over a small amount of deep residual rust (Fig. 11-27). Occasionally, the rust rises to the surface and is more amenable to removal at a later date.

More deeply embedded foreign bodies can often be removed at the slit lamp with fine forceps (Figs. 11-28 and 11-29). Ideally, the foreign body is removed through its entrance wound. When a deep corneal foreign body cannot be readily extracted at the slit lamp, it may require removal in the operating room (Figs. 11-30, 11-31, and 11-32). In a cooperative patient, the procedure may be performed under topical anesthesia, but local anes-

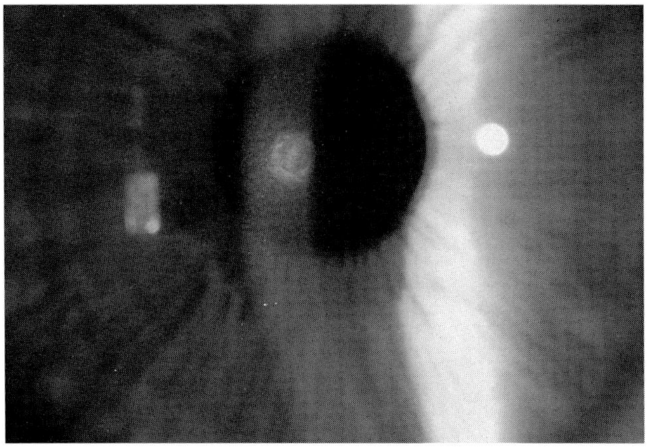

Fig. 11-27 Corneal rust ring. A small amount of residual rust remains in the stroma after rust ring removal. The epithelium has healed completely.

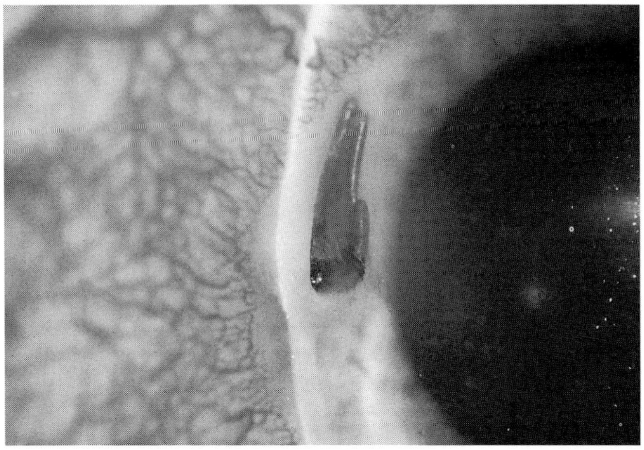

Fig. 11-28 Corneal foreign body. Because this large piece of nail in the peripheral cornea did not appear to involve full-thickness cornea, it was removed with fine forceps at the slit lamp.

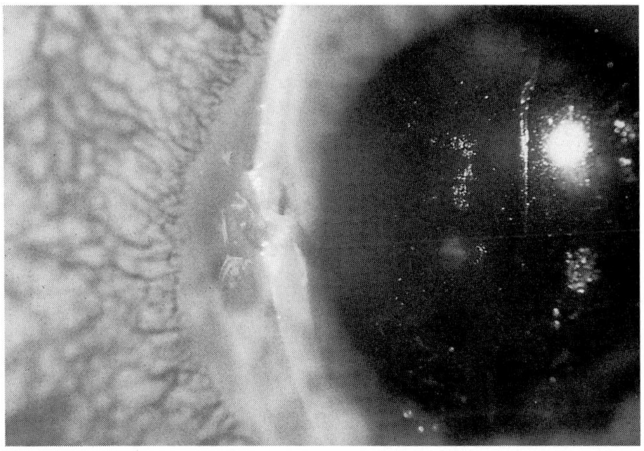

Fig. 11-29 Corneal foreign body. Immediately after the nail foreign body seen in Fig. 11-28 was removed from the cornea. The patient was treated with topical antibiotics and followed up as an outpatient because no leakage of aqueous developed.

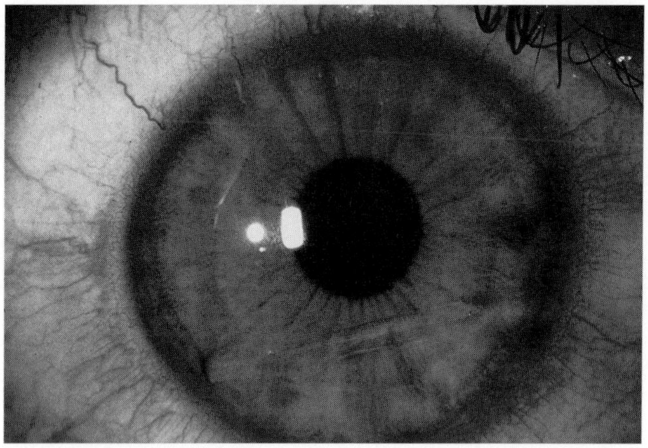

Fig. 11-30 Corneal foreign body. A large glass foreign body deeply embedded in the inferior cornea. Because it appeared to involve the deep, perhaps full-thickness, cornea, it was removed in the operating room.

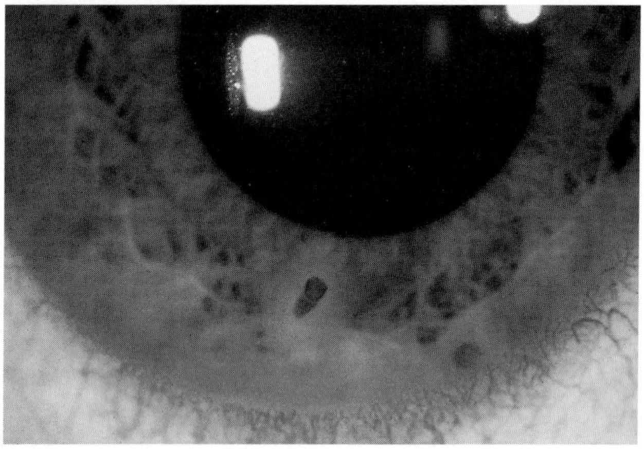

Fig. 11-31 Corneal foreign body. The end of a thorn is seen in the inferior cornea.

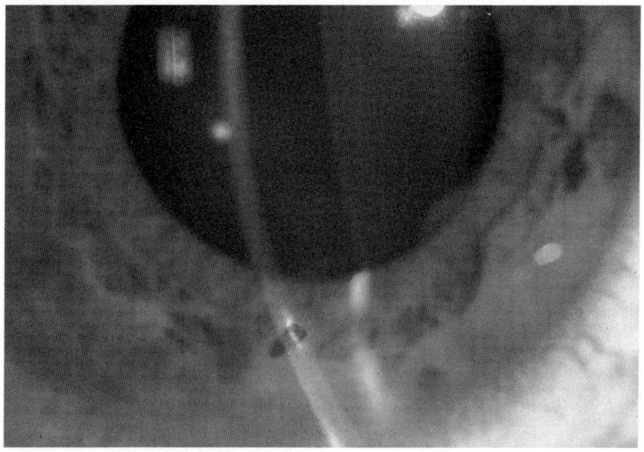

Fig. 11-32 Corneal foreign body. A slit-beam view of the thorn seen in Fig. 11-31 demonstrates its deep corneal location.

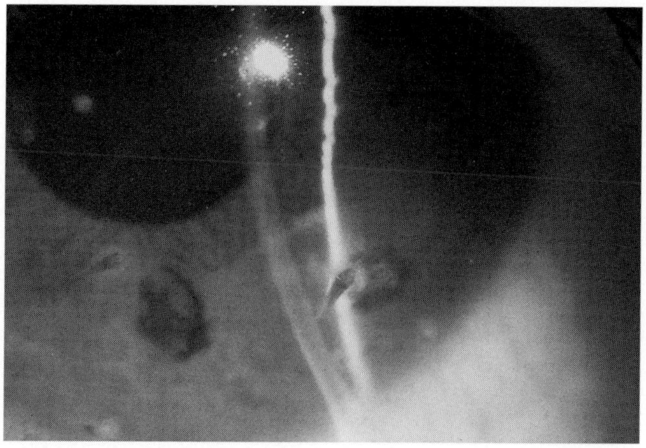

Fig. 11-33 Corneal foreign body. A spike from the outer shell of a chestnut is seen in the slit beam to be embedded in the cornea and to extend into the anterior chamber. A second spike can be seen at the inferior aspect of the pupil.

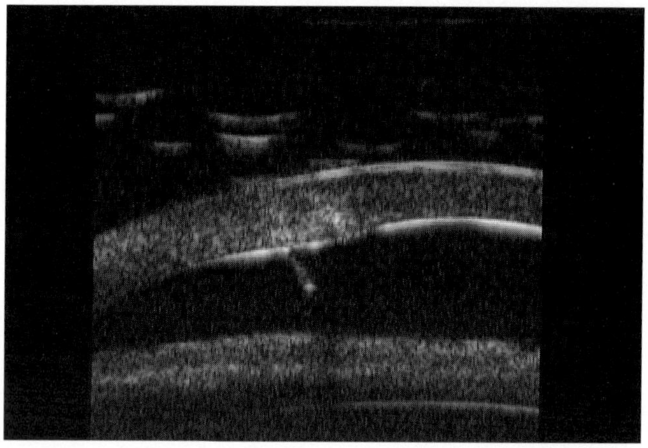

Fig. 11-34 Corneal foreign body. An ultrasound biomicroscopic examination demonstrates the protrusion of the spike seen in Fig. 11-33 into the anterior chamber.

thesia is often necessary. A rare earth magnet or a more powerful electromagnet may help to remove metallic foreign bodies. Deep foreign bodies may require a small enlargement of the entrance wound for removal (Figs. 11-33 and 11-34). Care must be taken not to push the material through Descemet's membrane and into the anterior chamber. Occasionally, a curved needle can be used to impale the foreign body and back it out of its entrance wound. Generally small wounds do not require suturing, but gaped wounds should be closed with fine suture (e.g., 10-0 nylon) and the knots buried.

Postoperative treatment after corneal foreign body or rust ring removal involves the use of cycloplegia and topical antibiotics such as for a corneal abrasion. Frequent follow-up is required until the epithelial defect has resolved. Corneal metallic foreign bodies in place for several days may be surrounded by small corneal infiltrates.

These are generally sterile, but require close follow-up. If an anterior chamber reaction occurs, the infiltrate may not be sterile and should be treated with frequent strong antibiotic drops as for infectious keratitis. After superficial metallic foreign body injury, a small amount of iron may remain in the anterior cornea and cause a small, dense, white opacity called a Coats' white ring.

CONJUNCTIVAL FOREIGN BODY AND LACERATION AND SUBCONJUNCTIVAL HEMORRHAGE

Trauma to the eye often involves the conjunctiva. One of the common sequelae of conjunctival trauma is a subconjunctival hemorrhage. It may be small or large and may even involve the entire bulbar conjunctiva (Figs. 11-35, 11-36, and 11-37). The blood initially appears bright red, but it may become deep maroon if it is dense and elevates the conjunctiva. As the blood clears over days to a few weeks, the conjunctiva becomes less elevated and appears less red and more pink, but the blood typically spreads out to involve a larger area of conjunctiva. Patients should be warned that the hemorrhage may appear to worsen before it resolves. No treatment is required unless the conjunctiva is so elevated that the eyelids have difficulty closing. This exposure should be treated with lubricating drops and ointments. Dellen, areas of corneal desiccation from poor spread of the tear film adjacent to conjunctival elevations, can also develop. Dellen also should be treated with aggressive lubrication with ointments.

Any patient with a subconjunctival hemorrhage after trauma requires a complete dilated ophthalmic evaluation. Fluorescein dye should be placed for careful examination of the conjunctiva for a superficial foreign body, abrasion, or laceration. Superficial foreign bodies should be removed at the slit lamp with a foreign-body spud or fine forceps. Conjunctival abrasions are treated with antibiotic drops or ointment. Conjunctival lacerations should be carefully examined for a subconjunctival foreign body or underlying scleral laceration (Fig. 11-38). Blunt trauma may result in scleral laceration without conjunctival laceration. Subconjunctival foreign bodies and scleral lacerations may be difficult to observe if significant subconjunctival hemorrhaging occurs. After the administration of topical anesthesia, a cotton-tipped applicator can often be used at the slit lamp to move a conjunctival laceration opening to inspect the underlying sclera and to rule out a scleral laceration or a foreign body. If a scleral laceration cannot be ruled out at the slit lamp, an exploration in the operating room may be

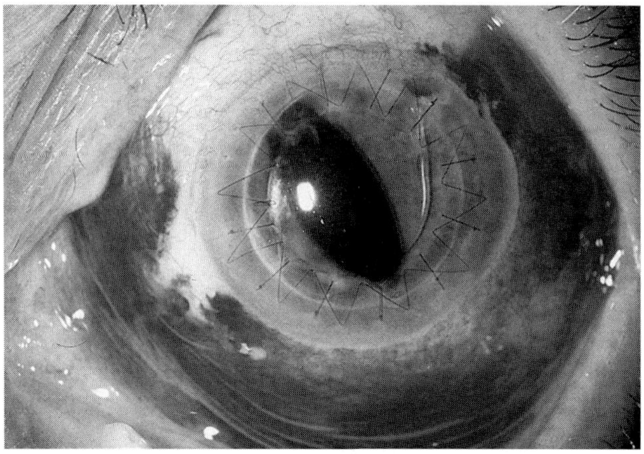

Fig. 11-36 Subconjunctival hemorrhage. A large nasal, inferior, and temporal subconjunctival hemorrhage can be seen. It most likely began inferiorly, and the blood tracked nasally and temporally. (See color plate.)

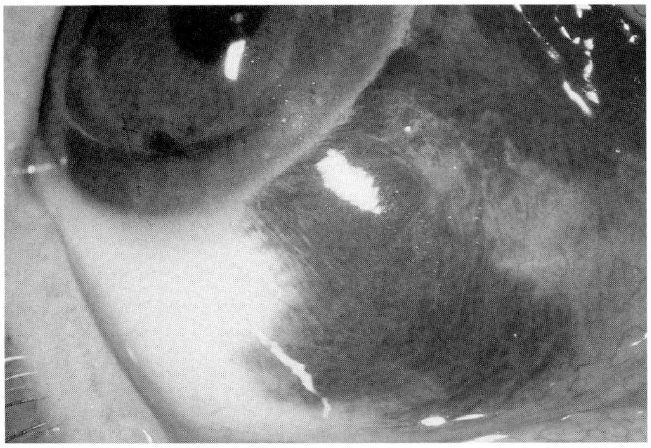

Fig. 11-35 Subconjunctival hemorrhage. An inferotemporal subconjunctival hemorrhage is seen. The blood reaches the limbus but does not involve the cornea.

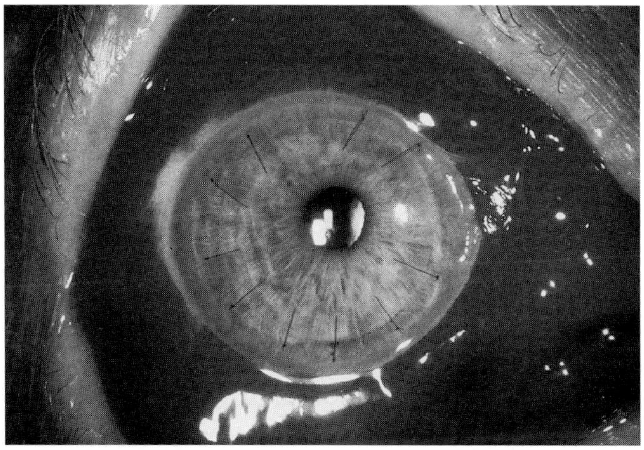

Fig. 11-37 Subconjunctival hemorrhage. A large, elevated, subconjunctival hemorrhage involving the entire bulbar conjunctiva is demonstrated. A subconjunctival clot can be seen inferonasally.

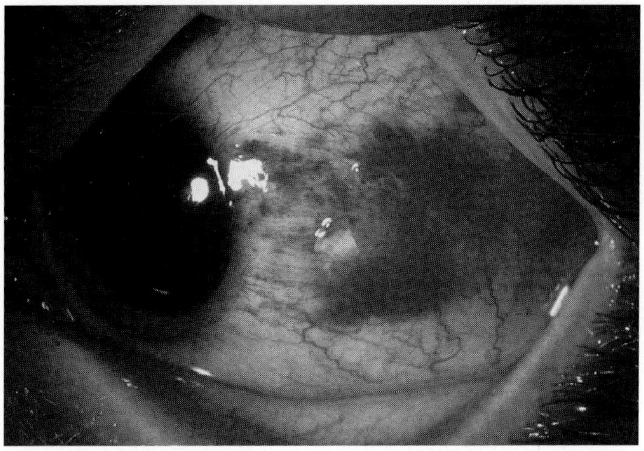

Fig. 11-38 Conjunctival laceration. A conjunctival laceration with surrounding conjunctival hemorrhage from a tree branch is seen. The pupil is dilated for the complete posterior segment examination required after trauma.

warranted. When a deep intraocular foreign body is suspected, a computed tomography is indicated (see Intraocular Foreign Body later in this chapter).

If a ruptured globe is not suspected after the slit-lamp examination, small conjunctival lacerations can be left alone. Subconjunctival foreign bodies can occasionally be removed at the slit lamp but may require an operating room setting. The conjunctival laceration may have to be enlarged to create access to the foreign body and to inspect the sclera to confirm the absence of a rupture. Large conjunctival lacerations, typically larger than 10 mm, can be sutured closed with absorbable suture (e.g., 8-0 Vicryl). Lacerations involving the plica semilunaris or the caruncle should be sutured closed to prevent irregular healing and a poor cosmetic result. Special care should be taken to avoid including underlying Tenon's capsule in the conjunctival wound repair. Additionally, the conjunctival edges should be well apposed to avoid epithelial cyst formation.

Surgical exploration to rule out a ruptured globe is indicated when a scleral laceration cannot be ruled out at the slit lamp. Signs of occult scleral laceration are listed in Box 11-3. Exploration is performed in the operating room, usually under general anesthesia and rarely under topical anesthesia if the chance for finding a rupture is low. Peribulbar and retrobulbar anesthesia are avoided to prevent increasing orbital pressure or a retrobulbar hemorrhage from extruding the intraocular contents through a rupture site. A limbal conjunctival peritomy can be created, or the existing conjunctival laceration can be extended to check the underlying sclera for a laceration. Once it is ruled out, the conjunctiva is closed.

After a ruptured globe is ruled out, the upper eyelids can be everted to examine for foreign bodies. A foreign body under the upper eyelid should be suspected if linear epithelial defects are present in the cornea. Foreign matter often embeds in the upper tarsal area, especially near the eyelid margin. Occasionally, double eversion of the upper eyelid with a Desmarres eyelid retractor is required to examine the upper fornix. All foreign bodies should be removed, usually with irrigation, a cotton-tipped applicator, foreign-body spud, or fine forceps under topical anesthesia. Antibiotic drops or ointment are used after foreign body removal, as after corneal abrasion.

Box 11-3 Signs of an Occult Ruptured Globe

Large or 360° subconjunctival hemorrhage
Conjunctival chemosis
Abnormally deep or shallow anterior chamber (compared with fellow eye)
Abnormally low or high intraocular pressure (compared with fellow eye)
Iris irregularity
Hyphema
Subluxed or dislocated lens
Limited extraocular motility
Vitreous hemorrhage

TRAUMATIC IRITIS

An anterior chamber reaction or iritis can occur after ocular trauma. It generally presents with photophobia, ocular pain, tearing, and often decreased vision within hours to days of the trauma. Patients may also report pain in the injured eye when light is shone into the uninjured eye.

Slit-lamp evaluation reveals white blood cells and flare in the anterior chamber. The red-free illumination of the slit lamp can be used to rule out hyphema because red blood cells disappear with red-free light. As with any significant ocular trauma, a complete dilated ocular examination should be performed. If iritis has developed, the pupil is often smaller (and dilates less well) and the intraocular pressure is often lower than the fellow eye. Occasionally, if significant inflammatory debris in the anterior chamber clogs the trabecular outflow tracts, the intraocular pressure is elevated. Frequently perilimbal conjunctival injection occurs. Before dilation, the iris sphincter should be evaluated carefully for tears. A single tear may appear as a V or a notch in an otherwise round pupil. Multiple iris sphincter tears can cause significant pupillary dilatation. Iridodialysis (separation of the iris root from the ciliary body) and cyclodialysis (separation of the ciliary body from the scleral spur) can also occur, but they are usually associated with severe injuries and hyphema.

Box 11-4 Evaluation and Treatment of Traumatic Iritis

Slit-lamp and dilated fundus examination to evaluate anterior chamber reaction and rule out other intraocular abnormalities
Cycloplegic drops (e.g., 1% to 2% cyclopentolate qid, 0.25% scopolamine tid)
Occasionally, corticosteroid drops (e.g., 1% prednisolone qid) if severe or not responding to cycloplegic agents

qid, Four times a day; *tid,* three times a day.

Traumatic iritis is generally treated with cycloplegic drops (e.g., 1% to 2% cyclopentolate qid or 0.25 scopolamine three times a day [tid]). These medications tend to improve patient comfort and stabilize the blood-aqueous barrier, allowing the iritis to improve. In eyes that have severe anterior chamber reactions or that do not respond to cycloplegic agents alone, topical corticosteroid drops can be added (e.g., 1% prednisolone qid) (Box 11-4). Patients using topical corticosteroid drops must be monitored closely for intraocular pressure elevations. Traumatic iritis generally improves within a few days to 1 to 2 weeks, depending on the initial severity. Approximately 1 month after the trauma, the anterior chamber angles of both eyes must be evaluated by gonioscopy to look for angle recession, which predisposes the eye to glaucoma.

HYPHEMA AND MICROHYPHEMA

Hyphema and microhyphema are defined as blood in the anterior chamber (Fig. 11-39). When a layer of blood or a clot is visible, it is termed *hyphema*. When there is no layering but suspended red blood cells are seen in the anterior chamber on slit-lamp examination, it is called *microhyphema* (Box 11-5). Occasionally, the suspended red blood cells of microhyphema may form a layer and become frank hyphema. Soon after the onset of hyphema, the iris may not be visible because of the large amount of blood in the anterior chamber. When the blood is bright red, this total (100%) hyphema may consolidate to become less than 100% with some superior iris visible. When the blood is black, it generally indicates a clot and is called "eight-ball" hyphema. Eight-ball hyphema generally occupies the entire anterior chamber and may extend around the iris and into the posterior chamber.

Most hyphemas are caused by blunt ocular trauma. Ocular surgery may also cause hyphema, but this type is generally managed by close follow-up. Patients with spontaneous (nontraumatic and nonsurgical) hyphemas should be evaluated for neovascularization of the iris or the anterior chamber angle, iris–intraocular lens chafing syndrome, and blood dyscrasia. Less common causes include iris tumors, herpes zoster iritis, leukemia, and, especially in children, juvenile xanthogranuloma and retinoblastoma.

Traumatic hyphemas typically cause immediate but variable visual loss. The vision clears as the blood settles. Occasionally, bleeding recurs within a few days, causing another decrease in vision. Other symptoms of hyphema include pain and photophobia.

A complete dilated ocular examination is required, and a ruptured globe must be ruled out, either on examination or in the operating room (Fig. 11-40). The amount of hyphema should be quantified and the intraocular pressure measured. Ocular damage such as iris sphincter tears, iridodialysis, cyclodialysis, and cataract

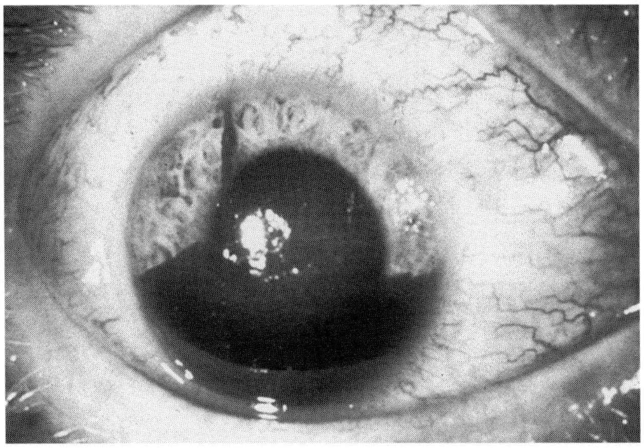

Fig. 11-39 Hyphema. A large hyphema is evident after blunt trauma. The bleeding may have originated superiorly where a strand of blood is present. A resolving central corneal abrasion is also seen. (See color plate.)

Box 11-5 Definition of Hyphema and Microhyphema

HYPHEMA

Layer of red blood cells in the anterior chamber
Amount of layering determines size of hyphema (e.g., 10% hyphema)

MICROHYPHEMA

Red blood cells suspended in the anterior chamber without layering

EIGHT-BALL HYPHEMA

A maroon or black clot of blood occupying the entire anterior chamber; may have extension around the iris and into the posterior chamber

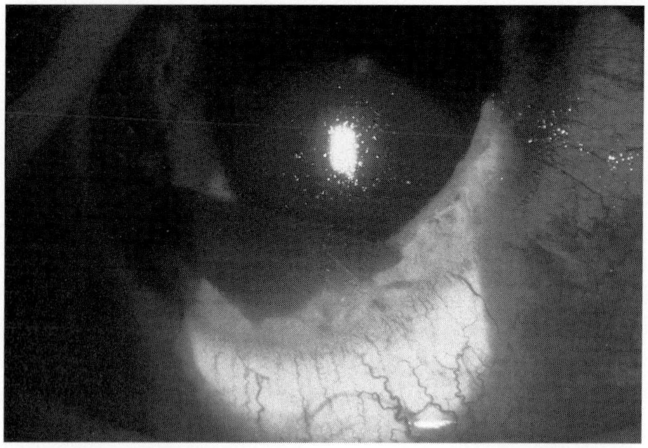

Fig. 11-40 Hyphema. A hyphema is present inferiorly. Additionally, a full-thickness corneal laceration has occurred, and a glass foreign body is embedded in the cornea inferiorly. A tiny iris defect can be seen in the peripheral iris at the 5 o'clock position. The hyphema does not reach the corneal periphery because of peripheral iris-cornea touch from a shallow anterior chamber.

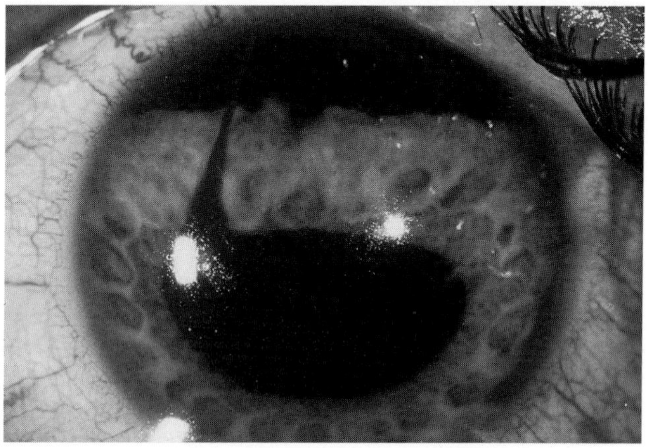

Fig. 11-41 Hyphema and iridodialysis. A large superior iridodialysis was caused by blunt trauma. Active bleeding occurred from the iris root superiorly. A small layered hyphema is seen from the 3 to 4 o'clock positions.

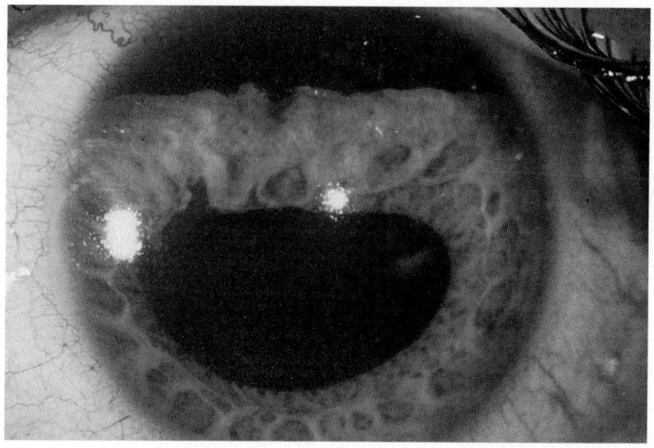

Fig. 11-42 Hyphema and iridodialysis. The active bleeding seen in Fig. 11-41 has stopped, and the layered blood has disappeared 2 days later. A small blood clot attached to the iris at the 10 o'clock position is in the process of resolving.

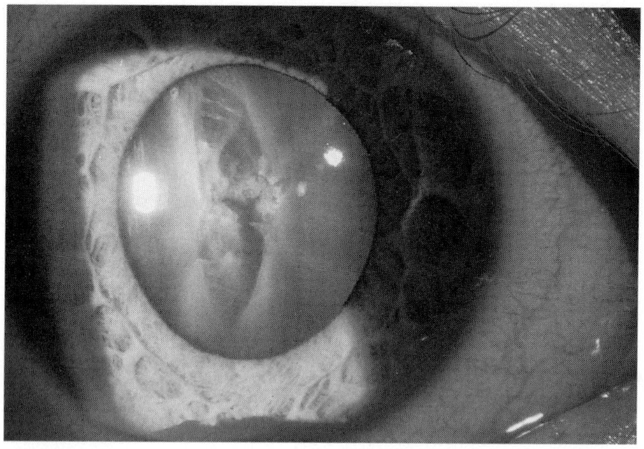

Fig. 11-43 Hyphema and cataract. A large, vertically oriented, fish-mouth tear in the anterior capsule causing a dense cataract is present after blunt trauma. No evidence of a ruptured globe is found. A small inferior hyphema can be seen.

should be documented (Figs. 11-41, 11-42, and 11-43). Ideally a dilated fundus examination should also be performed. B-scan ultrasonography may be helpful to rule out posterior damage if the retina cannot be visualized. Patients of African and Mediterranean descent should be screened for sickle trait and disease (through Sickledex, hemoglobin electrophoresis, or both).

No treatment for traumatic hyphema is universally accepted. The following is one reasonable approach. Hospital admission is considered for all children, all noncompliant patients with microhyphema, and all patients with hyphema, especially those at greater risk for visual loss (Box 11-6). Rebleeding, which occurs in 5% to 30% of patients with hyphema, is associated with a worse prognosis than the initial hemorrhage. Most episodes of rebleeding are larger than the original hyphema and pose an increased risk for secondary glaucoma and corneal blood staining. These eyes also require a higher rate of surgical intervention.

Initial treatment of hyphema consists of limited activity or bed rest with the head of the bed elevated 30°. The eye is shielded but not patched so the patient can recognize sudden worsening of vision, which may indicate a recurrence of bleeding. The treatment is 1% atropine drops tid. Aspirin and nonsteroidal antiinflammatory agents are contraindicated. If a severe anterior chamber reaction develops, topical corticosteroids (e.g., 1% prednisolone) 4 to 8 times a day can be given (Box 11-7).

Elevated intraocular pressure should be treated aggressively. Treatment is required if patients with sickle

Box 11-6 Risk Factors for Visual Loss for Patients with Hyphema and Microhyphema

Sickle trait or disease
Uncontrolled elevated intraocular pressure
Large (>50%) hyphema
Poor vision on presentation (<20/200)
Delayed presentation (after the first day)
Recurrence of bleeding

Box 11-7 Treatment of Patients with Hyphema

Consider hospital admission for children, noncompliant patients with microhyphema, and patients with hyphema at higher risk for visual loss
Bed rest or limited activity with head of bed elevated 30°
Eye shield but no patch
1% Atropine drops 3 times a day
No aspirin or nonsteroidal antiinflammatory drugs
If severe, topical corticosteroids (e.g., 1% prednisolone 4 to 8 times a day)
Treat elevated intraocular pressure aggressively
Hospitalized patients are treated with oral aminocaproic acid (50 mg/kg every 4 hours, maximum 30 g/day)
Consider oral prednisone (e.g., 0.75 mg/kg per day)

Box 11-8 Medical Treatment of Elevated Intraocular Pressure in Patients with Hyphema

Treat intraocular pressures greater than 24 mm Hg in patients with sickle trait or disease and greater than 30 mm Hg in most other patients
First-line treatment: topical beta-blocker (e.g., 0.5% timolol or levobunolol bid)
Second-line treatment: alpha-agonist (e.g., 0.2% brimonidine tid)
Third-line treatment: carbonic anhydrase inhibitor (e.g., 2% topical dorzolamide or 1% brinzolamide tid or 50 to 75 mg oral methazolamide bid to tid)
Last-line treatment: 20% intravenous mannitol (1 to 2 g/kg over 45 minutes)

bid, Twice a day; *tid,* three times a day.

Box 11-9 Indications for Surgical Evacuation of a Hyphema

Corneal blood staining (urgent surgery, especially in children at risk for amblyopia)
Persistent clot in most of the angle for 7 days
Elevated intraocular pressure:
- In patients without sickle trait or disease:
  - >50 mm Hg for 5 days or
  - >35 mm Hg for 7 days
- In patients with sickle trait or disease:
  - >25 mm Hg for 1 to 2 days

trait or disease have intraocular pressures greater than 24 mm Hg and if most other patients have intraocular pressures greater than 30 mm Hg. Beta-blockers are a first-line treatment. Alpha-agonists can also be used. Topical and systemic carbonic anhydrase inhibitors are safe in most patients but may lower anterior chamber pH and induce sickling in susceptible patients. If a systemic carbonic anhydrase inhibitor is required in a patient with sickle trait or disease, 50 mg methazolamide tid may induce less acidosis than acetazolamide. If medical treatment is unsuccessful, intravenous 20% mannitol (1 to 2 g/kg over 45 minutes) can be used (Box 11-8). If mannitol is necessary to control intraocular pressure, surgical evacuation may be needed.

Inpatients are treated with oral aminocaproic acid (50 mg/kg every 4 hours, maximum 30 g/day). This antifibrinolytic agent stabilizes clot formation at the site of the hemorrhage and reduces rebleeding, but it is associated with nausea, vomiting, and postural hypotension. The aminocaproic acid dose is reduced by half on posttrauma day 2 and stopped on posttrauma day 3 if bleeding has not recurred. If bleeding recurs, the aminocaproic acid is continued for an additional day or two. Topical aminocaproic acid gel may be as effective as the oral preparation with fewer systemic side effects. Once it is approved by the Food and Drug Administration, it can be used for outpatient therapy. Some physicians use oral prednisone (e.g., 0.75 mg/kg per day) to treat significant hyphema.

Inpatients are examined twice a day, and outpatients are observed daily for 3 days after the trauma or the last episode of bleeding. The examination should document evidence of rebleeding, corneal blood staining, and intraocular pressure. As the blood clears, other intraocular abnormalities such as iris or lens damage may become apparent.

Surgical evacuation of the hyphema should be considered for the conditions described in Box 11-9. Anterior chamber paracentesis to remove 0.1 ml aqueous can be performed to lower the intraocular pressure as a temporizing measure before more definitive surgery.

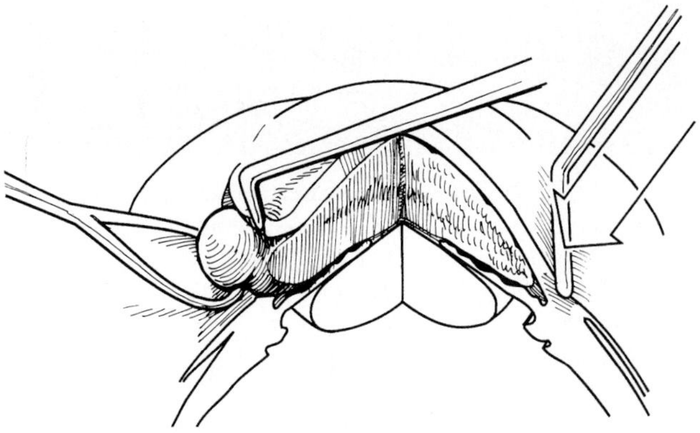

Fig. 11-44 Anterior chamber clot expression procedure. A large limbal conjunctival peritomy and entrance into the anterior chamber is created. Gentle pressure is placed at the limbus 180° away to express the clot.

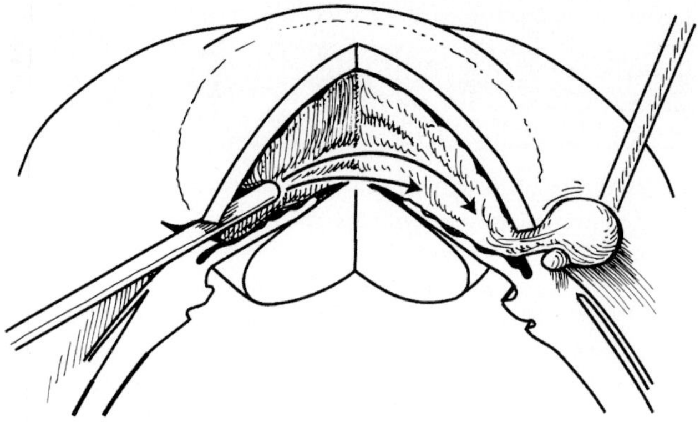

Fig. 11-45 Hyphema washout procedure. When primarily free blood cells are in the anterior chamber, a washout can be performed. Saline is irrigated into the anterior chamber through one incision, and the blood is released from another incision. Fluid should be directed into the anterior chamber angle because blood is often trapped there.

The clot and residual blood can be removed by expression or cutting. Expression is performed by creating a 3- to 5-clock hour conjunctival peritomy and limbal incision into the anterior chamber (Fig. 11-44). The posterior aspect of the wound is depressed, and the clot is manually expressed. Irrigation with saline or gentle extraction with a blunt instrument such as a muscle hook can aid in removal of the clot. Once the clot is expressed, the anterior chamber and angle are irrigated with saline to remove any residual blood. The wound is closed with 10-0 nylon sutures. Alternatively, if primarily free-floating red blood cells are present, they can be removed through two smaller incisions. Two 2-mm limbal incisions are created. Saline irrigation is placed through one while blood is released from the eye through the second (Fig. 11-45). If a clot exists, a vitreous cutting instrument can be inserted into the anterior chamber through one of the incisions while irrigation continues through the other (or one incision can be used for both irrigation and aspiration) (Fig. 11-46). The vitrector is used to cut out the clot. Visibility is often poor, and extreme care must be taken not to injure intraocular structures such as cornea, iris, and lens. Once the clot is removed, the anterior chamber angle should be cleared of as much blood as possible. The trabecular meshwork is blocked mostly by free red blood cells rather than by the clot, which tends to retract from the angle. Therefore clearance of the free blood is probably more important than removal of every bit of the clot. The incisions are closed with 10-0 nylon sutures as needed. If significant glaucoma has developed, trabeculectomy may be performed simultaneously with the clot removal. Additionally, peripheral iridectomy may be required to relieve pupillary block, which may be associated with an eight-ball hyphema (Box 11-10).

Once the acute hyphema has resolved, the patient should refrain from strenuous physical activity for 2 weeks. One month after the trauma, the eye should undergo gonioscopy to look for angle recession, which predisposes to glaucoma, and a dilated fundus evaluation. Patients should be examined yearly because of the increased long-term risk for glaucoma.

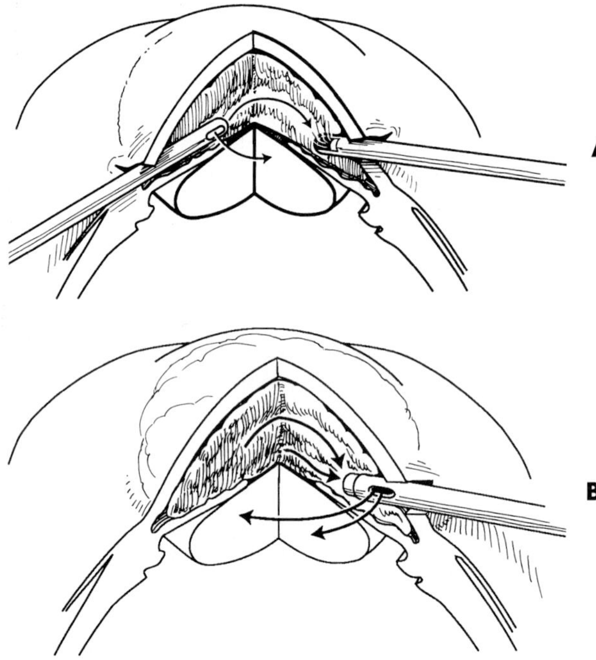

Fig. 11-46 Excision of an anterior chamber clot procedure. **A,** Two-port method. Two separate limbal incisions have been made. Irrigation is placed through one port, and a vitrector is used through the other port to excise the clot. Because the visualization of the vitrector cutter is often poor, extreme care must be taken to avoid damaging intraocular structures such as the iris and the lens. **B,** One-port method. A combined vitrector with an irrigating sleeve can be placed through a single port to excise the clot.

Box 11-10 Surgical Intervention Options for Hyphema

Anterior chamber paracentesis (temporizing measure)
Anterior chamber washout
Clot expression
Clot excision with an automated vitrectomy instrument
Trabeculectomy, peripheral iridectomy, or both can be performed simultaneously with hyphema removal as needed to control elevated intraocular pressure

CORNEAL/CORNEOSCLERAL LACERATION AND WOUND DEHISCENCE

Both blunt and sharp trauma can cause a ruptured globe, a full-thickness break in the cornea or sclera. Blunt trauma typically causes ruptures at the weakest portions of the eye (i.e., the limbus and just behind the extraocular muscle insertions). After ocular surgery, the weakest site is often the surgical incision (e.g., a cataract wound, a corneal transplant wound, or a radial keratotomy incision) (Box 11-11). Blunt trauma often causes wound dehiscence. Sharp trauma typically produces penetrating injury to the globe. If the responsible implement exits the other side of the eye, it is termed a *perforating injury of the globe*. The implement may then come out of the eye, or it may remain as an intraocular or intraorbital foreign body. Common instruments of penetrating trauma include nails, metal fragments, kitchen utensils, glass, and wood.

The history is extremely important when a ruptured globe is suspected. The exact nature of the injury and the composition of any possible foreign body should be elicited. As described previously, any significant ocular trauma requires a complete ophthalmic examination. Once a ruptured globe is found, however, the remainder of the ocular examination of the injured eye is deferred until after surgical repair to prevent further damage. Many ruptured globes can be easily diagnosed from simple penlight evaluation. The diagnosis, however, can be subtle. Signs of an occult ruptured globe (usually a scleral rupture) include severe 360° subconjunctival hemorrhage or chemosis, a deep or shallow anterior chamber (compared to the fellow eye), a subluxed or dislocated lens, and limitation of extraocular motility. Other signs include low intraocular pressure (compared to the fellow eye), though it may be normal or elevated, iris irregularity, hyphema, and vitreous hemorrhage.

Corneal lacerations vary from barely visible to grossly apparent. To distinguish between a partial-thickness and a full-thickness corneal laceration, a careful slit-lamp examination and a Seidel test should be conducted. Topical fluorescein is placed on the laceration, which is examined with cobalt blue light. If aqueous exits the eye through the laceration, it causes the fluorescein to appear bright yellow-green as the dark green fluorescein is diluted in a stream of aqueous (Fig. 11-47). When this stream is seen, it is termed *Seidel positive* (Box 11-12). Partial-thickness lacerations are Seidel negative. Self-sealed full-thickness lacerations also appear Seidel negative. To determine whether a wound is partial thickness or full thickness but is self-sealing, gentle digital pressure may be applied at the limbus to see if it is truly Seidel negative. Note that a full-thickness corneal laceration with a flat anterior chamber also appears Seidel negative if no aqueous is directed through the wound. If a ruptured globe cannot be ruled out on slit-lamp examination, surgical exploration should be performed. Computed tomography (axial and coronal views) should be obtained if an intraocular or intraorbital foreign body is suspected (see next section). Occasionally, gentle B-scan ultrasonography can be helpful in locating a scleral rupture or an intraocular foreign body.

Box 11-11 Most Common Sites of Globe Rupture Caused by Blunt Trauma

Previous ocular surgery site (e.g., cataract wound, corneal graft wound, radial keratotomy incision)
Just posterior to a rectus muscle insertion
Limbus

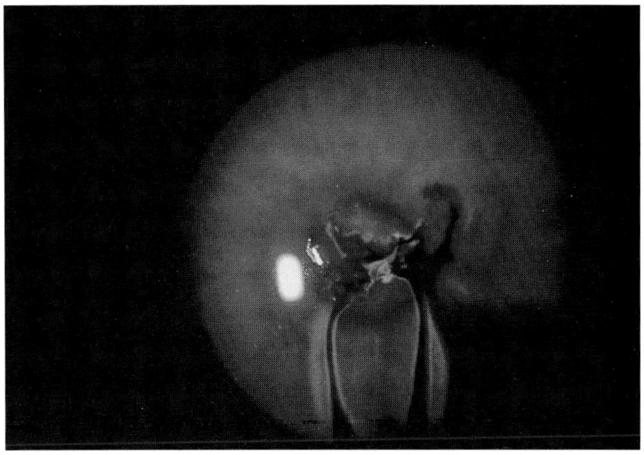

Fig. 11-47 Seidel test. Topical fluorescein dye is placed on the eye, which is viewed with a cobalt blue light. When aqueous leaks through a full-thickness corneal laceration, the dye is seen to be pushed out of the way by the aqueous fluid, termed *Seidel positive*. (See color plate.)

Partial-thickness corneal lacerations can be treated with topical antibiotics (e.g., ofloxacin or ciprofloxacin drops or ciprofloxacin ointment qid). If the wound edges are well apposed, no additional treatment is required (Figs. 11-48 and 11-49). If the wound is gaped (Fig. 11-50), it should be closed with fine sutures (e.g., 10-0 or 11-0 nylon) to reduce the corneal scarring and irregularity. Small, well-apposed, self-sealed or almost self-sealed corneal lacerations with a formed anterior chamber without extension into the sclera can often be managed medically with topical antibiotics (e.g., ofloxacin or ciprofloxacin 6 times a day) and systemic antibiotics (as described on p. 305) and twice daily follow-up at first. Shelved lacerations tend to self-seal more readily than perpendicular lacerations (Figs. 11-51 and 11-52). Often an aqueous suppressant is also used to decrease flow through the laceration. Pressure patching may be helpful, and topical corticosteroids should be avoided. Occasionally, a bandage soft contact lens can be used to keep the wound edges well apposed until healing has occurred for partial-thickness and self-sealed full-thickness corneal lacerations (Box 11-13).

Box 11-12 Seidel Test

PURPOSE

To determine whether a corneal laceration is full thickness.

PROCEDURE

Place fluorescein on the corneal wound and evaluate with a cobalt blue light.

SEIDEL POSITIVE

Aqueous flowing through the wound causes the fluorescein to turn yellow-green and stream away, indicating a full-thickness laceration.

SEIDEL NEGATIVE

The fluorescein does not change color, indicating a partial-thickness or self-sealed laceration. Often, a full-thickness laceration with a flat anterior chamber appears Seidel negative if no aqueous is exiting the laceration.

DISTINGUISH BETWEEN A PARTIAL THICKNESS AND SELF-SEALED LACERATION

If initially Seidel negative, gentle digital pressure can be placed at the limbus to see whether a small amount of aqueous will exit the wound, indicating that it is full thickness but self-sealing.

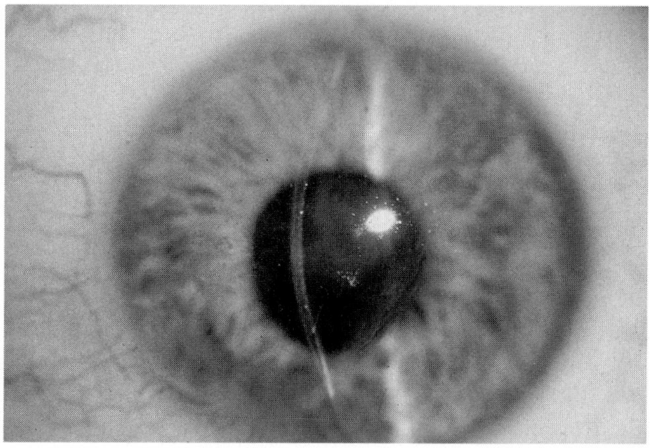

Fig. 11-49 Partial-thickness corneal laceration. This deep lamellar partial-thickness laceration was caused by windshield glass shattered in a car accident. The entrance can be seen at the edge of the pupil from the 3 to 6 o'clock positions. The slit beam at the 6 o'clock position best demonstrates the depth of the laceration.

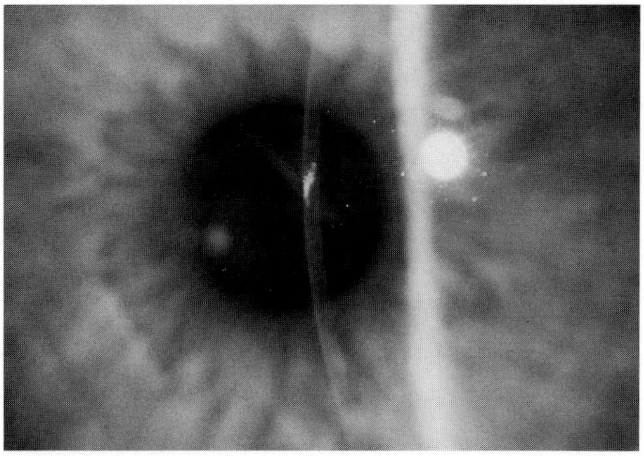

Fig. 11-48 Partial-thickness corneal laceration. The slit beam demonstrates a partial-thickness corneal laceration. It reaches approximately 80% corneal thickness.

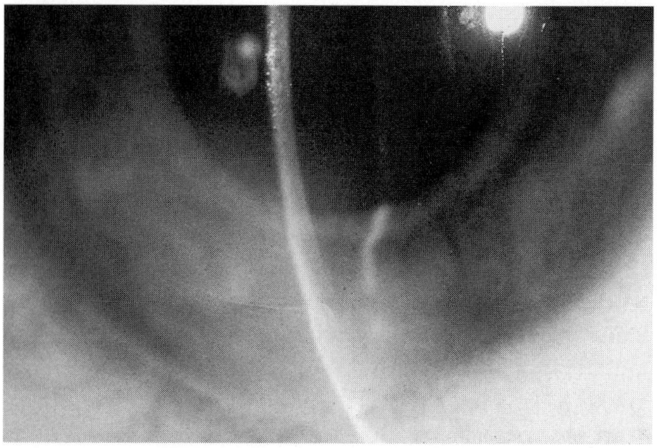

Fig. 11-50 Partial-thickness corneal laceration. A partial thickness laceration is evident inferiorly. The slit beam demonstrates moderate gaping of the incision, which is often best treated with surgical closure. The anterior chamber depth is normal.

Before repair of the ruptured globe, the eye should be shielded and the patient should receive nothing by mouth. Systemic antibiotics should be started in the emergency department (e.g., 1 g cefazolin IV q 8 h or 1 g vancomycin IV q 12 h plus gentamicin 6 mg/kg per day [use ideal body weight or real body weight, whichever is less] or 1 g ceftazidime IV q 8 h or 200 to 400 mg ciprofloxacin IV q 12 h in adults; 25 to 50 mg/kg per day cefazolin IV in 3 divided doses and 2 mg/kg gentamicin IV q 8 h in children). Vancomycin is used instead of cefazolin in patients allergic to penicillin or cephalosporin and in those with a higher probability of *Bacillus* spp infection (see the Intraocular Foreign Body section in this chapter). Tetanus prophylaxis and antiemetics are given as needed. Vomiting can cause a retrobulbar or a suprachoroidal hemorrhage that results in the extrusion of intraocular contents, so antiemetics should be used when necessary. Pain medication should be given, if necessary, after proper informed consent for surgery has been obtained (Boxes 11-14 and 11-15).

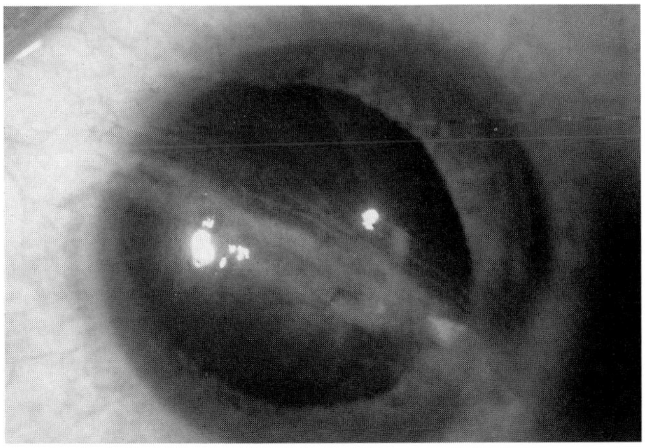

Fig. 11-51 Partial-thickness corneal laceration. A healed limbus-to-limbus corneal laceration scar is present in the visual axis.

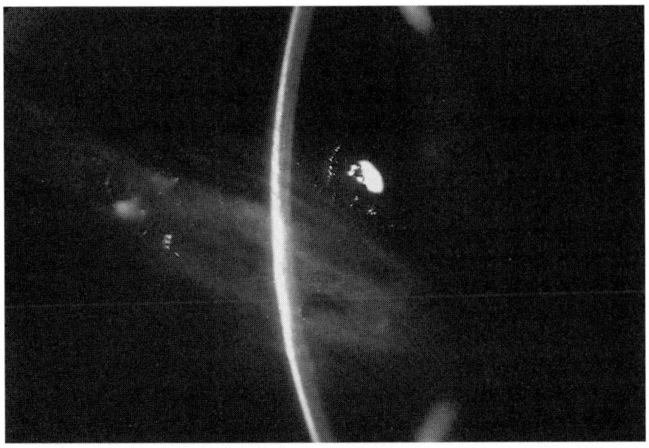

Fig. 11-52 Partial-thickness corneal laceration. Slit-beam view of the laceration seen in Fig. 11-51 demonstrates the anterior location of the scarring.

Box 11-13 Treatment of Partial-Thickness and Self-Sealed Full-Thickness Corneal Lacerations

If the edges are well apposed, topical antibiotics are used (e.g., ofloxacin or ciprofloxacin drops or ciprofloxacin ointment qid) until healed.
If the edges are gaped, the wound should be closed with sutures (e.g., 10-0 or 11-0 nylon).
Pressure patching, aqueous suppressants, and no topical corticosteroids are often helpful.
Rarely, a bandage soft contact lens can be used to obtain better wound apposition.
For self-sealed full-thickness corneal lacerations, use systemic antibiotics (see Box 11-14 below).

Box 11-14 Preoperative Treatment of Full-Thickness Corneal and Corneoscleral Lacerations

Shield the eye
Nothing by mouth
Tetanus prophylaxis as needed
Systemic antibiotics (described in Box 11-15)
Antiemetics and pain medication as needed
Obtain informed consent for surgery before giving significant pain medication
Obtain imaging studies (e.g., computed tomography) if an intraocular foreign body cannot be ruled out
Arrange for surgery as soon as possible, ideally within 12 to 24 hours

Box 11-15 Systemic Antibiotic Prophylaxis in Penetrating Ocular Trauma

- *Adults:* Cefazolin 1 g IV every 8 hours or vancomycin* 1 g IV every 12 hours plus gentamicin 6 mg/kg per day (use ideal body weight or real body weight if lower) or ceftazidime 1 g IV every 8 hours or ciprofloxacin 200 to 400 mg IV every 12 hours
- *Children:* Cefazolin 25 to 50 mg/kg per day IV in three divided doses and gentamicin 2 mg/kg IV every 8 hours

Oral antibiotics are used after 3 days of IV antibiotics for a total of 10 days

- *Adults:* Ciprofloxacin 500 mg twice a day or ofloxacin 400 mg twice a day
- *Children* (younger than 18 years): Cephalexin 25 to 50 mg/kg per day in four divided doses

*Note that *Bacillus* spp are best treated with vancomycin or clindamycin.

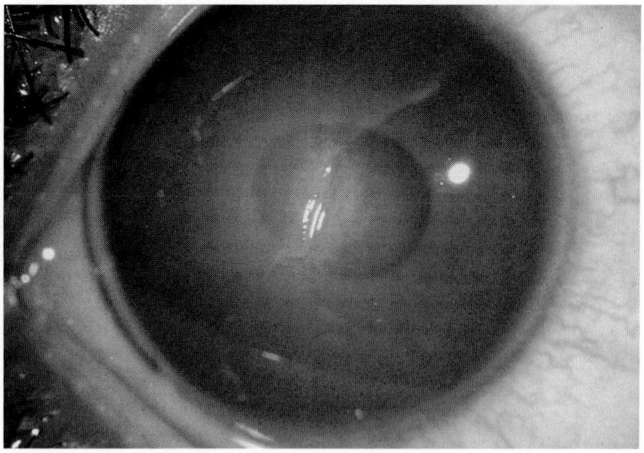

Fig. 11-53 Full-thickness corneal laceration. A full-thickness corneal laceration is evident centrally.

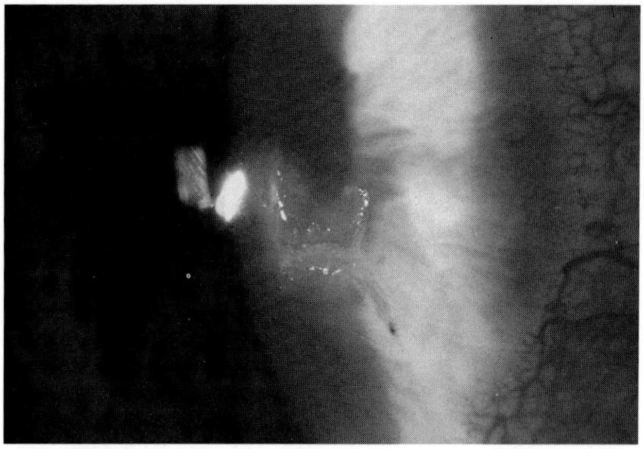

Fig. 11-54 Full-thickness corneal laceration. A stellate corneal laceration with moderate surrounding corneal edema is seen.

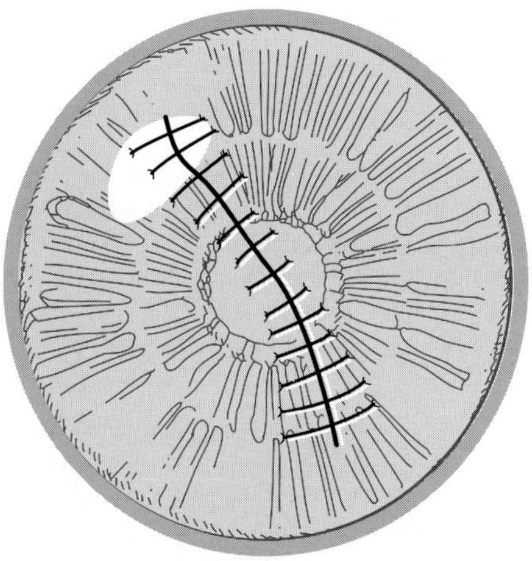

Fig. 11-55 Linear corneal laceration repair procedure. A linear corneal laceration should be repaired with multiple interrupted sutures. Ideally, to preserve a moderately normal corneal contour, the central sutures should be slightly shorter and the peripheral sutures slightly longer than average.

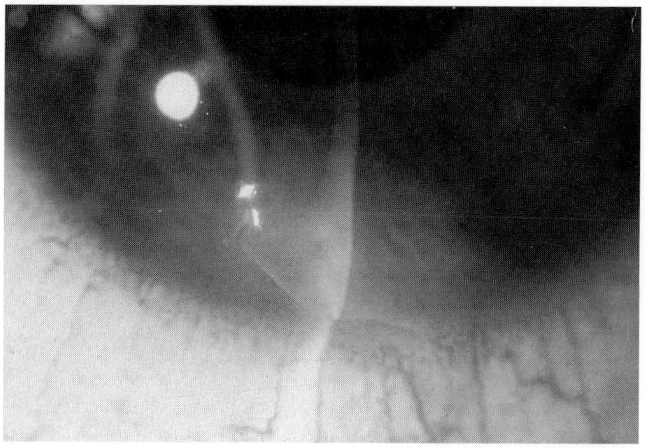

Fig. 11-56 Full-thickness corneal laceration. A full-thickness, inferior corneal laceration that reaches the limbus can be seen.

Surgical repair should occur as soon as feasible, ideally within 12 to 24 hours of the injury. It is performed under general anesthesia to avert the possibility of a retrobulbar hemorrhage or of increased intraorbital pressure causing additional damage. Depolarizing agents such as succinylcholine should theoretically be avoided because they may initially cause contraction of the extraocular muscles and extrusion of the intraocular contents. Occasionally, topical anesthesia can be used for small corneal lacerations without uveal prolapse in cooperative patients. Care should be taken to avoid pressure on the globe during the preparation and draping of the patient. When a scleral rupture is suspected but not yet identified, a 360° conjunctival peritomy is performed, and conjunctiva and Tenon's capsule are dissected away from the sclera in all four quadrants. Muscle hooks are used to elevate the muscles to inspect the entire sclera, especially the four rectus muscle insertion sites, which are thin and prone to rupture. If no rupture is found after careful inspection of the entire sclera, the conjunctiva is closed with absorbable suture (e.g., 8-0 Vicryl).

Corneal and corneoscleral lacerations are carefully explored with cellulose sponges and fine forceps to assess the extent of the corneal and intraocular damage (Figs. 11-53 and 11-54). Cultures should be taken (with a swab or in the same manner as for a corneal ulcer) if infection is suspected. If the anterior chamber is formed, a limbal paracentesis incision can be created with an angled blade, taking care not to damage the iris or the lens. The corneal wound is closed with interrupted 10-0 nylon sutures (Figs. 11-55, 11-56, and 11-57). The initial sutures are placed at readily identifiable landmarks in the laceration, such as the apex of a flap or the limbus. If the laceration is relatively straight, the first suture should bisect the lesion and additional sutures should bisect the remaining spaces until closed (Figs. 11-58 and 11-59). Sutures should be approximately

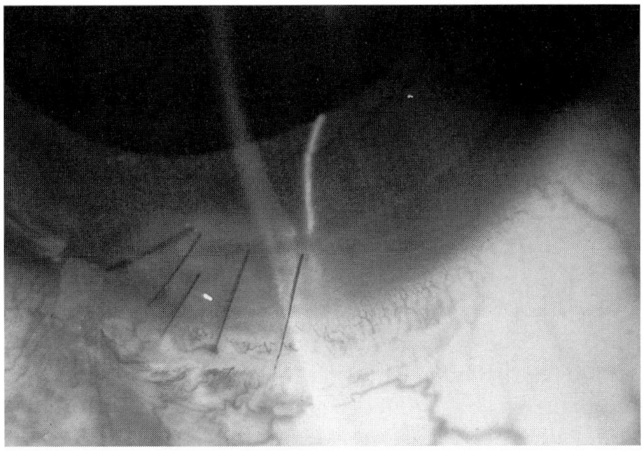

Fig. 11-57 Full-thickness corneal laceration. The laceration seen in Fig. 11-56 was repaired with five interrupted 10-0 nylon sutures. A small conjunctival peritomy was performed to explore for scleral extension of the laceration; none was present. The peritomy was closed with one 8-0 Vicryl suture.

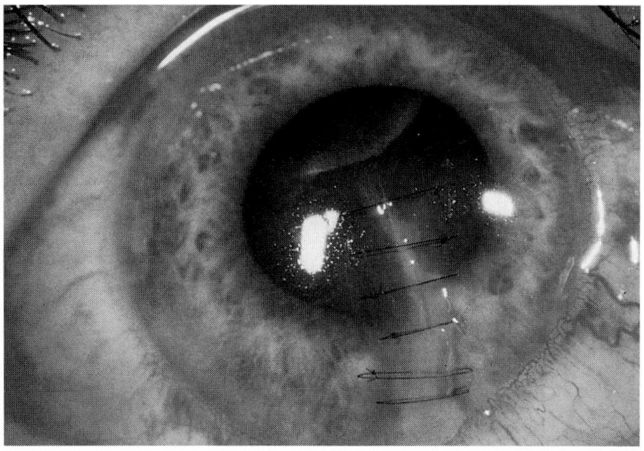

Fig. 11-59 Full-thickness corneal laceration with uveal prolapse. Five days after the eye seen in Fig. 11-58 was repaired with six 10-0 nylon sutures, the wound is secure and the hyphema has cleared. The iris was reposited at the time of the repair, and the pupil is relatively round. A small amount of iris pigment is found in the laceration wound.

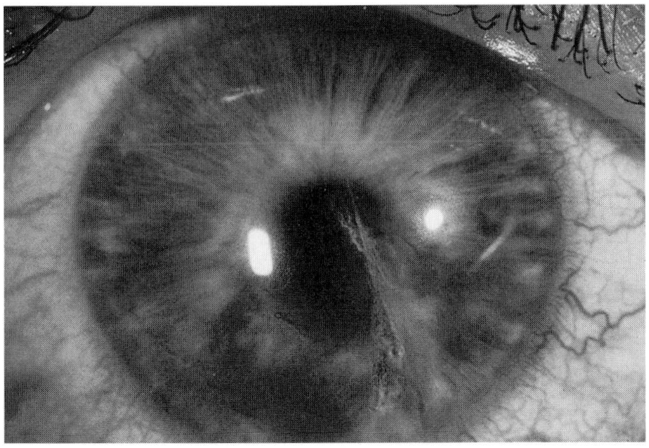

Fig. 11-58 Full-thickness corneal laceration with uveal prolapse. A linear full-thickness corneal laceration can be seen centrally. The pupil is distorted inferiorly because some of the iris has prolapsed from the wound. Mild hemorrhage is noted in the anterior chamber.

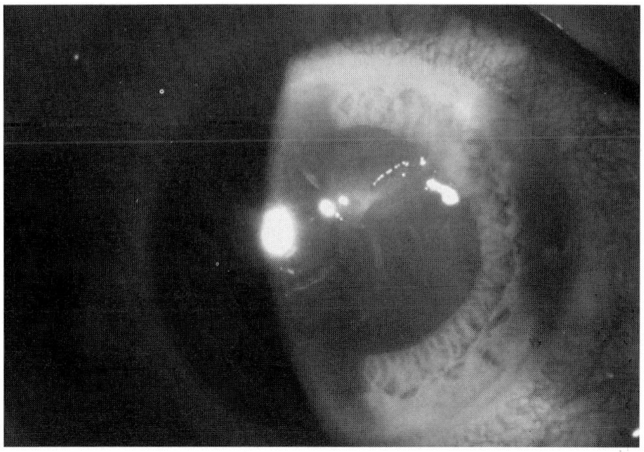

Fig. 11-60 Full-thickness corneal laceration. A small central corneal laceration can be seen. The anterior chamber is shallow, and Descemet's folds are present.

90% depth and 1.0 to 1.25 mm in length on either side of the laceration (Figs. 11-60 and 11-61). Whenever possible, the sutures should straddle the visual axis, and no sutures should be directly in the center of the line of sight. Ideally, to retain a relatively normal central corneal dome, sutures in the center of the cornea should be slightly shorter and sutures in the periphery somewhat longer than average. If the laceration extends to the limbus, a conjunctival peritomy should be performed to explore the adjacent sclera to check for scleral extension, which requires repair if present (Fig. 11-62). The limbus is closed with 9-0 or 10-0 nylon. Occasionally, viscoelastic substance aids in wound closure, but the bulk of the viscoelastic material must be removed from the eye before the end of surgery or the

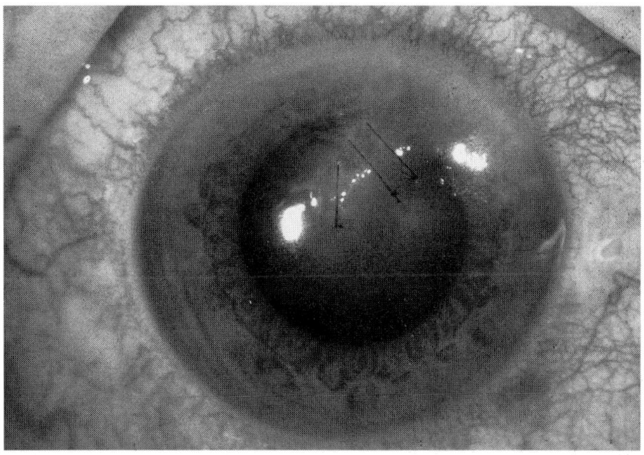

Fig. 11-61 Full-thickness corneal laceration. Postoperative day 1 of the eye seen in Fig. 11-60. Three 10-0 nylon sutures were used to close the wound. The knots are buried.

intraocular pressure may rise dramatically. Stellate lacerations can be extremely difficult to close. An X suture or a *purse-string-type* suture is occasionally required (Fig. 11-63). In the rare situation that a stellate laceration cannot be closed with sutures, a small drop of cyanoacrylate tissue glue can be applied to close the wound. The glue should not cover adjacent corneal sutures because the glue often separates from the cornea (but not the suture material) before the sutures are to be removed, causing significant irritation and inflammation. Whenever corneal glue is used, a bandage soft contact lens is placed on the eye. Occasionally, extensive tissue loss requires lamellar or penetrating corneal graft to close the wound (see Chapter 10). The suture knots should be buried, ideally away from the visual axis. The conjunctival peritomy can be closed if it is large (e.g., 8-0 Vicryl). The globe is reformed through the paracentesis site or the laceration site, and the wound security is tested with cellulose sponges, a Seidel test, or both.

When a scleral laceration is found, it is closed with interrupted 8-0 or 9-0 nylon sutures (Figs. 11-64 and 11-65). The suturing should begin anteriorly and progress posteriorly until the end of the laceration is visualized and then closed, if at all possible. A rectus bridle suture (e.g., 4-0 silk) or a limbal traction suture (e.g., 6-0 Vicryl) can be used to carefully generate greater exposure. Sometimes a rectus muscle must be disinserted to reach the laceration, and then it must be reattached (e.g.,

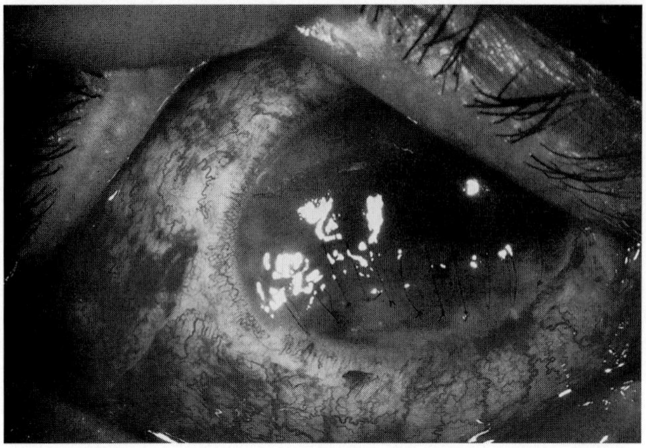

Fig. 11-62 Full-thickness corneoscleral laceration. A large corneoscleral laceration was repaired with multiple 10-0 nylon sutures in the cornea, and 8-0 and 9-0 nylon sutures were used in the sclera inferotemporally. The conjunctiva was closed with 8-0 Vicryl.

A

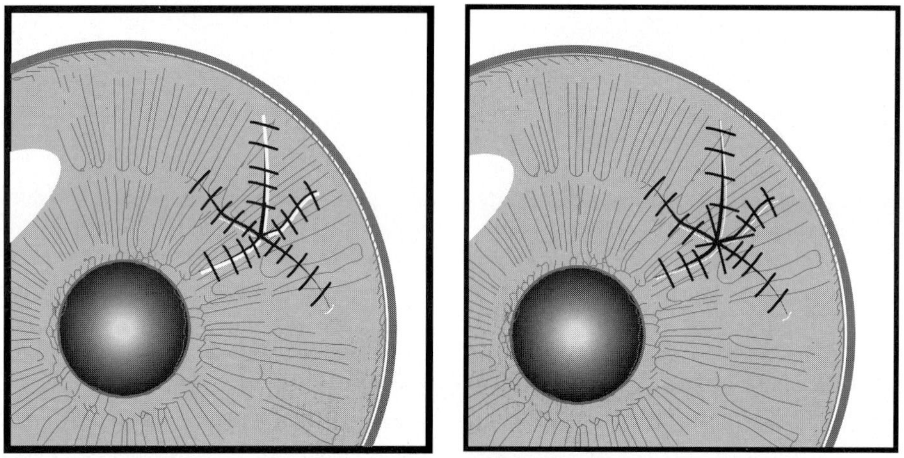

B

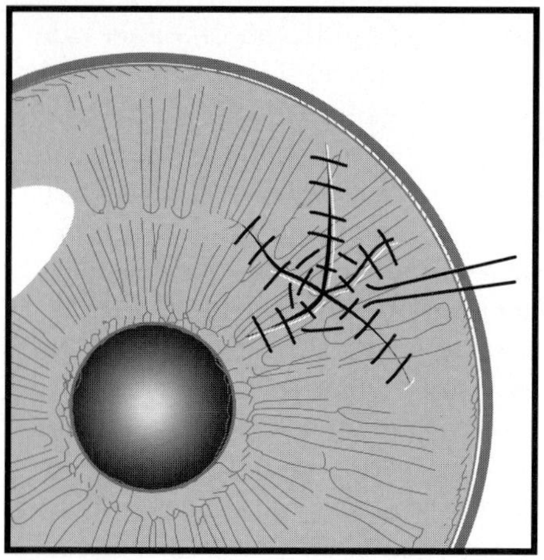

C

Fig. 11-63 Stellate corneal laceration repair procedure. **A,** Often multiple interrupted sutures are able to seal a stellate corneal laceration. **B,** An X suture may be required to achieve a watertight closure of a complicated stellate laceration. **C,** Occasionally, a *purse-string* suture is necessary to seal a stellate laceration wound.

with 6-0 Vicryl) once the laceration is repaired. Rarely, the most posterior extent of a laceration is left open because of lack of exposure. Fortunately, the orbital contents often tamponade these posterior lesions. Uveal material should be reposited in the eye whenever possible. If vitreous extrudes from a scleral rupture, it should be cut flush with the surface with scissors or an automated vitrector.

If the iris prolapses through a corneal laceration, all attempts should be made to reposit it (Fig. 11-66). Even small portions of iris can be used to restore iris architecture during subsequent anterior segment reconstruction. No epithelium should be adherent to the iris before it is replaced in the eye. Significant iris damage, such as iridodialysis (Figs. 11-67, 11-68, and 11-69) or cyclodialysis, is often repaired at a later date (Figs. 11-70, 11-71, and 11-72). Grossly necrotic or infected iris (rarely occurring less than 24 hours after the injury) should be amputated, as should completely shredded iris strands. Frequently, the iris must be swept out of the wound (in a limbus-to-pupil direction) through the paracentesis site with a cyclodialysis spatula or a 27- to 30-gauge irrigating canula (Fig. 11-73). Contact with the lens and corneal endothelium should be avoided. If vitreous protrudes through the wound, it should be excised with an automated vitrectomy machine before complete wound closure. A

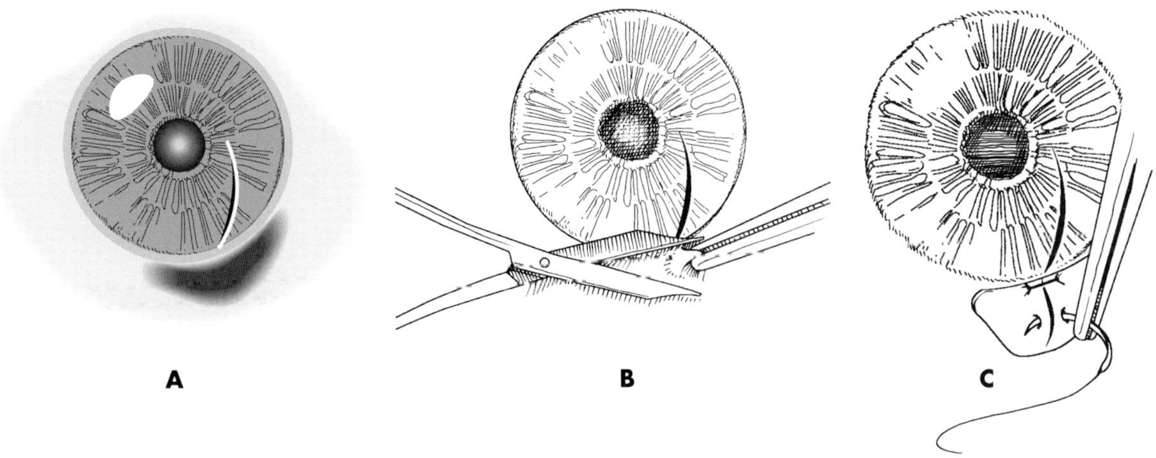

Fig. 11-64 Corneal laceration with scleral extension repair procedure. **A,** When a corneal laceration reaches the limbus, a surgical exploration for scleral extension must be performed. The scleral involvement is often hidden by conjunctival hemorrhage. **B,** A conjunctival peritomy is performed to expose the end of the laceration. **C,** Once the end of the laceration is identified, it should be repaired. A limbal suture is performed first because the limbal landmarks are easy to identify.

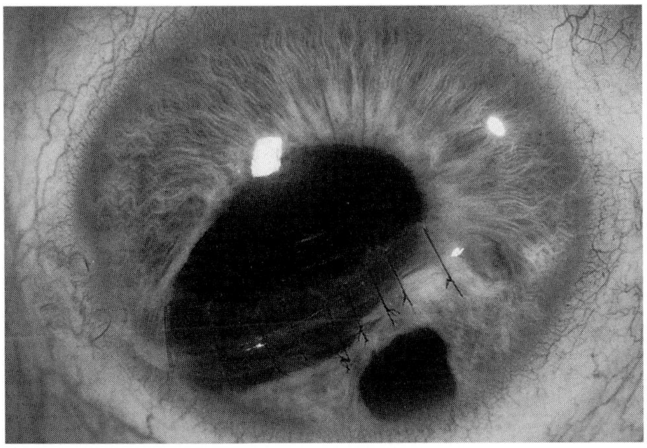

Fig. 11-65 Full-thickness corneoscleral laceration. This corneoscleral laceration was repaired 4 months ago. Cataract extraction was required at the time of the ruptured globe repair.

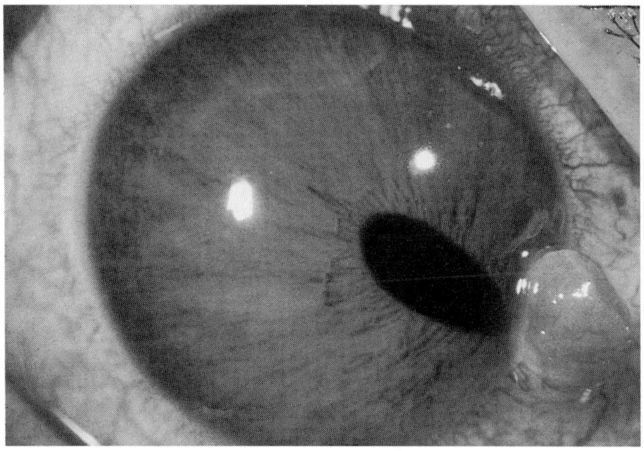

Fig. 11-66 Full-thickness limbal laceration with uveal prolapse. A puncture wound at the limbus with significant iris prolapse is seen. All attempts should be made to reposit viable, noninfected iris.

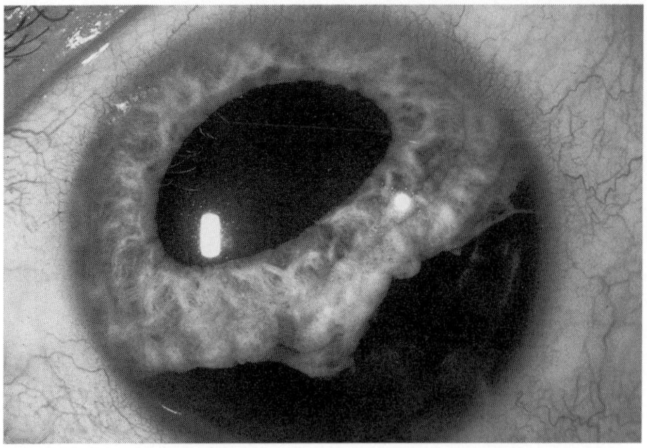

Fig. 11-67 Iridodialysis. A large iridodialysis can be seen from the 2 to 8 o'clock positions.

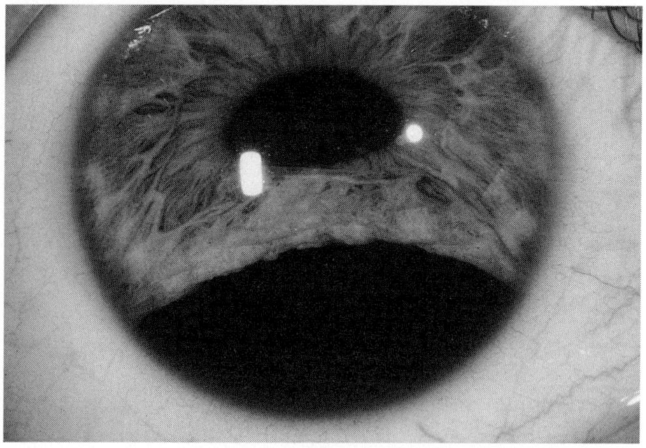

Fig. 11-68 Iridodialysis. One year after blunt trauma, a stable iridodialysis is seen. The patient's visual acuity remained excellent.

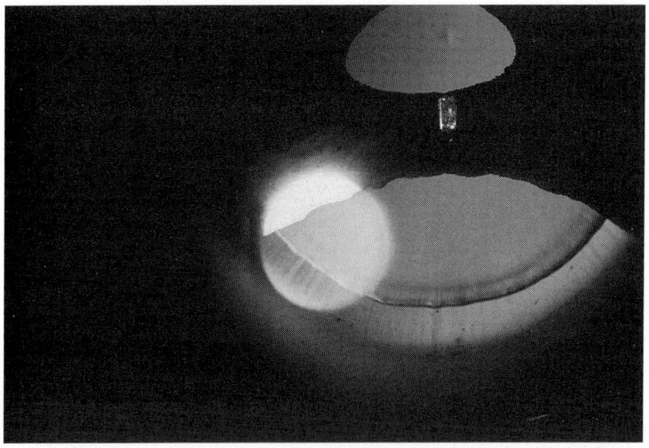

Fig. 11-69 Iridodialysis. Retroillumination off the retina in the eye seen in Fig. 11-68 demonstrates the edge of the crystalline lens with intact lens zonular attachments.

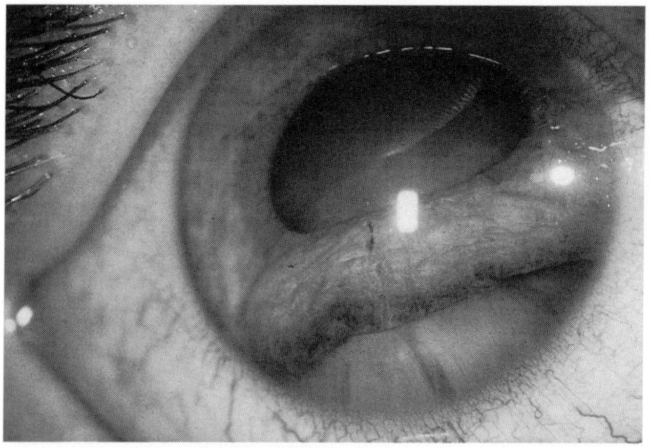

Fig. 11-70 Iridodialysis. Blunt trauma from a BB gun caused a large inferior iridodialysis and a traumatic cataract in this child.

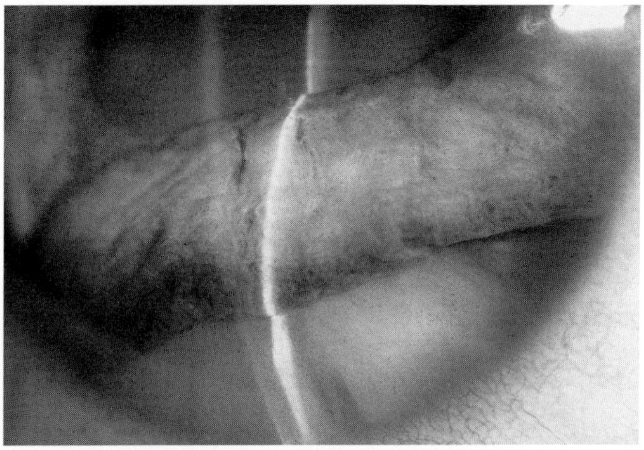

Fig. 11-71 Iridodialysis. Slit-beam view of the eye seen in Fig. 11-70 demonstrates that the lens is intumescent inferiorly and touches the corneal endothelium in that area.

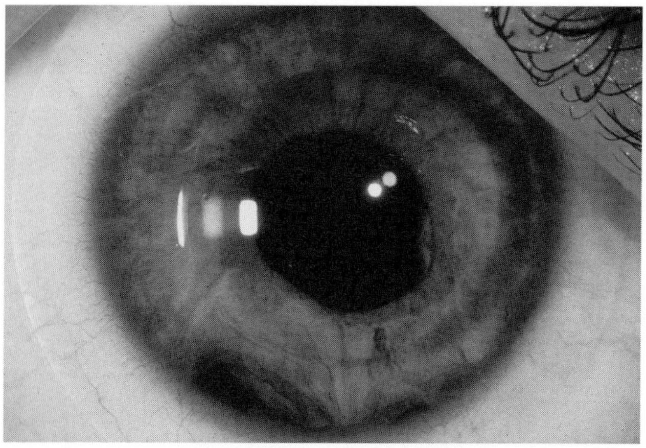

Fig. 11-72 Iridodialysis. Six months after a cataract extraction (without an intraocular lens implant) and repair of the iridodialysis with two 10-0 nylon mattress sutures attaching the iris to the sclera inferiorly, this patient's visual acuity is 20/20 with an aphakic soft contact lens.

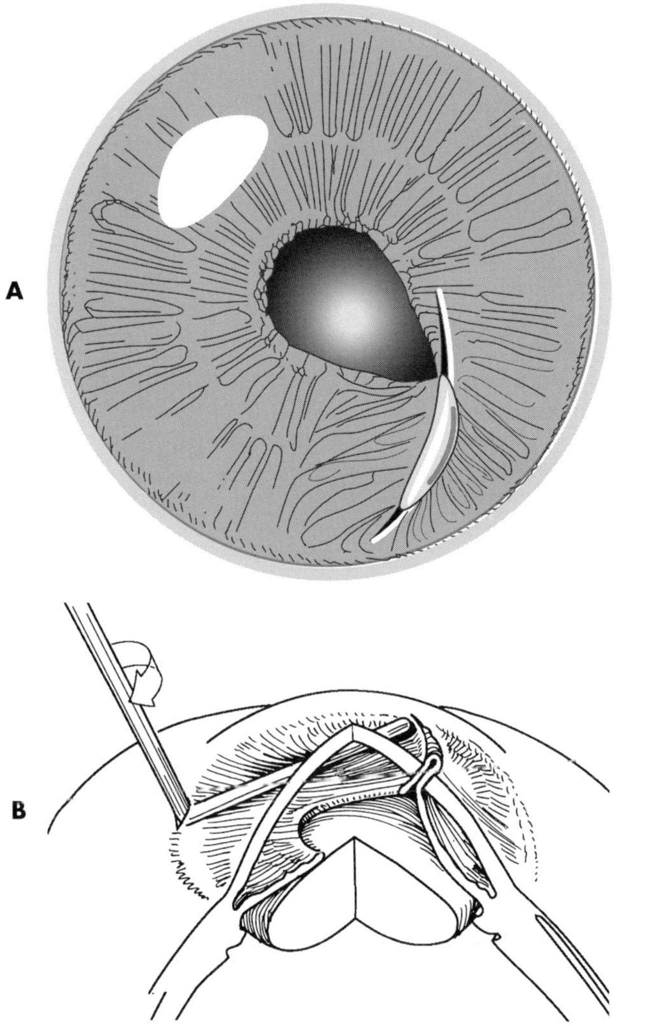

Fig. 11-73 Corneal laceration with iris prolapse repair procedure. **A,** A corneal laceration with iris prolapse often creates an irregular pupil. **B,** Through a limbal paracentesis, a cyclodialysis spatula can be used to sweep the iris out of the wound. The tip is placed at the peripheral extent of the prolapse, and the iris is gently pulled centrally to draw it back into the eye. Care should be taken not to create iris bleeding or iridodialysis.

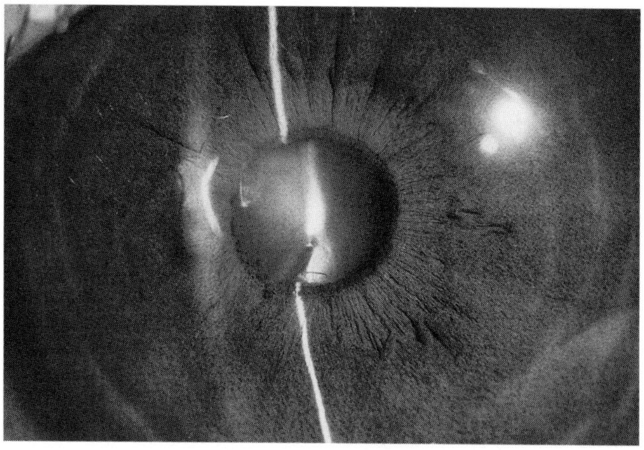

Fig. 11-74 Full-thickness corneal laceration and cataract. A large sewing needle caused a full-thickness corneal laceration and cataract. A break in the anterior capsule can be seen, but no cortex fluffs into the anterior chamber. Because the wound was self-sealing, it was not sutured.

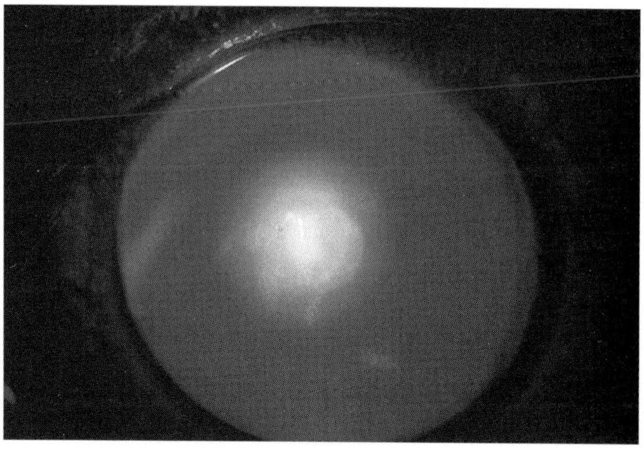

Fig. 11-75 Full-thickness corneal laceration and cataract. Cobalt blue light after fluorescein dye demonstrates the Seidel negative aspect of the self-sealing sewing needle wound seen in Fig. 11-74. The cataract was removed, and an intraocular lens implant was placed electively at a later date. (See color plate.)

peaked pupil is suggestive of vitreous in the anterior chamber and wound, and it should be cleared out with an automated vitrector if possible. Care should be taken to avoid incorporating any iris or vitreous in the wound.

If a traumatic cataract is present at the time of the laceration repair, it may be left alone or removed depending on the status of the lens. There are several reasons to delay cataract surgery until days or weeks after the laceration is repaired. Cataract extraction at the time of laceration repair is a technical challenge because the laceration and associated corneal edema often result in limited visibility. Additionally, posterior capsular rupture and vitreous loss often complicate cataract extraction. It is also more difficult to place an intraocular lens implant because accurate keratometry readings and axial length measurements are impossible to obtain. Not infrequently, fibrin on the anterior lens capsule can simulate a cataract, whereas the lens is really clear. Consequently, if the lens capsule is grossly intact and no cortical material appears in the anterior chamber, the cataract can usually be left alone and removed at a later date if it impairs vision (Figs. 11-74 and 11-75).

If the lens capsule is clearly disrupted and cortical material fluffs up into the anterior chamber, or if the swollen cataractous lens prevents reformation of the anterior chamber, the cataract should be removed at the time of laceration repair (Fig. 11-76). It is typically removed through a standard limbal cataract incision after

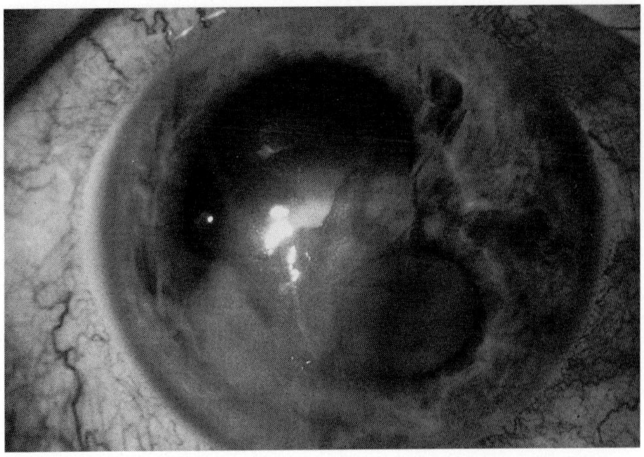

Fig. 11-76 Full-thickness corneal laceration and cataract. A large corneal laceration and cataract with cortex fluffing up into the anterior chamber is seen. The pupil is peaked at the 3 o'clock position as a small tag of iris is adherent to the wound. A small amount of blood is also present in the anterior chamber.

the laceration has been repaired. It is often possible to remove the entire nucleus with the use of a phacoemulsification tip with minimal to no ultrasound power. Cortical material is removed with irrigation and aspiration. In traumatic cataracts, disruption of the posterior capsule, lens zonule, or both, often develops, resulting in the need for anterior vitrectomy. The eye is usually left aphakic, and a secondary lens implant is placed if desired once the eye has healed and accurate keratometry readings and axial length measurements are obtained. Although controversial because of the potential increased risk for endophthalmitis from the foreign intraocular lens material, some surgeons place lens implants at the time of cataract extraction and laceration repair using keratometry readings and axial length measurements from the uninjured eye. The wound is closed with 10-0 nylon as necessary (Box 11-16).

Even after severe trauma all attempts should be made to repair a ruptured globe. Occasionally, the eye is so damaged that primary enucleation should be contemplated. Proper informed consent must be obtained before surgery for this extreme measure. In eyes with no potential for vision after primary ruptured globe repair, enucleation should be considered within 10 to 14 days of the trauma to reduce the chance for sympathetic ophthalmia.

After surgery corneal and corneoscleral lacerations are treated with subconjunctival antibiotics (e.g., gentamicin and cefazolin or vancomycin). Topical antibiotic drops (e.g., ofloxacin or ciprofloxacin 6 times a day) are given, and the patient is observed closely for evidence of infection, perhaps signaling early endophthalmitis. Any worsening of intraocular inflammation after corneal and corneoscleral laceration repair should raise suspicion for endophthalmitis. Intravenous antibiotics are continued for 3 days and are then changed to oral antibiotics (e.g., ciprofloxacin 500 mg twice a day [bid] or ofloxacin 400 mg bid in adults; cephalexin 25 to 50 mg/kg per day in 4 divided doses in children younger than 18 years) for a total 10-day antibiotic course. Patients must be observed closely to monitor for infection, glaucoma, and poor wound healing.

Corneal and limbal sutures are generally removed between 2 and 6 months after the repair, depending on healing and vision. Loose sutures require immediate removal. Chronic exposed sutures or knots can cause giant papillary conjunctivitis (Figs. 11-77 and 11-78). Minimal to significant residual corneal scarring may form (Figs. 11-79, 11-80, and 11-81). Initial visual rehabilitation consists of spectacle refraction and contact lens fitting. Contact lenses are a useful option for unilateral aphakia. Rigid contact lenses can correct high degrees of irregular astigmatism (Fig. 11-82). An iris-tinted contact lens can dramatically improve glare in patients with significant iris loss (Figs. 11-83 and 11-84). Occasionally surgery may be indicated. Aphakic patients who are intolerant of contact lenses can often undergo secondary lens implantation. Certain types of refractive errors are amenable to keratorefractive surgery. Penetrating keratoplasty with or without other anterior segment reconstruction proce-

Box 11-16 Surgical Treatment of Corneal and Corneoscleral Lacerations

Avoid ocular pressure when preparing the eye for surgery.
General anesthesia (without depolarizing agents) is typically used. Topical anesthesia can be used for small corneal lacerations without uveal prolapse in cooperative patients.
Potential scleral lacerations should be explored after a conjunctival peritomy.
Scleral lacerations should be closed with 8-0 or 9-0 nylon sutures.
Corneal lacerations should be closed with 10-0 nylon sutures.
Uveal tissue should be reposited in the eye if noninfected and viable.
Vitreous should be cut away from the wound and the anterior chamber, if possible, with an automated vitrectomy instrument.
Avoid incorporating uveal tissue and vitreous in the wound.
Remove a traumatic cataract if the anterior capsule is clearly broken and cortical material is fluffing up into the anterior chamber or if the swollen cataractous lens prevents reformation of the anterior chamber.

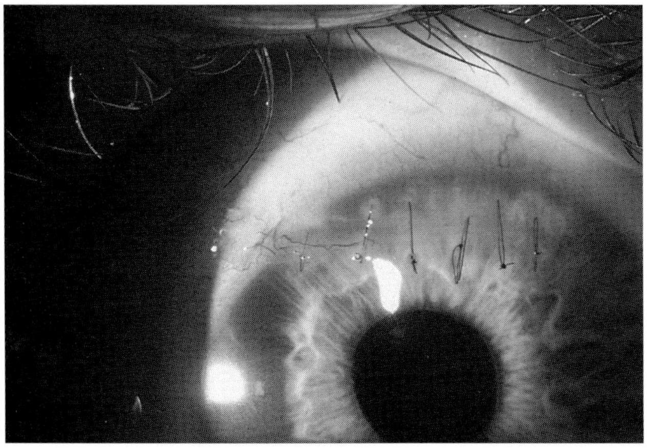

Fig. 11-77 Loose exposed corneal laceration sutures. Several corneal laceration sutures are loose and exposed, causing foreign-body sensation and discharge. Additionally, a few of the knots were not buried.

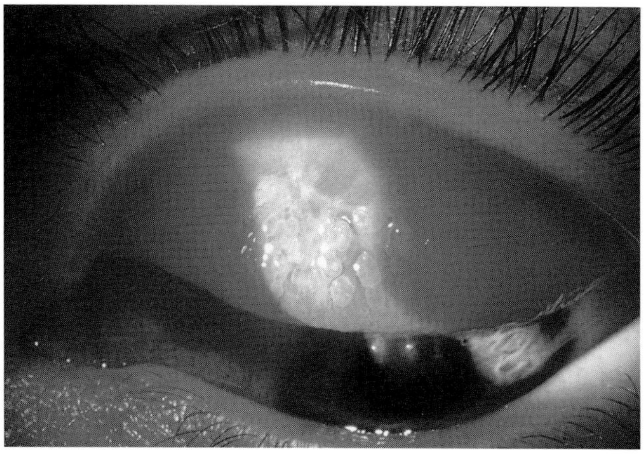

Fig. 11-78 Suture-related giant papillary conjunctivitis. The chronically exposed sutures seen in Fig. 11-77 have caused giant papillary conjunctivitis.

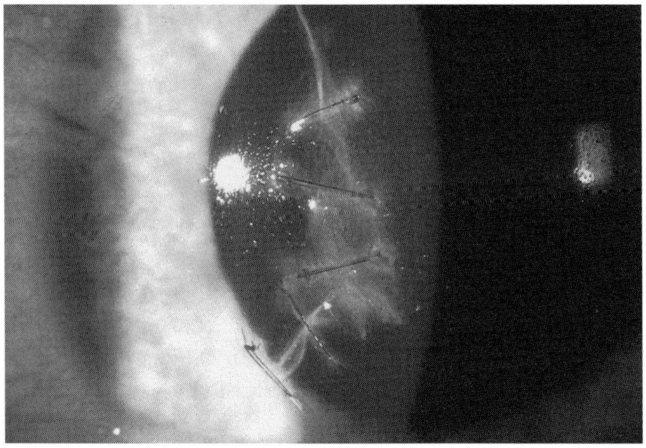

Fig. 11-79 Corneal laceration repair. Mild residual corneal scarring is seen several months after corneal laceration repair.

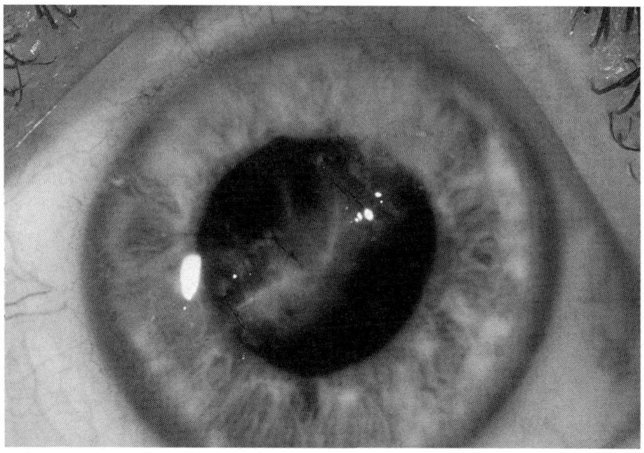

Fig. 11-80 Corneal laceration repair. Moderate residual corneal scarring is present centrally after corneal laceration repair.

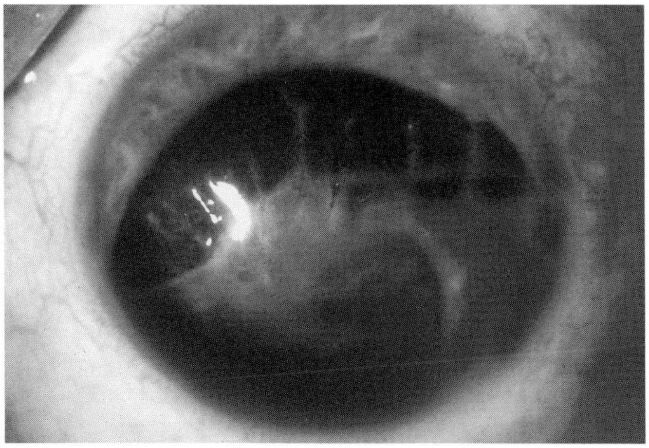

Fig. 11-81 Corneal laceration repair. Significant central corneal scarring is still present 6 months after a large corneal laceration repair and cataract removal.

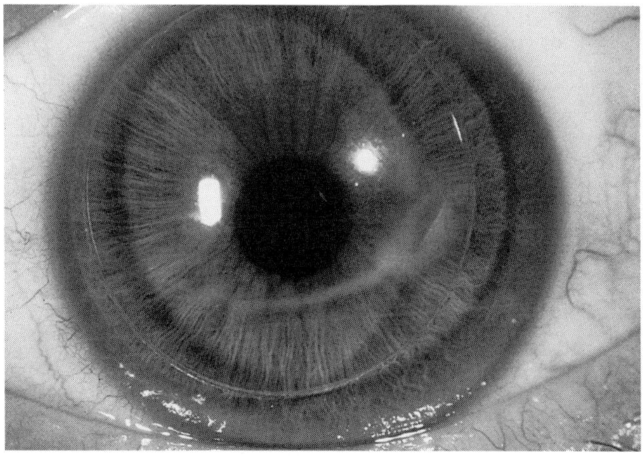

Fig. 11-82 Rigid contact lens. A rigid contact lens can correct high degrees of regular and irregular astigmatism common after corneal laceration repair. This eye, with a moderately large corneal laceration inferior to the pupil, achieved excellent vision with a rigid contact lens.

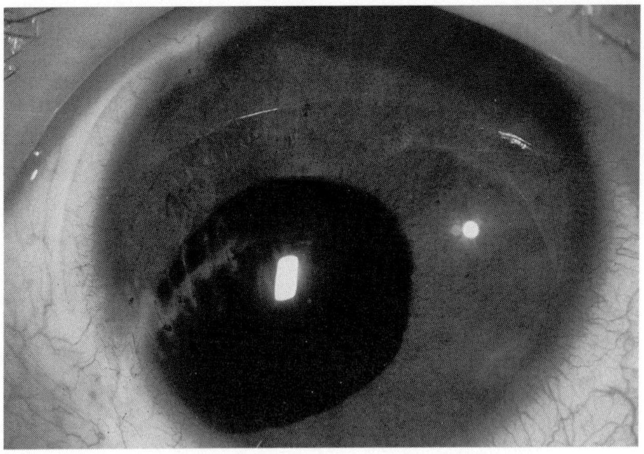

Fig. 11-83 Large irregular pupil. After a corneal laceration repair and traumatic cataract extraction, this patient had severe symptoms of glare with standard aphakic contact lenses because of the large irregular pupil.

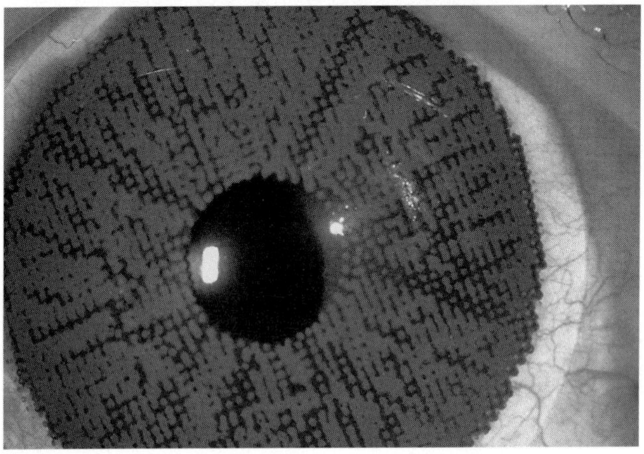

Fig. 11-84 Iris-tinted contact lens. An iris-tinted contact lens, placed on the eye seen in Fig. 11-83, cured the patient's glare symptoms.

Box 11-17 Visual Rehabilitation After Corneal and Corneoscleral Laceration Repair

- Suture removal
- Spectacle refraction
- Aphakic contact lens for unilateral aphakia
- Rigid gas-permeable contact lens for irregular astigmatism
- Iris-tinted contact lens for significant iris tissue loss
- Keratorefractive surgery for selected refractive errors
- Penetrating keratoplasty for central corneal scars
- Anterior segment reconstruction for severe intraocular abnormalities

dures, such as lysis of iridocorneal adhesions, iridoplasty, goniosynechiolysis, cataract or lens remnant removal, automated vitrectomy, and placement of an intraocular lens, may be effective for significant corneal scars and intraocular abnormalities when the posterior segment is healthy (Box 11-17).

INTRAOCULAR FOREIGN BODY

A foreign body in the eye often accompanies ocular trauma. The foreign body may be apparent on initial evaluation. Frequently, however, the foreign body is difficult, if not impossible, to visualize because it is hidden by normal ocular structures, such as limbus or iris, or by abnormalities such as corneal edema, cataract, or hyphema. A foreign body must be suspected in all cases of ocular trauma.

All penetrating ocular injuries should be evaluated for intraocular foreign bodies (Figs. 11-85 and 11-86). The slit-lamp examination should concentrate on finding the entrance wound and searching the anterior chamber and iris for a foreign body. Iris transillumination (checked by directing a small beam of light directly through the undilated pupil and looking for a red reflex coming through a defect in the iris) should be evaluated. Dilated examination should evaluate the lens for the disruption of the anterior capsule, a focal cataract, and an embedded foreign body. If the globe is well formed and the wound does not leak, gentle gonioscopy can be used to evaluate the anterior chamber angle, especially inferiorly, for an occult foreign body (Fig. 11-87). Delayed inferior corneal edema may be observed when a foreign body is present in the inferior angle. A dilated fundus examination should also be performed to rule out a posterior segment foreign body, but ocular manipulation should be avoided in an eye with an obvious laceration.

Unless the complete dilated ophthalmic examination can definitively exclude an intraocular foreign body, an imaging study should be performed. Generally computed tomography of the eye and orbit (axial and coronal views) is performed (Fig. 11-88). Wood, glass, and plastic may be difficult to visualize on CT imaging. Although magnetic resonance imaging may be helpful in such cases, it is contraindicated in the presence of a metallic foreign body or a foreign body of unknown composition. Ultrasound biomicroscopy is an effective tool to identify even small foreign bodies in the anterior one fifth of the globe (Fig. 11-89). B-scan ultrasonography can be helpful sometimes to detect a foreign body in the posterior segment (Fig. 11-90) or the anterior orbit, but intraocular air can mimic a foreign body during this imaging procedure.

Once an intraocular foreign body is located, its composition must be determined. Certain foreign bodies cause severe inflammatory reactions, whereas others

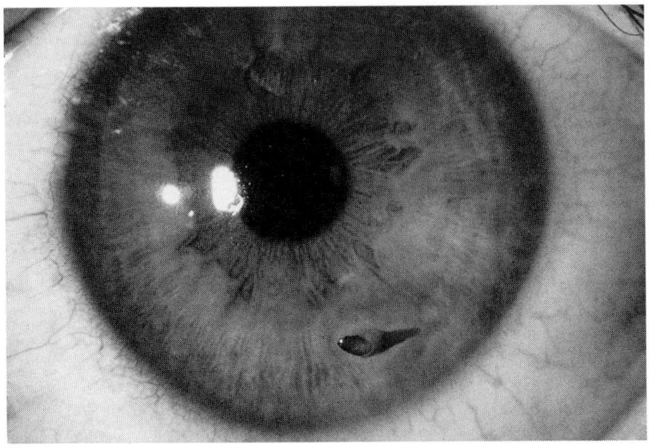

Fig. 11-85 Potential intraocular foreign body. A thorn is embedded deeply into the cornea.

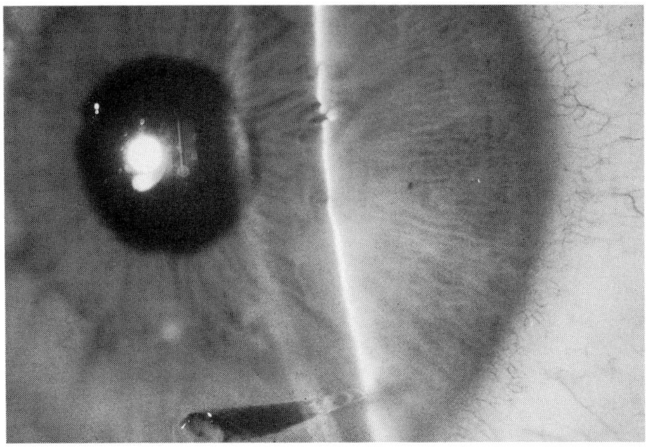

Fig. 11-86 Potential intraocular foreign body. A slit beam demonstrates that the thorn enters the anterior chamber. Other examination techniques, such as looking for iris transillumination defects and gentle gonioscopy, may be helpful in ruling out intraocular foreign bodies.

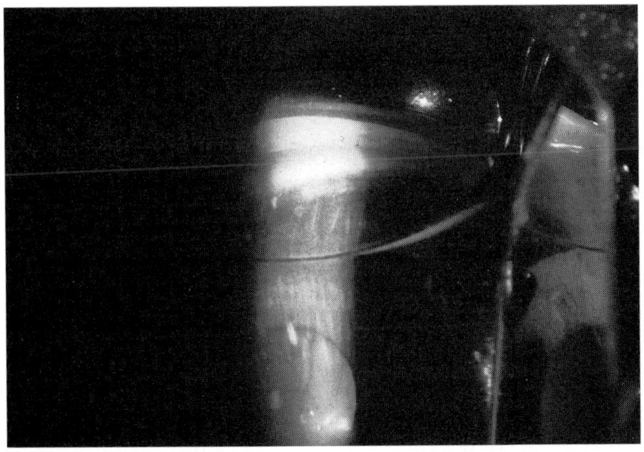

Fig. 11-87 Intraocular foreign body seen on gonioscopy. Gonioscopy revealed a metallic foreign body in the inferior angle.

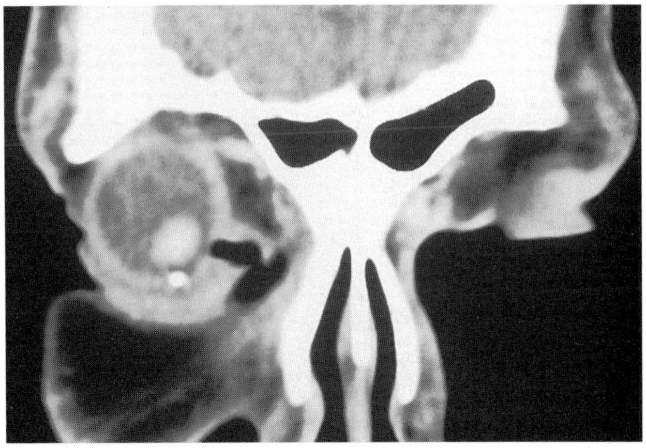

Fig. 11-88 Intraocular foreign body seen on computed tomography. Computed tomography of the eye seen in Fig. 11-87 demonstrates a radiodense foreign body in the anterior globe.

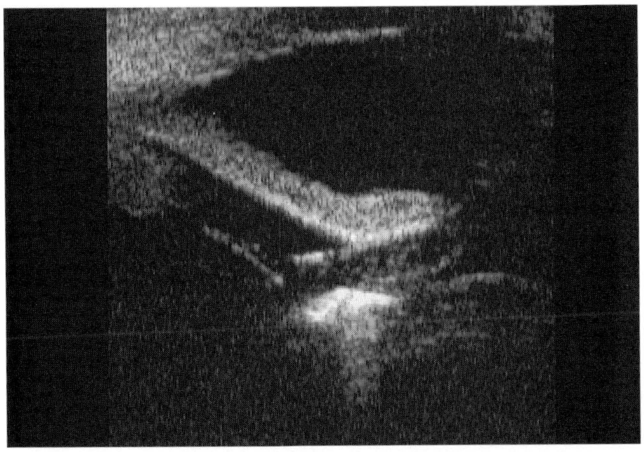

Fig. 11-89 Intraocular foreign body seen on ultrasound biomicroscopy. A foreign body was clearly identified in the anterior lens behind the iris on ultrasound biomicroscopic evaluation. It turned out to be a piece of metal, which was subsequently removed with an electromagnet during the cataract extraction. (Courtesy of Elizabeth L. Affel, M.S.)

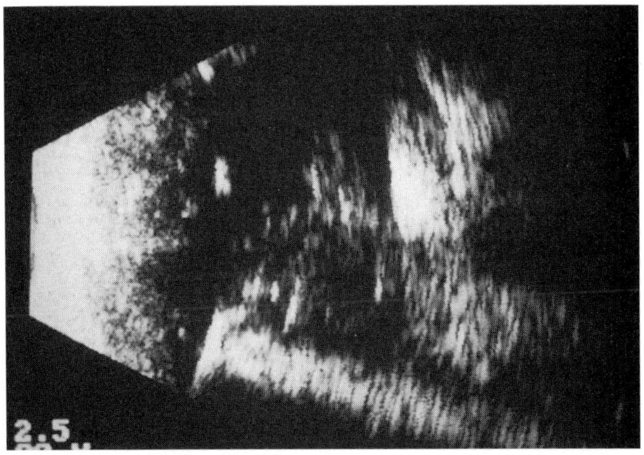

Fig. 11-90 Intraocular foreign body seen on B-scan ultrasonography. An intraocular foreign body was seen on B-scan ultrasonography. Note the shadowing caused by the BB inferiorly. (Courtesy of Deborah BenArosh, C.O.A.)

Box 11-18 Foreign Body and Inflammatory Reaction

SEVERE INFLAMMATORY REACTION

Magnetic: Iron
Steel

Nonmagnetic: Copper
Vegetable matter

MILD INFLAMMATORY REACTION

Magnetic: Nickel

Nonmagnetic: Aluminum
Mercury
Zinc

INERT (TYPICALLY PRODUCES NO INFLAMMATORY REACTION UNLESS A TOXIC COATING IS PRESENT)

Glass
Carbon
Coal
Cilia
Stone
Lead (most BB and gunshot pellets contain 80% to 90% lead and 10% to 20% iron)
Porcelain
Rubber
Plastic
Silver
Gold
Platinum

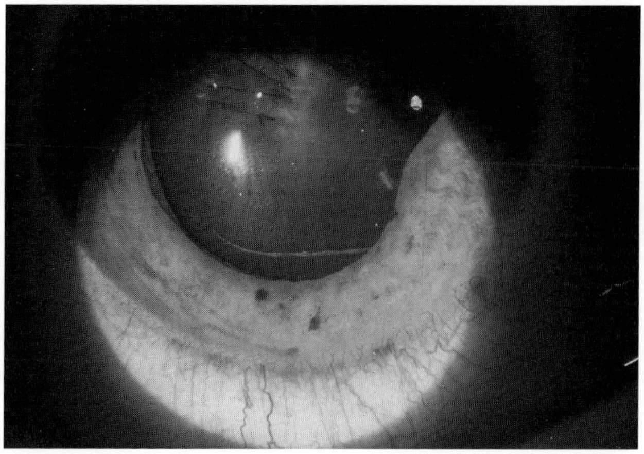

Fig. 11-91 Intraocular eyelash. One month after a ruptured globe repair, an eyelash was noted in the anterior chamber. It was probably not noticed previously because of a large hyphema that resolved. If an intraocular eyelash is not causing inflammation or touching the corneal endothelium, it can often be left in place.

produce mild reactions or are inert (Box 11-18). Even an inert foreign body can cause a significant inflammatory response if it is coated with a toxic substance. Vegetable and copper foreign bodies should be removed on an emergency basis. Iron, steel, nickel, aluminum, mercury, and zinc foreign bodies should be removed on an urgent basis. Inert foreign bodies are generally removed at the time of surgical repair of the ruptured globe, but they may be left in place if the surgical removal risks causing significant ocular damage. Eyelashes are not infrequently found in the eye after penetrating trauma. Cilia that cause inflammation or that touch the corneal endothelium should be removed, but most can be left in place without sequelae (Fig. 11-91). Any foreign material with a high risk for infection should be removed, as should any foreign body that causes a significant inflammatory reaction. Long-standing iron intraocular foreign bodies can lead to siderosis, causing a brown discoloration to the iris, corneal endothelium and epithelium, and lens. Siderosis can also cause pupillary mydriasis in addition to retinal degeneration and optic atrophy. Chalcosis, or copper deposition in the eye, results from a persistent intraocular copper-containing foreign body of less than 80% to 85% copper. Higher concentrations of copper lead to severe inflammatory reactions. Chalcosis can cause a green-brown discoloration of Descemet's membrane peripherally, similar to a Kayser-Fleischer ring in Wilson's disease, and a green-brown sunflower cataract.

The principles of preoperative treatment are similar to the treatment of a ruptured globe as described earlier. A shield should be placed on the eye. The patient should receive nothing by mouth. Tetanus prophylaxis should be performed as needed. Systemic antibiotics should be started. Antiemetics and pain medication should be given as needed. Informed consent should be obtained before giving significant pain medication.

General anesthesia should be used in patients with ruptured globes to prevent extrusion of the intraocular contents from increased orbital pressure or a retrobulbar hemorrhage from a local block. Care must be taken not to apply preoperative massage or pressure to the eye during preparation for surgery. No povidone-iodine solution should be placed in the eye. During the removal of an anterior chamber foreign body, no cycloplegic agent is used so the pupil can be kept small to protect the lens and to minimize the chance of the foreign body dislocating posteriorly. When a lenticular or posterior segment foreign body is present, cycloplegic agents are given.

An anterior segment foreign body can be removed through the wound or through a separate limbal incision after the wound is repaired (Fig. 11-92). Viscoelastic material is extremely helpful to secure the foreign body in position and to minimize its movement during attempted removal. Sharp-edged foreign bodies, such as shards of glass, can cause severe intraocular damage during removal. Paracentesis away from the wound allows easy placement of viscoelastic and reformation of the anterior chamber. A rare earth magnet or the much stronger elec-

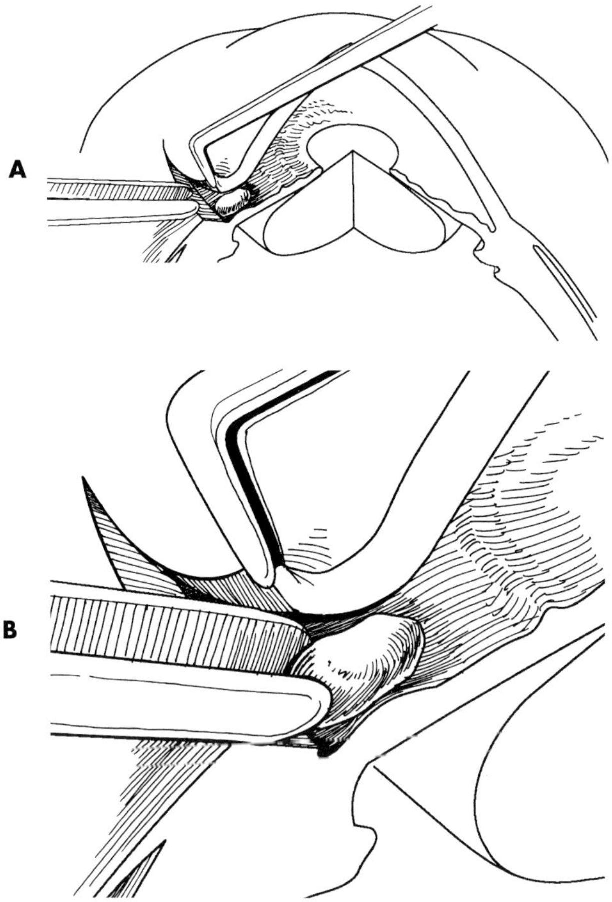

Fig. 11-92 Removal of an intraocular foreign body procedure. **A,** A foreign body in the anterior chamber angle generally requires removal. After a conjunctival peritomy, a posterior limbal incision is performed to reach the junction of the iris and cornea. **B,** Fine forceps can be used to remove the intraocular foreign body. Viscoelastic can often be helpful in stabilizing the foreign body and even "delivering it" through the wound.

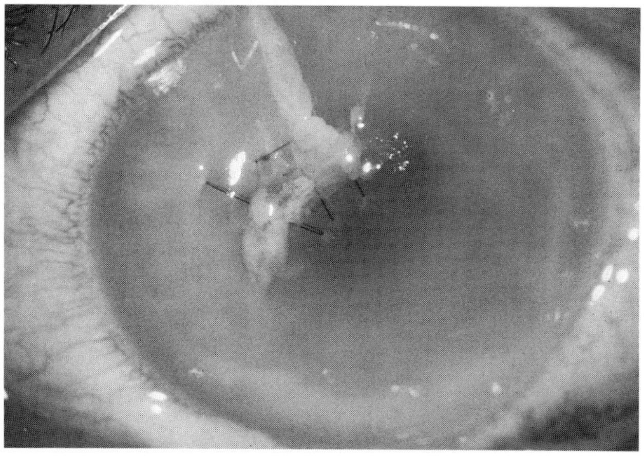

Fig. 11-93 Endophthalmitis. Twenty-four hours after a nail-induced corneal laceration was repaired, severe corneal and intraocular inflammation was noted. A vitreous tap was performed, and intravitreal antibiotics were injected. *Bacillus cereus* grew from the vitreous tap. The eye did poorly despite aggressive medical and surgical treatment.

Box 11-19 Treatment of an Intraocular Foreign Body

- Remove copper and vegetable foreign bodies on an emergency basis
- Remove other noninert foreign bodies on an urgent basis
- If possible, remove inert foreign bodies without causing more intraocular damage, at the time of laceration repair
- Do not dilate the pupil for anterior chamber foreign bodies
- Use viscoelastic material to stabilize the foreign body
- Remove metallic objects with forceps or a magnet either from the laceration wound or from a separate limbal incision
- Anterior chamber angle foreign bodies are best removed by limbal incisions over the foreign body

tromagnet may be useful in the removal of certain metallic foreign bodies. Foreign bodies can often be removed with fine forceps. Special diamond dust-studded foreign body forceps are also available for better grasping of objects.

Anterior chamber angle foreign bodies are often best removed by a separate limbal incision over the area of the foreign body. Generally, an incision much larger than the size of the foreign body is required for safe removal. Unlike a limbal cataract incision, this incision must enter the eye more posteriorly, at the apex of the anterior chamber angle without an underlying lip of cornea, to allow effective removal of the foreign body. Intraoperative gonioscopy may be necessary to determine the exact location of the foreign body before creation of the limbal incision. Once the limbal incision is completed, viscoelastic can be injected into the anterior chamber, away from the incision, and the foreign body "delivered" through the incision. A foreign body embedded in the lens superficially can be removed with forceps or a magnet. Foreign bodies deeper in the lens may require extracapsular cataract extraction (Box 11-19). The wounds and incisions are closed as described for corneal and corneoscleral lacerations above. Subconjunctival antibiotics are given.

After surgery patients are treated with intravenous antibiotics as described earlier. Visual rehabilitation is similar to that for corneal and corneoscleral lacerations. Patients are followed up closely for evidence of inflammation and infection, which may be delayed. Endophthalmitis is a concern in any ruptured globe. When an intraocular foreign body is involved, the incidence of endophthalmitis increases. A devastating infection can result from *Bacillus* spp, most commonly *Bacillus cereus* (Fig. 11-93). Vancomycin and clindamycin are

MAJOR POINTS

Perform an evaluation under anesthesia in any trauma patient (usually a child) in whom an adequate examination cannot be obtained.

Patients with contact lens-related corneal abrasions should be treated with topical antibiotics with good *Pseudomonas* coverage and should *not* be pressure patched.

Although chemical injuries from acids tend to cause less ocular damage than those from alkali (because acids precipitate corneal proteins, which act as a buffer and a barrier to additional acid entering the eye), severe acid injuries can be blinding.

Alkali denatures proteins and saponifies lipids in corneal cell membranes, allowing more alkali to enter the eye quickly and cause potentially devastating ocular damage.

The emergency treatment of ocular chemical burns is copious irrigation of the eye(s) with a neutral solution such as water or saline.

If used after chemical burns, topical corticosteroids should be tapered and discontinued approximately 7 to 10 days after a chemical injury to reduce the potentiation of collagenases and subsequent corneal melting.

Foreign bodies under the upper eyelid often cause linear corneal abrasions. This finding should prompt eversion of the upper eyelid and the search for and removal of any foreign material.

Subconjunctival hemorrhages often spread out as they resolve, making them look worse during the first several days.

All patients with traumatic subconjunctival hemorrhages should undergo complete dilated ophthalmic examination to rule out more extensive ocular damage.

Signs of an occult traumatic scleral rupture include 360° subconjunctival hemorrhage, significant chemosis, abnormally deep or shallow anterior chamber, abnormally high or low intraocular pressure, subluxed or dislocated lens, limited extraocular motility, and vitreous hemorrhage.

If a scleral laceration or a rupture cannot be ruled out during clinical examination, surgical exploration is generally warranted.

Hyphema is a layer of blood in the anterior chamber. Microhyphema is suspended red blood cells in the anterior chamber without layering.

Patients with hyphema or microhyphema who are of African or Mediterranean descent should be screened for sickle trait and disease.

Patients with hyphema at highest risk for poor outcome include those with sickle disease or trait, uncontrolled elevated intraocular pressure, large (>50%) hyphema, poor (<20/200) visual acuity on initial examination, and delayed presentation. Rebleeding is associated with a worse outcome than initial hemorrhage.

Initial treatment of hyphema and microhyphema consists of bed rest or limited activity, an eye shield (but no patch), 1% atropine drops tid, and occasionally topical corticosteroids. Oral aminocaproic acid can be used for inpatients. Intraocular pressure must be carefully monitored and treated if elevated, especially in patients with sickle trait or disease.

Surgical evacuation of hyphema should be considered for corneal blood staining, persistent clot in most of the angle, and elevated intraocular pressure for several days.

A Seidel test is useful to distinguish a partial-thickness from a full-thickness corneal laceration. It is also helpful in following up potentially self-sealing full-thickness corneal lacerations.

If an intraocular foreign body cannot be ruled out on clinical examination, computed tomography or another imaging study should be performed for that purpose.

Full-thickness corneal and scleral lacerations are treated with systemic antibiotics to prevent endophthalmitis.

Surgical repair of a ruptured globe should occur as soon as feasible after the injury, ideally within the first 12 to 24 hours.

General (rarely topical) anesthesia is used for ruptured globe repair because a local block risks increasing intraorbital pressure and a retrobulbar hemorrhage, potentially causing extrusion of intraocular contents through the wound.

Scleral lacerations are sutured with interrupted 8-0 or 9-0 nylon, whereas corneal lacerations are closed with 10-0 nylon.

Attempts should be made to reposit uveal tissue. Grossly infected, necrotic, or shredded iris tissue should be amputated.

Vitreous should be excised from the wound and anterior chamber if possible. Care should be taken not to incorporate iris or vitreous in the wound closure.

Most traumatic cataracts do not have to be removed at the time of ruptured globe repair. If the lens capsule is clearly disrupted and cortical material is fluffing up into the anterior chamber or if the swollen cataractous lens is preventing reformation of the anterior chamber, the cataract should be removed at the time of the ruptured globe repair.

In eyes with no potential for vision after repair of a ruptured globe, enucleation should be considered within 10 to 14 days of the trauma to reduce the chance for sympathetic ophthalmia.

Vegetable and copper intraocular foreign bodies require emergency removal, but most other foreign bodies can be removed at the time of routine ruptured globe repair. Certain inert foreign bodies (e.g., glass, cilia, plastic, others) can be left in place if removal is considered too risky.

Viscoelastic agents, diamond-studded foreign body forceps, and magnets can be extremely useful in the removal of intraocular foreign bodies.

Bacillus spp can cause devastating endophthalmitis in eyes after trauma, especially when an intraocular foreign body is involved. Vancomycin and clindamycin are effective agents against *Bacillus* spp, but an aggressive surgical approach is often necessary to save the eye.

If significant inflammation is present after a ruptured globe repair, it is more likely to be caused by infection than by retained lens material.

especially effective for treating *Bacillus* spp. The patient should be examined carefully each day after surgery for several days to rule out acute endophthalmitis. The incidence of posttraumatic endophthalmitis is highest when the lens or vitreous cavity has been violated, when a retained intraocular foreign body is present, and when the injury occurred outdoors. When an intraocular metallic foreign body has been left in the eye, an electroretinogram should be performed routinely to look for toxic retinal metallosis. This retinal toxicity may be reversible once the foreign body is removed.

CONCLUSION

With increasing interest in measures to prevent ocular trauma at work, in sports, and at home, it is hoped that the incidence of eye injuries decreases with time. However, a certain amount of ocular trauma is inevitable. Even patients with seemingly mild injuries should undergo complete ocular examinations to rule out more extensive damage. If an adequate examination cannot be performed, an evaluation under anesthesia should be seriously considered. Additional testing with B-scan ultrasonography, ultrasound biomicroscopy, and computed tomography may be required. Appropriately managed, even severe eye injuries can result in good visual outcomes.

SUGGESTED READINGS

Endophthalmitis Vitrectomy Study Group: Results of endophthalmitis vitrectomy study: a randomized trial of immediate vitrectomy and of intravenous antibiotics for the treatment of postoperative bacterial endophthalmitis, *Arch Ophthalmol* 113:1479-1496, 1995.

Hersh PS, Kenyon KR: Anterior segment reconstruction following ocular trauma, *Int Ophthalmol Clin* 28:57-68, 1988.

Kuhn F, Morris R, Witherspoon CD, et al: A standardized classification of ocular trauma, *Ophthalmology* 103:240-243, 1996.

Kutner B, Fourman S, Brein K, et al: Aminocaproic acid reduces the risk of secondary hemorrhage after traumatic hyphema, *Arch Ophthalmol* 105:206-208, 1987.

Lin DTC, Webster RG, Abbott RL: Repair of corneal lacerations and perforations, *Int Ophthalmol Clin* 28:69-75, 1988.

Napier SM, Baker RS, Sanford DG, Eastbrook M: Eye injuries in athletics and recreation, *Surv Ophthalmol* 41:229-244, 1996.

Power WJ, Foster CS: Update on sympathetic ophthalmia, *Int Ophthalmol Clin* 35:127-137, 1995.

Rowsey JJ, Hayes JC: Refractive reconstruction for acute eye injuries, *Ophthalmic Surg* 15:569-574, 1984.

Thoft RA: Chemical and thermal injury, *Int Ophthalmol Clin* 19:243-256, 1979.

Wagoner MD: Chemical injuries of the eye: current concepts in pathophysiology and therapy, *Surv Ophthalmol* 41:275-313, 1997.

Index

A

Page numbers in *italic* indicate illustrations; page numbers followed by *b* indicate boxes; page numbers followed by *t* indicate tables.

B

C

I